Sixth Edition

Articulation and Phonology in Speech Sound Disorders

A Clinical Focus

Jacqueline Bauman-Waengler

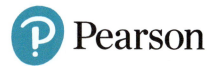

Pearson

Director and Publisher: Kevin Davis
Portfolio Manager: Aileen Pogran
Managing Content Producer: Megan Moffo
Content Producer (Team Lead): Faraz Sharique Ali
Content Producer: Deepali Malhotra
Portfolio Management Assistant: Maria Feliberty
Development Editor: Krista McMurray
Executive Product Marketing Manager: Christopher Barry
Executive Field Marketing Manager: Krista Clark
Procurement Specialist: Deidra Headlee

Cover Design: Pearson CSC, Jerilyn Bockorick
Cover Art: Tetra Images/Shawn O'Connor/Brand X Pictures/Getty Images
Full Service Vendor: Pearson CSC
Full Service Project Management: Pearson CSC, Prince John William Carey
Editorial Project Manager: Pearson CSC, Carmina Jimenez
Printer-Binder: LSC Communications
Cover Printer: LSC Communications
Text Font: 10/12 Charis SIL Regular

Library of Congress Cataloging-in-Publication Data
Names: Bauman-Waengler, Jacqueline Ann, author.
Title: Articulation and phonology in speech sound disorders : a clinical
    focus / Jacqueline Bauman-Waengler.
Description: Sixth edition. | Boston : Pearson Education, [2018] | Includes
    bibliographical references and indexes.
Identifiers: LCCN 2018046080 | ISBN 9780134990576 | ISBN 0134990579
Subjects: LCSH: Articulation disorders. | English language—Phonetics.
Classification: LCC RC424.7 .B378 2018 | DDC 618.92/855—dc23
LC record available at https://lccn.loc.gov/2018046080

10 2023

ISBN 10:   0-13-499057-9
ISBN 13: 978-0-13-499057-6

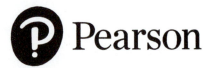

To all the speech-language pathologists who are working hard to make a difference to the children and adults they serve.

About the Author

JACQUELINE BAUMAN-WAENGLER has been a professor for more than 25 years. Her main teaching and clinical emphases are phonetics and phonology, including disorders of articulation and phonology in children and child language disorders. She has published and presented widely in these areas both nationally and internationally. In addition to the sixth edition of *Articulation and Phonology in Speech Sound Disorders: A Clinical Focus*, Bauman-Waengler has also published *Introduction to Phonetics and Phonology: From Concepts to Transcription* (2009) with Pearson. A new book, coauthored with Diane Garcia, will be available at the end of November from Plural Publishing, San Diego, CA. It is titled *Phonological Treatment of Speech Sound Disorders in Children: A Practical Guide.*

Preface

The concept for this book grew out of a perceived need to create a bridge between theoretical issues in speech-language pathology and their clinical application. The goal for the sixth edition has remained the same: to tie strong academic foundations directly to clinical applications. To this end, every chapter contains suggestions for clinical practice as well as clinical examples and clinical applications. These features will assist the reader in developing an understanding of how basic concepts and theoretical knowledge form the core for clinical decision making in the assessment and remediation of speech sound disorders. Learning aids located throughout the chapter include video clips and clinical applications. Those learning aids at the end of every chapter include case studies, critical thinking, and multiple-choice questions.

New to This Edition

With the publication of this sixth edition, this book will have been in use for 20 years. Therefore, this edition of *Articulation and Phonology in Speech Sound Disorders: A Clinical Focus* has had a serious overhaul with significant changes.

- *Chapter Applications: Case Study at the beginning of each chapter.* These applications focus on real-life experiences that beginning students and clinicians will be confronted with. For example, what does a beginning clinician need to know to be able to choose one therapy approach versus another? They are all directly related to the content of the specific chapter.

- *American Speech-Language Hearing Association's (ASHA) position statements, definitions, and practice policies.* Several of the chapters have sections delineating new definitions, such as the current definition of speech sound disorder; practice policies, such as the alignment with ASHA and the World Health Organization's diagnostic practices; ASHA's position on dialects and cultural competence; and specific treatment overviews, such as for dysarthria. This will aid students as they transition into competent clinicians.

- *More user-friendly phonetic descriptors.* This edition has also seen a shift from describing and, in cases, transcribing vowels and consonants in a more user-friendly manner. An attempt has been made to align the descriptive process according to the International Phonetic Alphabet chart in its new 2015 revision. This will aid students in learning the specific descriptions without being unnecessarily burdened with cumbersome terminology.

- *New topic: Anatomy and physiology.* New to this edition is a brief overview of the anatomy and physiology of the speech mechanism (Chapter 2). This is applicable to the discussion of normal speech production as well as those disorders, for example, cleft palate, cerebral palsy, and acquired dysarthria, in which characteristic deviations of the processes underlying speech production are a portion of the clinical picture.

- *New topic: Principles of motor learning.* A new section has been added that discusses the conditions of practice and feedback for motor learning (Chapter 9). Therapeutic applications specific to articulation disorders are given as well as research documenting the efficacy of such principles in childhood apraxia of speech, for example.

- *New topic: Classification of speech sound disorders (Dodd, 2013).* This diagnostic classification system is now introduced (Chapter 1) and expanded upon in several chapters. For example, in Chapter 7 the characteristics of four of the categories—articulation disorder, phonological delay, consistent phonological disorder, and inconsistent phonological disorder—are noted. A case study example is given for each to provide the student with more information on how each of these categories could look clinically. This will give students a much needed structure of how to organize their diagnostic data. A clinical application is also given of a child demonstrating an articulation *and* a phonological disorder. This is often difficult for students to understand.

- *Expanded and reorganized topics: Diagnostic protocols.* Chapter 6, Assessment and Appraisal, provides expanded information on contextual testing and the use of multisyllabic words within the diagnostic process. Specific measures are noted that a clinician could use to assess these variables. In addition, updated lists of standardized speech assessment, language screening measures, prosodic assessment protocols, the testing or screening of phonological and phonemic awareness, and the assessment of a child's communicative participation are given. The student or practitioner will have resources for a large number of formal and informal measures to assess each of these areas.

- *Expanded and reorganized topics: Summarizing data.* The analysis of collected data from a standardized speech assessment and spontaneous speech sample have been completely redone for Chapter 7. Thus, the analysis of the inventory, distribution, stimulability, and determining phonemic contrasts has been streamlined. New analysis forms and a new case study have been used to organize these data and demonstrate their use. Results have been tied to the previously noted classification of speech sound disorders. This will be especially valuable to beginning clinicians as they attempt to organize and categorize the data they have collected. Also new to this edition are measures of whole-word accuracy and variability. A case study is provided so that students can understand how to apply and calculate these measures.

- *Expanded and reorganized topics: Theoretical foundations and their clinical application.* Several of the theoretical constructs have been deleted from this chapter (Chapter 4), while others, such as feature geometry and optimality theory have been expanded to include more practical clinical applications that the student can work through easily. Sonority theory and implicational universals have also been included in this chapter as well as distinctive features and their use in maximal oppositions target selection. These principles are a major portion of specific phonological target selection and therapies which are presented in Chapter 10.

- *Expanded and reorganized topics: Treatment of Phonological Disorders (Chapter 10).* This chapter has been expanded to include more information on several of the therapies that are considered to be phonological in respect to the target selection or treatment options. However, this chapter has also been streamlined so that a clinician is able to obtain an overview of the treatment process. This includes returning to the classification system noted in Chapter 1, utilizing variables such as the age of the child and the severity of the disorder to determine who would maximally benefit from each type of treatment possibility. Also new to this chapter is the categorization "inconsistent speech disorder." Diagnostic criteria and the treatment process are discussed. For each of these phonological treatment methods a case study new to this edition demonstrates how this child's error patterns might be implemented to establish treatment targets and goals.

- *Expanded and reorganized topics: Speech Sound Disorders in Selected Populations (Chapter 11).* This chapter now includes a section on Down syndrome, which contains general as well as articulatory/phonological characteristics. In addition, when possible, the therapy section examines treatment efficacy studies that are based on reviews of controlled studies to determine which treatment protocols demonstrate maintenance and generalization of the treatment effects and increased performance. This is important information for clinicians as they are faced with a large number of treatment choices.
- *Categorical learning objectives.* These have been fine-tuned in each chapter so that the reader begins each chapter with a set of easily identifiable goals for the chapter's learning process. Each set of learning objectives provides the scaffolding for major divisions of the chapter and leads directly to quizzes and critical thinking components that compartmentalize key concepts.
- *New clinical exercises.* This text includes a number of new or revised clinical exercises to allow the student to master theoretical concepts by applying them to real-life situations. The eText edition of this text also contains embedded videos that can be used in conjunction with these clinical exercises, allowing for additional analysis opportunities.
- *Updated references.* References in each chapter have been updated to reflect the most recent research in the field.

The eText edition of this text offers interactive digital features, including:

- *Digital functionality.* The digital eText version of this title provides interactive tools to enhance students' experience with the material, including tools that allow students to search the text, make notes online, print important activities, and bookmark passages for later review.
- *Video Examples.* Video Examples have been added to the eText edition. They give students an inside look at the world of communication disorders. These videos, chosen specifically for this text, illustrate critical concepts in easily digestible 2- to 3-minute clips.
- *Video Tool Exercises.* One Video Tool Exercise per chapter in the eText edition offers students an opportunity to engage with chapter content further. These activities consist of a video accompanied by short-answer questions to promote deeper understanding of key concepts.
- *Linked glossary.* Key terms throughout the text are linked, giving students one-click access to crucial definitions.

Instructor's Resource Manual

To help instructors in preparing their courses, we have provided an Instructor's Resource Manual. This supplement is available online or can be obtained by contacting a Pearson sales representative. To download and print the Instructor's Resource Manual, go to www.pearsonhighered.com and then click on "Educators."

Acknowledgments

Preparing the sixth edition—as with previous editions—might appear at first to be a simple process but it actually was a large time investment supported by many people. I have to admit, based on past experience, I was a bit skeptical about a "team". However, this team has been wonderful, helpful, knowledgeable, and efficient. First, I would like to thank Aileen (Berg) Pogran, who is the Executive Portfolio Manager of this sixth edition and relatively new to Pearson. Her support has been amazing. Other team members include Krista (Slavicek)

McMurray, Development Editor, whose eye for detail has been really very helpful; Faraz Sharique Ali, Content Producer US (Team Lead), who has been a behind the scenes person but could be relied on for all sorts of needs, thank you; Carmina Jimenez, Editorial Project Manager, who is so quick and efficient, great; Prince John William Carey, Project Manager, who has been so kind and helpful in spite of my having to change deadlines constantly; and Jon Theiss, Digital Development Editor, always providing a top notch video. A special thanks to Deepali Malhotra, Content Producer, who recently took a vague concept of mine and turned it into a cover design which is so perfect: a child who is happy and hopeful, representing to me the future and the possibilities. Thank you to Deepali and her team. All of these amazing people have been so supportive and helpful as I proceeded through this task.

For this edition, I would like to say a special thanks to my reviewers: Christine Fiestas from Texas A&M -Kingsville; Carol Tessel from Florida Atlantic University; Haralambia Kollia from William Paterson University; Maria Grigos from New York University; Peter Richtsmeier from Oklahoma State University; Tim Brackenbury from Bowling Green State University. I hope that you can recognize many of the wonderful suggestions that guided me through these revisions.

Brief Contents

Contents

Chapter 1
Clinical Framework

Basic Terms and Concepts

⌄ Learning Objectives

When you have finished this chapter, you should be able to:

1.1 Define communication, speech, and language.

1.2 Define disorders of communication, speech, and language.

1.3 Distinguish between articulation and speech sounds (phones), phonology, and phonemes.

1.4 Define speech sound disorder and understand its relationship to articulation and phonological disorders.

1.5 Classify speech sound disorders according to specific parameters.

Communication, Speech, and Language

Communication is central to our lives. We communicate in a number of ways—from text messaging to facial expressions. Simply defined, communication is the process of sharing information between individuals (Pence Turnbull & Justice, 2017). When we think about the diversified population that we encounter within the discipline of communication disorders, a broader definition might be helpful. **Communication** is a process that consists of two or more people sharing information, including facts, thoughts, ideas, and feelings. Communication includes how to interact with other people and things, how to understand spoken language, and how to exchange information with others using gestures or symbols. Communication does not have to involve language and does not have to be vocalized (Justice & Redle, 2014; National Joint Committee for the Communicative Needs of Persons with Severe Disabilities, 2010). Communication refers to any way that we convey information from one person to another. For example, we use Twitter, Skype, and FaceTime as ways to communicate. In addition, smiling, waving, and raising your eyebrows at a comment are all examples of nonverbal communication. Sign languages, such as American Sign Language or Seeing Essential English, are nonverbal conventional linguistic systems used to communicate.

However, the most widely used means of communication is speech. **Speech** is the expression of thoughts in spoken words, that is, in oral, verbal communication. Speech can be further divided into *articulation*, the motor production of speech sounds; *fluency*, the flow of speaking, including rate and rhythm; and *voice*, including vocal quality, pitch, loudness, and resonance (American Speech-Language-Hearing Association [ASHA], 1993). The term *speech* is used in various ways. Speech can be a more formal, spoken communication to an audience. For example: *Having to give a speech to her class was always frightening for Andrea.* Speech can also indicate a manner of speaking: *Her speech was marked by a distinct Australian accent.* Speech is also used together with the term *language* to indicate the mental faculty of verbal communication: *The child's speech and language skills were tested as a portion of the diagnostic.* Based on this last example, it seems important to differentiate between speech and language. What are the distinctions between these two terms: *speech* versus *language*?

Figure 1.1 Subdivisions of Language

Phonology	• Study of the sound system of a language; includes arrangement, systematic organization, and rule system of vowels and consonants (Parker & Riley, 2010). • Example: The phonology of English contains "sh," /ʃ/; Spanish does not.
Morphology	• Study of the structure of words; analyzes how words can be divided into units labeled as morphemes, which are the smallest meaningful units of language (Crystal, 2010). • Example: The word *bicycle* has two morphemes, "bi" = two, and "cycle" = circular or wheel.
Syntax	• Study of organizational rules denoting word, phrase, and clause order; sentence organization; and the relationship between sentence elements (Owens, 2016). • Example: "I like chocolate ice cream" has appropriate syntax, but "Ice cream I chocolate like" does not.
Semantics	• Study of linguistic meaning; includes the meaning of words, phrases, and sentences (Parker & Riley, 2010). • Example: Semantics includes the fact that certain words, such as "bat," have more than one meaning and that certain words, such as "dog" and "canine," have similar meanings.
Pragmatics	• Study of language used to communicate within various situational contexts; includes such things as conversational skills and the flexibility to modify speech for different listeners and social situations (Paul, Norbury, & Gosse, 2018). • Example: Among other things, pragmatics includes facial expressions, body gestures, and word emphases to communicate specific meanings.

According to the American Speech-Language-Hearing Association (ASHA), **language** can be defined as a complex and dynamic system of conventional symbols that is used in various modes for thought and communication (American Speech-Language-Hearing Association Committee on Language, 1983). This definition further states that language is rule governed and is described by at least five linguistic parameters: phonological, morphological, syntactical, semantic, and pragmatic. Language is intricate and includes variability and change. In addition, all members of a language agree on the symbolic system that is used, and language is used to communicate in a variety of ways.

Within our definition of language are the terms **phonology**, **morphology**, **syntax**, **semantics**, and **pragmatics**. Definitions and examples of each of these parameters are contained in Figure 1.1. One of these parameters, phonology, is of major importance in this text.

To summarize, communication is the process of sharing information between and among individuals. Communication can be broadly divided into speech and language. Speech is the expression of thoughts in spoken words; it is oral, verbal communication. On the other hand, language is a complex, dynamic, and rule-based system of conventional symbols that is used in diverse modalities for thought and communication. However, as practitioners, we deal with communication, speech, and language *disorders*. What characteristics would a disordered system demonstrate?

▶ Video Example 1.1
This video features a short explanation of communication. What do you think? Do we communicate with computers?
https://www.youtube.com/watch?v=JdbL7jJb3JE&t=

Disorders of Communication, Speech, and Language

According to the 1993 guidelines of ASHA, a **communication disorder** is the impairment in the ability to receive, send, process, and comprehend concepts, including verbal, nonverbal, and graphic symbol systems. Communication disorders are further subdivided into speech, language, hearing, and central auditory processing difficulties. A **speech disorder** is used to indicate oral, verbal communication that is so deviant from the norm that it is noticeable or interferes with communication. Speech disorders are divided into articulation, fluency, and voice disorders. On the other hand, a **language disorder** involves the impaired comprehension and/or use of spoken, written, and/or other symbol systems. A language disorder may involve one or more of the following areas: phonology, morphology, syntax, semantics, and pragmatics. Impaired auditory sensitivity leads to a **hearing impairment**. Individuals with hearing impairments are typically classified as either hard of hearing or deaf. The final area within this classification system is a **central auditory processing disorder**. These deficits result in difficulties with information processing of auditory signals that are not related to impaired sensitivity of the auditory system. Thus, these difficulties are not the result of a hearing impairment. Refer to Figure 1.2 for the subdivisions of communication disorders.

For the purpose at hand, we are primarily interested in speech disorders related to the impairment of the articulation of speech sounds and language disorders related to the category of phonology. In this context, it is important to examine the terms *articulation* and *speech sounds (phones)* as well as *phonology* and *phonemes*. The following section defines and gives examples of how these words are used in our clinical practice within communication disorders.

Figure 1.2 Subdivisions of Communication Disorders

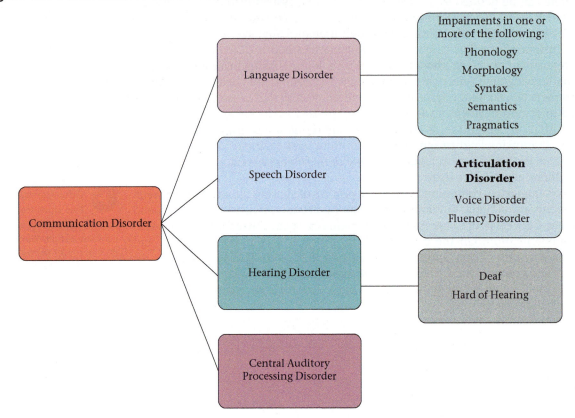

Articulation and Speech Sounds (Phones): Phonology and Phonemes

The term *articulation* and its derivations are often used to describe an individual's speech. They might appear in a referral statement or within a diagnostic report; for example:

> Sandy was referred to the clinic because her parents were concerned about her *articulation* skills.
>
> Bob could *articulate* the sound correctly in isolation but not in word contexts.
>
> Joe's *articulation* disorder affected his speech intelligibility.

For the purpose at hand, **articulation** refers to the totality of motor movements involved in production of the actual sounds that comprise speech (Bauman-Waengler, 2009). The learning of articulatory skills is a developmental process involving the gradual acquisition of the ability to move the **articulators** (those structures that are important in forming the individual sounds) in a precise and rapid manner. Thus, *learning to articulate is a specific kind of motor learning.* Just as children become more adept at certain motor skills as they grow older, their articulation skills develop as well. For example, a 2-year-old child and a 6-year-old child differ in their articulatory abilities. Errors in articulation can result from difficulty with the motoric aspects of speech production (Small, 2020). Thus, the peripheral motor processes involved in the planning and execution of articulation are impaired; the central language capabilities of the individual remain intact. In summary, articulation is a specific, gradually developing motor skill that involves motor processes.

Speech sounds are central units in any discussion of disordered speech. Although the human vocal tract is capable of producing a wide array of sounds, including coughing and burping, speech sounds are special sounds because they are associated with speech. **Speech sounds**, which can also be labeled as **phones**, represent physical sound realities; they are end products of articulatory motor processes. When talking about a child's s-production in the context of an articulation test, for example, we refer to the *speech sound* or *phone* production of [s].

Speech sounds or phones are real, physical sound entities used in speech. However, in addition to their *articulatory form*, they also have a linguistic function. *Linguistic function* includes, for example, the rules that address how specific sound units can be arranged to produce appropriate words and the phoneme concept. A **phoneme** is the smallest linguistic unit that is able, when combined with other such units, to distinguish meaning between words (Bauman-Waengler & Garcia, 2020). For example, "tick" has three phonemes: /t/, /ɪ/, and /k/. We know that these are phonemes of American English because the word they form is meaningful. In contrast, /s/ is also a phoneme of American English, as can be seen in "sick," /s/, /ɪ/, /k/, which differs from "tick" by one phoneme: /t/ versus /s/. As far as notation is concerned, speech sound (phone) productions are usually placed within brackets in phonetic transcription, whereas phoneme values are symbolized by slanted lines, or virgules. For example, [s] indicates that it was a sound someone actually pronounced in a specific manner. On the other hand, /s/ signifies the phoneme "s."

The idea of the phoneme is considered to be an abstraction. A phoneme is not a single, concrete, unchanging entity. A phoneme as an abstraction is based on the many variations that occur for a particular sound unit as it changes in differing contexts of conversational speech. This does not necessarily make the phoneme concept complex or difficult to understand. We constantly deal with abstractions. Take, for example, the concept "cat." A cat is not a single, unchanging entity. There are big cats and small cats, cats that are striped or solid colored of various shades. However, we accept certain characteristics as being typical to the concept of "cat." We could say that the *cat concept* embraces a whole family of units that are related yet somehow distinct. Even two cats of the same size, color, and build will have slight variations that could be detected most certainly by the owners. If we apply this to the phoneme concept, we find a similar abstraction. So when we speak of a particular phoneme, /t/ for example, we are referring to the typical "t" but we also take into consideration the varieties of "t" that are used in various contexts and by different speakers. The term *allophone* is used to refer to the changes that occur in a phoneme when produced by speakers in differing contexts. **Allophones** are variations in phoneme realizations, in phones, that do not change the meaning of a word when they are produced in differing contexts. Allophones are phonetic variations of a phoneme (Crystal, 2010). Within the phonological system of American English, there are many examples of allophones.

Several allophonic variations can occur with the /p/ phoneme, for example. At the beginning of a word as a single sound unit, /p/ is typically aspirated. Aspiration is that slight puff of air that you hear if you pronounce the word "pie" or "pot." This is transcribed as [pʰ], the small raised ʰ representing the puff of air or aspiration in phonetic transcription. However, /p/ is typically unaspirated following "s,"

Clinical Exercises In American English, [t] and [d] phones between two vowels are often produced as a flap (or referred to as a tap), [ɾ]. For example, say the word "butter" or "ladder" casually and note the quick movement of the tip of the tongue as it briefly taps the ridge on the roof of the mouth. Sometimes this movement is so casual that the tongue does not even touch the roof of the mouth. This is an acceptable production of [t] or [d]. It is an allophonic variation in this particular context. Does this change the meaning of the previously noted words? What would you think if a child said "ladder" this way on an articulation test?

Say the word "leap" and then the word "cool" slowly. Concentrate on the production of [l]. Do you notice any differences between the first and the second [l] productions? These two different productions are termed light "l" (leap) and dark "l" (cool) to denote the different ways "l" is articulated. Discuss why this would be an allophonic variation in American English. In Russian, these two types of [l] productions have phonemic value.

as in "spy" or "spot," for example. If you pronounce these words, you will find that the puff of air, the aspiration that you noticed in "pie," is not present. However, these allophonic variations exemplified by aspiration or lack of aspiration do not have phonemic value within the phonological system of American English. In other words, we can hear these differences, but both aspirated and unaspirated p-sounds are considered one phoneme, /p/.

As will be noted later, a current ASHA definition of "speech sound disorder" uses "speech sound" as an umbrella term to designate both the physical realities or forms (phones) and the linguistic functional abstraction of the phoneme. To not confuse this issue any further, within this text physical form realities will be referred to as phones and linguistic functional entities will be referred to as phonemes.

Phonology is the study of how phonemes are organized and function in a language. Phonology includes the inventory of phonemes of the language in question, thus a list of all the vowels and consonants that function in American English to differentiate meaning. However, phonology also focuses on how these phonemes are *organized* to convey meaning within a language system. Such a description would include how the phonemes can and cannot be arranged to form meaningful words. **Phonotactics** refers to the description of the allowed combinations of phonemes in a particular language.

Phonotactics of General American English includes the fact that some phoneme combinations do not occur in American English words. An example would be "sh" + "v." General American English does have other "sh" combinations, such as "sh" + "r" (e.g., *shrink*) or "sh" + "t" (e.g., *wished*). The "sh" + "v" combination does, however, occur in the phonological system of German. Words such as *Schwein* (for "pig") document this as a *phonotactic* possibility in German.

Phonotactics also restricts some consonant clusters in General American English to their use in certain word positions, for example, the clusters /sk/ and /ks/. Words or syllables can begin or end with /sk/ (e.g., *skate, risk*), but this is not the case with /ks/. This cluster can occur only at the end of a syllable or word (e.g., *kicks*). This is a *phonotactic* characteristic of the phonological system of General American English. A more complete discussion of the phonotactics of American English will be presented in Chapter 2.

▶ **Video Example 1.2**
American Sign Language (ASL) also has a phonological system. In this video, Dr. Crain explains the phonology of ASL and gives examples of allophonic variations. Can you demonstrate one example of ASL phonology?

https://www.youtube.com/watch?v=f2Yk48uvhtY

Table 1.1 Phoneme Versus Phone

Phoneme	Phone
The smallest unit within a language that is able, when combined with other units, to establish word meanings and distinguish between them	Actual realizations of phonemes; also referred to as *allophonic variations* or *phonetic variations*
Linguistic unit, an abstraction	Concrete, produced, transmitted, and perceived
Used in reference to a particular language system	Can be examined without referring to a specific language system
Basic unit within phonology	Basic unit within phonetics
Notation is within virgules (e.g., "the /s/ phoneme")	Notation is within brackets (e.g., "the [f] phone")

From early to contemporary publications, phoneme realizations have also been labeled **phonetic variations**. Phones or phonetic variations can be examined without reference to a given language system. This is not the case with phonemes. When using the term *phoneme*, we refer exclusively to the function of the sound in question: to its ability to signify differences in word meaning within a *specific* language (refer to Table 1.1). Two words that differ in only one phoneme value are called **minimal pairs**. Examples of minimal pairs are *dog* versus *log* and *dog* versus *dot.*

How do these terms relate to our clinical decision making? Phones as end products of articulatory motor processes are the units we are describing when we use phonetic transcription to capture an individual's actual productions on a standardized speech test or a spontaneous speech sample. Phones and their errors relate to articulatory deviations. However, what if we notice that a child's productions of *swing, sing, ring,* and *wing* all sound the same, for example, that they all sound like *wing*? The child is not using the necessary phonemic contrasts to signal differences between these words. Both listener and speaker will probably not be able to differentiate between these words because they sound identical. Now we are analyzing the child's phoneme system, the child's ability to use phonemes to establish and distinguish between word meanings. If this occurs consistently throughout the child's speech, we could conclude that the child's phoneme system is limited—that is, restricted when compared to the norm. Difficulties when using phonemes contrastively to distinguish meanings relate to *linguistic* abilities, to the individual's phonological system as one subcategory of language.

Phones, then, are related to motor, articulatory skills. On the other hand, phonemes represent an understanding of the phonological system of a particular language. Table 1.1 summarizes the differences between the phoneme and the phone. The next section will examine disorders that are related to phone production and phonemic differentiation. Current definitions as well as clinical examples will be provided.

Defining Speech Sound Disorders: Articulation and Phonological Disorders

The term **speech sound disorder** has been defined in various ways depending on the date and the source of the definition. To stay current with ASHA, its more recent definition of speech sound disorder will be used. This definition is located

Figure 1.3 Definition of Speech Sound Disorders

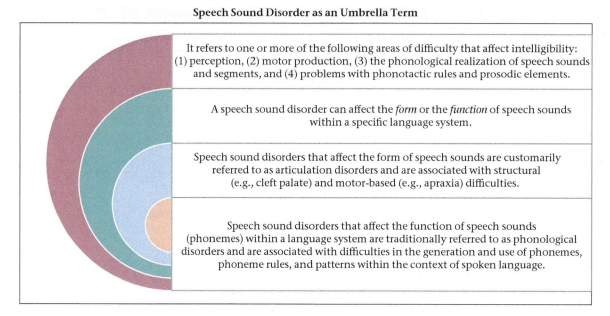

Speech Sound Disorder as an Umbrella Term

It refers to one or more of the following areas of difficulty that affect intelligibility: (1) perception, (2) motor production, (3) the phonological realization of speech sounds and segments, and (4) problems with phonotactic rules and prosodic elements.

A speech sound disorder can affect the *form* or the *function* of speech sounds within a specific language system.

Speech sound disorders that affect the form of speech sounds are customarily referred to as articulation disorders and are associated with structural (e.g., cleft palate) and motor-based (e.g., apraxia) difficulties.

Speech sound disorders that affect the function of speech sounds (phonemes) within a language system are traditionally referred to as phonological disorders and are associated with difficulties in the generation and use of phonemes, phoneme rules, and patterns within the context of spoken language.

(Based on ASHA practice portal, n.d.-b American Speech-Language-Hearing Association)

on the Practice Portal of ASHA, which is a site intended to provide audiologists and speech-language pathologists with current information that can be used in their daily clinical practice. The goal of this website is to offer the best available evidence and expertise in client care by identifying resources that are relevant and credible. A portion of the definition of speech sound disorder is adapted from the website and contained in Figure 1.3.

First, according to this definition, a speech sound disorder is an umbrella term. Therefore, as a label, "speech sound disorder" is not just one entity but a term used to represent several variations of deviant "speech." Different domains can affect intelligibility, and any one child may demonstrate difficulties in several of these areas. For example, perceptual difficulties may affect the child's ability to accurately perceive the distinctions between "s" and "sh," and motor production inconsistencies may also hinder the accuracy of articulating these two phones. Also inherent in the definition is the fact that a child could demonstrate motor problems together with phonological realization and phonotactic, rule-based usage problems.

An important distinction still contained within the definition is the form and function dichotomy. Although there seems to be some argument that this is not a valid dichotomy (Buckingham & Christman, 2006, 2008), it does provide a framework that can be useful for practitioners. Disorders that affect the form of speech sounds (phones) are historically referred to as articulation disorders, whereas phonemic functional difficulties are referred to as phonological disorders. Let's examine articulation versus phonological disorders to see how they have been typically defined.

An **articulation disorder**, as a subcategory of a speech disorder, is the atypical production of phones characterized by substitutions, omissions, additions, or distortions that may interfere with intelligibility (ASHA, 2014). Articulation errors are typically classified relative to a child's age, which translates into stages within this developmental process. Younger children are at an earlier stage in this

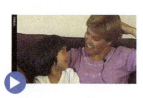

Video Example 1.3
This video features a 4-year-old named Caitlin. Do you notice any phones that she is still having trouble producing?

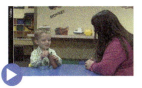

development, whereas older children are at a later stage or may have completed the process. Depending on the age of the child, certain articulation errors may be considered to be typical (age-appropriate errors) or atypical (non–age-appropriate errors). When assessing an individual, we often gather information on the inventory of phones used. The **phonetic inventory** is a list of all phones, including their variations.

On the other hand, a **phonological disorder**, as a subcategory of a language disorder, refers to the impaired comprehension of the sound system of a language and the rules that govern these sound combinations (American Speech-Language-Hearing Association Ad Hoc Committee on Service Delivery in the Schools, 1993; ASHA, 2008). When an individual's phonological system deviates enough from the norm, this could lead to a phonological disorder.

Phonology is closely related to other components of the language system, such as morphology, syntax, semantics, and pragmatics. A child's phonological system, therefore, can never be regarded as functionally separate from these aspects of the child's language growth. Several studies (e.g., Cummings, 2009; Edwards, Beckman, & Munson, 2004; Krueger & Storkel, 2017; Mortimer, 2007; Munson, Edwards, & Beckman, 2005a; Roberts, 2005) have documented that delayed phonological development can occur concurrently with delayed lexical and grammatical development. Although the direct relationship between phonological and grammatical acquisition remains unclear, interdependencies certainly exist between these areas.

Assessment of a child with a phonological disorder would include gathering information about all phonemes that the child uses to distinguish meaning—the phonemic inventory. The **phonemic inventory** is the repertoire of phonemes used by the child to contrastively differentiate meaning. When compared to the phonemic inventory of General American English, we might find that certain phonemes are not used contrastively in the child's speech—that is, the child's phonemic inventory is restricted.

In addition, we might analyze the child's phonotactics by examining the organization of her phoneme system. Children who have difficulties with the organization of their phoneme system might not realize the phonotactics that are typical for American English. Their speech may demonstrate **phonotactic constraints**; in other words, the phoneme use is restricted, and the phonemes are not used in all possible word positions. **Constraints** are any patterns noted that seem to limit or restrict the productional possibilities of our clients (Blache, 2000). Phonotactic constraints could be evidenced if a child uses only certain vowels or consonants in specific word positions. Thus, [k] could be used at the beginning of a word but not at the end: "cat" would be [kæt], but "cake" would be [keɪ]. Phonotactic limitations when producing consonant clusters could also be a constraint. For example, consonant clusters are used occasionally by a child at the end of a word but never at the beginning: "clown" would be [kaʊn], but "trains" would be [teɪnt]. Constraints can vary; therefore, the clinician will have to look at the transcription and see if any patterns of restrictions or limitations are specifically noted.

Although the distinction between an articulation disorder and a phonological disorder is important, it is not an either/or dichotomy. Many of the children with speech sound disorders will evidence characteristics of both types of difficulties. These two types of speech sound disorders should not be considered mutually exclusive, but rather consideration should be given to the impact that both articulatory and phonological difficulties may have in a child's distinctive profile. A child may demonstrate problems with physically producing phones *and* using phonemes contrastively to differentiate words. Both articulatory and phonological features

Video Example 1.4
In this video, 4-year-old Ben explains how he constructed an art project. Do you hear any phones that are distorted? Listen carefully to his s-sounds and "j" [ʤ] (the sound at the beginning and end of "judge").

are merely different sides of the same coin. It is the clinician's task to identify the child's possibly changing and evolving areas of deficit and select strategies that will teach this child the necessary skills.

However, this dichotomy is theoretically useful and can be applied practically to diagnostic and intervention procedures. Therefore, for the purpose at hand, a distinction is made between articulation disorders, those in which the peripheral motor processes are disturbed, and phonological or phonemic-based disorders, those in which the organization and function of the phonological system are impaired. Although this division between articulation and phonological disorders may remain at times unclear, a systematic attempt to distinguish between them is one important aspect of clinical decision making. This dichotomy is used throughout this text and developed more fully in later chapters. Other classification systems of speech sound disorders have been developed and expanded upon over the years. The following section examines two of the prominent classification systems.

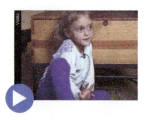

Video Tool Exercise 1.1

Listening to the Sound Productions of a 4-Year-Old

Complete the activity based on this video.

Classifying Speech Sound Disorders

There are many ways to classify speech sound disorders. That said, there is no universally agreed-upon system. One thing is agreed upon, however: Children with speech sound disorders represent a heterogeneous group. There is support for a broad-based division into those disorders with a known cause versus those with an unknown cause (e.g., Ruscello, 2008). Known causes include, among others, cerebral palsy, cleft lip/palate, and sensorineural hearing loss. However, this type of classification leaves most children in the "unknown" category. This diverse group of children, representing the majority of children with speech sound disorders, differs in disorder severity, speech characteristics, involvement of other aspects of the linguistic system, and response to treatment, to mention just a few factors (Baker, 2006; Bowen, 2009; Dodd, 2011). This type of broad-based etiological classification fails to subdivide this large and varied group of children.

Other systems have been developed to classify speech sound disorders. This section proposes to briefly discuss the classification of speech sound disorders according to two descriptions: (1) subtypes and etiologies of speech sound disorders, represented by the Speech Disorders Classification System (e.g., Shriberg et al., 2010) and (2) a descriptive-linguistic framework, represented by the Differential Diagnosis System (e.g., Dodd, 2013).

Subtypes and Etiological Factors: Speech Disorders Classification System

The Speech Disorders Classification System is a product of systematic research. It has evolved as a research tool and has been described by Shriberg and colleagues (e.g., Shriberg, 1980, 2010; Shriberg & Kwiatkowski, 1982a, 1982b; Shriberg et al., 2010). This classification system is divided into types of speech sound disorders and possible etiologies.

TYPES OF SPEECH SOUND DISORDERS.　In addition to the categorization of normal speech acquisition, there are three types of speech sound disorders.

1. *Speech delay.* Onset between 3 and 9 years of age, represented by significant speech sound substitutions and deletions that may become age appropriate with treatment.

2. *Motor speech disorder.* Onset between 3 and 9 years of age, represented by significant speech sound distortions, deletions, and substitutions that may not be age appropriate even after treatment.

3. *Speech errors.* Onset between 6 and 9 years of age, represented by speech sound distortion errors that occur primarily on s- and r-sounds. Although these problems may persist throughout the lifespan, they are not associated with the social and academic consequences that are noted in (1) speech delay or (2) motor speech disorder.

For children over 9 years of age, the term *persistent speech disorder* is used.

ETIOLOGIES OF SPEECH SOUND DISORDERS. This list attempts to describe the causes of the various types of speech sound disorders.

1. *Speech delay.* Consists of three subcategories: (a) a speech delay associated with cognitive-linguistic difficulties that may be transmitted genetically, (b) a speech delay marked by auditory-perceptual processing problems that result from the fluctuating hearing loss associated with otitis media with effusion at a very early age, and (c) a speech delay with psychosocial involvement. This last group of children may be either aggressive or withdrawn, and it is hypothesized that their temperaments may make it more difficult for them to obtain the feedback they need to develop appropriate speech skills.

2. *Motor speech disorder.* Includes two subtypes of speech delay: (a) speech motor involvement with planning and/or programming restraints, which is consistent with apraxia of speech, and (b) speech delay-dysarthria.

3. *Speech errors.* Consists of two subtypes for English speakers: (a) the distortion of s-sounds and (b) the distortion of r-sounds. In their need to communicate, these children attempt to master some aspects of speech before they are ready to do so. They adopt a communication pattern (s- or r-sound distortions) that continues into the school years. This has been labeled as a phonological attunement causation factor. Refer to Figure 1.4 for an overview of this classification system.

However, Shriberg and colleagues (2010) point out that the noted etiological classification system is not intended for clinical practice until more research can validate these initial findings. In addition, the authors identify that the subtypes noted are not mutually exclusive. These complex developmental disorders could demonstrate difficulties in several of the domains. The overlapping and indistinct boundaries between subgroups, specifically the speech delay subgroups, is one reported problem of the Speech Disorders Classification System (Waring & Knight, 2013). Waring and Knight (2013) also note that these diagnostic labels provide little information about the nature, severity, or type of therapy indicated for children with these specific speech difficulties. Finally, it appears that the clinical feasibility of this system is questionable. In an attempt to label children within these parameters, Fox, Howard, and Dodd (2002) noted that more than half of the children within their study could not be classified. As more research is conducted with this classification system, the parameters will hopefully become clearer and this system could be more widely used with clinical populations.

Figure 1.4 Speech Disorders Classification System (SDCS)

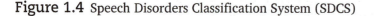

Types

- Speech delay: significant speech sound substitutions and deletions; may become age appropriate with treatment
- Motor speech disorder: speech sound distortions, deletions, and substitutions; may not be age appropriate even after treatment
- Speech errors: speech sound distortion errors on primarily s and r-sounds
- Persistent speech errors: term used after 9 years of age

Etiologies

- Speech delay associated with (1) cognitive-linguistic problems that may be genetic, (2) auditory-perceptual processing problems caused by early occurrence of otitis media with effusion, and (3) psychosocial involvement
- Motor speech disorder with (1) planning and/or programming constraints (childhood apraxia of speech) or (2) dysarthria
- Speech errors with persistent s- or r-sound problems caused by "phonological attunement"

(Adapted from Shriberg, 1980, 2010; Shriberg et al., 2010.)

The following section examines the second classification system, which is based on a descriptive-linguistic framework: the Differential Diagnosis System (e.g., Dodd, Holm, Crosbie, & McCormack, 2013).

Examining Error Patterns: The Differential Diagnosis System

The descriptive-linguistic framework consists of describing children's speech sound difficulties according to the error patterns they demonstrate. The system is developmental and compares the child's deviant productions to those of children of the same age with normal speech sound acquisition. This type of categorization caused a major shift in diagnosing children with speech sound disorders. Rather than labeling children as having multiple individual sound errors, clinicians began to talk about patterns and sound class errors (refer to Grunwell, 1997).

Dodd (1995, 2005) proposed a classification system that was based on the descriptive-linguistic model and consisted of five subgroups of speech sound disorders.

1. *Articulation disorder.* This is an inability to pronounce certain phones, typically s- and r-sounds. The child uses a consistent substitution or distortion for the target sound in both spontaneous and imitated productions.
2. *Phonological delay.* These children demonstrate phonological patterns that are evidenced in normal development but are typically noted at an earlier chronological age.

3. *Consistent phonological disorder.* This involves consistent use of some non-developmental error patterns. These children may demonstrate atypical and idiosyncratic error patterns.

4. *Inconsistent phonological disorder.* The phonological systems of these children show at least 40% variability of production when asked to name 25 pictures on 3 separate trials within a single session. Thus, multiple errors are demonstrated for the same word.

5. *Childhood apraxia of speech.* This is seen as a multi-deficit motor-speech disorder involving phonological planning, phonetic, and motor programming difficulties (Ozanne, 2013).

Refer to Figure 1.5 for an overview of the Differential Diagnosis System.

It appears that this system is useful clinically. Studies have demonstrated that children can be consistently classified according to these parameters (e.g., Broomfield & Dodd, 2004). Dodd and colleagues (2013) have constructed speech sound profiles that summarize the major features of the subgroups, the impact of intelligibility, and possible treatment strategies. Although additional research findings would further authenticate this model—especially the validity of inconsistent phonological disorder and its distinction from childhood apraxia of speech (Waring & Knight, 2013)—the model does provide clinical possibilities.

To summarize, Table 1.2 outlines several terms that are used clinically and in research in reference to speech sounds and speech sound disorders.

Figure 1.5 Differential Diagnosis System

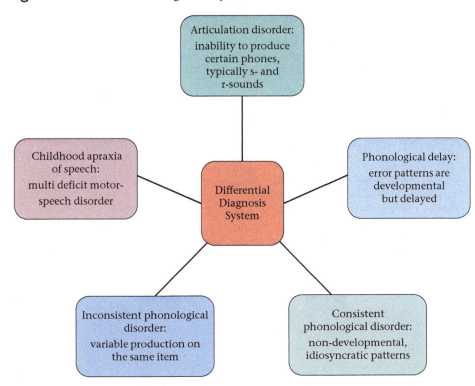

(Adapted from Dodd, 1995; Dodd et al., 2013.)

Table 1.2 Speech Sounds and Speech Sound Disorders: Terminology

Term	Definition	Examples
Articulation	The totality of motor processes involved in the planning and execution of speech.	Describes the phone production of individuals (e.g., "The *articulation* of [s] was incorrect."). Describes tests that examine the production of phones (e.g., "The clinician administered a standardized speech assessment, an *articulation* test.").
Articulation disorder	Difficulty with the motor production aspects of speech or an inability to produce certain speech sounds.	A diagnostic category that indicates that an individual's phone productions vary widely from the norm (e.g., "Tony was diagnosed as having an *articulation* disorder.").
Phonology	The study of the sound system of a language; examines the sound units of that particular language, how these sounds are arranged, their systematic organization, and the rule system.	Describing the inventory and arrangement of sound units (e.g., the Spanish *phonological system* has fewer vowels than American English. The phoneme /s/ is present in Spanish, but /z/ is not.).
Phonological disorder	Impaired comprehension and/or use of the sound system of a language and the rules that govern the sound combinations.	The inventory of phonemes may be restricted (e.g., "Jonathan used the phoneme /t/ for /d, k, g, s, z, ʃ, ʒ, tʃ, dʒ/.").
Speech sound disorder	An umbrella term that refers to disordered form (articulation) and/or function (phonological) of speech sounds within a specific language system (ASHA, n.d.-b).	The child's speech sound disorder affected the articulation of his phones and the phonemic function of phonemes.
Persistent speech sound disorders	Errors that persist past the typical age of acquisition (9 years old).	Children with this disorder show little spontaneous improvement, and their response to intervention is poor. There is commonly no known cause (Wren, Roulstone, & Miller, 2012).
Inconsistent speech disorder/inconsistent phonological disorder	Phonological systems that demonstrate variability of production on the same item. This is determined by at least 40% variability on the production of 25 words repeated 3 times in a single session (Dodd, 1995, 2005).	These children do not respond to typical pattern-based treatment but seem to respond to first decreasing variability of their productions.
Speech sound delay	Speech sound errors that are often noted as "normal" errors found in young children as they acquire specific sounds. A "delay" usually has the premise that the child will catch up and achieve normal development.	A category that is typically used in young children to denote a mismatch between the child's speech sound acquisition and what is considered to be a norm reference.
Deviant speech sound development	Speech sound errors that are not typically observed in the development of most young children.	A term that typically indicates a process that is not delayed but different (e.g., "Lindsey demonstrated substitutions, such as [s] for [p, b, t, d]. Her speech sound development appeared deviant.").

Term	Definition	Examples
Speech or phonological disability	*Disability* is a complex phenomenon reflecting the interaction between features of a person's body and features of the society in which she lives (World Health Organization [WHO], 2014). *Disability* is an umbrella term including impairments.	In reference to speech or phonology, this would indicate a serious speech sound/phonological difficulty that affects the child's or person's functioning in society.
Speech or phonological impairment	An *impairment* is any loss or abnormality of physiological or anatomical structure or function (WHO, 2014).	In reference to speech or phonology, *impairment* is typically used synonymously with *disorder*. The anatomical/physiological basis for the term is typically not a primary consideration.

Summary

This chapter introduced the reader to several terms that are fundamental to the assessment and treatment of speech sound disorders. As an introduction, the terms *communication*, *speech*, and *language* were provided, as were the five subcategories of language: *phonology*, *morphology*, *syntax*, *semantics*, and *pragmatics*. Definitions and clinical applications were noted for *articulation*, *phonology*, *phone*, and *phoneme* as a foundation for this understanding. Speech sound forms versus linguistic function were used to distinguish between the phone and the phoneme. Based on these definitions, differentiations between speech sound, articulation, and phonological disorders were presented, as was nomenclature that is widely used in clinical practice and research relative to these terms.

Case Studies

Speech Sound Disorder: Articulation

Sandy is a 6-year-old child who was seen in a diagnostic session at the speech and hearing clinic. Her parents are concerned about her inability to produce [s]. Based on an analysis of a spontaneous speech sample and a standardized speech assessment, it was found that Sandy misarticulated [s] and [z] in all transcribed situations: Her tongue placement was too far forward during the productions. The child was able to differentiate her mispronunciations from norm productions of [s] and [z]. No other speech sounds were in error, and language skills were found to be within normal limits. Sandy used her distorted realizations in every position in which [s] and [z] should occur. Thus, she seemed to understand the organization of /s/ and /z/ within the language system. The clinician hypothesized that this child is having difficulties with the actual production level only, with the speech sounds [s] and [z], whereas the understanding of their phoneme function was intact.

Phonology: Phonological Disorder

Travis, a 6-year-old first-grader, was referred by his classroom teacher to the speech-language pathologist. The teacher said that although Travis's speech was fairly intelligible, she was concerned about speech and language problems she had noticed in class. Her second concern was that these difficulties might be affecting Travis's emerging literacy skills. According to the teacher, Travis was having difficulty distinguishing between certain sounds and words as the class progressed with elementary reading and writing tasks.

A standardized speech assessment and a spontaneous speech sample were analyzed with the following results: Travis had difficulties with s-production. At the end of a word or syllable, [s] was always deleted. At the beginning of a word or syllable, [s] was produced as "sh," [ʃ]. Interestingly enough, when the clinician analyzed other words, she found that Travis could produce [s], but not in its proper context. Thus, several words that contained [ʃ] were articulated with normal sounding [s] realizations. Testing of minimal pairs containing /s/ and /ʃ/ revealed that Travis was having difficulty distinguishing between the phonemic values of the two sounds.

On language tests and in spontaneous conversation, Travis deleted the plural -s and the third-person singular -s (e.g., "He, she, it walk"). Comprehension of these grammatical forms was often in error.

The clinician hypothesized that Travis had a phonological disorder—that he had difficulties with the phoneme function and the phonotactics of /s/. This problem was affecting his morphological development. Because of the noted problems in discrimination, this could also have an effect on his beginning reading and writing skills.

Think Critically

The following small speech sample is from Tara, age 7 years 7 months.

$[r] \rightarrow [w]$
$[ð] \rightarrow [d]$
$[gr] \rightarrow [gw]$

rabbit	[wæbət]	ready	[wɛdi]
feather	[fɛdɚ]	arrow	[ɛwoʊ]
green	[gwin]	toothbrush	[tutbwəʃ]
this	[ðɪs]	thinking	[θɪŋkɪŋ]
that	[ðæt]	round	[waʊnd]
rope	[woʊp]	bridge	[bwɪdʒ]
rooster	[wustɚ]	street	[stwit]
bathing	[beɪdɪŋ]	thin	[θɪn]
nothing	[nʌtɪŋ]	them	[ðɛm]
bath	[bæt]	breathe	[bwid]

1. Which speech sound errors are noted in this sample?
2. Which sounds are substituted for the sounds in error?
3. Can any phonotactic restraints be noted in the correct productions of "th" and "r"?

 Chapter Quiz 1.1 Complete this quiz to check your understanding of chapter concepts.

Chapter 2
Articulatory Phonetics

Speech Sound Form

 ## Learning Objectives

When you have finished this chapter, you should be able to:

2.1 Define and classify phonetics and the branches of phonetics.

2.2 Briefly review the anatomical-physiological foundations of speech production.

2.3 List the differences in production and function of vowels versus consonants.

2.4 Identify the descriptive parameters used for vowels of General American English and categorize the vowels accordingly.

2.5 Identify the descriptive parameters used for the consonants of General American English and classify the consonants accordingly.

2.6 Define coarticulation and assimilation, and list the different types of assimilatory processes.

2.7 Identify the various types of syllable structures, including phonotactic restraints that might be noted in children.

Chapter Application: Case Study

Harry is a 7-year-old first-grader. He has a noticeable r-sound problem. Harry's parents thought that he would grow out of the speech problem. However, Harry is beginning to be very self-conscious of the difficulty, especially since the r-sound is in his name. At the beginning of words with "r," he uses a "w" sound; at the end of words, "r" sounds like a type of "uh" (as in "come") or "oo" (as in "look"). Harry is showing some difficulties in spelling. Since r-sounds are so frequent in General American English, Harry's teacher wonders if his articulation might be affecting his spelling. Does he hear the difference between "ring" and "wing," for example, if the context isn't provided when spelling out words to dictation? Harry is now enrolled in speech-language therapy. Considering his "r" problems, what would you do?

   Are there specific placement techniques you could use to establish an r-sound? Since there are three ways in which r-sounds can be produced, is one

(continued)

better to try to achieve versus the others? Knowledge of the production features of speech sounds is important for clinicians as they evaluate and treat children with specific sound errors.

Phonetics: Definitions and Classification

The description and classification of speech sounds or phones is the main aim of phonetics. Sounds may be identified with reference to their production (or "articulation"), their acoustic transmission, or their auditory reception. The most widely used description is articulatory, which is the emphasis of this chapter.

Generally stated, phonetics is the science of speech. However, it might be useful to delineate speech in its entirety while also indicating the various divisions of phonetics. Thus defined, **phonetics** is the study of speech emphasizing the description and classification of speech sounds (phones) according to their production, transmission, and perceptual features. Speech production is exemplified by articulatory phonetics; speech transmission by acoustic phonetics; and speech perception by auditory phonetics. In this chapter, the terms *speech sounds* and *phones* will be used interchangeably. However, it should be remembered that according to the American Speech-Language-Hearing Association (ASHA, n.d.-b) definition, speech sounds and their disorders are represented by both form (phone) and function (phoneme) difficulties.

Articulatory phonetics deals with the production features of phones, their categorization, and arrangement according to specific details of their production. Central aspects include the way they are actually articulated, their objective similarities, and their differences. *Articulation* is typically used as a more general term to describe the overall speech production of individuals. Articulatory phonetics as a field of study attempts to document phones according to specific parameters, such as their manner or voicing features. Articulatory phonetics is closely aligned with speech sounds/phones and speech sound disorders.

Acoustic phonetics deals with the transmission properties of speech. Here, the frequency, intensity, and duration of phones are described and categorized, for example. If you have ever analyzed specific sounds according to their frequencies, this would be classified as one aspect of acoustic phonetics.

Within **auditory phonetics**, investigators focus on how we perceive sounds. Our ears are not objective receivers of acoustic data. Rather, many factors, including our individual experiences, influence our perception. Such factors are examined in the field of auditory phonetics.

In this text, we are primarily interested in articulatory phonetics and in articulation. An integral portion of articulatory phonetics is the description and classification of speech sounds, in other words, the actualities of how phones are formed. This knowledge is important for both the assessment and treatment of speech sound form errors. Knowledge of the production features of speech sounds guides clinicians when they are evaluating the various misarticulations noted in a clinical evaluation. Thus, one important step in our diagnostic process involves gathering phonetic information on the exact way an individual misarticulates sounds.

Thus, articulatory phonetics *categorizes* and *classifies* the production features of speech sounds. A thorough knowledge of how vowels and consonants are generated remains essential for successful assessment and remediation of speech sound disorders. Although contemporary phonological theories have provided new ways

▶ **Video Example 2.1**
This short video presents the definition and scope of phonetics. What is the difference between phonetics and phonology? How do the three basic areas of study in phonetics align with what you have just read in this text? Can you add anything to the definitions noted on this page?

https://www.youtube.com/watch?v=nG_tcUlp634

of viewing the diagnosis and intervention of these disorders, knowledge of the speech sounds' production features provides a firm basis for using such procedures. Without this knowledge, phonological process analysis, for example, is impossible.

This chapter discusses articulatory-phonetic aspects of the speech sounds of General American English. The specific goals are to:

1. Provide a brief review of the anatomical-physiological foundation of speech production.
2. List the production features of vowels and consonants of General American English.
3. Introduce the concepts of coarticulation and assimilation as a means of describing how sounds change within a given articulatory context.
4. Examine the structure of syllables, including the phonotactics of General American English.

The production of vowels and consonants as well as their subsequent language-specific arrangements into syllables and words depends on articulatory-motor processes. If these processes are impaired, speech sound production will be disordered. Articulatory motor processes depend in turn on many anatomical-physiological prerequisites, which include respiratory, phonatory, or resonatory processes. For example, the speech problems of children with cerebral palsy often originate in abnormal respiration, resonance, and/or phonation prerequisites for articulation. Therefore, the proper function of these basic systems must first be secured before any articulatory improvement can be expected. Articulatory-motor ability is embedded in many different anatomical-physiological requisites, which are of fundamental importance to speech-language pathologists.

Anatomical-Physiological Review of the Foundations of Speech Production

This section provides an overview of the anatomical and physiological prerequisites for speech production. The structures involved in producing speech are cumulatively labeled the **speech mechanism**. The speech mechanism is further divided into the respiratory, phonatory, resonatory, and articulatory systems. Refer to Figure 2.1 for a representation of these four systems. In addition, further references for anatomy and physiology texts are provided in Appendix 2.1.

The Respiratory System

The respiratory system consists of the lungs, rib cage, thorax, abdomen, trachea, and those muscles associated with breathing. The primary function of the respiratory system is the vital exchange of gases for life support. The secondary function of this system is to generate a stream of air for the production of speech. Without this airflow, voice is not possible and speech sounds are not audible.

The principal muscle of inhalation is the diaphragm. The diaphragm consists of a strong fibrous central tendon as well as a peripheral muscular section. The muscular portion of the diaphragm is connected anteriorly and laterally to the lower edges of the ribs. Its posterior connection is to the upper lumbar vertebrae located toward the lower back area. These attachments of the diaphragm create a

Figure 2.1 Overview of the Respiratory, Phonatory, Resonatory, and Articulatory Systems

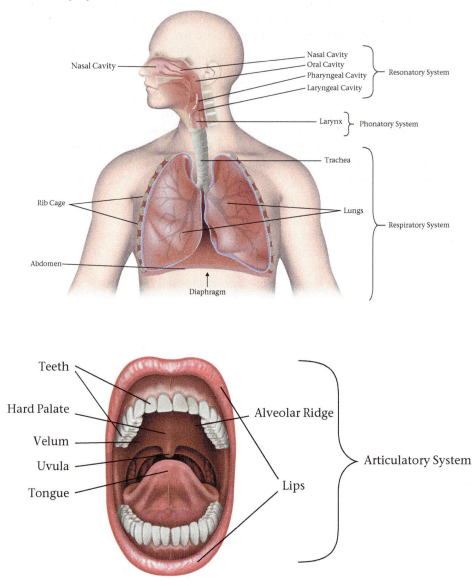

continuous sheet that divides the torso of the body into the thoracic cavity (above the diaphragm) and the abdominal cavity (below the diaphragm). Several muscles aid inhalation; the more important ones are the external and internal intercostals.

As inhalation begins, the muscular portion of the diaphragm contracts. Contraction shortens the muscular fibers, which then pull the central tendon down and somewhat forward. As the diaphragm moves downward, the up-and-down dimensions of the thoracic cavity increase and the contents of the abdominal cavity are compressed. Therefore, the saying "take a breath deep in the belly" does not mean that the air is going into your belly but rather that the deeper the inspiration, the more the abdominal contents are compressed and the belly is somewhat extended. At the same time, contractions of specific thoracic muscles attached to the ribs cause the ribs to swing up and outward. This increases the front-to-back and side-to-side dimensions of the thoracic cavity (refer Figure 2.2).

For respiration to occur, the lungs must increase their volume during inspiration and decrease their volume during expiration. Because the lungs do not contain skeletal muscle tissue, this process must be mediated by what has been termed **pleural linkage**. Two pleurae accomplish this pleural linkage, one covering the outer surface of the lungs and one covering the inner surface of the thorax and the top portion of the diaphragm. The two membranes are airtight and fused together, producing a small amount of fluid that provides smooth, lubricated movement of the lungs during respiration. There is a powerful negative pressure between the two membranes, which links the membranes so closely that the lungs cohere (stick) to the thoracic walls. Thus, any movement of the thoracic cavity results in movement of the lungs. As the dimensions of the thoracic cavity increase, these airtight membranes cause the lungs to follow the thoracic walls as they enlarge; thus, the lungs are forced to expand.

Figure 2.2 Changes in the Dimensions of the Thoracic Cavity During Inhalation

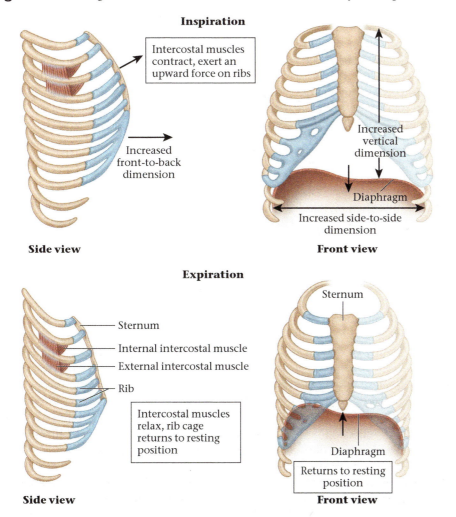

During rest, the pressure within the lungs, the so-called **alveolar pressure**, is equal to the outside air pressure. However, as inspiration begins, the increase in the thoracic dimensions and the consequent expansion of the lungs as they follow the expanding thoracic cavity results in a negative alveolar pressure. The consequence is that the outside air rushes in until the alveolar pressure again equals the outside air pressure. As outside air rushes into the lungs, the muscles of inhalation gradually cease their activity. At this point, exhalation begins. The diaphragm starts to relax to its uncontracted state, moving upward; the thoracic cavity's dimensions decrease. Both actions, the upward movement of the diaphragm and the relaxation of the extended wall of the thorax, increase the alveolar pressure to the degree that air is forced out of the lungs; thus, exhalation occurs. Generally, one can state that thoracic muscles support inhalation, whereas abdominal muscles can support exhalation. Under normal circumstances, exhalation is rather passive, however; if we want to make a prolonged utterance (or try to prolong "ah" for 20 seconds), then we might use the abdominal muscles to assist.

The task of the respiratory system during speech production is even more complex. Speech production necessitates a regulated amount of subglottal pressure over a rather wide range of volumes. **Subglottal air pressure** refers to the pressure below the vocal folds, the glottis being the space between the vocal folds. If you take a deep breath, but only say a word or two, this pressure will have to be regulated if normal but not excessive loudness is to be maintained. On the other hand, if you utter a longer sentence, a relatively constant amount of subglottal pressure must be maintained from the beginning of the utterance, when there is clearly more air in the lungs, to its end, when there is far less air. To maintain a constant loudness level during the whole utterance, the outflow of air must somehow be equalized. This equalization of various lung volumes and pressure levels is accomplished through an interplay of inspiratory and expiratory muscles. Based on this interplay of balancing actions between inspiratory and expiratory muscles, the respiratory system is able to constantly supply the laryngeal system with precisely regulated subglottal pressures.

The Phonatory System

The next important system for speech production is the phonatory system. We have noted that, through controlled expiration, the respiratory system provides a relatively even flow of pressurized air from the lungs. This air moves through the passage from the lungs to the larynx. The vocal folds, the most important part of the larynx, provide the source of sound for speech. However, the primary function of the larynx and vocal folds is not speech but rather preventing foreign substances from entering the respiratory system. We have all had the experience of "swallowing the wrong way" or "something going down the wrong tube." One can probably recall that this resulted in coughing, sometimes rather forcefully. This powerful reflex entails the vocal folds coming together so that air is trapped under them, which results in a buildup of air pressure. A sudden release of this closure produces an explosive expulsion of air sufficient enough to hopefully expel the foreign substance from the respiratory tract.

When not fulfilling the previously mentioned primary function, the larynx can serve as a sound generator for speech. The larynx is suspended from the hyoid bone, a horseshoe-shaped bone located at the base of the tongue, above the thyroid cartilage. Several of the laryngeal muscles are attached to this bone. The larynx itself consists of nine cartilages (one thyroid, one cricoid, one epiglottis, two arytenoid, two corniculate, and two cuneiform) as well as connecting membranes and ligaments.

Extrinsic muscles of the larynx (those having at least one attachment to structures outside the larynx) are primarily responsible for support and fixation of the larynx, whereas **intrinsic muscles of the larynx** (those having both attachments within the larynx) are necessary for control during voice production. The extrinsic muscles surround the larynx and anchor it in its position. The intrinsic muscles are far more interesting during voice production. Two muscles help to **adduct**, or close, the vocal folds, one opens the vocal folds, one tenses the vocal folds, and one comprises the main mass of the vocal folds. These muscles and their functions are summarized in Table 2.1 and Figure 2.3.

Looking at vocal fold vibration in a simplistic manner, we see that during quiet breathing the vocal folds are drawn away from the midline. The onset of phonation is marked by the vocal folds moving toward the midline, into an adducted position. In this adducted position, the vocal folds obstruct expiratory airflow, and subglottal pressure begins to build up. At a critical point of pressure buildup, the vocal folds are "blown apart"; the glottis is now open, with the natural consequence of an immediate decrease in subglottal pressure. The folds come together again due to their inherent elasticity, the sudden pressure drop between the folds, and aerodynamic properties.

The average number of glottal openings per second is known as a person's **fundamental frequency**. Although every speaker is capable of producing a wide range of fundamental frequencies, females typically have a higher range of fundamental frequencies than males (the fundamental frequency for females is approximately 200 to 260 cycles per second, whereas for males it is between 120 and 145 cycles per second; Zemlin, 1998). Changes in the *tension* of the vocal folds are primarily responsible for variations in fundamental frequency. On the other hand, changes in vocal loudness result from *variations in subglottal air pressure*, which varies the *amplitude of the vocal folds' vibratory cycle*. When more subglottal air pressure is present, the vocal folds move farther away from the midline during their vibratory cycles. We perceive this as an increase in loudness.

Table 2.1 The Function and Attachments of the Intrinsic Muscles of the Larynx

Muscle	Specific Function	Attachments
ADDUCTORS		
Lateral cricoarytenoid	Closes the vocal folds	Upper border of cricoid to the anterior surface of the arytenoid cartilage
Interarytenoid	Closes the vocal folds: two portions, transverse and oblique	Transverse: lateral margin and posterior portion of one arytenoid, runs horizontally to the lateral margin and posterior portion of the opposite arytenoid cartilage
		Oblique: from the base of one arytenoid to the apex of the opposite one.
ABDUCTOR		
Posterior cricoarytenoid	Only one abductor of the vocal folds. It opens the vocal folds	Runs obliquely from the posterior portion of the cricoid lamina to the upper surface and the posterior surface of the arytenoid cartilage
ELONGATING/TENSING		
Cricothyroid	Regulates longitudinal tension: two portions, pars recta and pars oblique	Both portions originate on the lateral edges of the cricoid cartilage; pars recta inserts into the bottom edge of the thyroid cartilage, pars oblique inserts into the top portion of the body of thyroid cartilage
Thyroarytenoid	**MAIN MASS OF VOCAL FOLDS**	From the inner surface of the thyroid cartilage to two different portions of the arytenoid cartilages

Figure 2.3 Intrinsic Muscles of the Larynx: Transverse and Oblique Interarytenoid Muscles, Posterior Cricoarytenoid Muscle, Cricothyroid Muscle (Pars Recta and Pars Oblique), and the Lateral Cricoarytenoid Muscle

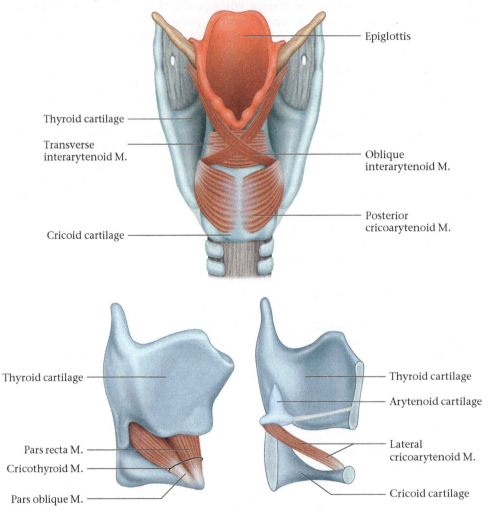

The consistent cyclic vibration of the vocal folds also plays a role in the quality or timbre of the voice. The term **timbre** refers to the tonal quality that differentiates two sounds of the same pitch, loudness, and duration (Crystal, 2010). If you produce "ah" and your friend then says "ah," trying to match your pitch, loudness, and duration, the two utterances will still sound different. This is due to the characteristic vocal quality, or timbre, of each person's voice.

The Resonatory System

The resonatory system is composed of three cavities within the vocal tract: the pharyngeal, oral, and nasal cavities. (The **vocal tract** consists of all speech-related systems above the vocal folds.) The **pharyngeal cavity**, a muscular and membranous tube-like structure, extends from the epiglottis to the soft palate. The **oral cavity**, or mouth area, extends from the lips to the soft palate. The **nasal cavities**, or nose area, consist of two narrow chambers that begin at the soft palate and end at the exterior portion of the nostrils. The floor of the nasal cavities is the hard palate.

Sound energy generated by the larynx is modified as it travels through the pharyngeal, oral, and/or nasal cavities. This portion of the speech mechanism is called the resonatory system because the modification of sound energy is primarily the result of resonance principles. **Resonance** is the selective reinforcement and absorption of sound energy at specific frequencies. In other words, certain frequencies are amplified or intensified (reinforced), whereas others are suppressed or damped out (absorbed). Resonance is one major component in determining our characteristic vocal qualities as well as in providing the basis for specific speech sounds. The pharyngeal, nasal, and oral areas could be described as differently shaped cavities that are variable in size and form. For example, protruding the lips would change the shape of the oral cavity, whereas muscular action lowering the larynx would change the dimensions of the pharyngeal cavity. In addition, variations in the walls of the resonating cavity (i.e., certain structures are softer and more pliable, whereas others are harder and denser) contribute to the resonating properties.

One structure within this system that does have a direct impact on the resonance quality of specific sounds in General American English is the velopharyngeal mechanism. It directly affects speech sound quality by channeling airflow through either the oral or the nasal cavities. The **velopharyngeal mechanism** consists of the structures and muscles of the velum (soft palate) and those of the pharyngeal walls (refer Figure 2.4). The **velopharyngeal port**, the passage that connects the oropharynx and the nasopharynx, can be closed by (1) elevation and posterior movements of the velum and (2) some forward and medial movements of the posterior and lateral pharyngeal walls. These combined movements resemble the action of a sphincter. Closure of the passageway between the oral and nasal cavities is important for three reasons. First, during the primary function of swallowing, the velopharyngeal port closes as the bolus of food or drink passes from the oral cavity to the pharyngeal cavity. This closure prevents the food or drink from entering the nasal cavity. Second, as a secondary function, closure of the velopharyngeal port is important for the production of specific groups of speech sounds, namely nasal versus non-nasal sounds. Nasal sounds are those produced with an open velopharyngeal port allowing airflow through the nasal cavity. In

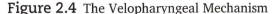

Figure 2.4 The Velopharyngeal Mechanism

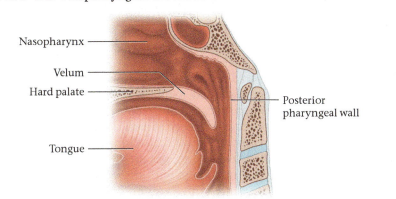

General American English, there are only three nasal sounds: "m," "n," and "ng." Non-nasal sounds are those produced with the velopharyngeal port closed; airflow passes through the oral cavity only. Third, accurately timed and adequate closure of the velopharyngeal port is necessary for normal vocal timbre. Without this, voice quality may sound hypernasal.

The Articulatory System

The articulatory system is directly involved in forming individual speech sounds. The structures within this system consist of the lips, tongue, mandible, teeth, hard palate (including the alveolar ridge), velum, and uvula, which are called articulators. Due to their importance for speech realization, a brief review of each of these structures will be helpful for later discussions about specific speech sound productions.

The lips consist primarily of the orbicularis oris muscle. However, many facial muscles insert into the lips. The lips are, therefore, very flexible for both facial expression as well as for speech sound production. The lips are the main articulators in sounds such as "b," "p," and "m," for example.

The next articulator, the tongue, is the most important and most active one for speech sound production. Due to the manner of its attachments and the number of intrinsic and extrinsic muscles involved, the tongue is capable of a wide range of movements. The body of the tongue, which is known as the **dorsum** (Zemlin, 1998), can move horizontally backward and forward and vertically up and down, can assume a concave or convex shape relative to the palate, can demonstrate central grooving, and can be spread or tapered in its appearance. Horizontal (forward and backward) and vertical (closer and farther away from the palate) movements are primarily responsible for vowel articulations. In addition, the shape of the tongue plays a major role in both vowel and consonant productions. There are many sounds for which various portions of the tongue are considered main articulators.

The mandible or lower jaw houses the lower teeth. Inadequate, inappropriate, or sluggish mandibular movement may contribute to articulatory difficulties (Zemlin, 1998).

The primary function of the teeth is to process food before it is swallowed and continues on its digestive route. For speech sound production, the secondary function of the teeth is their role as articulators for speech sounds such as "f" and "v" and the th-sounds in "the" or "with."

The next group of articulators consists of structures of the roof of the mouth: the hard palate, alveolar ridge, soft palate (velum), and uvula. If you glide your tongue posteriorly from behind the front teeth, you will encounter a prominent ridge-like structure known as the **alveolar ridge**. This protuberance is formed by the alveolar process, which is a thickened portion of the maxilla (upper jaw) housing the teeth. Moving past the alveolar ridge, the hard, bony structure is the hard palate. Farther back, there is a softer muscular portion, which is referred to as the soft palate or velum. An appendage-like extension of the soft palate is the uvula. All of these structures—alveolar ridge, hard palate, velum, and uvula—play a role in the qualitative end product of speech sounds. For example, "t" and "d" are produced by the tongue tip coming in contact with the alveolar ridge. The last sound in "wing," the so-called "ng" sound, has articulatory features that involve the back of the tongue coming in contact with the velum. In General American English, there are no uvular sounds. However, in French and German there is a uvular trilled-r-type sound where the uvula is actually brought into motion.

This section has provided a very brief review of the structure and function of the respiratory, phonatory, resonatory, and articulatory systems. The next section examines speech sounds, specifically the characteristics of vowel and consonant productions.

Vowels Versus Consonants

Speech sounds are commonly divided into two groups: vowels and consonants. **Vowels** are produced with a relatively open vocal tract; *no significant constriction* of the oral (and pharyngeal) cavities is required. The airstream from the vocal folds to the lips is relatively unimpeded. Therefore, vowels are considered to be *open sounds*. In contrast, **consonants** have *significant constriction* in the oral and/ or pharyngeal cavities during their production. For consonants, the airstream from the vocal folds to the lips and nostrils encounters some type of articulatory obstacle along the way. Therefore, consonants are considered to be *constricted sounds*. For most consonants, this constriction occurs along the sagittal midline of the vocal tract. The **sagittal midline** *of the vocal tract* refers to the median plane that divides the vocal tract into right and left halves. This constriction for consonants can be exemplified by the first sound in *top* or *soap*. For "t," the contact of the front of the tongue with the alveolar ridge (the ridge behind the front teeth) occurs along the sagittal midline, whereas the characteristic s-quality is made by airflow at the sagittal midline as the tongue approximates the alveolar ridge. By contrast, during all vowel productions, the sagittal midline remains free.

In addition, under normal speech conditions, vowels in General American English are always produced with vocal fold vibration; they are voiced speech sounds. Only during whispered speech are vowels unvoiced. Consonants, on the other hand, may be generated with or without simultaneous vocal fold vibration; they can be voiced or voiceless. The transcription of various vowels and consonants with examples of words in which these sounds can be heard are provided in Table 2.2. Note that various phonetic texts might transcribe sounds in somewhat different ways. Examples are provided to guide you with the transcription that is used in this text. Refer Appendix 2.2 for a list of how several texts vary in the transcription of vowels.

Vowels can also be distinguished from consonants according to the patterns of acoustic energy they display. Vowels are highly resonant, demonstrating at least two formant areas. Thus, vowels are more intense than consonants; in other words, they are typically louder than consonants. In this respect, we can say that vowels have greater sonority than consonants. **Sonority** of a sound is its loudness relative to that of other sounds with the same length, stress, and pitch (Ladefoged & Johnson, 2010). Because of the greater sonority of vowels over consonants, vowels are also referred to as **sonorants**. Certain groups of consonants are also labeled sonorants. When contrasted to other consonants, **sonorant consonants** are produced with a relatively open expiratory passageway. The sonorant consonants include the nasals ([m, n, ŋ]) and the approximants ([l, ɹ, w, j]). The sonorants are distinguished from the **obstruents**, which are characterized by a complete or narrow constriction between the articulators hindering the expiratory airstream. The obstruents include the plosives ([p, b, t, d, k, g]), the fricatives ([f, v, s, z, θ, ð, ʃ, ʒ, h]), and the affricates ([tʃ, dʒ]).

There are also functional distinctions between vowels and consonants. In other words, vowels and consonants have different linguistic functions. This has often been referred to as the *phonological difference* between vowels and consonants (Crystal, 2010). The term *consonant* indicates this relationship: *con* meaning "together with" and *sonant* reflecting the tonal qualities that characterize vowels. Thus, consonants are those speech sounds that function linguistically *together with* vowels. As such, vowels serve as the center of syllables, or as syllable nuclei. Vowels can constitute syllables by themselves—for example, in the first syllable of *a-go* or *e-lope*. Vowels can also appear with one or more consonants, exemplified by *blue, bloom,* or *blooms*. Although there are many types of syllables, the vowel is always the center of the syllable, its nucleus. A small group of consonants can serve as the nucleus of syllables. A consonant that functions as a syllable nucleus is referred to as a **syllabic**. These form and functional differences are summarized in Table 2.3.

Table 2.2 International Phonetic Alphabet (IPA) Symbols

Consonant Symbol	Word Example	Consonant Symbol	Word Example	Consonant Symbol	Word Example	Vowel Symbol	Word Example	Vowel Symbol	Word Example
[p]	<u>p</u>ay	[b]	<u>b</u>oy	[m]	<u>m</u>oon	[i]	<u>ea</u>t	[ɝ]	gi<u>r</u>l
[t]	<u>t</u>oy	[d]	<u>d</u>oll	[n]	<u>n</u>ot	[ɪ]	<u>i</u>n	[ɚ]	winne<u>r</u>
[k]	<u>c</u>oat	[g]	goat	[ŋ]	si<u>ng</u>	[ɛ]	<u>e</u>nd	[ʌ]	c<u>u</u>t
[f]	<u>f</u>ace	[v]	<u>v</u>ase	[j]	<u>y</u>es	[æ]	<u>a</u>t	[ə]	<u>a</u>bove
[θ]	<u>th</u>ink	[ð]	<u>th</u>ose	[l]	<u>l</u>eap	[a]	f<u>a</u>ther[3]	[eɪ]	<u>a</u>pe
[s]	<u>s</u>ip	[z]	<u>z</u>ip	[ɹ][2]	<u>r</u>ed	[u]	m<u>oo</u>n	[oʊ]	b<u>oa</u>t
[ʃ]	<u>sh</u>op	[ʒ]	bei<u>g</u>e	[h]	<u>h</u>op	[ʊ]	w<u>oo</u>d	[aɪ]	t<u>ie</u>
[tʃ]	<u>ch</u>op	[ʤ]	job			[ɔ]	f<u>a</u>ther[3]	[aʊ]	m<u>ou</u>se
[w]	<u>w</u>in	[ʍ]	<u>wh</u>en[1]			[ɑ]	h<u>o</u>p	[ɔɪ]	b<u>oy</u>

[1]Historically, the [ʍ] was used in "wh" words such as "where" and "when"; it was a voiceless sound. It has now merged with [w] throughout much of the United States (Wolfram & Schilling-Estes, 2006).

[2]The symbol [ɹ] will be used throughout this text for "r"-sounds. This reflects the usage of the International Phonetic Alphabet for the General American English "r." Refer "Approximants" (page 35) for further explanation.

[3]May be regional or individual pronunciation.

Table 2.3 Features Differentiating Vowels and Consonants

Vowels	Consonants
No significant constriction of the vocal tract	Significant constriction of the vocal tract
Open sounds	Constricted sounds
Sagittal midline of the vocal tract remains open	Constriction occurs along sagittal midline of the vocal tract
Voiced	Voiced or unvoiced
Acoustically more intense	Acoustically less intense
Demonstrate more sonority	Demonstrate less sonority
Function as syllable nuclei	Only specific consonants can function as syllable nuclei

General American English Vowels: Descriptive Parameters

Vowels are commonly described according to certain parameters (Abercrombie, 1967; Crystal, 2010; Heffner, 1975; Kantner & West, 1960; Shriberg, Kent, McAllister, & Preston, 2019):

1. The height of the tongue relative to the palate—for example, high versus low vowels.
2. The portion of the tongue involved in the articulation—for example, front versus back vowels.
3. The degree of roundedness of the lips—for example, rounded and unrounded or spread.

The four-sided form called a *vowel quadrilateral* is often used to demonstrate schematically the front–back and high–low positions. The form roughly represents the tongue position in the oral cavity (refer Figure 2.5).

There are two types of vowels: monophthongs and diphthongs. The quality of **monophthongs** remains the same throughout their entire production. They are pure vowels (Abercrombie, 1967). **Diphthongs** are vowels in which there is a change in quality during their production (Ladefoged & Johnson, 2010). The initial segment, the beginning portion of such a diphthong, is phonetically referred to as the **onglide**, and its end portion as the **offglide**.

Figure 2.5 Vowel Quadrilateral of General American English Vowels

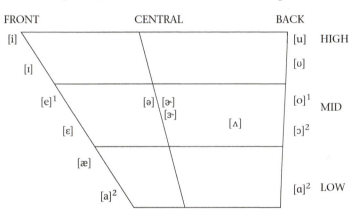

[1]These vowels can be transcribed as [eɪ] and [oʊ], as they are typically diphthongs in stressed syllables.
[2]The three vowels [a], [ɑ], and [ɔ] vary from speaker to speaker and word situation. They are allophonic variations.

Clinical Exercises The vowel quadrilateral is a rough sketch of the inside of the oral cavity. As can be noted, the right axis is at a 90-degree angle, whereas the left axis is at a much wider angle. In relationship to the mouth and tongue, this difference relates to the movement capabilities of the front versus the back of the tongue. The front of the tongue can move not only up and down but also somewhat forward and back. The back of the tongue is restricted to a relatively up and down movement. If you work with a child who has vowel difficulties, could you use this information clinically?

Using this notation system—(1) tongue height (high, mid, low), (2) tongue portion (front, central, back), and (3) roundedness (rounded, unrounded, spread)—descriptions of the most common vowels of General American English follow.

Front Vowels

All front vowels show various degrees of unrounding (lip spreading), with the high-front vowels showing the most. The lip spreading becomes less as one moves from the high-front vowels to the mid-front vowels, finally becoming practically nonexistent in the low-front vowels.

[i]	A high-front vowel, unrounded.
[ɪ]	A high-front vowel, unrounded.
[e]	A mid-front vowel, unrounded. In General American English, this vowel is typically produced as a diphthong, especially in stressed syllables or when articulated slowly.
[ɛ]	A mid-front vowel, unrounded.
[æ]	A low-front vowel, unrounded.
[a]	A low-front vowel, unrounded. In General American English, the use of this vowel depends on the particular regional dialect of the speaker. In the New England dialect of the Northeast, one might often hear it.

Back Vowels

Back vowels display different degrees of lip rounding in General American English. The high-back vowels [u] and [ʊ] often show a fairly high degree of lip rounding, whereas the low-back vowel [ɑ] is commonly articulated as an unrounded vowel.

[u]	A high-back vowel, rounded.
[ʊ]	A high-back vowel, rounded.
[o]	A mid-back vowel. This vowel is typically produced as a diphthong, especially in stressed syllables or when articulated slowly.
[ɔ]	A low mid-back vowel, rounded. The use of this vowel depends on regional pronunciation.
[ɑ]	A low-back vowel, unrounded. There seems to be some confusion in transcribing [ɔ] and [ɑ], although acoustic differences certainly exist. One distinguishing feature is that [ɔ] shows some degree of lip rounding, whereas [ɑ] does not.

▶ **Video Example 2.2**

This video outlines the descriptive features of vowels of General American English. Is it similar to the description provided in this chapter? Do you note any differences between the speaker's explanation of vowels and what you have just read?

https://www.youtube.com/watch?v=u7jQ8FELbIo

Central Vowels

[ɝ]	A central vowel, rounded, with r-coloring. Rounding may vary from speaker to speaker, however. [ɝ] is a stressed vowel. It is typically more intense acoustically, has a higher fundamental frequency, and has a longer duration when it is compared to similar unstressed vowels, such as [ɚ].
[ɚ]	A central vowel, rounded, with r-coloring. Again, lip rounding may vary from speaker to speaker. This is an unstressed vowel.
[ɜ]	A central vowel, rounded. [ɜ] is very similar in pronunciation to [ɝ], but it lacks any r-coloring. This vowel is heard in certain dialects. For example, [ɜ] might be heard in a Southern dialect pronunciation of *bird* or *worth*. Also, it could be heard in the speech of children having difficulties producing "r"-sounds.
[ʌ]	A central vowel, unrounded. It is a stressed vowel.
[ə]	A central vowel, unrounded. It is an unstressed vowel.

Clinical Application

Do Children Have Difficulties Producing Vowels?

Vowel errors in children who are developing phonological skills in a normal manner are relatively uncommon. However, children with phonological disorders may show deviant vowel patterns. Several studies (e.g., Davis, Jacks, & Marquardt, 2005; Pollock, 2013; Pollock & Berni, 2003; Reynolds, 2013; Stoel-Gammon & Herrington, 1990) have documented the presence of specific vowel problems in phonologically disordered children. Although certain vowel substitutions seem to be articulatory simplifications that could also occur in normal development, other errors appear to be idiosyncratic. Assessment of vowel qualities should be a portion of every diagnostic protocol. This can easily be achieved with any standardized speech assessment by transcribing the entire word rather than just the sound being tested if one of the sounds is in error.

Diphthongs

As previously defined, a diphthong is a vowel sound that demonstrates articulatory movement resulting in a qualitative change during its production. Its initial portion, the onglide, is acoustically more prominent and usually longer than the offglide. **Rising diphthongs** are common in General American English. This means that when producing these diphthongs, essential portions of the tongue move from a lower onglide to a higher offglide position; thus, relative to the palate, the tongue moves in a rising motion. This can be demonstrated on the vowel quadrilateral as well.

Certain diphthongs are referred to as **centering diphthongs**. These diphthongs have the same characteristics as the ones previously noted: a louder and typically longer onglide and a less intense and shorter offglide. However, in these diphthongs, the offglide, or less prominent element of the diphthong, is a central vowel, typically [ə] or [ɚ]. In British English and in some dialects of American English, one could hear [bɪə] for the word "beer," with the vowel [ɪ] as onglide and [ə] as offglide. More common in General American English is the use of the central vowel with r-coloring [ɚ] as an offglide. Thus, *fear* is often pronounced as [fɪɚ], *far* as [fɑɚ], and *bear* as [bɛɚ] (Ball & Rahilly, 1999). Theoretically, any vowel may be combined with [ə] or [ɚ] to form the onglide of a centering diphthong; however, in General American English, certain centering diphthongs are more common than others. Thus, [ɪɚ], [ɛɚ], and [ɑɚ], which can be heard in *dear* [dɪɚ], *bear* [bɛɚ], or *farm* [fɑɚm], are far more prevalent than [iɚ] or [uɚ]. Lowe (1994) refers to diphthongs that are paired with [ɚ] as **rhotic diphthongs**. In this case, **rhotic** refers to the r-coloring noted in specific vowels or consonants of General American English. Rhotic vowels are [ɝ] as in "b<u>ir</u>d" and [ɚ] as in "fath<u>er</u>," whereas rhotic consonants are [ɹ] as in "<u>r</u>abbit." The word "farm," [fɑɚm], contains a rhotic diphthong with the rhotic vowel [ɚ] as offglide. Thus, centering diphthongs may contain either [ə] or [ɚ] as offglides, whereas rhotic diphthongs are limited to the r-vowel [ɚ] as an offglide. These diphthongs are also seen transcribed with [r]. Thus, *dear* is transcribed as [dɪr], *bear* as [bɛr], and *farm* as [farm].

Discrepancies may be noted between the transcriptions of diphthongs offered in this text and the ones offered in other texts. Because phonetic transcription is purely *descriptive*, never *prescriptive*, any transcription will, of course, vary according to the actual pronunciation. Refer Shriberg et al. (2019) for a thorough discussion of the various ways diphthongs have been transcribed. Appendix 2.2 offers various ways in which diphthongs and rhotic diphthongs are transcribed in current phonetic texts.

[eɪ]	A **nonphonemic diphthong**.
	Nonphonemic diphthongs are those that the meaning of the word would *not* change if the vowel were to be pronounced as a monophthong [e] versus a diphthong [eɪ]. Therefore, no change in meaning would result if just the onglide were realized. Words pronounced [beɪk] or [bek], for example, would be recognized as the same word.
[oʊ]	A nonphonemic diphthong.
[aɪ]	A **phonemic diphthong**.
	Phonemic diphthongs are those that the meaning of the word *would* change if only the vowel onglide were produced—that is, if the vowel was realized as a monophthong. A realization of [a] instead of [aɪ] will change the meaning in General American English, as the words *sod* [sad] versus *sighed* [saɪd] demonstrate.
[ɔɪ]	A phonemic diphthong.
	The opposition [dʒɔ], *jaw*, versus [dʒɔɪ], *joy*, exemplifies its phonemic value as a meaning-differentiating sound feature of English.
[aʊ]	A phonemic diphthong.
	Oppositions such as [mas], *moss*, versus [maʊs], *mouse*, exemplify its phonemic value.

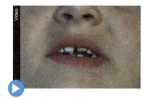

Video Tool Exercise 2.1
Identifying Central Vowels and Diphthongs
Complete the activity based on this video.

Clinical Application

Analyzing the Vowel System of a Child

Occasionally, the vowel system of a client may be restricted or show deviant patterns. In this case, a more in-depth analysis of the vowel productions may be necessary. Vowel systems can be examined by using the vowel quadrilateral and knowledge of the diphthongs as guiding principles. Front, back, and central vowels as well as diphthongs can be checked in relationship to their accuracy and their occurrence in the appropriate contexts.

George, age 5 years 3 months, is a child with a deviant vowel system. George was being seen in the clinic for his phonological disorder. He was a gregarious child who loved to talk and would try to engage anyone who would listen in conversation. The only problem was that George was almost unintelligible. This made dialogue difficult, possibly more so for those who would patiently and diligently try to understand his continuing attempts to interact.

In addition to his many consonant problems, the following vowel deviations were noted:

VOWEL ERRORS

Intended Production	→	Actual Production	Word Examples	Transcriptions		
[eɪ]	→	[ɛ]	grapes	[gɹeɪps]	→	[dɛ]
			table	[teɪbl̩]	→	[tɛboʊ]
[i]	→	[ɪ]	feet	[fit]	→	[fɪ]
			teeth	[tiθ]	→	[tɪ]
			three	[θɹi]	→	[dwɪ]
[ɛ]	→	[æ]	bed	[bɛd]	→	[bæt]
			feather	[fɛðɚ]	→	[fædə]
[u]	correct	[u]	shoe	[ʃu]	→	[tu]

Intended Production	→	Actual Production	Word Examples	Transcriptions		
			spoon	[spun]	→	[mun]
[ʊ]	correct	[ʊ]	book	[bʊk]	→	[bʊ]
[oʊ]	correct	[oʊ]	stove	[stoʊv]	→	[doʊ]
			nose	[noʊz]	→	[noʊ]
[ɑ]	correct	[ɑ]	mop	[mɑp]	→	[mɑ]
			blocks	[blɑks]	→	[bɑ]

George's productions of the back vowels [u], [ʊ], [oʊ], and [ɑ] are on target. The front vowels do show a deviant pattern, however. Not only is the diphthong [eɪ] produced as a monophthong, but the articulatory position of the vowel substitution for [eɪ] is realized lower, as [ɛ]. This tendency to lower vowels is also noted in the other productions with front vowels, in which [i] becomes [ɪ] and [ɛ] becomes [æ].

General American English Consonants: Descriptive Parameters

Three phonetic categories are used to characterize consonants: (1) voicing features, (2) place of articulation, and (3) manner of articulation. According to the International Phonetic Alphabet, additional features are occasionally used. For example, [f and [v] are described as labiodental sounds. Thus, lips (labio) and teeth (dental) are indicated in the descriptor. For the purpose of this text, the International Phonetic Alphabet descriptions are used. Since this is the standard for our transcription, it is important to use this categorization as much as possible. Figure 2.6 is an example of a chart that delineates these parameters.

Voicing is the term used to denote the presence or absence of simultaneous vocal fold vibration, resulting in voiced or voiceless consonants. The voiced and voiceless consonants of General American English are noted by the shaded boxes in Figure 2.6. Pairs of similar sounds, such as [t] and [d], that differ only in their voicing feature are referred to as **cognates**.

Figure 2.6 General American English Consonants According to Voicing, Place, and Manner

MANNER	PLACE													
	Bilabial		Labiodental		Dental		Alveolar		Postalveolar		Palatal		Velar		Glottal
Plosive	p	b					t	d					k	g	
Nasal		m						n						ŋ	
Fricative			f	v	θ	ð	s	z	ʃ	ʒ					h
Affricate									tʃ	dʒ					
Approximant		w						ɹ				j			
Lateral approximant								l							

Shaded areas indicate a voiced sound.

Place of articulation describes where the constriction or narrowing occurs for the various consonant productions. The upper lip, upper teeth, palate, and velum are the main stationary places of articulation when describing the consonants of General American English. The bottom lip and the tongue are the movable portions involved in articulating consonants. Thus, the bottom lip moves to meet the top lip in bilabial [p] and [b], whereas the tongue comes very close to the alveolar ridge for [s] and [z], for example. You may read that certain sounds are labeled as lingua-alveolar or lingua-dental, but it is understood that the primary articulator is the tongue; thus, "lingua-" is often omitted. Refer Figure 2.7 for the structures of articulation and their resulting phonetic descriptors.

Manner of articulation refers to the type of narrowing that the articulators produce for the realization of a particular consonant. There are various manners of articulation, ranging from complete closure for the production of plosives to a far more open, less constricted vocal tract for the production of approximants. The following manners of articulation are used to account phonetically for the consonants of General American English.

Plosives (sometimes referred to as stops). During the production of **plosives**, complete blockage is secured at specific points in the vocal tract. Simultaneously, the velum is raised so that no air can escape through the nose. The expiratory air pressure builds up naturally behind this closure

Figure 2.7 Structures of the Oral Cavity as Places of Articulation for General American English Consonants

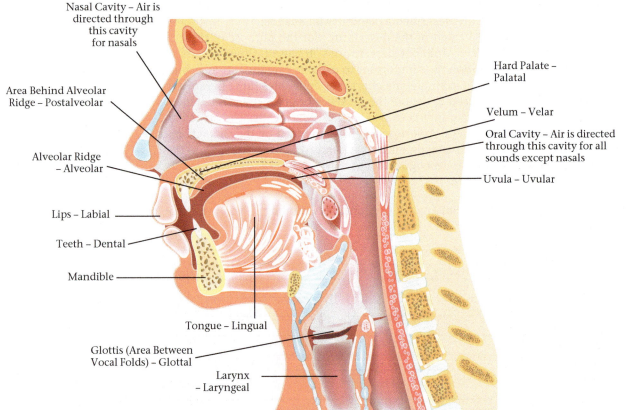

(**stop**), an increase in air pressure results, and then this air is suddenly released (**plosive**). Examples of plosives are [p], [b], [t], [d], [k], and [g].

Fricatives. Fricatives result when the articulators approximate each other so closely that the escaping expiratory airstream causes an audible friction noise. As with the stops, the velum is raised for all fricative sounds. Examples of fricatives are [f], [v], [θ], [ð], and [h]. The other fricatives, referred to as **sibilants**, have a higher amplitude and pitch due to the presence of high-frequency components. In General American English, [s], [z], [ʃ], and [ʒ] belong to the sibilants.

Nasals. Nasal consonants are produced with the velum lowered so that air can pass freely through the nasal cavity. However, there is a complete blockage within the oral cavity between the articulators. These sounds have been called *nasal stops* because of the closure of the articulators and the ensuing free air passage through the nasal cavity (Ball & Rahilly, 1999). The nasals in General American English are [m], [n], and [ŋ].

Affricates. In **affricate** sounds, two phases can be noted. First, a complete closure is formed between the articulators, and the velum is raised. Because of these articulatory conditions, expiratory air pressure builds up behind the blockage formed by the articulators—the stop phase, which is considered the first portion of the affricate. Second, the stop is then slowly (in comparison to the plosives) released orally, resulting in the friction portion of the speech sound. Affricates are sometimes described as a stop plus fricative combination. However, affricates are different than other consonant blends or clusters, such as [ks] or [ps]. Consonant clusters are those in which the stop portion and the fricative portion differ in their place of articulation. In contrast, affricates are single, uniform speech sounds characterized by a slow release of a stopping phase into a homorganic (*hom* = same) friction element. The two most prominent affricates in General American English are [tʃ] and [dʒ].

Approximants. Approximants are a manner of articulation in which the articulators come close to each other (they approximate each other), but the constriction is far less than for the fricatives. The opening is wider, and there is a much broader passage of air. According to the International Phonetic Alphabet, the consonants [w], [j], [ɹ], and [l] are approximants. The consonant [l] is considered a lateral approximant due to the midline closure and lateral release of air during its production. The sounds [l] and [ɹ] have also been termed **liquids**, whereas [w] and [j] are also labeled as **glides**.

Rhotics (r-sounds). Three variations of "r" exist: (1) The tongue tip is raised toward the alveolar ridge. This type of production is officially transcribed by the International Phonetic Association as [ɹ], an upside-down "r." (2) The retroflexed rhotic is produced with the tongue tip bent backward in a "retroflexed" position. It is officially transcribed as [ɻ], an upside-down "r" with a retroflexed diacritic. (3) The "bunched" rhotic is produced by raising the middle of the tongue toward the palate while the tongue tip is relatively low, near and behind the front lower teeth. There is no official transcription marker for the bunched rhotic. Although many texts use [r] to characterize the General American English rhotic, according to the International Phonetic Alphabet, the [r] symbol is officially reserved for the alveolar trilled "r" sound, which can be heard in Spanish, for example. For the purposes of this text, the r-sound will be transcribed as [ɹ]. Unless otherwise specified, this transcription will include all three types of r-productions.

The phonetic characteristics of the r-sounds are especially difficult to describe. First, there are different types of rhotic productions. Second, the actual production of these sounds is highly context dependent. Thus, the production easily changes, based on the surrounding context. In addition, the positioning of the tongue for individual speakers is highly variable. Clinicians should be aware that the rhotics can be produced in a number of ways when attempting a correct production in therapy. Refer Chapter 9 for more details.

Table 2.4 summarizes the manner of articulation for the consonants of General American English, and Table 2.5 lists the consonants of General American English with voicing, place, and manner features.

> **Clinical Exercises** Consider the manner of articulation: If a child produces [t] for [s], what does the child need to understand to achieve [s]? What is the difference between a plosive and a fricative in their manner of articulation? Can you think of any ways to demonstrate this to the child?

Table 2.4 Phonetic Description: Manner of Articulation

Manner of Articulation	Phonetic Descriptor	Examples
Complete blockage	Plosive	[p], [b], [t], [d], [k], [g]
Very narrow opening between articulators	Fricative	[f], [v], [s], [z], [ʃ], [ʒ], [θ], [ð], [h]
Nasal emission	Nasal	[m], [n], [ŋ]
Release of stop portion to a homorganic fricative portion	Affricate	[tʃ], [dʒ]
Articulators come close to one another but not nearly as much as for fricatives	Approximant	[w], [j], [l], [ɹ]
Lateral airflow of an approximant	Lateral approximant	[l]

Video Example 2.3

This video provides a description of the voicing, place, and manner characteristics of General American English consonants. Is this phonetic description similar to what was explained in the text? What differences do you note between the video and the text?

https://www.youtube.com/watch?v = dfoRdKuPF9I

Table 2.5 Phonetic Descriptions of the Consonants of General American English: Voicing, Place, and Manner Features

[p]	Voiceless bilabial plosive
[b]	Voiced bilabial plosive
[t]	Voiceless alveolar plosive
[d]	Voiced alveolar plosive
[k]	Voiceless velar plosive
[g]	Voiced velar plosive
[f]	Voiceless labiodental fricative
[v]	Voiced labiodental fricative
[s]	Voiceless alveolar fricative
	The [s] (and [z]) can be produced in one of two ways: with the tongue tip up or with the tongue tip resting behind the lower front teeth.
[z]	Voiced alveolar fricative

[ʃ] Voiceless postalveolar fricative usually with lip rounding

[ʒ] Voiced postalveolar fricative typically with lip rounding

[θ] Voiceless dental fricative

The [θ] and [ð] are typically produced with either the tongue tip resting behind the upper incisors or the tongue tip slightly between the upper and lower incisors.

[ð] Voiced dental fricative

[m] Voiced bilabial nasal

[n] Voiced alveolar nasal

[ŋ] Voiced velar nasal

[w] Voiced labio-velar approximant

The first portion of this description, labio-, refers to the lip rounding of this sound; the second portion, velar, refers to the body of the tongue being raised toward the velum, similar to [u].

[j] Voiced palatal approximant

[l] Voiced alveolar lateral approximant

[ɹ] Voiced alveolar approximant (bunched or tongue directed toward the alveolar ridge) or voiced retroflexed approximant

[h] Voiceless glottal fricative

Although this sound is classified as a glottal fricative, in General American English there is normally no constriction at the laryngeal, pharyngeal, or oral levels. Refer Heffner (1975) for a discussion of the [h] production in General American English.

[tʃ] Voiceless alveolar plosive portion followed by a voiceless postalveolar fricative portion

[dʒ] Voiced alveolar plosive portion followed by a voiced postalveolar fricative portion

---

Clinical Application

Rhotic Errors Versus Central Vowels with R-Coloring

Children with "r" problems, often produce the central vowels with r-coloring ([ɜ˞] and [ə˞]) in error as well. However, that is not always the case. Note the following patterns seen in Latoria's speech.

Intended Production	→	Actual Production	Word Example			Transcriptions
[tɹ]	→	[tw]	tree	[tɹi]	→	[twi]
[bɹ]	→	[bw]	bridge	[bɹɪdʒ]	→	[bwɪʒ]
[ɹ]	→	[w]	ring	[ɹɪŋ]	→	[wɪŋ]
[bɹ]	→	[bw]	zebra	[zibɹə]	→	[zibwə]
[ɹ]	→	[w]	garage	[gəɹɑʒ]	→	[dʒəwɑ]
[θɹ]	→	[θw]	thread	[θɹɛd]	→	[θwɛd]
[tɹ]	→	[tw]	treasure	[tɹɛʒə˞]	→	[twɛʒə˞]

(continued)

Intended Production	→	Actual Production	Word Example			Transcriptions
		Central Vowels with R-Coloring				
[ɚ]	correct	[ɚ]	feather	[fɛðɚ]	→	[fɛdɚ]
[ɚ]	correct	[ɚ]	soldier	[souldʒɚ]	→	[souʒɚ]
[ɚz]	correct	[ɚz]	scissors	[sɪzɚz]	→	[sɪzɚz]
[ɝ]	correct	[ɝ]	birthday	[bɝθdeⁱ]	→	[bɝdeⁱ]

On the one hand, Latoria has a [w] for [ɹ] substitution ([ɹ] → [w]) for the consonant [ɹ]. On the other hand, she can produce the central vowels with r-coloring accurately.

Clinical Exercises Which type of [s] do you use: [s] with the tongue tip up or the tongue tip down? Say a few words with [s] and note the position of your tongue. Try producing both types of [s]-productions.

Some clinicians use only the tongue-tip-down version of [s] to remediate [s] difficulties. If the child produces [θ] as a substitution for [s], why might the tongue-tip-down production be advantageous?

Sounds in Context: Coarticulation and Assimilation

Until now, this text has discussed articulatory characteristics of speech sounds as discrete units. However, the articulators do not move from sound to sound in a series of separate steps. Speech consists of highly variable and overlapping motor movements. Sounds within a given phonetic context influence one another. For example, if the [s]-production in *see* is contrasted to the one in *Sue*, we can observe that the [s] in *see* is produced with some spreading of the lips, whereas there is lip rounding in *Sue*. This difference results from the influence of the following vowel articulations: [i], a vowel with lip spreading, facilitates this feature in the [s]-production in *see*, whereas the lip rounding of [u] influences the production of [s] in *Sue*. These types of modifications are grouped together under the term *coarticulation*. **Coarticulation** describes the concept that the articulators are continually moving into position for other segments over a stretch of speech. The result of coarticulation is referred to as *assimilation*. The term **assimilation** refers to adaptive articulatory changes through which one speech sound becomes similar, sometimes identical, to a neighboring sound segment. Such a change may affect one, several, or all of a sound's phonetic constituents; that is, a sound may change the place, manner, and/or voicing properties under the articulatory influence of another sound. Assimilation processes can be perfectly natural consequences of normal speech production and are by no means restricted to developing speech in young children. Because the two segments become more alike, assimilatory processes are also referred to as **harmony processes**.

There are different *types* and *degrees* of assimilatory processes:

1. *Contact versus remote assimilation:* When directly adjacent sounds are modified, this is called **contact** (or **contiguous**) **assimilation**. If at least one other segment separates the sounds in question, especially when the two sounds are in two different syllables, one speaks of **remote** (or **noncontiguous**) **assimilation**.

2. *Progressive versus regressive assimilation:* In **progressive assimilation**, a segment influences a following sound in a linear manner. This is also referred to as **perseverative assimilation** (Crystal, 2010; Ladefoged & Johnson, 2010). In **regressive assimilation**, a sound segment influences a preceding sound.

3. *Total versus partial assimilation:* **Total assimilation** occurs when the changed segment and the source of the influence become identical. **Partial assimilation** exists when the changed segment is close to, but not identical to, the source segment.

Refer Table 2.6 for examples of the different assimilation processes.

Children at different stages of their speech-language development tend to use assimilation processes in systematic ways. Typical assimilation processes and the ages at which these processes occur in children are discussed in Chapter 5. This is of obvious interest to clinicians whose task is to separate normal from impaired phonological development. In normally developing children and those with disordered phonology, syllable structure can also affect their production possibilities. This is discussed in the next section.

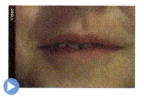

Video Example 2.4
Listen to 6-year-old Sandy as she says eight words. Notice the lip rounding (and smile) on the words "poo" and "toot." This is an example of coarticulation. What causes the lip rounding on these two words?

Table 2.6 Examples of Assimilation Processes The following examples were noted in the results of a standardized speech assessment or a spontaneous speech sample.

Word	Intended Production	Child's Production	Changes Noted	Assimilation	Type of Assimilation
jumping	[d͡ʒʌmpɪŋ]	[d͡ʒʌmbɪŋ]	[mp] → [mb]	The [p] changes to a [b] due to the influence of the voicing of the nasal [m].	Contact, progressive, partial
skunk	[skʌŋk]	[stʌŋk]	[sk] → [st]	The [k] changes to a [t] due to the influence of the place of articulation for [s]. Now both [s] and [t] have the same place of articulation.	Contact, progressive, partial
yellow	[jɛlou]	[lɛlou]	[j] → [l]	The [j] changes to an [l] due to the influence of the [l] in the second syllable. Now the sounds are identical.	Remote, regressive, total
telephone	[tɛləfoun]	[tɛdəfoun]	[l] → [d]	The [l] changes to a [d] due to the manner of articulation of the beginning [t]. Now both sounds have the same manner of articulation.	Remote, progressive, partial
ice cream	[aɪskrim],	[aɪstrim]	[k] → [t]	The [k] changes to a [t] due to the influence of the place of articulation of the [s]. Now they have the same place of articulation.	Contact, progressive, partial
bathtub	[bæθtʌb]	[θæθtʌb]	[b] → [θ]	The [b] changes to a [θ] due to the influence of the [θ] in the second syllable. The two become the same sound.	Remote, regressive, total

Syllable Structure

If we are asked to break words into component parts, syllables seem to be more natural than sounds. For example, speakers of unwritten languages characteristically use syllable, not sound, divisions. They may even resist the notion that any further breakdown is possible (Ladefoged & Johnson, 2010). Also, preschool-age children use syllabification when they try to analyze a word. It is only after children are exposed to writing that they begin to understand the possibility of dividing words into sounds. Thus, syllables appear to be easily recognizable units.

Counting the number of syllables in a word is a relatively simple task. Probably all will agree on the number of syllables in the words "away" and "articulation," for example. What we might disagree on are the beginning and end points of the syllables in question. To arrive at a consensus, it is first necessary to differentiate between written and spoken syllables.

A dictionary has written syllabification rules. There, we learn that the word "cutting" is to be divided as cut-ting. However, differences may, and often do, exist between written and spoken syllables. The written syllabification rules for *cutting* do not reflect the way we would syllabify the word when speaking. The divisions [kʌ tɪŋ] would be more probable during normal speech. An awareness of existing differences between spoken and written syllable boundaries is important for speech-language specialists.

Determining spoken syllables can be especially problematic because a dictionary of rules for the boundaries of *spoken* syllables does not exist. Thus, two competent speakers of a given language may syllabify the same word in different ways. Words such as *hammer* and *window* would probably not cause problems. However, how should one syllabify *telephone*, as [tɛ lə foʊn] or [tɛl ə foʊn]? That is, does [l] belong to the second or the first syllable? Variations in the syllabification of spoken words do indeed exist between speakers. To understand this, a look at the syllable structure is a good way to begin.

Structurally, the syllable can be divided into three parts: *peak, onset,* and *coda.* The **peak** is the most prominent, acoustically most intense part of the syllable. Although vowels are clearly more prevalent as syllable peaks, consonants are not strictly excluded. Consonants that serve as the syllable peak are referred to as *syllabics.* A peak may stand alone, as in the first syllable of the word *a-way,* or it can be surrounded by other sounds, as in *tan* or *bring.*

The **onset** of a syllable consists of all the segments prior to the peak, whereas the **coda** is made up of all the sound segments of a syllable following its peak. The segments that comprise the onset are also termed **syllable releasing sounds**, and those that comprise the coda are termed **syllable arresting sounds**. Thus, the onset of *meet* [mit] is [m]; that is, [m] is the syllable releasing sound. The coda, or syllable arresting sound, of *meet* is [t]. This also applies to consonant blends within one syllable. The onset of *scratched* is [skɹ], its peak is [æ], and the coda is [tʃt]. Not all syllables have onsets or codas. Both syllables of *today* [tudeɪ] lack a coda, whereas *off* [ɑf] does not have an onset. The number of segments that an onset or a coda may contain is regulated by the phonotactic rules of the language in question. General American English syllables can have one to three segments in an onset (<u>r</u>ay, <u>st</u>ay, <u>str</u>ay) and one to four segments in a coda (si<u>t</u>, si<u>ts</u>, six<u>th</u> [sɪksθ], six<u>ths</u> [sɪksθs]). When referring to sounds within a syllable or word, a specific notation is often used: C refers to a consonant, while V refers to a vowel. Thus, the word "eat" [it] has a VC structure while "around" [əɹɑʊnd] has a VCVCC structure.

The peak and coda together are referred to as the **rime**. Therefore, in the word "sun," the onset is "s" and the rime is "un." Syllables that do not contain codas are called **open** or **unchecked syllables**. Examples of open, unchecked syllables are *do* [du], *glee* [gli], or the first syllable of *rebound* [ri baʊnd]. Syllables that do have codas are called **closed** or **checked syllables**, such as in *stop* [stɑp] or the first syllable in *window* [wɪn].

The words "sheep" and "keep" have the same rime. Therefore, these words "rhyme." The word "rime" is used to mean specifically syllable rime, to differentiate it from the concept of "poetic rhyme." For the purpose at hand, when we are referring to the nucleus + coda, the term *rime* will be used. Refer to the diagram of the CVC words "sheep" and "keep."

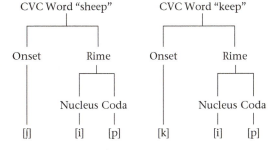

Clinical Significance

The use of specific syllable structures is often neglected when analyzing the speech characteristics of children. However, they do seem to play an important developmental role. A child's first words typically consist of open or unchecked syllables, such as [bɑ] for *ball* or [mɪ] for *milk*. If children start to produce closed syllables, they usually contain only single-segment codas. Similarly, two-syllable words at this stage of development usually consist of open syllables (e.g., Ingram, 1976; Menn, 1971; Velten, 1943). Productions such as [beɪ bi] for *baby* or [ti pɑ] for *teapot* are examples.

As can be noted, children often have limitations on their syllable and word shapes, especially young children and those with speech sound disorders. In this context, a child's phonotactic restrictions might be analyzed as one diagnostic measure. This type of assessment includes (1) the number of syllables a child uses, (2) whether the child uses a vowel as a nucleus of the syllable, (3) the demonstration of both open and closed syllable structures, and (4) the use of consonant clusters (Bauman-Waengler & Garcia, 2020; Velleman, 2016).

The length of a word influences the accuracy of speech production. Thus, shorter words are easier for children. Children's production of consonants and vowels in one-syllable words are more accurate than in words with more than one syllable (James, van Doorn, McLeod, & Esterman, 2008). As words get longer, the natural tendency for children is to omit the unstressed syllable. Thus, "potato" becomes "tato" and "pajamas" becomes "jamas."

Most children also include a vowel as the nucleus of a word. However, some children with speech sound disorders, especially those with childhood apraxia of speech, may have difficulty producing consonant + vowel syllables. These children may use a high number of words that consist of a single consonant without a vowel as the nucleus or a single vowel without a consonant onset (Velleman, 2016).

Although most very young children produce predominantly open syllables, that does not mean that closed syllables (i.e., those with a final consonant) are not used. For example, Stoel-Gammon (1987a) found that 67% of the 34 two-year-old children she studied used two-syllable words ending in a final consonant. Thus, very young children do use closed syllables. That may not be the case with children with speech sound disorders, however.

The final phonotactic restriction relates to the use of consonant clusters. Here, we need to differentiate between use and mastery. Many consonant clusters are not mastered until possibly 8 or 9 years of age. However, onset and coda consonant clusters are used by 2- and 3-year-old children. Word-initial clusters seem to contain [w], such as [pw] or [bw]; therefore, they are substitutions for [pɹ]/[pl] or [bɹ]/[bl] (McLeod, van Doorn, & Reed, 2001). Also, word-final clusters are demonstrated. McLeod and colleagues (2001) noted [-nd] and [-ts] in children 30 months old.

In summary, if we want to make a production easier for a child, the ease of syllable production can be affected by at least three circumstances: (1) the *number of syllables* in an utterance, (2) the *type of syllable* (open versus closed), and (3) the *degree of syllable stress* (stressed or unstressed). Generally, fewer syllables, open syllables, and stressed syllables facilitate accurate productions of specific target sounds. Another concept that could be included is (4) the *number of consonants grouped together*. Single consonants (singletons) are easier to produce than consonant clusters. Therefore, a word with just a single consonant is easier to produce than a similarly structured word with consonant clusters. The following diagram represents these four factors based on ease of production.

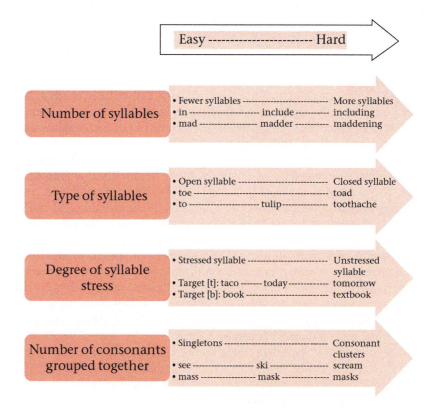

Easy ------------------------ Hard

Number of syllables
- Fewer syllables ------------------------ More syllables
- in --------------------- include ---------- including
- mad ------------------ madder ---------- maddening

Type of syllables
- Open syllable ------------------------ Closed syllable
- toe ----------------------------------- toad
- to --------------------- tulip------------ toothache

Degree of syllable stress
- Stressed syllable ------------------------ Unstressed syllable
- Target [t]: taco ------- today------------ tomorrow
- Target [b]: book ------------------------ textbook

Number of consonants grouped together
- Singletons ------------------------------ Consonant clusters
- see ------------------- ski ---------------- scream
- mass ----------------- mask -------------- masks

Clinical Exercises Claire has an [s] problem and is beginning to work on two-syllable words. Can you create a list of 5 two-syllable words that would be easier for her to produce based on the principle of open versus closed syllables? Can you create another list of 5 two-syllable words that would be easier based on syllable stress?

Summary

This chapter presented a broad definition of phonetics and its three subdivisions: articulatory, acoustic, and auditory phonetics. Within articulatory phonetics, an overview of vowels and consonants was given, and the form and function of the vowels and consonants of General American English were discussed. Both vowels and consonants were classified according to their articulatory production features and their linguistic functions. Phonetic descriptors were given to provide the clinician with a detailed account of articulatory action during normal production of vowels and consonants. These features can later be contrasted to those noted in the impaired sound realizations of children and adults with speech sound disorders.

In the second portion of this chapter, coarticulation, assimilation processes, and syllable structure were defined and examined. Coarticulation and resulting assimilatory processes were described as normal articulatory consequences that regularly occur in the speech of individuals. Assimilatory processes were defined according to the type and degree of sound modification. Examples of assimilatory processes noted in children were provided. The final section, on syllable structure, defined the parts of the syllable and examined some phonotactic constraints that occur in young children and those with speech sound disorders. It was suggested that an analysis of syllable structures could provide the clinician with additional knowledge when evaluating individuals with speech sound disorders.

Case Study

The following sample is from Tina, age 3 years 8 months.

dig	[dɛg]	cat	[tæt]
house	[haʊθ]	bath	[bæt]
knife	[naf]	red	[led]
duck	[dʊt]	ship	[sɪp]
fan	[vɛn]	ring	[wɪŋ]
yes	[wɛt]	thumb	[dʌm]
boat	[boʊt]	that	[zæt]
cup	[tʊp]	zip	[wɪp]
lamp	[wæmp]	key	[di]
goat	[doʊt]	win	[jɪn]

[θ] → [d]

[θ] → [z]

Compare the typical vowel productions to those noted in the sample according to the following:

1. The portion of the tongue involved in the articulation (front, central, back)
2. The tongue's position relative to the palate (high, mid, low). For example:

    dig → [dɛg]   A high-front vowel changed to a mid-front vowel

Compare the typical consonant productions to those noted in the sample according to voicing, place, and manner characteristics. For example:

house → [haʊθ]   A voiceless alveolar fricative [s] is changed to a voice-less dental fricative [θ]

Continue to analyze the vowel and consonant changes for the other words in the sample.

Think Critically

1. Some young children have trouble producing [s] and [z]; they substitute [θ] and [ð] for these sounds. Thus, the word "Sue" would be pronounced [θu] and "zoo" would be pronounced [ðu]. Compare the two articulations and see whether you might be able to describe to a child of age 6 what he or she would have to do to change the articulation from [θ] and [ð] to [s] and [z].

2. Identify the following assimilation processes according to the parameters: contact versus remote and progressive versus regressive.

news	[nuz̲]	however	newspaper	[nus̲peɪpɚ]
panty	[pænti]	→	[pændi]	
did you	[dɪd ju]	→	[dɪd ʒu]	
incubate	[ɪnkjubeɪt]	→	[ɪŋkjubeɪt]	
misuse	[mɪsjuz]	→	[mɪʃ juz]	

3. Identify the following syllable structures according to (a) onset, peak, and coda and (b) closed or open syllables. For example:

   win.dow → [wɪn.doʊ]

   1st syllable: onset-peak-coda, closed syllable

   2nd syllable: onset-peak, open syllable

   telephone

   wagon

   shovel

   banana

4. You are testing [k] sounds in the initial and final positions with a child who is 4 years old and has a [t] for [k] substitution. You would like to keep the syllable structure consistent for all the words used. Therefore, all words should be one syllable in length, and syllable structures should be comparable. Find six words that could be used for a 4-year-old child and that would test [k] under these conditions.

 Chapter Quiz 2.1 Complete this quiz to check your understanding of chapter concepts.

Appendix 2.1 Selected Readings in Anatomy and Physiology of the Speech and Hearing Mechanisms

Culbertson, W. R., Cotton, S. S., & Tanner, D. C. (2015). *Anatomy and physiology study guide for speech and hearing.* Dubuque, IA: Kendall Hunt Publishing.

Fuller, D. R., Pemental, J. T., & Peregoy, B. M. (2012). *Applied anatomy and physiology for speech-language pathology and audiology.* Baltimore, MD: Lippincott Williams & Wilkins.

Hoit, J., & Weismer, G. (2017). *Foundations of speech and hearing: Anatomy and physiology.* San Diego, CA: Plural Publishing.

Mulroney, S. E., & Myers, A. K. (2016). *Netter's physiology flash cards* (2nd ed.). Philadelphia, PA: Elsevier.

Netter, F. H. (2014). *Atlas of human anatomy* (6th ed.). Philadelphia, PA: Saunders-Elsevier Health Sciences.

Seikel, J. A., King, D. W., & Drumwright, D. G. (2005). *Anatomy and physiology for speech and language* (5th ed.). Boston, MA: Cengage Publishing.

Zemlin, W. R. (1998). *Speech and hearing science: Anatomy and physiology* (4th ed.). New York, NY: Allyn and Bacon Pearson.

Appendix 2.2 Phonetic Symbols Used in Current Phonetic Transcription Texts

Word Example: Diphthongs	Bauman-Waengler (2009)	Edwards (2003)	Garn-Nunn and Lynn (2004)	Shriberg et al. (2018)	Small (2020)
buy, my	[aɪ] or [ɑɪ], depending on pronunciation	[aɪ]	[aɪ]	[a͞ɪ]	[aɪ]
bay, may	[e] monophthong, [eɪ] diphthong	[e]	[e] monophthong, [eɪ] diphthong	[e] monophthong, [e͞ɪ] diphthong	[e] monophthong, [eɪ] diphthong
boat, home	[o] monophthong, [oʊ] diphthong	[o]	[o] monophthong, [oʊ] diphthong	[o] monophthong, [o͞ʊ] diphthong	[o] monophthong, [oʊ] diphthong
cow, loud	[aʊ]	[aʊ]	[aʊ]	[a͞ʊ]	[aʊ]
boy, hoist	[ɔɪ]	[ɔɪ]	[ɔɪ]	[ɔ͞ɪ]	[ɔɪ]
Word Example: Rhotic Diphthongs					
fear, beer	[ɪɚ]	[ɪr]	[ɪr]	[ɪr]	[ɪr]
bear, mare	[ɛɚ]	[ɛr]	[ɛr]	[ɛr]	[ɛr]
more, floor	[oɚ] or [ɔɚ], depending on pronunciation	[ɔr]	[ɔr]	[ɔr]	[ɔr]
bar, far	[ɑɚ]	[ɑr]	[ɑr]	[ɑr]	[ɑr]

Chapter 3
Phonetic Transcription and Diacritics

∨ Learning Objectives

When you have finished this chapter, you should be able to:

3.1 Define phonetic transcription as a notational system.

3.2 Explain the use and value of phonetic transcription for speech-language therapists.

3.3 Define diacritics.

3.4 Identify the diacritics used to delineate consonant sounds.

3.5 Categorize the diacritics used to describe vowel sounds.

3.6 Characterize the diacritics used to mark stress, duration, and syllable boundaries.

Chapter Application: Case Study

This was Kelly's first time in clinic that she was the only clinician in her own diagnostic session. She knew that the child she would be diagnosing, 5-year-old Ava, had several speech sound errors. For example, Ava had a lateral lisp; this had been noted by Kelly's supervisor. Kelly started by asking Ava to talk about her day in kindergarten. Ava was very hard to understand in conversational speech, so Kelly asked Ava to look at some pictures and talk about them. Kelly noted that, yes, Ava had a lateral s-sound problem. However, in addition, she saw that Ava produced [t] and [d] with her tongue tip protruding slightly between her teeth. At first, it sounded as if Ava was deleting the plosives at the end of words, but as Kelly watched, she could see that the articulators came into contact—for example, for the [p] in the word "cup"—but then the release phase did not seem to be present—the lips remained closed and together. Kelly wondered if this might be an unreleased plosive production.

How would you transcribe these errors: lateral s-sounds (both with [s] and [z]); [t] and [d] produced with the tongue tip too far forward, actually between the teeth; and unreleased plosives? Phonetic transcription and diacritics are important in your diagnosis of speech sound disorders. Without the accuracy and knowledge of the appropriate symbols, it is very difficult to document our diagnostic findings so that our therapy can be as goal directed as possible.

VIRTUALLY every book on speech sound disorders contains a brief discussion of phonetic transcription. Typically, the symbols and diacritics of the International Phonetic Alphabet (IPA) are listed with a comment on the importance of accurate transcription in the assessment procedure. This underplays its importance, however; accurate transcription is *the* basis for the diagnosis of speech sound disorders. If clinicians cannot correctly identify and transcribe the speech productions of their clients, their therapy will not be as focused as it should be. Transcribing words phonetically is also an invaluable aid in documenting change as therapy progresses. It is a vital skill in assessing and treating speech sound disorders.

Nevertheless, in training and in clinical practice, phonetic transcription seems to be one of the most neglected areas of study. Although transcription skills are as indispensable as they are difficult to master, the chance to learn them is often limited to one undergraduate course. This meager knowledge base is seldom systematically expanded or revisited in other courses or in most clinical experiences. Many practicing clinicians simply are not comfortable with phonetic transcription and, therefore, unfortunately use it as infrequently as possible.

Phonetic transcription is more than just transposing perceived sounds into "strange" symbols; it is above all a process of fine-tuning one's auditory perception for the purpose of successful clinical intervention. Perceptual skills improve with systematic efforts to listen carefully to, and differentiate accurately among, subtle changes in sound quality. Although this is not a workbook on phonetic transcription (this section does not offer nearly enough information for such a course), it does emphasize and treat phonetic transcription in considerably more detail than most textbooks on speech sound disorders.

The first goal of this chapter is to introduce the IPA as a notational system used to document norm productions of vowels and consonants of General American English. However, the transcription of disordered speech requires more than that. It needs supplemental signs, diacritical marks that can be added to basic transcription symbols to indicate specific production features and sound values. These provide a means of documenting irregular articulatory events. Therefore, this chapter's second goal is to present and discuss some of the more common diacritical marks. Clinical comments are included to exemplify the use of these diacritics. The third goal of this chapter is to examine the clinical application of phonetic transcription, including the use of diacritics. Examples are provided to demonstrate how phonetic transcription can be used in the assessment and treatment process.

Phonetic Transcription as a Notational System

Speech is a fleeting event, existing for only the shortest period—so short, in fact, that if artificial means are not used, its existence cannot be documented even immediately after it occurs. Historically, all writing systems were invented to make speech events last longer—to preserve them.

Traditional writing systems do a great job in preserving *what* has been said, but they fall grossly short in indicating *how* it has been said, even though this can be just as important. For example, a speech-language specialist needs to document the details of a child's aberrant sound realizations. There are no letters in our alphabet for laterally produced s-sounds, for instance. Professionals clearly need more information about *how* a specific speech event has been executed than about *what* has been said. For these special purposes, traditional writing systems are useless and special systems had to be invented to serve these needs. *Phonetic transcription* systems were devised to document real actualizations of speech events.

Today, the frequently revised IPA is probably the most widely accepted transcription system in the world (Figure 3.1). The International Phonetic Association, founded in 1886, published the first IPA in 1888. It offers a one-to-one correspondence between phoneme realizations and sound symbols. However, at the same time, many additional signs can be used to identify modifications in the original production. Generally, the IPA serves the professional interests of speech-language pathologists well. Its symbols capture much of what we are interested in. Professionals will need to add to the inventory of available symbols to characterize an irregular production. That, though, is to be expected because phonetic transcription systems are typically designed to transfer standard (but highly impermanent) speech events adequately into (more durable) readable signs. In *aberrant* speech, just about anything can happen, and this may well necessitate additional characters to indicate unusual articulatory events. If such additional characterization becomes necessary, the specific phonetic value of any added sign must, of course, be described precisely and in detail. If other professionals cannot reliably "read" the transcribed materials, they cannot accurately transform the symbols into the original phonetic events; that is, they will not know how the sound was actualized. Under such circumstances, any phonetic transcription becomes pointless.

Transcription is separated into two types: broad and narrow. The more general type of transcription is referred to as **broad transcription**, which is based on the phoneme system of the particular language; each symbol represents a phoneme. Because phonemes within a language system are noted, this type of transcription is also referred to as **phonemic transcription**. For broad transcription, the symbols are placed within slashes / /, which are termed *virgules*. Thus, /p/ would indicate phonemic transcription.

A second type of transcription is **narrow transcription**. This type records the sound units with as much production detail as possible. This notation encompasses the use of both the broad classification system noted in the IPA and extra symbols, which can be added to give a particular phonetic value—in other words, to characterize specific production features. This type of transcription is also denoted as **phonetic transcription** because it includes phonetic (i.e., production feature) details. For narrow transcription, the symbols are placed within brackets [ ]. For example, [tʰ] would be a narrow transcription exemplifying a sound unit [t] with aspiration [ʰ]. Another way to look at broad and narrow transcription is to refer back to the definitions of *phoneme* and *allophone* (refer page 5). Broad transcription notes the differences in *phonemes*, whereas narrow transcription exemplifies *allophones*. As clinicians, we are often analyzing disordered speech; therefore, additional symbols may be added to the basic sound units to characterize allophonic variation. These notations are termed *diacritics* and are discussed later in the chapter. At times, the actual speech production may be so different that another phoneme symbol will be needed. For example, a child may produce "th" for "s" in all words. We could summarize this as a difference in a child's phonemic system; broad transcription exemplified by /θ/ for /s/ could be used. On the other hand,

Video Example 3.1
In this video, an explanation of how to navigate the International Phonetic Alphabet chart is given. According to this video, why do we need the International Phonetic Alphabet? Which parameters are used to order the consonants and vowels on the chart?

https://www.youtube.com/watch?v=g_SHfoUDj8A

Figure 3.1 The International Phonetic Alphabet (revised 2015)

THE INTERNATIONAL PHONETIC ALPHABET (revised to 2015)

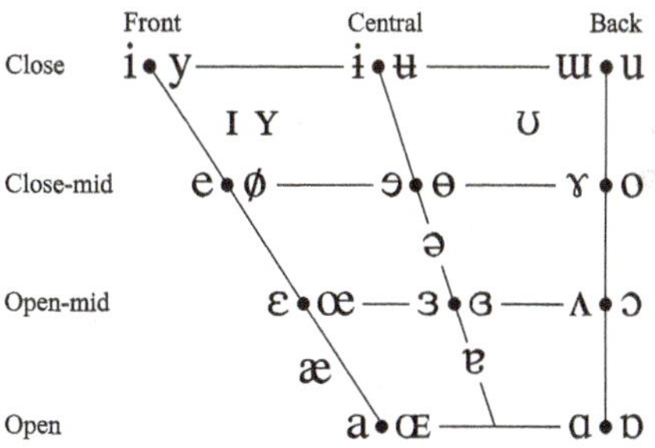

Source: Copyright 2005 International Phonetic Association. Reproduced by permission. Available http://www.internationalphoneticassociation.org/content/ipa-chart

Clinical Comments

This dichotomy between broad and narrow transcription, or phonemic versus phonetic transcription, relates directly to the difference between a phonemic and a phonetic inventory. A *phonemic inventory* contains all the phonemes that a child uses contrastively. Because /θ/ and /s/ are two different phonemes, if a child uses both contrastively—for example, contrasting "sink" and "think"—both would be included in the phonemic inventory. However, if the child uses /θ/ for all /s/ phonemes, then only /θ/, and not /s/, would be included in the phonemic inventory. On the other hand, the phonetic inventory includes, but is not limited to, the phonetic details that are categorized by the use of diacritics. Therefore, if a child says [sʷ] (lip-rounded [s]), [s̪] (dentalized [s]), and [sʲ] (palatalized [s]) for /s/, then /s/ is part of the phonemic inventory, but all three variants—[sʷ], [s̪], and [sʲ]—would be contained in the phonetic inventory. Related to [s] productions, the lateral "s" [ɬ] is considered to be so different in its production from /s/ that it is considered a separate phoneme. This is due to the fact that lateralization is considered to be a *primary* articulation. Therefore, if a child says [ɬ] for *all* /s/ phonemes, then /ɬ/ is in the phonemic and phonetic inventories, but /s/ would not be included in either.

narrow transcription is used if a child's tongue placement of "s" is just a bit too far forward, and the result does not sound like "th" but rather like a distorted "s." A marker, a diacritic, is added to "s." This narrow transcription is [s̪], the small symbol under the "s" indicating a dentalized production, one in which the tongue is approaching the front teeth; that is, the tongue is slightly forward, giving the "s" a distorted quality.

The dichotomy between phonetic and phonemic transcription often leads to transcribers using brackets, [ ], and slashes, / /, interchangeably. However, as noted in the previous chapter, brackets, [ ], should be used when listening to and transcribing actual productions. This notation indicates actual realizations, the concrete productions of a speech sound. Therefore, if we are transcribing a child's speech, brackets, [ ], should be used. If we are summarizing a phonemic inventory, then phonemic or broad transcription might be sufficient. As speech-language clinicians, however, we often assess disordered speech. In this case, narrow transcription will probably be used to note as much detail as possible. Narrow transcription is a necessity when the individual's speech patterns demonstrate errors that cannot be perceptually classified as phonemes of the given language.

Phonetic transcription is a purely *descriptive* enterprise. Occasionally, beginning transcription materials consist of lists of orthographically presented words (*book, table, snail,* and so on) that students then have to transfer into phonetic symbols. Such a practice can be misleading. It supports the mistaken notion that there is a *prescriptive* part to phonetic transcription that provides some guiding principle about how words are supposed to be pronounced. This is also suggested by dictionaries: Each entry tells the reader how to spell a word correctly, and the symbols that follow indicate how the word "should be" pronounced. There is, of course, nothing wrong with indicating how words are commonly pronounced, but the jump from how they *are* pronounced to how they *should be* pronounced has nothing to do with the idea behind or practice of phonetic transcription.

The Use and Value of Phonetic Transcription for Speech-Language Therapists

Accurate phonetic transcription is an indispensable clinical tool for speech-language pathologists. That is why it has to be taken so seriously, especially when it is used to assess and remediate impaired articulation and phonology. Without a reliable record of how a child or adult realized a particular speech sound, we simply do not have enough information for goal-directed intervention, nor can we document changes in production that might occur during therapy. Phonetic transcription provides a reasonably accurate written record of what was said and what it sounded like.

Admittedly, phonetic transcription is somewhat troublesome and time consuming. In addition, it certainly has its own problems. Some rules have to be strictly observed to overcome these problems. The first thing any aspiring transcriber has to understand is that the human ear is not without bias. We are unable to *receive* only; we must always *perceive* as well. That is, people automatically judge and interpret incoming acoustic signals based on their experience with those signals. In respect to spoken language, this means that when listening to the incoming acoustic signal, the listener unwillingly "distorts" it in the direction of former experiences, including how the listener would have produced it. This "built-in" tendency is the greatest danger to any serious transcription effort. Any higher degree of accuracy is very difficult to attain if perceptual biases rule transcription efforts. To overcome the tendency to "interpret" what was heard requires considerable goodwill, patience, and special training.

Several other problems must be considered when using phonetic transcription. For example, many circumstances, such as the age of the client or an unusual vocal quality, can affect our transcription. Other factors may produce large variations in the inter- and intrajudge reliability of transcriptions, including the intelligibility of the client, the position of the sound in the word, and whether narrow or broad transcription is used (Shriberg & Lof, 1991). Shriberg, Kent, McAllister, and Preston (2019) provide an excellent overview of the sources of variation and the factors that affect the reliability of phonetic transcription. These problems are very real, and caution must be exercised when using phonetic transcription. On the other hand, we cannot simply disregard transcription because of its inherent problems or use a private system of noting sound realizations. Instead, the importance of developing good, reliable transcription skills should be stressed. These skills will prove to be an invaluable resource in the assessment and treatment of speech sound disorders.

Defining Diacritics

Diacritics are marks added to sound transcription symbols to give them a particular phonetic value. The set of basic phonetic transcription symbols represents language-specific typical productions. Because speech-language pathologists deal mostly with aberrant articulatory events, it follows that diacritical marks are of special importance when characterizing the speech of their clients. Diacritics are often needed to note the clients' deviant sound qualities.

Numerous diacritics are noted in Figure 3.1. Although these diacritics have functioned fairly effectively, extensions to the International Phonetic Alphabet

Video Example 3.2
In this video, a brief overview of diacritics on the International Phonetic Alphabet chart is provided. According to the video, what is the definition of diacritics? Can you give an example of a diacritic? Note the diacritic for syllabics, which will be covered later in the chapter.

https://www.youtube.com/watch?v=bpxtxYC3jqs

(extIPA) were developed specifically to address the transcription of disordered speech. The extIPA symbols, first published in 1990, were revised in 2002 and more recently in 2015. Refer to Figure 3.2 for a list of the extIPA symbols. The following discussion of diacritics includes only those frequently used by clinicians. Readers should refer to Figures 3.1 and 3.2 for special transcription needs as they develop their skills.

Figure 3.2 ExtIPA Symbols for Disordered Speech (revised 2015)

extIPA SYMBOLS FOR DISORDERED SPEECH
(Revised to 2015)

CONSONANTS (other than those on the IPA Chart)

	Bilabial	Labio-dental	Labio-alveolar	Dento-labial	Bidental	Linguo-labial	Inter-dental	Alveolar	Retroflex	Palatal	Velar	Velo-pharyngeal	(Upper) pharyngeal
Plosive		p̪ b̪	p̺ b̺	p̟ b̟			t̪ d̪						Q ɢ
Nasal			m̺ n̺	m̟ ṃ		n̼ n̼	n̪ n̪						
Trill						r̼	r̪					f̬ŋ f̬ŋ	
Fricative, median			f̺ v̺	f̟ v̟	h̪ h̪	θ̼ ð̼	θ̪ ð̪	θ̺ ð̺				f̬ŋ f̬ŋ	
Fricative, lateral						ɬ̼ ɮ̼	ɬ̪ ɮ̪		ɬ̢ ɮ̢	ʎ̥ ʎ̬	ʟ̥ ʟ̬		
Fricative, lat. + med.								ls lz					
Fricative, nasal	m̥ m̃	m̥ m̃					n̪ ñ	n̥ ñ	n̥ ñ	n̥ ñ	ŋ̥ ŋ̃		
Approxt., lateral						l̼	l̪						
Percussive	ʬ ʬ				ʭ								

DIACRITICS

ş	labial spreading	ş	ð̃, ð̃	denasal, partial denasal	m̃ ñ	ş	main gesture offset right	ş
ş	strong articulation	f̬	ð̃	fricative nasal escape	ṽ	ş	main gesture offset left	ş
ş	weak articulation	v̬	ð̃	velopharyngeal friction	ş ʒ̃	ş	whistled articulation	ş
\	reiteration	p\p\p	↓	ingressive airflow	p↓	oo	sliding articulation	θs

CONNECTED SPEECH, UNCERTAINTY ETC.

(.) (..) (...)	short, medium, long pause
f, ff	loud(er) speech: [{f laʊd f}]
p, pp	quiet(er) speech: [{p kwaɪət p}]
allegro	fast speech: [{allegro fɑst allegro}]
lento	slow speech: [{lento sloʊ lento}]
crescendo, ralentando etc. may also be used	
Ⓞ, Ⓒ, Ⓥ	indeterminate sound, consonant, vowel
Ⓕ, Ⓟ etc.	indeterminate fricative, probably [p] etc.
( )	silent articulation, e.g. (ʃ), (m)
(( ))	extraneous noise, e.g. ((2 sylls))

VOICING

ₒ	pre-voicing	ₒz	
ₒ	post-voicing	z̬	
ş	partial devoicing	z̥ ʒ̥	
ş	initial partial devoicing	z̥ ʒ̥	
ş	final partial devoicing	z̥ ʒ̥	
ş	partial voicing	ş	
ş	initial partial voicing	ş	
ş	final partial voicing	ş	
ₒ⁼	unaspirated	p⁼	
ʰₒ	pre-aspiration	ʰp	

OTHER SOUNDS

ɹ̺	apical-r
ɹ̈	bunched-r (molar-r)
ş ʒ̺	laminal fricatives (incl. lowered tongue tip)
kᶯ etc.	[k] with lateral fricated release etc.
tˡˢ dˡᶻ	[t, d] with lateral and median release
tʰ̪	[t] with interdental aspiration etc.

t̼θ	linguolabial affricate etc.
ʞ p̅ ɱ̅	velodorsal oral and nasal stops
ˌ	sublaminal lower alveolar percussive
ǃ̬	alveolar click with sublaminal percussive release
⊙r̼	buccal interdental trill (raspberry)
*	sound with no available symbol

© ICPLA 2015

Source: Reprinted by permission of the International Clinical Phonetics and Linguistics Association.

Diacritics Used with Consonants

These symbols describe deviations from normal tongue placement for consonants.

Dentalization. This term refers to an articulatory variation in which the tongue approaches the upper incisors. It is marked by [̪] placed under the IPA symbol. For example, the symbol [d] stands for a voiced alveolar stop. A dentalized realization results when a child places the tip of the tongue not against the alveolar ridge, as the IPA symbol indicates, but against the inside of the upper incisors. A *dentalized realization* is transcribed as:

[d̪] = dentalized [d]

[d̪] occurs quite often as the result of coarticulation. Compare [d]-productions in the words "widow" and "width." The articulatory influence of the following [θ], a dental or even interdental sound, will probably "dentalize" normally alveolar [d] realizations. Dentalized s-sounds, [s̪] and [z̪], frequently occur in the speech of children (Smit, 1993b).

Palatalization. Another modification of consonant articulation is *palatalization*. Only sounds for which the palate is *not* the place of articulation can be palatalized. However, if the place of articulation is the alveolar ridge or the upper incisors, palatalization occurs if the anterior portions of the tongue approach the front or middle of the palate—that is, when the articulators are positioned somewhat posteriorly. For velar consonants, palatalization indicates the movement of the articulators in the direction of the palate to a more anterior articulation. Palatalization causes a typical change in the quality of the sounds in question. The diacritical mark for palatalization is a superscript j added to the right of the basic IPA symbol:

[sʲ] = palatalized [s]
[tʲ] = palatalized [t]

Velarization. This term refers to a more posterior tongue placement (in the direction of the velum) for palatal sounds. The diacritical mark for velarization is a superscript ɣ placed to the right of the IPA symbol. Thus [tˠ] is a velarized [t]. An exception is the so-called dark [l], a velarized [l], which may be transcribed in two different ways. In General American English, the velarized [l] production, the so-called dark [l], is usually heard in word-final positions, for example, in *pull* or *shawl*; as a syllabic, such as in *little* or *bottle*; preceding a consonant, exemplified by *salt* or *build*; and preceding high-back vowels [u] (*loop*) and [ʊ] (*look*) (Small, 2020). The velarization in these cases is often so prominent that even main phonetic characteristics of [l], the articulation of the tongue tip against the alveolar ridge, are sometimes no longer present. In such a case, the velarization actually replaces the typical alveolar l-articulation. The velarized production is an allophonic variation of [l]; it does not change the meaning of the word in question. Velarized [l]-productions are transcribed as [ɫ] or [lˠ]:

[fuɫ] = velarized [l]-sound
[kulˠ] = velarized [l]-sound

The so-called dark and light l-sounds are discussed in more detail in Chapter 9.

Lateralization. [l] is the only lateral in General American English. It cannot be lateralized because it is a lateral already. If during any consonant production other than [l] air is released laterally, we speak of *lateralization*. For example, [s] can become lateralized. Articulations of [s] and [z] require a highly accurate placement of frontal parts of the tongue *approximating* the alveolar ridge, not touching the alveolar ridge. This precarious position must be maintained throughout the entire sound duration, a motorically difficult task, especially for young children. To make things easier, children sometimes establish direct contact between the articulators at the alveolar ridge. Under these circumstances, the airstream cannot, of course, escape centrally any longer. In an attempt to maintain the fricative effect of [s], children then release the air laterally into the cheeks. The result is a conspicuous [s] variation, a lateral lisp. Lateralization is considered a primary articulation; therefore, the production features are changed so much that a different phoneme results. For example, the voiceless lateral "s" is a phoneme of the Navajo language, whereas the voiced lateral has phonemic value in Mongolian (Ladefoged & Maddieson, 1996). The lateral "s" production is categorized as an alveolar lateral fricative. According to the IPA, [ɬ] is the voiceless lateral alveolar fricative, and [ɮ] is its voiced lateral counterpart:

[sɪp] → [ɬɪp] = a lateralized [s]
[zɪp] → [ɮɪp] = a lateralized [z]

The extIPA also provides symbols to distinguish among productions that demonstrate *both* lateral and central airflow (as opposed to just lateral airflow). The symbols for those are:

[su] → [ꞎsu] = a voiceless alveolar fricative with lateral and central airflow
[zu] → [ɮzu] = a voiced alveolar fricative with lateral and central airflow

Clinical Comments

Problems with s-Sounds

Dentalized, palatalized, and lateralized [s] realizations are frequent distortions noted in children. In some children, the dentalized [s] may co-occur with "th" for "s" substitutions ([s] → [θ] or [s] → [s̪]), as in the following productions:

"Santa Claus" [θæn tə klɑs̪] for [sæn tə klɑz]

The tongue position that is too far forward for children's [s]-productions may fluctuate slightly, so that the production is perceived at times as [s̪] and at other times as [θ]. When it is perceived as [s̪], it is an allophonic variation of [s]. However, if it is heard as [θ], the production has crossed phonemic boundaries; it is now perceived as a different phoneme. It is interesting to note that certain children may also use this dichotomy systematically: For example, [θ] may be realized at the beginning of a word or syllable, whereas [s̪] may be produced at the end of a word or syllable. Such a possibility should be considered in our assessment.

Differentiating among dentalized, palatalized, and lateralized [s]-productions may seem difficult at first. However, clear perceptual qualities distinguish the three forms. Dentalized [s]-sounds, [s̪], have a "dull" quality; they lack the sharp, high-frequency characteristic of typical [s]-productions. On the other hand, lateralized [s]-sounds, [ɬ], have a distinct noise component to them that is typically rather conspicuous. If the airflow is just on one side (either right or left), a speech-language specialist typically observes a distortion of the lips and even the jaw to the side of the air escape. Palatalized [s] variations, [sʲ], perceptually approach a [ʃ] quality. Palatalization of [s] is marked by the anterior portions of the tongue approaching parts of the palate, resulting in a slightly posterior placement of the articulators. If [s] is compared to [ʃ], one notes that [ʃ] realizations also require a more posteriorly placed articulation (alveolar [s] versus prepalatal [ʃ]).

Voice Symbols

Devoicing of Voiced Consonants.   Under normal circumstances, vowels and more than half of our consonants are voiced. If these sounds become completely devoiced in a speech sample, the speech needs to be marked. In cases of total devoicing, the IPA symbol for the voiceless counterpart of the voiced sound, its unvoiced cognate, is usually indicated:

[ʃus] for "sho<u>es</u>"
[tip] for "<u>d</u>eep"

In this case, the phonemic value has changed from /z/ to /s/ in "shoes" and from /d/ to /t/ in "deep."

Partial Devoicing.   Often, however, the sound in question is only partially devoiced. This is considered an allophonic variation of the voiced consonant. The diacritic for partial devoicing is a small circle in parentheses placed under the sound symbol:

[ʃuz̥]

[d̥ɪp]

These examples are transcribed according to the extIPA, which differentiates initial devoicing [₍̥] (the parenthesis is on the left) and final devoicing [̥₎] (the parenthesis is on the right).

Voicing of Voiceless Consonants.   Voiceless consonants may also be voiced, especially if they occur between two vowels. A casual pronunciation of *eighteen* might serve as an example. If voiceless consonants become totally voiced, the phoneme value has changed and the segment is transcribed with the respective symbol:

[eɪtin] → [eɪdin]

Partial Voicing.   If voiceless consonants become partially voiced—that is, are allophonic variations of the consonant—the diacritical mark is a lowercase v in parentheses under the respective sound symbol:

[eɪt̬in] for "eighteen"

Initial and final partial voicing are [₍̬] and [̬₎], respectively.

Clinical Comments

Partial Voicing and Devoicing

Partial voicing and devoicing are difficult to discern and to transcribe correctly. The first impression of transcribers is often some minor qualitative variance—the sound is somehow "off." Such a first impression is usually a good reason to focus subsequently on the voicing–devoicing opposition. This two-step procedure makes it easier to arrive at the difficult judgment: partially voiced or partially devoiced.

Also, General American English has a tendency to devoice (or partially devoice) final consonants. The following are examples from Daniel, age 4 years 7 months.

(continued)

"stove"	[stoʊv]	→	[stoʊf]	total devoicing
"slide"	[slaɪd]	→	[slaɪd̥]	partial devoicing
"flag"	[flæg]	→	[flæg̥]	partial devoicing
"nose"	[noʊz]	→	[noʊs]	total devoicing

The general devoicing tendency in final positions in American English suggests that realizations like these should probably not be considered aberrant productions.

Aspiration and Nonaspiration of Plosives.   The strong burst of breath that accompanies the release of the articulatory closure in plosives typically leads to aspiration. This aspiration is noted by using a small superscript h following the voiceless plosive sound:

"table" [tʰeɪbəl]

Voiceless plosives are usually aspirated at the beginning of words; however, they are not aspirated in consonant clusters. Word-final aspiration is variable (Edwards, 2003). Plosives, which are normally aspirated, are not marked unless the aspiration is excessive.

Voiceless plosives that are normally aspirated may be produced without this aspiration. In this case, the diacritic for unaspirated productions, [⁼], could be added:

"pie" [p⁼aɪ]

This example indicates that a normally aspirated [p] has occurred without aspiration. This may not appear significant; however, if you have ever tried to learn French, with its unaspirated voiceless plosives (such as in "Paris"), you might understand the difficulty. Children may also not aspirate plosives when they are usually aspirated. This can lead to the clinical impression of a voiced plosive.

Unreleased Plosives.   Plosives can be modified in another manner. Unreleased plosives result when the articulatory closure is maintained and not—as usual—released. Although voiceless unreleased stops are more obvious because of their loss of aspiration, voiced stops can be unreleased as well. Unreleased stops typically occur at the end of an utterance or at the end of one-word responses. To indicate an unreleased articulation, the diacritical mark [˺] is added:

Boy, was it hot.
[bɔɪ wʌz ɪt hɑt˺]

Clinical Comments

Transcribing Unreleased Plosives

Unreleased plosives should be noted *during* the simultaneous transcription of a client's speech. Listening to and transcribing from recordings can be misleading because, when recorded, unreleased plosives can sound similar to consonant omissions. During live transcriptions, we can hear and at least partially see the actual articulation. This provides a much better basis for our judgment regarding an unreleased plosive production or a deletion.

The following transcriptions come from a standardized speech test of Billy, age 4 years 3 months:

"cup"	[kʌp]	→	[tʌp˺]
"music"	[mjuzɪk]	→	[mudɪk˺]
"book"	[bʊk]	→	[bʊk˺]
"feet"	[fit]	→	[fit˺]
"watch"	[wɑtʃ]	→	[wɑt˺]
"sandwich"	[sænwɪtʃ]	→	[gæmɪt˺]

Unreleased plosives seldom warrant therapeutic intervention. Billy's case was different, however. In addition to his many articulation errors, unreleased consonants contributed substantially to a decrease in his intelligibility.

Syllabic Consonants. Unstressed syllables easily become *reduced syllables*. This means that their vowel nucleus practically disappears. If the vowel nucleus is reduced, the following consonant becomes a syllabic; that is, it becomes the peak of that syllable. This is especially the case in unstressed final syllables when a nasal or the lateral follows the preceding vowel. The proper diacritic mark for such an occurrence is a straight line directly under the syllabic consonant:

fɪʃɪŋ → fɪʃən → fɪʃn̩

Clinical Comments

Syllabics

In spontaneous speech, adults often reduce the unstressed final syllable, as in the following example:

He broke the bottle.
[hi bɹoʊk ðə bɑtl̩]

Children can also demonstrate the use of syllabics. For example:

"little" [lɪtl̩]
"scratching" [skɹæ tʃn̩]
The boy is fishing; he has a fishing pole.
[ðə bɔɪ ɪzˈfɪʃn̩ hi hæz əˈfɪʃn̩ poʊl]

Although such syllabics obviously need to be noted and transcribed, they are considered norm realizations.

Labialization and Nonlabialization of Consonants. Consonants, with the exception of [ʃ] and [w], are typically produced without lip rounding. Lip rounding is a production feature of both of the consonants that are exceptions. If a normally unrounded consonant—for example, a normally unrounded [s]—is produced with lip rounding, this is referred to as *labializing the sound in question*. The diacritic for labialized consonants is a superscript w placed to the right of the symbol in question. When consonants that are normally rounded (such as [ʃ] and [w]) are produced without lip rounding, this is considered nonlabialization. The diacritic for labial spreading [↔] is placed under the symbol in question [ʃ̬] to indicate nonlabialization. Labialized consonants can be the result of assimilation processes, as in the following example:

"soup" [sʷup] = labialized [s] due to the influence of the rounded [u] vowel

Labialization from assimilation of normally unrounded consonants is noted, but it is not considered a speech sound problem. On the other hand, [ʃ] is usually produced with at least some degree of lip rounding. The following example indicates [ʃ] without lip rounding:

"ship" [ʃ̬ɪp] = nonlabialized [ʃ]

Unrounded [ʃ] realizations can also result from assimilation; however, some children unround [ʃ] in all contexts. This is considered an aberrant production and should be noted. It usually affects the quality of the [ʃ], making it sound somewhat "off," qualitatively different from a typical production.

Derhotacization. Derhotacization is the loss of r-coloring typically for the central vowels with r-coloring, [ɝ] and [ɚ]. Derhotacized central vowels are transcribed as [ɜ] and [ə]. However, [ɹ], as in *rabbit*, can lose its characteristic r-coloring as well. Children often substitute a [w] for this sound. Another possibility is the substitution of [ʋ], which is a voiced labiodental approximant. For [ʋ], the lower lip approximates the upper teeth. It is very similar to the voiced [w] but with the teeth and lips held in the position used to articulate the letter "vee." The [ʋ] sound, in contrast, also lacks the high-back tongue position of [w], which is considered a labio*velar* approximant.

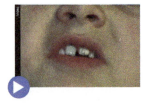

Video Example 3.3
In this video, 6-year-old Summer says eight different words three times each. Listen to and transcribe this child's speech. Is there lip rounding on the "sh" words? Try to transcribe them accordingly. Also note the differences in lip rounding for [ʧ], "ch" on "matches" versus "church." Does Summer demonstrate any other speech sound difficulties?

Clinical Comments

Rounding and Unrounding of [ʃ]

Rounded [s]- and unrounded [ʃ]-sounds are frequent sibilant realizations of children. These may be aberrant productions or context-based assimilation processes. The following is an excerpt from a transcription of Matt, age 4 years 6 months:

The boy is swinging really high.
[ðə bɔɪ ɪz sʷwɪŋən rili haɪ]
My mommy made vegetable soup.
[maɪ mɑmi meɪd vɛdʒəbəl sʷup]

In addition to Matt's unorthodox pronunciation of *vegetable*, we note that his [s]-sounds are rounded. In the given context, they may be regressive assimilation processes influenced by the rounding of the following [w] or [u].

This does not seem to be the case in Chris's transcription, which is based on a standardized speech assessment and a spontaneous speech sample.

"fish"	[fɪʃ]	→	[fɪʃ̬]
"watch"	[wɑtʃ]	→	[wɑʃ̬]
"chicken"	[tʃɪkən]	→	[ʃ̬ɪkən]
"shovel"	[ʃʌvəl]	→	[ʃ̬ʌvəl]

At lunch I ate a peanut butter sandwich.

[æt lʌnʃ aɪ eɪt ə pinət bʌtɚ ʃænɪʃ]

I wish I had some new tennis shoes, like Michael Jordan.

[aɪ wɪʃ aɪ hæd sʌm nu tɛnəs ʃuz laɪk maɪkəl ʃoɚdən]

Chris, in contrast to Matt, *un*rounds his "sh"-sounds even when they precede a rounded vowel, as in the word "shoes." He also occasionally uses [ʃ] for [s]-, [tʃ]-, and [dʒ]-sounds.

Diacritics Used with Vowels

Rounding and Unrounding of Vowels.   Some vowels have lip rounding as one of their production features, and others are typically produced with no lip rounding—[u] versus [i], for example. The rounding or unrounding of the lips is an important feature of vowel realizations. However, for several reasons, some clients may delete or inappropriately add these characteristics. This results in a distortion of the respective sound quality. The IPA offers one symbol to indicate lip rounding in normally unrounded vowels and another symbol to indicate unrounding of vowels typically produced with lip rounding. The signs are placed directly under the vowel symbol in question and consist of a small *c*-type notation, which indicates unrounding (or less rounding than is considered normal) when open to the right. When this *c* is reversed, creating an opening to the left, it denotes rounding (or more rounding than is normally the case):

[u̜] = unrounded [u]
[ɛ̹] = rounded [ɛ]

Changes in Tongue Placement for Vowels.   Deviations in tongue positioning affect vowel as well as consonant articulations. Different vowel qualities are established essentially by different sizes and forms of the vocal tract. Two main factors determining these sizes and forms pertain to the location of the raised portion of the tongue (front and back dimensions) and the extent to which the tongue is raised in the direction of the hard or soft palate (high and low dimensions).

Raised or Lowered Tongue Position.   The IPA offers a set of diacritics that signals the direction of tongue heights on the vertical plane, leading to deviations from norm vowel productions. The diacritic [˕] under the vowel symbol marks a lower elevation, whereas the diacritic [˔] under the character marks a higher elevation of the tongue than is normally the case for the production of the vowel in question. For example,

[sɪ̞t]

would state that the high-front elevation of the tongue for standard [ɪ] articulation has not been reached in this realization; that is, the tongue articulation was lower than normal, resulting in a perceptible distortion for [ɪ]. Trying to describe our auditory impression of this sound, we would say that it shifted in the direction of (but did not reach) the sound quality of [e].

Similarly, the transcription

[bɪ̝t]

would indicate a higher-than-normal elevation of the tongue for [ɪ], resulting in a quality that approaches [i] characteristics.

The same principle applies to all vowels. A question that logically follows is whether it makes a difference which symbol we use if the vowel is somewhere between two qualities. In other words, do a raised [e] ([e̝]) and a lowered [ɪ] ([ɪ̞]) signify the same vowel quality? The answer is no. In our previous example, the speech-language specialist must decide whether this vowel realization sounded more like an [e]- or an [ɪ]-type vowel. Based on the transcriber's auditory perception, the basic vowel quality first must be chosen, and then the modifying diacritic mark should be added to it. This is easier to understand if you refer again to the definitions of *phoneme* and *allophone*. These symbols are indicating allophonic variations in a vowel. Therefore, the phoneme that you understood must first be selected and then the diacritic is added to indicate an allophone.

Think of the symbol as a pointer with its base the top of the T-type notation. If the pointer projects down [˕], the tongue has been lowered; if it points up [˔], the tongue has been raised.

Advanced or Retracted Tongue Position.   There are also diacritics signaling tongue variations on the horizontal plane that lead to deviations from norm productions. They indicate a tongue position that is too far forward or too far back for a normal production of the vowel in question. The diacritic for vowels produced with a tongue more advanced than usual is [+]. More retracted protrusions are marked by the diacritic [−]. Both are placed under the vowel symbol.

[ɛ̟] is an [ɛ] vowel with an advanced tongue articulation; the tongue placement is more forward than is typically the case.

[ʊ̠] is an [ʊ] vowel with a retracted tongue articulation; the tongue placement is too far back.

Clinical Comments

Noting Changes in Tongue Positions for Vowels

Changes in the position of the tongue for vowel realizations are often perceptually difficult to target. Although transcribers are aware that the vowel quality is slightly distorted, they may not be sure what has caused this deviation. If the tongue has been lowered or raised, the vowel quality will sound somehow similar to the neighboring vowel on the vertical plane of the vowel quadrilateral. Thus, a lowered [ɛ] will have a certain [æ] quality, or a raised [ʊ] will approach [u]. The best reference source in these cases is the vowel quadrilateral. However, this is not so simple if the tongue movements pertain to the horizontal plane—that is, to a tongue position too advanced or retracted. One point of reference is that front vowels that demonstrate a retracted tongue position and back vowels that demonstrate a tongue position that is too far forward, sound somewhat "centralized"—that is, their distinct qualities appear reduced. Therefore, although the vowel can still be identified as the respective front or back vowel, it approaches a [ʌ]-type quality.

Nasality Symbols. During the production of most General American English speech sounds, the velum is tensed to block the escape of the expiratory air through the nasal cavity. The only exception to this rule is for the nasals. This is—quite correctly—what the textbooks tell us. However, in reality, the conditions are not always so clear-cut. If a nasal follows a vowel, for example, nasality often seeps into the vowel segment; the preceding vowel becomes nasalized:

[tæn] → [tæ̃n]

As long as the nasality does not overstep the boundary of natural assimilatory processes, this nasality remains unmarked. Speakers and listeners perceive these variations as normal. However, if the nasality is perceived as being excessive, or hypernasal, we need to place the "tilde" [~] (which you may have encountered in Spanish language classes) over the respective sounds. As speech-language specialists, we encounter hypernasality prominently in the speech of clients with dysarthria and cleft palates.

Denasality is also encountered in the speech of our clients. The symbol for denasality is the tilde with a slash through it, placed above the nasal consonant:

ni →ñ̷i

This symbol refers to a reduction of nasal quality. Only nasal consonants can be denasalized. If nasal consonants are perceived as having a total lack of nasal quality (i.e., having a completely oral quality), then the symbol for the resulting homorganic voiced plosive is used:

ni → di

Clinical Comments

Assimilation and Dialect

One characteristic of African American dialect is the total regressive assimilation of postvocalic nasals (e.g., Moran, 1993; Wolfram, 1989). The assimilation process is regressive in that the nasal following the vowel changes the characteristic of the preceding vowel into a nasalized vowel. It is considered a *total* assimilation process because the postvocalic nasal consonant is totally gone. The following examples demonstrate this process:

"pen"	[pɛn]	→	[pɛ̃n]	→	[pɛ̃]
"thumb"	[θʌm]	→	[θʌ̃m]	→	[θʌ̃]

These pronunciations were noted on a standardized speech test from a child, age 4 years 3 months, speaking African American dialect:

"broom"	[brum]	→	[brũ]
"gum"	[gʌm]	→	[gʌ̃]
"sandwich"	[sæn wɪtʃ]	→	[sæ̃ wɪtʃ]
"ice cream"	[aɪs krim]	→	[aɪs krĩ]

The total regressive assimilation process is dialectal in nature. In the African American dialect, it represents a pronunciation possibility.

Video Example 3.4
In this video, phonetic descriptions of "annoying sounds" that teenagers make are given. Try to follow the phonetic descriptions of the sounds that are made. There are explanations for specific vowels and consonants using the diacritics that have been covered. Can you follow the video speaker's descriptions and possibly replicate them?
https://www.youtube.com/watch?v = ZY2R_K3NFPo

Diacritics for Stress, Duration, and Syllable Boundaries

Stress Markers. Every multisyllabic word has its own stress pattern, which our clients may or may not realize in a regular manner. The main purpose of all stress realizations is to emphasize certain syllables over others, thus creating a hierarchy of prominence among them.

Primary Stress. The order of prominence is actualized by differences in loudness, pitch, and duration, the loudness differences being the most striking of the three. Generally, two different loudness levels are observed. The loudest syllable is said to have the *primary stress*. It is marked by a superscript short straight line in front of the respective syllable.

"syllable"	[ˈsɪ lə bəl]
"railway"	[ˈɹeɪl weɪ]
"superior"	[sə ˈpɪɚ i ɚ]

Secondary Stress. The next loudest syllable bears the *secondary stress*. It is indicated by a subscript short straight line in front of the syllable in question.

"supermarket"	[ˈsu pɚ ˌmɑɚ kət]
"signify"	[ˈsɪg nə ˌfaɪ]
"phonetic"	[ˌfə ˈnɛ tɪk]

Clinical Comments

Displacement of Stress

Clients with dysarthria typically have difficulties with stressing. The following transcription exemplifies such a possible displacement of stress:

"birthday"	
Norm speaker:	[ˈbɝθ ˌdeɪ]
Dysarthric speaker:	[ˌbɝθ ˈdeɪ]
"umbrella"	
Norm speaker:	[ˌəm ˈbrɛ lə]
Dysarthric speaker:	[ˈʌm ˌbrə lə]

Some people find it difficult to distinguish among specific stressed versus unstressed syllables in words. For them, it may be helpful to know that in General American English, different loudness levels characterizing stress usually (but not always) go hand in hand with changes in pitch; thus, the louder the syllable, the higher the pitch. Paying attention to pitch differences first, may therefore aid in discriminating among differing levels of loudness in stressing. It is also helpful to know that many (but again, not all) words in General American English have their primary (or secondary) stress emphasis on the first syllable. A third possibility for those having difficulty distinguishing stress differences is to vary systematically the loudness in each of the syllables of the word in question, [ˈdʒɛˌloʊ] versus [ˌdʒɛˈloʊ], for example. Typically, one version of that particular word will sound clearly more acceptable than the other. By a process of elimination, one can often determine the appropriate stress pattern.

Duration Symbols. Sounds take up different amounts of time in continuous speech. We are so used to these measurable differences in sound duration that we register changes in these typical lengths automatically as "too short" or "too long." If that is our perceptual impression, we have to indicate it by means of diacritic markers. Normal (i.e., inconspicuous) sound duration remains unmarked.

Lengthening. Longer than normal duration is signaled by either one or two dots following the sound symbol in question. The more dots, the longer the sound.

[fit]	standard vowel duration
[fi·t]	slightly longer than normal vowel duration
[fi:t]	clearly longer than normal vowel duration

Shortening. Shorter than normal speech sound productions also occur. Different degrees of shortening are, as a rule, not indicated. The diacritic mark for any shortened sounds is [˘] placed above the respective sound symbol.

Shortening sounds can lead to cutting off a portion of their phonetic properties. Young children with unstable [s]-sounds sometimes shorten the normally fairly long s-segments to something that may sound like the release portion of [t]. If onset and holding portions of [t] are also identifiable, the obvious transcription would be [t]. However, if that is not the case—that is, if we indeed have an [s]-impression—we would transcribe this as [š].

Syllable Boundaries. Syllable boundaries are indicated by a period placed between the syllables.

"reliable"	[ɹi.laɪ.ə.bəl]
"attention"	[ə.tɛn.ʃən]

Additional Symbols

The following symbols are not diacritics but are often used when transcribing aberrant speech.

Glottal Stop. The glottal stop ([ʔ]) is produced when a closed glottis (i.e., the space between the vocal folds) is suddenly released after a buildup of subglottal air pressure. The release of air pressure creates a popping noise. The glottal stop is considered an allophonic variation of some plosive productions and can serve to release vowels in stressed syllables or separate successive vowels between words:

"oh"	[ʔoʊ]	releasing a vowel
"Anna asks"	[ænə ʔæsks]	separating successive vowels

Some children with articulatory or phonological impairments use the glottal stop as a sound substitution.

Bilabial Fricatives. The voiceless ([ɸ]) and voiced ([β]) bilabial fricatives are not phonemes of General American English but can be used as sound substitutions in aberrant speech. For example, a child might substitute a bilabial fricative for the labiodentals [f] or [v] or possibly produce the [p] and/or [b] as a fricative, resulting in [ɸ] or [β]. Both sounds are produced by approximating the lips so that a horizontally long but vertically narrow passageway is left between them for the voiceless or voiced breath stream to pass. The bilabial fricatives are phonemes in several languages. For example, [ɸ] is a phoneme of Japanese, and [β] has phonemic value in Spanish.

Palatal Fricatives. The voiceless [ç] and voiced [ʝ] palatal fricatives may be heard as substitutions for [ʃ] and [ʒ]. These aberrant productions are characterized by a more posterior positioning of the articulators than for [ʃ] or [ʒ]. Thus, the place of constriction for the articulators shifts from postalveolar to this palatal position. The voiceless [ç] sounds similar to a voiceless [j].

Velar Fricatives. When attempting to produce the velar stops [k] and [g], some children may not raise the tongue sufficiently to create a complete closure. In this case, a fricative may result. The symbols for the velar fricatives are [x] for the voiceless sound and [ɣ] for its voiced cognate.

Uvular Plosives. These sounds may again be heard in a child who is attempting to produce [k] or [g]. In this case, the client produces a plosive, but the place of articulation is too far back in the mouth, resulting in a sound that might be perceived as having a "guttural" quality. The voiceless uvular plosive is transcribed as [q], and its voiced counterpart is noted as [G].

Flap, Tap, or One-Tap Trill. The flap, tap, or what is also known as the one-tap trill [ɾ] is a frequent allophonic variation of [t] and [d]. This variation often occurs when plosives are preceded and followed by vowels, as in *city* or *butter*. The flap, tap, or one-tap trill is articulated with a single tap of the tongue tip against the alveolar ridge or possibly with only a movement of the tongue tip in the direction of the alveolar ridge. This is considered a normal and acceptable allophonic variation of [t] and [d].

| "butter" | [bʌɾɚ] |
| "ladder" | [læɾɚ] |

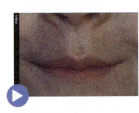

Video Tool Exercise 3.1

Identifying Devoicing and Interdental Articulations Complete the activity based on this video.

Clinical Application

The ExtIPA and Multiple Interdentality

Multiple interdentality, a label dating back to at least the 1930s (Froeschels, 1931, 1937), can be seen in our clinical population. It is used to describe an immature speech habit in which children produce [t], [d], [l], and [n] with their tongue tip too far forward. In other words, the tongue tip is between their teeth, resulting in an interdental production. According to the extIPA chart (refer to Figure 3.2), we see that these sounds can be transcribed in the following manner:

$$[t̪], [d̪], [n̪], [l̪]$$

Children with multiple interdentality often have difficulty with [s] and [z] as well. These sounds are also produced interdentally and end up sounding like "th" sounds, thus [θ] and [ð].

Clinical Implications

Phonetic transcription and, especially, its diacritic marks appear at first glance to be complicated to handle and difficult to remember. The obvious question arises as to how these diacritics could be helpful in our assessment and therapeutic process.

- First, accurate phonetic transcription involves ear training, a sharpening of our auditory discrimination abilities. These skills are indispensable for clinical expertise, something that cannot be emphasized enough.

- Second, phonetic transcription and, especially, the use of diacritic marks provide a generally agreed-upon, professional way to note certain deviations from typical productions. This system allows clinicians to communicate freely with other professionals in the field of communication sciences and disorders. Transcription symbols can be translated back into actual speech events in the same way that musicians can read notes and translate them back into tunes.

- Third, by being aware of the many variations that can occur, accurate phonetic transcriptions allow for additional diagnostic complexity that would not be considered otherwise. If we do not know what to listen for—unreleased plosives or partial devoicing, for example—we might not identify some of these variations.

- Fourth, diacritics can be used very effectively to document change over time during a remediation process. Often, therapy involves a systematic change of a child's articulation, which evolves slowly into a standard production in more complex environments such as words or sentences, for example. A child's articulation of [s] might evolve from [θ] to [s̬] and finally to a typical [s]-production. Diacritics can be used to document this change. By not using diacritics and simply saying that the [s] is "distorted," we are not documenting the systematic nature of the change.

The realizations of [s] illustrate well how the use of diacritics can have valuable practical consequences for assessment and intervention. Knowing what to listen for, we find that what once sounded like simply a distorted [s] can now be specified as the actual aberrant form presented: a palatal versus a lateral versus a dentalized [s]-distortion, for example. All these variations can be noted using the respective diacritic marks. In addition to the clarification that the notation system provides, detailed knowledge about actual realizations is indispensable for assessing and successfully remediating [s] errors. By establishing that the [s] appears distorted, we are saying only that it is an atypical production. We have addressed the *acceptability* issue of the sound realization but not its aberrant *production* features, the most important information for clinical purposes. However, by comparing a child's actual articulatory features with the known features for typical [s]-productions, we will know precisely which placement characteristics need to be changed therapeutically.

Identifying an [s]-distortion as a palatal [s], for example, gives detailed information that can be used when planning therapy. A palatal [sʲ] is produced with the tongue tip too far back in the direction of the palatal area. Because of this tongue position, the palatal [s] has a [ʃ]-like quality. All other production features are usually in accordance with norm [s]-articulations; the lateral edges of the tongue are raised, and the sagittal grooving necessary for the [s] is present as well. It may be possible, therefore, that a child needs only to move the tongue tip to a more anterior position to produce a more normal sounding [s]. By applying this knowledge, therapy becomes not only more goal directed but also much simpler—with the consequence of saving time and possible frustration.

The advantage of knowing how children actually produce distorted speech sounds becomes even more obvious if we compare two distorted sound productions, one palatal [s] ([sʲ]) and one dentalized [s] ([s̪]). The [s̪] is characterized by a tongue placement that is too far forward. In this case, children need to move the tongue posteriorly to obtain [s]. This would be in direct contrast to the procedure necessary for the [sʲ], in which a more frontal placement for the articulators becomes necessary. Detailed knowledge of a client's production features then proves to be an important asset leading to expedient therapeutic intervention.

Theoretically and practically, the importance of the preceding discussion seems rather obvious. Its essential ingredient is our ability to note and differentiate among changes in sound quality as the basis for our remedial task. By fine-tuning transcription skills, not only do the listener's discrimination and transcription capabilities increase, but also the effectiveness of the whole intervention process improves.

Based on the author's clinical experience, Table 3.1 offers the most frequently used transcription symbols.

Table 3.1 Commonly Used Transcription Symbols

Phonemic Symbol	Definition	Use
[ɬ]	Voiceless alveolar lateral fricative	Indicates a lateral [s].
[ɮ]	Voiced alveolar lateral fricative	Indicates a lateral [z].
[ʋ]	Voiced labiodental approximant	May be used as a substitution for [ɹ].
[ɜ]	Central vowel without r-coloring heard in a stressed word position	Used to demonstrate lack of r-coloring in the stressed central vowels.
[ə]	Central vowel without r-coloring heard in an unstressed word position	Used to demonstrate lack of r-coloring in the unstressed central vowels.
[ʔ]	Glottal stop	May be used as a substitution for plosives (or other consonants).
ˌ	Dentalized; tongue approaches the upper incisors	[s̪], [z̪] An s-production in which the articulators are too far forward and the s-production approaches a [θ] or [ð] quality.
j	Palatalized; articulators approach the palate for nonpalatalized sounds	[sʲ], [zʲ] For [s] and [z], these productions sound more qualitatively like [ʃ].
[↔]	Unrounded production	[ʃ̹] No lip rounding on production, and may occur with affricate productions.
˺	Unreleased plosive	[t˺] May at first sound like a consonant deletion, but movement of the articulators to a closed position is noted.
[t̪], [d̪], [n̪], [l̪]	Interdental productions	Some young children may show interdental productions on any or all of these sounds that may also be evident in s-productions.

Clinical Application

Using Diacritics in the Assessment Process

Andy, age 6 years 2 months, was referred to the speech-language specialist by his classroom teacher. According to the teacher, his main problem seemed to be his "speech," which she described as being somewhat difficult to understand and containing many sound errors. After a thorough appraisal, the speech-language specialist was concerned that Andy might have a phonemic-based disorder. When first listening to Andy's spontaneous speech, in addition to his [w/ɹ] substitutions, she thought that he used [θ] realizations for [θ]-, [s]-, [z]-, and [ʃ]-sounds. The clinician was worried that Andy was not able to differentiate between these phonemes. She had to admit, though, that there were some qualitative differences among the productions that she could not quite describe. She decided to continue with her assessment, paying special attention to these sounds. She also used some pictures that pinpointed these sounds in an elicited speech sample. After carefully listening to Andy's actual productions and later to the video recordings, the clinician arrived at the following results:

One-Word Articulation Test Results

Intended Production	→	Actual Production	Word Examples	Transcriptions
[s], [z]	→	[s̪], [z̪]	sun	[sʌn] → [s̪ʌn]
			bus	[bʌs] → [bʌs̪]
			zoo	[zu] → [z̪u]
			All consonant clusters with [s]	[s] + consonant → [s̪] + consonant
[ʃ]	→	[sʲ]	shoe	[ʃu] → [sʲu]
			fish	[fɪʃ] → [fɪsʲ]
			dishes	[dɪʃəz] → [dɪsʲəz]
[θ]	Correct	[θ]	thumb	[θʌm] → [θʌm]
[ð]	Correct	[ð]	feather	[fɛðɚ] → [fɛðə]

Selected Spontaneous Speech Sample

I have a red toothbrush. My mommy tells me every night to brush my teeth.

[aɪ hæv ə wɛd tuθbwəsʲ maɪ mɑmi tɛlz̪ mi ɛvɹi naɪt tu bwʌsʲ maɪ tiθ]

Today in school we made an art picture.

[tudeɪ ɪn s̪kul wi meɪd ən ɑt pɪks̪ʲə]

We cut out all sorts of things with scissors and pasted them on this sheet of paper.

[wi kʌt aʊt ɑl s̪ɔəts̪ ʌv θɪŋkz̪ wɪθ s̪ɪz̪əz̪ ænd peɪs̪təd ðɛm ɑn ðɪs̪ sʲit ʌv peɪpə]

Andy did actually differentiate among [θ], [s], [z], and [ʃ] with a dentalized production—[s̪, z̪] for /s/ and /z/, a palatalized [sʲ] for /ʃ/, and correct "th" realizations. In this case, careful transcription and the use of diacritics made a difference in the outcome of this assessment.

Summary

Assessment procedures and results should be accurate, professional, and accomplished in a manner that is accountable. This chapter introduced the International Phonetic Alphabet as a widely used system that can provide these requisites for the assessment of speech sound disorders. The IPA was developed to document actual phonetic realizations of speech events. It is a means of transferring highly impermanent speech events into more durable graphic representations. Such a system offers the speech-language specialist a way to substantiate assessment results, document changes in therapy, and communicate effectively with other professionals. Transcription should never be considered optional; accurate transcription is a necessity for professional evaluations.

To increase the effectiveness of the IPA, certain diacritic marks are used to add production details to the meaning of the basic symbol. These marks are indispensable to the documentation of many of the unusual realizations of our clients. In addition to those diacritics noted on the IPA chart, the extensions to this chart, the extIPA, can be used for disordered speech. Such diacritics were itemized, explained, and exemplified in the second section of this chapter. This section also offered clinical comments on many of the diacritics and actual phonetic transcriptions using these marks.

The final section of this chapter demonstrated how phonetic transcription and the detailed knowledge acquired through its use in assessment procedures benefit the intervention and remediation processes. First, the accuracy needed for the transcription task promotes the fine-tuning of perceptual skills, a clinical proficiency that will, by its very nature, enhance the likelihood of successful intervention. Second, the specificity gained through phonetic transcription, including diacritics, leads to a far more goal-directed treatment approach, which increases clinical efficacy. Third, phonetic transcription and diacritics can be used to document systematic changes in therapy that can evolve in children's speech during the course of treatment.

Case Study

The following transcription is from Jordan, age 5 years 6 months. The first transcription is broad transcription; the second one is narrow transcription.

Broad Transcription: Phonemic inventory

sit	[sɪt]	soap	[soʊp]
sing	[sɪŋ]	soup	[sup]
sock	[sɑk]	summer	[sʌmɚ]
sun	[sʌn]	bus	[bʌθ]
miss	[mɪs]	toss	[tɑs]
goose	[gus]	race	[ɹeɪs]
house	[haʊs]	pass	[pæs]
zoo	[zu]	zap	[zæp]
bees	[biz]	news	[nuz]
rose	[ɹoʊz]	trees	[tɹiz]

Narrow Transcription: Phonetic Inventory

sit	[sɪt]	soap	[sʲoʊp]
sing	[sɪŋ]	soup	[sʲup]
sock	[sʲɑk]	summer	[sʲʌmɚ]
sun	[sʌn]	bus	[bʌθ]
miss	[mɪs]	toss	[tɑsʲ]
goose	[gusʲ]	race	[ɹeɪs]
house	[haʊsʲ]	pass	[pæs]
zoo	[zʲu]	zap	[zæp]
bees	[biz]	news	[nuzʲ]
rose	[ɹoʊzʲ]	trees	[tɹiz]

Based on this small sample, make a list of the consonants contained in the phonetic versus the phonemic inventories. What additional information do the diacritics provide? Do you see a pattern for the palatalized versus dentalized [s] and [z]?

Think Critically

1. What is the difference in production between [s̪] and [θ]? Which articulatory features would you need to change to produce a standard [s]? How would you explain this to a child?

2. What are the production features of [ʃ]? What would you do to change the production to a typical [ʃ]? Are there any vowel contexts you could use to assist in acquiring this production?

3. The following transcription is from a child, age 4 years 2 months. Label the diacritics and state which ones are context related and which ones would be considered aberrant productions.

[aɪ wʌnt t̪u go t̪u s̪ʌ bitʃ]
I want to go to the beach.

[sʲæli ɫɛd wi kʊd̚ goʊ]
Sally said we could go.

[dærɪ wʌnts̪ tu sʷwɪm]
Daddy wants to swim.

[ɪt wɪl bi f̬ʌn]
It will be fun.

4. Add the syllable boundaries and the primary stress markers to the following words:

outspoken

inspiration

national

monumental

October

5. Identify the following symbols. Which sound(s) might be the actual target(s) for a child who produces these sounds?

[x]	[ʔ]	[ʒ]	[ʋ]

 Chapter Quiz 3.1 Complete this quiz to check your understanding of chapter concepts.

Chapter 4
Theoretical Considerations and Practical Applications

 ## Learning Objectives

When you have finished this chapter, you should be able to:

4.1 Describe the evolution of the phoneme concept and its clinical application.

4.2 Define distinctive features and classify sounds according to these parameters.

4.3 Describe generative phonology and how it can be applied to disordered speech.

4.4 Identify naturalness, markedness, implicational universals, and their clinical application.

4.5 Define natural phonology and give examples of phonological processes.

4.6 Differentiate nonlinear phonologies, specifically feature geometry and optimality theory.

4.7 Introduce the sonority sequencing principle and its application to selecting targets.

Chapter Application: Case Study

Tanya thought that theories were very impractical. They often seemed complicated and not relevant to what she was going to be doing as a speech-language therapist. However, she was trying to learn about some of the current phonological models that were being used to select targets and structure therapy. She had just received the diagnostic report for a child that she was going to see in therapy. Her client was a 4-year-old boy, Luke, who was rather unintelligible. He had been evaluated using a constraint-based approach due to the limitations of his phonological system. One of the suggestions was that this child possibly could benefit from target selection using a complexity approach. Tanya had no knowledge of constraint-based models nor the complexity approach, which was somehow related to sonority principles. What should she do? *(continued)*

> There are current diagnostic and treatment protocols that use distinctive features (maximal oppositions), sonority and implicational universals (complexity approaches), natural process analysis (phonological processes), and constraint-based analysis (optimality theory) to describe a child's errors or to establish a treatment paradigm. This chapter on theoretical considerations is a starting point to understanding these various concepts.

THEORIES are very practical. They are based on confirmed observations or systematic experiments. As such, they try to abstract from many practical experiences, attempting to find order and rules amid seemingly entangled details. Theories can also serve as blueprints for practical tasks. For example, phonological theories attempt to explain the structure and function of phonemic systems and have been applied to both normal and disordered phonological systems. Various theories, such as natural phonology, which generated phonological processes, have resulted in analysis procedures that are often used to evaluate the phonological systems of children.

Theories guide and direct clinical work; they are fundamentally important to the diagnostic and therapeutic process. For example, the concept of phonological processes evolved from the theory of natural phonology (Donegan & Stampe, 1979; Stampe, 1969, 1972, 1973). The theory of natural phonology applied certain principles of generative grammar, itself another theory that has revolutionized the way professionals view language. These theories, and others, have resulted in major changes in the way we view diagnostics and therapy within communication disorders. Different types of analyses are now used diagnostically, and a major shift in therapy has occurred because of the impact of these theories.

Theories also offer a *variety* of clinical possibilities. Each theory provides a somewhat different perspective on the problem to be solved. Therefore, if one theory is used, assessment and treatment will vary from those suggested by a second theory. This gives clinicians several possible directions and approaches from which they can choose. Each theory and its application provide clinicians with unique problem-solving advantages. Thus, theories provide a means of maximizing diagnostic and therapeutic skills. They are significant to clinicians' professional work.

While Chapters 2 and 3 dealt primarily with production features of articulation, the focus in this chapter shifts to phonology—to speech sound function. This shift occurs because contemporary theories in our field are phonological theories; they clearly emphasize the function of the phoneme as a meaning-differentiating unit. The first goal of this chapter is to introduce the reader to some of the basic terminology and principles underlying many of the contemporary phonological theories. To this end, a brief review of phonology and its historical development begins this chapter. The second goal is to present several phonological theories that have been applied clinically within the discipline. Each phonological theory is discussed in relationship to its theoretical framework, how it developed, and how it functions. Finally, clinical implications are suggested for each of the presented theories.

The discussion of theoretical considerations in this edition is a fairly radical departure from that in previous editions. Several theories discussed in previous editions have been eliminated due primarily to their lack of applicability to speech sound disorders and their use within the discipline. Those that remain have been expanded so that readers can gain a better understanding of the conceptual framework and its applicability. In addition, models that are currently being used within therapy, such as the sonority sequencing principle, have been added.

The Evolution of the Phoneme Concept

As a review, *phonology* can be defined as the description of the systems and patterns of phonemes that occur in a language. It involves determining the language-specific phonemes and the rules that describe the changes that take place when these phonemes occur in words (Ladefoged & Johnson, 2014). Within this system, the smallest entity that can be distinguished by its contrasting function within words is called the *phoneme*. The phoneme is, thus, the central unit of phonology.

Many different theoretical frameworks for phonological investigations exist. However, these various approaches all have one fundamentally important commonality, the differentiation between the following two levels of sound presentation:

1. The *phonetic level*, with sounds (phones, allophones) as central units
2. The *phonemic level*, represented by phonemes.

Phonology as a concept and discipline has undergone considerable changes. The original French and German terms *phonologie* (Baudouin de Courtenay, 1895) and *Phonologie* (Trubetzkoy, 1931), respectively, were under the influence of structuralism. These terms were replaced by *functional phonetics* (Jakobson, 1962; Martinet, 1960). The term *functional phonetics* emphasized the functional aspect of speech sounds. Phonology has also been called *phonemics* (Sapir, 1925), underlining the linguistic function of the phoneme. The term *phonology* is presently preferred and used by most professionals within the field of communication disorders.

How Did the Concept of the Phoneme Develop?

Phoneme, as a term, first appeared in publications toward the end of the nineteenth century when linguists and phoneticians found it necessary to expand the former single-sound concept into a two-dimensional concept:

1. Speech sounds as production realities
2. Speech sounds in their meaning-establishing and meaning-distinguishing function, as "phonemes."

In their works, the British phonetician Henry Sweet (1845–1912), the German Eduard Sievers (1850–1932), and the Swiss Jost Winteler (1846–1929) laid the foundation for the understanding of this duality. However, historically, Baudouin de Courtenay deserves the credit for introducing the *concept of the phoneme* in 1870. (The word "phoneme" existed prior to this time, but it was used as another label for speech sound.) Baudouin de Courtenay interpreted the proposed sound duality as differences between a physiologically concrete sound realization and its mental image. Influenced by the thinking of his time, Baudouin de Courtenay interpreted phonemes as primarily *psychological* sound units, as "psychic equivalents of the sound" (Lepschy, 1970, p. 60), as the sound "intended" by the speaker and "understood" by listeners. This contrasted with the articulated sound, which was considered a physiological fact. Similarly, the Russian linguist L. V. Ščerba, who succeeded Baudouin de Courtenay, defined the phoneme as "the shortest general sound image of a given language which can be associated with meaning images, and can differentiate words" (Lepschy, 1970, p. 62).

The British phonetician Daniel Jones presented a more language-based phoneme concept in the first half of the twentieth century (Jones, 1938, 1950). He defined the phoneme as a "family of sounds in a given language which are related in character" (Jones, 1950, p. 10). According to Jones's definition, as long as speech sounds are understood as belonging to the same category, they constitute a phoneme of that language. For example, as long as [s]-productions, with all of their verifiable phonetic differences (e.g., different speakers, various circumstances), are evaluated by listeners as being the same (i.e., as belonging to the s-category), these allophonic variations represent the single phoneme /s/ in that language.

Today's prevalent phoneme concept is still more functionally oriented. The specific *use* of the phoneme in a language is the primary emphasis. Nikolai S. Trubetzkoy and Roman Jakobson introduced this strictly functional phoneme concept (strongly influenced by Ferdinand de Saussure's [1916/1959] revolutionary new "structuralistic" way of looking at language). Trubetzkoy wrote that "the phoneme can be defined satisfactorily neither on the basis of its psychological nature nor on the basis of its relation to the phonetic variants, but purely and solely on the basis of its function in the system of language" (Trubetzkoy, 1939/1969, p. 41).

One important aspect of a language's phonological system is its *phonemic inventory*. However, this is not the only variable used in characterizing different phonological systems. Edward Sapir (1921) pointed out that two languages having the same phoneme inventory can, nevertheless, have very different phonologies. Thus, although the inventories may be identical, the way these sound segments can and cannot be arranged to form words (phonotactics) may be quite different. Consequently, the *phonotactics*, or "permissible" sound arrangements within a language, is an important aspect of phonemes' "function" and is therefore an integral part of the phonology of a given language.

Speech Sound Versus Phoneme: Form and Function as a Unity

Every utterance has two facets: an audible sequence of speech sounds and their specific meaning conveyed through this sequence. For example, if someone says, "Hey, Joe, over here," there is an audible sequence of sounds, [heɪ dʒoʊ oʊvɚ hɪɚ], that conveys a specific meaning. Both the physical form of the speech sound and its language-specific function need to be realized for the utterance to be meaningful. If only one aspect, either speech sound form or function, is realized, a breakdown in the communicative process will occur. To apply this clinically, although a child may have the correct speech sound form—in other words, be able to produce [p]–[b], [t]–[d], and [k]–[g]—the child might leave out these sounds at the end of a word. Thus, form is accurate, but the child's realization of the function is inadequate. In this case, "beet" sounds like "bee" and "keep" becomes "key." A breakdown in communication would probably occur.

Adequate form and function of all segments are basic requirements for meaningful utterances in any language. Form is established by the way the segment in question is produced (i.e., by articulatory events). Segment function presupposes the observance of the language-specific rules regarding the arrangement of the speech sound segments. During an utterance, *form* and *function* are combined into meaning-conveying entities.

Segmental form and function largely depend on one another. Without acceptable production features, sound segments cannot fulfill their functional task. If, for example, the word "key" is realized as *tea*, a frequent error made by children with t/k substitutions, elements of sound production have interfered with sound function. In this case, the phonological opposition between /t/ and /k/ has been eliminated. Segment function depends on normal segment form.

Also, segment form depends on proper segment function. Without observing the phonotactic rules governing the language, an acceptable sound production will not relay the intended message. If, for example, a child produces a correct [s] but does not realize the phonotactic rules combining this [s] with other consonants in clusters, the meaning will be impaired. *Stop* might become *top*, or *hats* is realized as *hat*. For effective verbal communication to occur, regular segment form and function are indispensable.

Historically, "correct" single-sound realizations were often the central focus of articulation work. Mastering how sound segments can and cannot be joined together to establish and convey meaning within the respective language was largely neglected. The underlying assumption was that speakers with defective articulation either "know" these rules already or will "learn" them through various exercises that incorporated the sound in various contexts, for example. Articulation therapies focused on the realization of acceptable speech sound forms.

Today, it is often the other way around. The main orientation is the mastering of the phonological rules that govern the language-specific use of the sound segments. Children with phonological disorders demonstrate difficulties with the function of the sound segment, with the rule-governed arrangement of these units. Thus, mastery of the phonological rules, not the speech sound realization, becomes the main goal. This can be exemplified by the multiple oppositions approach to therapy, which is based on developing these functional contrasts that differentiate the meaning between words. (The multiple oppositions approach is described in detail in Chapter 10).

Both intervention approaches have contributed substantially to the treatment of speech sound disorders. They represent outgrowths of different theoretical viewpoints. However, their high degree of mutual dependency implies that, for successful articulation work, these two approaches are not clinically a matter of "either/or" but of "as well as." Of course, based on the specific clinical characteristics of an individual client, one approach may take precedence. If, for example, emphasis on speech sound form is the chosen approach, functional aspects would nevertheless also have to be considered. For example, a child who has just learned the speech sound [ʃ] (i.e., the form is learned) will practice this correct production in various syllable shapes according to phonotactic principles. In this example, function follows form. On the other hand, if speech sound function is the main goal, there might be a point in therapy when the clinician would need to consider aspects of speech sound form as well. For example, a child produces a speech sound that appears to be a correctly articulated [f]. However, the child uses this [f] as a substitution for [θ]. The word "bath" is articulated [bæf], and "thing" is articulated as [fɪŋ]. However, in words that normally are articulated with [f], the child uses a [p]; "fan" becomes "pan" and "fig" is articulated as "pig." The child can produce the form, but the function of the [f] would need to be taught. Contrasting the phonemes /f/ and /p/ in word pairs might help to establish the function of these two phonemes as meaning-differentiating units.

Clinical Application

Phonological and Articulation Therapies Working Together

Toby was 5 years 2 months when he was seen by the new speech-language specialist. Although he had previously received speech therapy, his speech was still considered very difficult to understand. A thorough assessment revealed that all fricative sounds were produced as plosives. Thus, [f] and [v] were articulated as [p] and [b], and the voiceless and voiced [s] and [z], [ʃ] and [ʒ], and [θ] and [ð] were articulated as [t] and [d]. Toby often had difficulty discriminating words containing these phonemic oppositions. Thus, if the clinician asked him to point to the picture of a "pin" versus a "fin" or of a "vase" versus a "base," Toby would often respond incorrectly. After completing the evaluation, the clinician decided that Toby had a phonological disorder: He did not understand the function of these phonemes in the language system.

The clinician began to work on differentiating and establishing these oppositions in meaningful contexts. Pictures and objects that contained these oppositions were used. The clinician noted that as Toby's discrimination abilities improved, he attempted to produce [f] and [v]; however, these realizations were consistently incorrect. As Toby struggled to correct the aberrant productions, the clinician realized that he was quickly becoming frustrated. The clinician used her knowledge of speech sound form to show Toby how to produce [f] and [v] in an acceptable manner. Toby was interested, responded quickly to this instruction, and soon could produce regular [f] and [v] sounds. He was very proud of his achievement and responded, [naʊ aɪ kæn teɪ ɪt waɪt].

In summary, effective verbal communication always mirrors both aspects of speech sounds: acceptable form and function. Remediation must consider both sides of this duality, as they represent two sides of the same coin.

The next part of this chapter addresses specific phonological theories. Each section defines, exemplifies, and provides clinical examples when applicable to demonstrate the relevance of these theories to clinical assessment and treatment.

Distinctive Feature Theories

Distinctive feature theories are attempts to determine the specific properties of a sound that serve to signal meaning differences in a language. The task is to determine which features are decisive for the identification of the various phonemes within a given language. Phonetic constituents that distinguish among phonemes are referred to as **distinctive features**.

How does one differentiate between apparent likenesses? For example, how do we distinguish among similar cars, houses, or streets? On a street where all the houses are somewhat similar, we might direct someone's attention to the location of the house (right-hand side, five houses from the corner), the color of the house (a sea-green color), or one distinguishing feature (there is a high wooden fence in front). "A distinctive feature is any property that separates a subset of elements from a group" (Blache, 1978, p. 56).

A sound component is said to be a *distinctive feature* if it serves to distinguish one phoneme from another. These units, which are smaller than sound segments, are considered "atomic" constituents of sound segments that cannot be broken down any further (Jakobson, 1949). Theoretically, an inventory of these properties would allow the analysis of phonemes not only of General American English but also of all languages. Thus, distinctive features are considered universal properties of speech segments.

How Do Distinctive Features Work?

Distinctive features are the smallest indivisible sound properties that establish phonemes. An inventory of distinctive sound features would demonstrate similarities and dissimilarities among phonemes. These similarities and differences are marked by the presence of certain properties in some phonemes and the absence of these properties in others. The term *binary* is used in most distinctive feature analyses to indicate these similarities and differences. A **binary system** uses a plus (+) and minus (−) system to signal the presence (+) or absence (−) of certain features. This may seem rather elementary, but other distinctive feature systems used multivalued features ranging from one to four; for example, refer to Ladefoged and Johnson (2014).

Many different distinctive features must be considered to arrive at those that distinguish among phonemes. For example, consonants must be distinguished from vowels, voiced consonants must be distinguished from voiceless consonants, and nasals must be distinguished from non-nasals, to mention just a few. If /k/ and /g/ are considered, the following binary oppositions could be established:

/k/	/g/
is a consonant = +consonantal	is a consonant = +consonantal
is not a vowel = −vocalic	is not a vowel = −vocalic
is not voiced = −voice	is voiced = +voice

In this representation of similarities and dissimilarities, voicing is the only feature that distinguishes /k/ from /g/. Two sound segments are considered distinct and can therefore serve as phonemes *if at least one of their features is different.*

To expand slightly on this feature system, consider the phonemes /k/, /g/, and /ŋ/. As previously noted, /k/ and /g/ are distinguished from each other by the feature of voicing. How could this feature system be expanded to include the distinctive features that distinguish among /k/, /g/, and /ŋ/?

/k/	/g/	/ŋ/
+ consonantal	+ consonantal	+ consonantal
− vocalic	− vocalic	− vocalic
− voice	+ voice	+ voice
− nasal	− nasal	+ nasal

Although voice distinguishes /k/ from /g/ and /ŋ/, nasality is the feature that differentiates /g/ and /ŋ/, all of their other features being the same. In this example, nasality is the distinctive feature that creates an opposition between the phonemes /g/ and /ŋ/.

The original distinctive feature matrix created by Jakobson, Fant, and Halle (1952) used 12 *acoustic* features based on the sound segments' spectrographic display. Such descriptions soon proved unsatisfactory for use because similar acoustic representations can be the result of several different articulatory gestures. This led to a revision of the original system. The distinctive feature system used most widely, especially in textbooks for speech-language pathologists, is the one in Chomsky and Halle's *The Sound Pattern of English* (1968), which is the major work in generative phonology. However, the concept of distinctive features did not change from the original version to Chomsky and Halle's (1968) distinctive features. Because some of the features were constructed to examine many different languages, these features are not always applicable to work in communication disorders. Therefore, the features presented here represent an abbreviated list of the distinctive features described in *The Sound Pattern of English*. Refer to Table 4.1.

In *The Sound Pattern of English*, the authors describe five features that establish and distinguish among phonemes: (1) major class features, (2) cavity features, (3) manner of articulation features, (4) source features, and (5) prosodic features.

The **major class features** characterize and distinguish among three sound production possibilities that result in different basic sound classes:

Table 4.1 General American English Consonant Matrix According to the Chomsky and Halle (1968) Distinctive Features

	p	b	t	d	k	g	θ	ð	f	v	s	z	ʃ	ʒ	tʃ	dʒ	m	n	ŋ	ɹ	l	w	j	h
Sonorant	−	−	−	−	−	−	−	−	−	−	−	−	−	−	−	−	+	+	+	+	+	+	+	+
Consonantal	+	+	+	+	+	+	+	+	+	+	+	+	+	+	+	+	+	+	+	+	+	−	−	−
Approximant[1]	−	−	−	−	−	−	−	−	−	−	−	−	−	−	−	−	−	−	−	+	+	−	−	−
Coronal	−	−	+	+	−	−	+	+	−	−	+	+	+	+	+	+	−	+	−	+	+	−	−	−
Anterior	+	+	+	+	−	−	+	+	+	+	+	+	−	−	−	−	+	+	−	−	+	−	−	−
Nasal	−	−	−	−	−	−	−	−	−	−	−	−	−	−	−	−	+	+	+	−	−	−	−	−
Lateral	−	−	−	−	−	−	−	−	−	−	−	−	−	−	−	−	−	−	−	−	+	−	−	−
High	−	−	−	−	+	+	−	−	−	−	−	−	+	+	+	+	−	−	+	−	−	+	+	−
Low	−	−	−	−	−	−	−	−	−	−	−	−	−	−	−	−	−	−	−	−	−	−	−	+
Back	−	−	−	−	+	+	−	−	−	−	−	−	−	−	−	−	−	−	+	−	−	+	−	−
Round	−	−	−	−	−	−	−	−	−	−	−	−	−	−	−	−	−	−	−	−	−	+	−	−
Continuant	−	−	−	−	−	−	+	+	+	+	+	+	+	+	−	−	−	−	−	+	+	+	+	+
Delayed release	−	−	−	−	−	−	−	−	−	−	−	−	−	−	+	+	−	−	−	−	−	−	−	−
Voiced	−	+	−	+	−	+	−	+	−	+	−	+	−	+	−	+	+	+	+	+	+	+	+	−
Strident	−	−	−	−	−	−	−	−	+	+	+	+	+	+	+	+	−	−	−	−	−	−	−	−

[1] The original term *vocalic* was changed to *syllabic* in *The Sound Pattern of English* (Chomsky & Halle, 1968). However, more current nonlinear approaches to phonology use the term *syllabicity* in a different manner (refer to Ball, 2016). Therefore, the term *approximant* is preferred. It expresses the same relationship as *syllabic*.

1. *Sonorant.* "Open" vocal tract configuration promoting voicing. General American English vowels, nasals, and approximants belong to this category.

2. *Consonantal.* Sounds produced with a high degree of oral obstruction, such as plosives, fricatives, affricates, approximants [ɹ] and [l], and nasals.

3. *Approximant.* Sounds produced with a low degree of oral obstruction (not higher than required for the high vowels [i] and [u]), such as vowels and approximants [l] and [ɹ].

Cavity features refer to the place of articulation:

1. *Coronal.* Sounds produced with "the blade of the tongue raised from its neutral position" (Chomsky & Halle, 1968, p. 304). The blade of the tongue refers to the front portion of the tongue, directly behind the tip of the tongue. This cavity feature marks several consonants—for example, [t], [d], [s], [z], [n], and [l]. Refer to Table 4.1 for additional consonants.

2. *Anterior.* Sounds produced in the frontal region of the oral cavity with the alveolar ridge being the posterior border—that is, labial, dental, and alveolar consonants. [m], [n], [b], [p], [f], [v], [d], and [t] are examples.

3. *Distributed.* Sounds with a relatively long oral-sagittal constriction, such as [ʃ], [s], and [z].

4. *Nasal.* Sounds produced with an open nasal passageway—exemplified by the nasals [m], [n], and [ŋ].

5. *Lateral.* Sounds produced with lowered lateral rim portions of the tongue (unilateral or bilateral). The only example in General American English is [l].

6. *High.* Sounds produced with a high tongue position, vowels as well as consonants. Thus, [i], [u], [k], and [ŋ] would be [+ high].

7. *Low.* Vowels produced with a low tongue position—[ɑ], for example. The only consonants that qualify for this category are [h], [ʔ] (the glottal stop), and pharyngeal sounds. The latter are produced with the root of the tongue as an articulator.

8. *Back.* Vowels and consonants produced with a retracted body of the tongue—for example, back vowels, velar and pharyngeal consonants.

9. *Round.* Production of vowels and consonants by rounding lips. [u] and [w] are [+ round].

Manner of articulation features specify the way the articulators work together to produce sound classes, signaling production differences between stops and fricatives, for example:

1. *Continuant.* "Incessant" sounds produced without hindering the airstream with any blockages in the oral cavity. Vowels, fricatives, and approximants are [+ continuant]; plosives, nasals, and affricates are [− continuant].

2. *Delayed release.* Sounds produced with a slow release of a total obstruction within the oral cavity. Affricates such as [tʃ] and [dʒ] are [+ delayed release].

Source features refer to subglottal air pressure, voicing, and stridency:

1. *Voiced.* Produced with simultaneous vocal fold vibration. All General American English vowels, approximants, nasals, voiced plosives, fricatives, and affricates are [+ voiced]. [p], [t], [k], [f], [s], and [ʃ], by contrast, are [− voiced].

2. *Strident.* The term *strident* (making a loud or harsh sound) is a feature of General American English voiceless and voiced fricatives and affricates. In General American English, the strident feature is used to distinguish interdental

fricatives [– strident] from alveolar fricatives. The interdental fricatives [θ] and [ð] are [− strident].

Chomsky and Halle (1968) named *prosodic features* but did not discuss them.

To summarize, the distinctive feature system is an attempt to document specific sound constituents that establish phonemes. Distinctive feature theories organize sound constituents according to some productional (or, in some cases, acoustic) properties that might be used in languages to establish meaning differences. The result is a system of contrastive, linguistically relevant elements. Historically, many different feature systems exist, and many of the newer phonological theories, such as feature geometry, use their own somewhat different distinctive features. No one feature system has clear advantages over another. All distinctive feature systems reflect the authors' concept of those characteristics that most aptly define the phoneme.

Clinical Application

Distinctive Feature Theories

Distinctive feature systems were originally developed to analyze the regular realization of phonemes within and across languages. However, the use of distinctive features to analyze disordered speech could not be overlooked. When sound substitution features were compared to target sound features, similarities and differences could be noted.

Distinctive feature systems offered several advantages over the previous analysis systems of classifying errors according to substitutions, deletions, and distortions. First, they provided a more complete analysis. For example, sound substitutions could be broken down into several feature components, which could then be compared and analyzed. Second, and perhaps more important, distinctive feature systems concentrated on the features that distinguish phonemes within a language. Previous analysis procedures had at best focused on phonetic production aspects of phones. With the impact of phonology on the field of communication disorders, this emphasis shifted to the phoneme and its function within the language system.

In relationship to disordered speech, distinctive feature analysis contrasted the features of the target sound with the substitution, resulting in a list of distinctive features that differentiated the two. This analysis could show whether (1) error sounds shared common features and (2) specific error patterns existed.

Therapeutic implications followed logically. If a child can be taught to discriminate between the presence and absence of these differentiating distinctive features, the aberrant sound productions should be easily remediated. However, can children really understand and differentiate between distinctive features? Jakobson's (1968) hypothesis that children acquire features rather than sounds seems to support this assumption. If this is the case, therapy could facilitate this developmental process. In addition, if children acquire features rather than sounds, a certain amount of generalization should occur. Consequently, children should be able to generalize features from sounds that they can realize to others they cannot. This could be therapeutically useful. Children who can produce, for example, + voicing in one phonemic context should be able to generalize this + voicing to other phonemic contexts. Therefore, treatment of one phonemic opposition with specific distinctive features should lead to the norm production of other phonemic oppositions with the same distinctive feature oppositions. This would be a means of treating more than one phoneme in a time-efficient manner. Based on this principle, several distinctive feature therapy programs were developed (Blache, 1989; Compton, 1976; McReynolds & Engmann, 1975; Weiner & Bankson, 1978). However, for children with speech sound disorders, both the analysis procedures and the clinical applicability of distinctive features have been difficult to use.

Clinical Application

Maximal Oppositions Approach and Distinctive Features

The maximal oppositions approach is a more current phonological method that uses distinctive features as one way to select targets. It is based on the premise that by selecting target phonemes that are maximally distinct (using either production or distinctive features), more change in the child's phonemic inventory will result. Research has documented the effectiveness of subsequent therapy when selecting targets in this manner. (Refer to for example, Gierut, 1989, 1990, 1991, 1992; Gierut & Neumann, 1992).

This approach using distinctive features first establishes which phonemes are *not* in the child's inventory. Phonemes for therapy are selected based optimally on those not in the inventory but that have one major class feature difference and those with the most distinctive feature differences. To establish a treatment target, a clinician must first look at the major class features noted in Table 4.1: sonorant, consonantal, and approximant. Table 4.2 looks at those consonants grouped accordingly.

Table 4.2 Consonants of General American English Grouped According to the Major Class Features

Sonorant		Consonantal		Approximant	
+ nasals [m, n, ŋ]	– plosives [p, b, t, d, k, g]	+ plosives	– approximants [w] and [j]	+ approximants [ɹ] and [l]	– approximants [w] and [j]
+ approximants [w, j], [ɹ, l]	– fricatives [f, v, s, z, ʃ, ʒ, θ, ð]	+ fricatives	– [h]		– plosives
+ [h]	– affricates [ʧ, ʤ]	+ affricates			
		+ nasals			– fricatives
		+ approximants [ɹ] and [l]			– nasals
					– affricates
					–[h]

(continued)

The first step is to order the sounds according to which ones show at least one major class feature difference. This would be depicted by a + for one sound class and a – for another within the specific major class feature. This can be done by looking at the right and left sides of each column. For example, for the sonorants, we find:

Sonorants:	
+ nasals	– plosives
+ approximants	– fricatives
+ [h]	– affricates

This also could be done for the features *consonantal* and/or *approximant*.

The second step is to determine which two sounds have the most feature differences. Let's use sonorants for our example. To calculate the number of distinctive feature differences, one would go down the chart and note which column has a + and which has a – for the two sounds. Table 4.3 sets the – sonorants along the horizontal axis and the + sonorants along the vertical axis. The number of feature differences are then placed in the respective boxes. The number of features *excludes* the one for the major class feature.

What does this tell us clinically about maximal oppositions? Let's say that Lillian does not have /s, z, θ, ð, ʃ, ʒ ɹ, l/ in her inventory. We want to address two sounds that are not in Lillian's inventory. According to our major class feature sonorant, a + and – feature sound class would be approximants and fricatives. Both /ɹ/ and /l/ are approximants and are not in Lillian's inventory. We could look for /ɹ, l/ in the first column versus the fricatives /s, z, θ, ð, ʃ, ʒ/ in the top row to see which sound or sounds would have the highest number of distinctive features. We see that /l/ versus /ʃ/ has five distinctive feature differences. These two phonemes might be targeted for treatment according to maximal oppositions. More about maximal oppositions will be discussed in Chapter 10, pages 353–357. However, this is one example of how distinctive features can be used clinically.

Table 4.3 Distinctive Feature Differences for + (Vertical Axis) and – (Horizontal Axis) Sonorants

	p	b	t	d	k	g	f	v	s	z	ʃ	ʒ	θ	ð	tʃ	dʒ
m	2	1	3	2	5	4	4	3	5	4	7	6	4	3	7	6
n	3	2	3	2	6	5	5	4	4	3	6	5	3	2	6	5
ŋ	5	4	6	5	2	1	7	6	8	7	5	4	7	6	6	5
ɹ	4	3	3	2	5	4	4	3	3	2	3	2	2	1	5	4
l	4	3	3	2	7	6	4	3	3	2	5	4	2	1	7	6
w	6	5	7	6	3	2	6	5	7	6	5	4	6	5	7	6
j	4	3	5	4	3	2	4	3	5	4	3	2	4	3	5	4
h	3	4	4	5	4	5	3	4	4	5	4	5	3	4	6	7

Generative Phonology

Generative phonology is an outgrowth of distinctive feature theory that represents a substantial departure from previous phonological theories. Pregenerative theories of phonology—that is, those occurring prior to generative phonology (e.g., by Jakobson et al., 1952; Jakobson & Halle, 1956)—distinguished between two levels of realization: phonetic and phonemic. However, in pregenerative theories, both the phonetic and the phonemic levels were analyzed by means of the actual productions, or the concrete realizations of speech—for example, by using tape recordings of different languages to assess the systems. Thus, pregenerative theories were developed around the *surface forms*. Surface forms, sometimes referred to as **surface-level representation**, are the actual end products of production. For example, if you transcribe a child's utterances, you are examining the surface form. The surface form is a phonetic sequence of units that have characteristic features. On the other hand, generative phonologies expanded this concept decisively to include what has been called the **underlying form** or **deep structure**. This is a purely theoretical concept that is thought to represent a mental reality at the core of language use (Crystal, 2010). Underlying forms exemplify the person's language competency as one aspect of his or her cognitive capacity. The underlying forms also serve as points of orientation to describe regularities of speech reality as they relate to other areas of language, notably morphology and syntax. Generative phonology assumes two levels of sound representation, an abstract underlying form called **phonological representation** and its modified surface form, **phonetic representation**. **Phonological rules** govern how this phonological representation (underlying representation or deep form) is transformed into the actual pronunciation (surface form).

Video Example 4.1
The first two minutes and thirty seconds of this video gives an overview of what is meant by surface and deep structure of language. The speaker gives an example to demonstrate the concept using a sentence's surface and deep structure. Can you think of ways you could apply this to phonology? What would be the surface structure if the child says "wabbit" for "rabbit"? What might that imply about the deep structure? Would you assume that the child has the /ɹ/ in her deep structure or not?

https://www.youtube.com/watch?v=cnygrKrQvY0

How Does Generative Phonology Work?

According to generative phonology, phonological rules explain the differences between phonological (deep-form) and phonetic (surface-level) representations. These rules are usually stated in a formalized notation system.

Some helpful notations include the following:

A → B	Indicates that A changes to B
/	Indicates the context
__	Underlining by itself indicates the location of the changed segment
#__	Indicates changes that occur at the beginning of a word
__#	Indicates changes that occur at the end of a word
∅	Indicates the deletion of a segment.

C, CC, and CCC can be used to indicate a consonant or consonant cluster.

Now, let's try this notation with an example. A child deletes [s] and [z] at the end of a word; "toss" becomes [tɑ] and "nose" becomes [noʊ]. The notation would look like this:

A → B/__# [s, z] → ∅/___# [s] and [z] are deleted at the end of a word.

In generative phonology, these rules are stated according to distinctive features where the + or – features are placed in a column with brackets. The distinctive features noted would be only those that distinguish that particular sound or sound class from the substituted sound or pattern. Not all distinctive features are listed, only those that would be used to differentiate that sound or sound pattern. Our previous example of [s] and [z] would look like this:

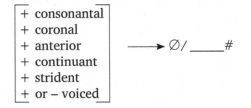

If all word-final consonants are deleted, the rule would look like this:

$$[+ \text{consonantal}] \longrightarrow \emptyset / \underline{\hspace{1cm}} \#$$

Note that the only – consonantal phonemes are /w, j, h/, which do not occur at the end of words in General American English. Some more common rules would be:

All fricatives and affricates are realized as stops:

$$[+ \text{continuant}] \longrightarrow [- \text{continuant}] / \begin{bmatrix} - \text{sonorant} \\ + \text{consonantal} \end{bmatrix}$$

The fricatives are + continuant, whereas the plosives are – continuant. However, now we need to *include* the affricates (which are – continuant) and *exclude* the nasals and the approximants. Therefore, the – sonorant and the + consonantal include affricates and exclude nasals and approximants.

Velars /k, g/ are realized as stops /t, d/:

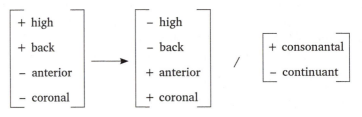

The first bracket (+ high, + back, – anterior, – coronal) defines the /k, g/, whereas the second bracket (– high, – back, + anterior, + coronal) defines /t, d/. The approximants /w, j/ and /h/ are eliminated with + consonantal, and the fricatives, nasals and approximants which are -high (in the second bracket) such as /s, z, m, n, ɹ, l/ are eliminated with – continuant.

Here is an example using the "C" notation. All initial two- and three-consonant clusters are reduced to one consonant:

CC or CCC → C/ #__

How Did Generative Phonology Develop?

Generative phonology represents the application of principles of generative (or transformational) grammar to phonology. As noted previously, generative phonology assumed two levels of representation, the more abstract underlying phonemic level and the more concrete surface phonetic level. It was a revolutionary approach for analysis that grew out of the in-depth study of English phonology represented by Chomsky and Halle's (1968) *The Sound Pattern of English*. The principles of generative phonology abandoned the prior version of phonemic analysis and introduced the concept of underlying phonological representations, which are mapped onto the surface-level pronunciations by a set of formal rules. The rules formulated previously serve as examples. The rules were the means used to go from the underlying representation to the surface-level pronunciation. These formalized rules provided the description of this process.

The concept that postulated not only a *deep* level of phonemic understanding but also a *surface* level of phonetic pronunciation was also termed *competence and performance*—competence representing the deep level and performance relating to the surface level. Competence was viewed as the individual's knowledge of the phonemic rules of a language, whereas performance was actual phonetic use in real situations.

Naturalness, Markedness, and Implicational Universals

If we were to examine toddlers' speech, we would obviously find that toddlers do not pronounce all words correctly. However, if one listens to a group of toddlers, one might find that many of the errors made are similar. Therefore, a toddler might say "wabbit" for "rabbit" and "dis" for "this." But you would probably not find a group of toddlers who say "jeep" for "peep." It appears that certain sounds are consistently used as substitutions when children are developing and are thus thought to be easier to produce than others. **Naturalness** and **markedness** are aspects of distinctive feature theory that seem to explain this possibility and have more direct clinical applicability. Markedness theory comes from the concept in phonology in which certain aspects—in this case, phonemes—are more common, or more natural, than others. These phonemes are labeled **unmarked**. Therefore, there are unmarked and marked phonemes. Thus, unmarked units are more natural, whereas marked units are less natural. According to *The Sound Pattern of English* (Chomsky & Halle, 1968), in which this concept was reintroduced, the two concepts—marked versus unmarked—can be seen as two ends of a continuum. Marked features are those that are (1) seemingly impossible to produce (those features on the International Phonetic Alphabet chart that are in the shaded areas, such as bilabial lateral fricatives) or (2) language-specific universals and tendencies that have demonstrated that certain phonemes occur infrequently in languages around the world (Roca, 1994). On the other hand, unmarked, more natural phonemes are found more frequently in languages around the world. This has been further extrapolated to include the idea that natural, unmarked features are easier to articulate and are likely to be acquired earlier in the phoneme development of children (Johnson & Reimers, 2010). For example, [p] is considered a natural sound (and therefore is unmarked). It occurs early in acquisition and in many languages around the world. On the other hand, the affricate [ʤ] is a marked sound: It is relatively more difficult to produce and is found infrequently in other languages. Table 4.4 ranks the phonemes used in languages around the world.

Table 4.4 Ranking of Consonants in Languages Around the World (University of California Los Angeles Phonological Segment Inventory Database [UPSID])

Consonant	m	k	j	p	w	b	h	g	ŋ	ʔ	n	s	tʃ	ʃ	t	f	l
Rank	1	2	3	4	5	6	7	8	9	10	11	12	13	14	15	16	17
Number of languages	425	403	378	375	332	287	279	253	237	216	202	196	188	187	181	180	174
Percentage of languages (from 451)	94.2	89.4	83.8	83.2	73.6	63.6	61.9	56.1	52.6	47.9	44.8	43.5	41.7	41.5	40.1	39.9	38.6

This Database was compiled by Ian Maddieson and Kristin Precoda (cf. Maddieson, 1984) and contains information on 451 languages. The languages for UPSID have been grouped according to families of languages. Approximately 7000 different languages are spoken around the world, but 90% of these languages are used by less than 100,000 people (Simons & Fennig, 2018).

Marked and unmarked features are typically used when referring to cognate pairs, such as /t/ and /d/, and sound classes, such as nasals. Sloat, Taylor, and Hoard (1978) describe the following sounds and sound classes according to markedness parameters:

Voiceless obstruents (plosives, fricatives, and affricates) are more natural (unmarked) than voiced obstruents.

Obstruents are more natural (unmarked) than sonorants (nasals, approximants, /h/).

Plosives are more natural (unmarked) than fricatives.

Fricatives are more natural (unmarked) than affricates.

After examining linguistic universals, trends in the phonological acquisition of children, and the loss of phonological skills in aphasics, Jakobson (1968) postulated that the presence of a marked trait in a language implied an existence of an unmarked counterpart. Referring to the above-mentioned sounds and sound classes, that would mean that the presence of voiced obstruents would imply voiceless obstruents (the marked implying the unmarked) in a specific language.

Implicational universals describe sound properties in which one property is, according to theoretical constructs, predictive of another. In this case, the presence of certain sound classes is predictive of another sound class. This predictive property could be stated as the presence of X implies Y. However, this cannot be turned around and be accurate; the existence of Y does not imply X. As an example, fricatives within a phonological system imply that there are stops (X implies Y), but the presence of stops does not mean that fricatives are within the system (Y does not imply X). The implicational universals for the sound classes of General American English consonants are listed in Table 4.5. If we look at their predictive possibilities, examples would be "fricatives imply stops" and "voiced plosives imply voiceless plosives." This would mean that if a language has fricatives, that language has plosives as well, and that if a language has voiced plosives in its inventory, the language also has voiceless ones. Application of these two examples to children's speech would mean that if a child has fricatives in his inventory, this implies that he has plosives. Also, if a child has voiced plosives, this implies the voiceless cognate. According to Jakobson (1968), the breakdown of speech in those with aphasia would be characterized by the loss of the later-acquired sounds before the earlier-acquired ones. Thus, individuals with aphasia would lose fricatives

Table 4.5 Implicational Universals

Predicting Property	Implies	Predicted Property
Affricates /tʃ, dʒ/	→	Fricatives /f, v, s, z, θ, ð, ʃ, ʒ/
Fricatives /f, v, s, z, θ, ð, ʃ, ʒ/	→	Plosives /p, b, t, d, k, g/
Liquids /l, ɹ/	→	Nasals /m, n, ŋ/
Voiced obstruents /b, d, g, v, z, ð, ʒ and dʒ/	→	Voiceless obstruents /p, t, k, f, s, θ, ʃ, tʃ/

Source: Adapted from Gierut, J., & Hulse, L. E. (2010).

before (homorganic) plosives and voiced plosives before voiceless ones. Whether these universal "laws" are generally valid under all conditions has been questioned repeatedly. However, these concepts clearly exemplify naturalness, markedness, and implicational universals as clinically relevant.

Clinical Application

Distinctive Features, Markedness, and Implicational Universals

The concept of naturalness versus markedness became a relevant clinical issue when it was observed that children with phonemic-based disorders tend to substitute more unmarked, natural classes of segments for marked ones. For example, children substituted stops for fricatives and deleted the more marked member of a consonant cluster (Ingram, 1989b). Although the results of at least one investigation demonstrated contrary findings (McReynolds, Engmann, & Dimmitt, 1974), most investigations supported the notion that children and adults with speech disorders more frequently showed a change from marked segments to unmarked substitutions (Kirk, 2008; Menn & Velleman, 2010; Taps Richard & Barlow, 2011). Markedness is also an important variable in newer theoretical models such as optimality theory.

The construct of implicational universals has been used in selecting targets for the complexity approach (refer to Chapter 10 for more detail). True to its name, the complexity approach targets more complex phonemes. Target selection is based in part on selecting marked targets that, according to the authors (e.g., Gierut, 1999, 2001; Gierut & Champion, 2001), create more change in the total phonological system of the children rather than selecting less complex, more natural unmarked targets.

To summarize, generative phonology as a portion of generative grammar has contributed to the field of linguistics and phonology. The generative phonological model has laid the foundation for other phonological theories. The theory of natural phonology, for example, also has its basis in generative phonology.

Natural Phonology

"[Natural phonology] is a natural theory . . . in that it presents language as a natural reflection of the needs, capacities, and world of its users, rather than as a merely conventional institution" (Donegan & Stampe, 1979, p. 127). **Natural phonology** incorporates features of naturalness theories and was specifically designed to explain the normal development of children's phonological systems. The theory of natural phonology postulates that patterns of speech are governed by an innate, universal set of phonological processes. **Phonological processes** are innate and universal; therefore, all children are born with the capacity to use the same system of processes. Phonological processes, as natural processes, (1) are easier for a child to produce and are substituted for sounds, sound classes, or sound sequences when children's motor capacities do not yet allow their normal realization, (2) are operating as all children attempt to use and organize their phonological systems so that they can progress to the language-specific system that characterizes their native language, and (3) are used to constantly revise existing differences among the innate patterns and the adult standard production. The theory points out prominent *developmental steps* that children go through until the goal of adult phonology is reached in the children's early years. Stampe (1969) thought that phonological processes explained the replacement of the difficult property of the sound or sound class with a simpler form. Disordered phonology is seen as an inability to realize this "natural" process of goal-oriented adaptive change.

How Does Natural Phonology Work?

The theory of natural phonology assumes that a child's innate phonological system is continuously revised in the direction of the adult phonological system. Stampe (1969) proposed three mechanisms to account for these changes: (1) limitation, (2) ordering, and (3) suppression. These mechanisms reflect properties of the innate phonological system as well as the universal difficulties children display in the acquisition of the adult sound system.

Limitation occurs when differences between a child's and an adult's systems become *limited* to only specific sounds, sound classes, or sound sequences. Limitation can be exemplified by the following: A child might first use a more "natural" sound for a more marked one. For example, all fricatives might be replaced by homorganic plosives (e.g., [f] → [p], [θ] → [t], [s] → [t]). Later, this global substitution of all fricatives by plosives might become *limited* to only [s] and [z], so that *sun* becomes [tʌn] and *zoo* becomes [du], for example, but *fun* and *pig* are accurate.

Ordering occurs when substitutions that appeared unordered and random become more organized. Ordering can be exemplified by the following: A child's first revisions may appear unordered. To stay with the plosive for fricative example, a child might at first also devoice the voiced plosives of the substitution; thus, ([s] → [t] and [z] → [t]). Thus, *Sue* is pronounced [tu], but *zoo* is also articulated as [tu]. Later, the child might begin to "order" the revisions by voicing initial voiced plosives but still retaining the plosive substitution. Now *Sue* is [tu] and *zoo* is [du].

The term **suppression** refers to the abolishment of one or more phonological processes as children move from the innate speech patterns to the adult patterns. Suppression occurs when a previously used phonological process is not used any longer.

According to Stampe (1979), all children embark on the development of their phonological systems from the same beginnings. Stampe sees children as possessing a full understanding of the underlying representation of the adult phoneme system: That is, from the very beginning, children's perceptual understanding of the phonemic system mirrors that of adults. Children simply have difficulties with the peripheral, motor realization of the phonetic surface form. This means that the underlying and surface-level representations would be the same. Many authors (e.g., Fey, 1992; Stoel-Gammon & Dunn, 1985) have questioned the validity of this idea. In addition, Stampe's account of phonological development presents children as passively suppressing these phonological processes. Other contemporary authors, notably Kiparsky and Menn (1977), see children as being far more actively involved in the development of their phonological systems.

Despite such shortcomings, Edwards (1992) states that "it is not necessary to totally discard the notion of phonological processes just because we may not agree with all aspects of Stampe's theory of Natural Phonology, such as his view that phonological processes are 'innate' and his assumption that children's underlying representations are basically equivalent to the broad adult surface forms" (p. 234). Phonological process analysis has found widespread clinical application, although it is not used to *explain* developmental speech events, which was the original intent of natural phonology, but to *describe* the deviations noted in the speech of children.

Because phonological processes are so central to the workings of natural phonology and to its clinical application, some of the more common processes are listed here with some explanatory remarks.

PHONOLOGICAL PROCESSES. Phonological processes are categorized as syllable structure processes, substitution processes, and assimilatory processes. **Syllable structure processes** describe those sound changes that affect the structure of the syllable. **Substitution processes** describe those sound changes in which one sound class is replaced by another. **Assimilatory processes** describe changes in which a sound becomes similar to, or is influenced by, a neighboring sound of an utterance.

Syllable Structure Processes

____ *Cluster reduction.* The articulatory simplification of consonant clusters into a single consonant.

Example: [pun] for *spoon.*

____ *Reduplication.* This process is considered a syllable structure process because the syllable structure is "simplified"; that is, the second syllable becomes merely a repetition of the first. *Total reduplication* refers to the exact reduplication of the first syllable. In *partial reduplication*, the vowel in the second syllable is varied (Ingram, 1976).

Examples:

Total reduplication: [wɑwɑ] for *water.*

Partial reduplication: [babi] for *blanket.* ____ isolleate

Weak syllable deletion. An unstressed syllable is omitted.

Example: [næne] for *ba'nana.*

Final consonant deletion. A syllable-arresting consonant, a coda, is omitted.

Example: [hɛ] for *head.*

Substitution Processes

Changes in Place of Articulation

Fronting. Sound substitutions in which the place of articulation is more anteriorly located than the intended sound. Prominent types include *velar fronting* (t/k substitution) and *palatal fronting* (s/ʃ substitution).

Examples: [ti] for *key*; [su] for *shoe.*

Labialization. The replacement of a nonlabial sound by a labial one.

Example: [fʌm] for *thumb.*

Alveolarization. The change of nonalveolar sounds, mostly interdental and labiodental sounds, into alveolar ones.

Example: [sʌm] for *thumb*.

Changes in Manner of Articulation

Stopping. The substitution of stops for fricatives or the omission of the fricative portion of affricates.

Examples: [tʌn] for *sun*; [dus] for *juice*.

Affrication. The replacement of fricatives by homorganic affricates.

Example: [tʃu] for *shoe*.

Deaffrication. The production of affricates as homorganic fricatives.

Example: [ʃiz] for *cheese*.

Denasalization. The replacement of nasals by homorganic plosives.

Example: [dud] for *noon*.

Gliding of liquids or fricatives. The replacement of liquids or fricatives by glides.

Examples: [wɛd] for *red*; [ju] for *shoe*.

Vowelization. The replacement of syllabic liquids and nasals, foremost [l], [ɚ], and [n], by vowels.

Examples: [teɪbo] for *table*; [lædʊ] for *ladder*.

Derhotacization. The loss of r-coloring in central vowels with r-coloring, [ɜ˞] and [ɚ].

Examples: [bɜd] for *bird*, [lædə] for *ladder*.

Changes in Voicing

Voicing. The replacement of a voiceless sound by a voiced sound.

Example: [du] for *two*.

Devoicing. The replacement of a voiced sound by a voiceless sound.

Example: [pit] for *beet*.

Assimilation processes can also be classified according to the type of assimilatory changes. For definitions and examples, refer to "Sounds in Context: Coarticulation and Assimilation" in Chapter 2.

Assimilatory Processes (Harmony Processes)

Labial assimilation. The change of a nonlabial sound into a labial sound under the influence of a neighboring labial sound.

Example: [fwɪŋ] for *swing*.

Velar assimilation. The change of a nonvelar sound into a velar sound under the influence of a neighboring velar sound.

Example: [gɑg] for *dog*.

Nasal assimilation. The influence of a nasal on a non-nasal sound.

Example: [mʌni] for *bunny*.

Note: The place of articulation is retained; only the manner is changed.

Liquid assimilation. The influence of a liquid on a nonliquid sound.

Example: [lɛloʊ] for *yellow*.

According to natural phonology, phonological processes are recognizable steps in the gradual articulatory adjustment of children's speech to the adult norm. This implies a chronology of phonological processes, specific ages at which the process could be operating and when the process should be suppressed. As useful as a chronology of normative data might seem for clinical purposes, tables of established age norms can easily be misleading. Individual variation and contextual conditions may play a large role in the use and suppression of phonological processes. However, based on standardized speech assessments, ages of suppression of the various processes are discussed in Chapter 5.

To summarize, natural phonology specifies an innate phonological system that is progressively revised during childhood until it corresponds with the adult phonological output. Limitation, ordering, and suppression are the mechanisms for the revisions that manifest themselves in phonological processes. Phonological processes are developmentally conditioned simplifications in the realization of the phonological system in question. As these simplifications are gradually overcome, the phonological processes become suppressed.

How Did Natural Phonology Develop?

David Stampe introduced natural phonology in 1969. However, several of its basic concepts had been established considerably earlier, most prominent among them being naturalness (markedness) and underlying versus surface forms, which are important aspects of generative phonology.

Markedness theory also plays a central role in generative phonology and optimality theory (McCarthy & Prince, 1995; Prince & Smolensky, 1993). According to generative phonologists, markedness values are universal and innate. Thus, Jakobson, with his concept of universal naturalness, and Chomsky and Halle, with their understanding of universal and innate naturalness, set the stage for Stampe's natural phonology. Stampe incorporated the conceptual framework of naturalness into his theory of natural phonology.

At the same time, the meaning and use of the term *underlying form* changed drastically as it was incorporated into natural phonology. Within generative grammar, underlying forms—lexical as well as phonological—are highly abstract entities. They represent *assumed points of reference* that are necessary for the explanation of the many possible surface forms. In contrast, within the context of natural phonology, underlying forms as "models" for surface realizations suddenly gained some concrete reality. The underlying form is *the adult norm* that is the intended goal for children's production efforts.

Clinical Application

Natural Phonology

The concept of phonological processes within natural phonology has affected both the assessment and the treatment of children with disordered phonological systems. Assessment procedures using phonological processes consist of contrasting the target word to a child's production. Aberrant productions are identified and labeled according to the phonological process that most closely matches the sound change. Typically, the processes are listed and the frequency of occurrence of individual processes is noted. Frequency of occurrence and the relative age of suppression play a role in targeting a process or processes for therapy. Depending on the age of the child, more frequent processes that should have been suppressed are commonly targeted for therapy.

(continued)

Unlike other analysis procedures, phonological processes can account for changes in syllable or word structures and those that result from assimilations. Although phonological processes are not commonly used to identify sound distortions, they could be. For example, [ʂ] could be labeled fronting and [sʲ] labeled backing. **Backing** refers to a substitution in which the place of articulation is located more posteriorly than the intended sound. It is considered an idiosyncratic process that can be found in the speech of children with phonemic-based disorders.

Phonological Process Analysis

A phonological process analysis is a means of identifying substitutions, syllable structure, and assimilatory changes that occur in clients' speech. Each error is identified and classified as one or more of the phonological processes. Patterns of errors are described according to the most frequent phonological processes present and/or to those that affect a class of sounds or sound sequences. Also, phonological processes that affect a large number of sounds are noted due to their probable impact on intelligibility. The processes used to identify substitutions are again primarily based on production characteristics; however, they do account for sound and syllable deletions as well as many assimilation processes.

Several assessment protocols analyze phonological processes in a standardized speech test or in spontaneous speech (e.g., refer to Bankson & Bernthal, 1990; Hodson, 2004; Khan & Lewis, 2015; Lowe, 1996). All of them identify each aberrant production according to the phonological process or processes that best represent the changes that have occurred. Most protocols also summarize the phonological processes by counting the total number of specific processes.

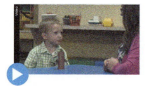

Video Example 4.2

In this video, 4-year-old Ben's sound substitutions are inconsistent. Transcribe a couple of his errors and note some of the phonological processes he uses. For example, listen to his consonant clusters and his "th" sounds. What do you hear with [l]? How would you classify his /l/-production as a phonological process?

Clinical Exercises A child demonstrates a high degree of fronting (velar only), cluster reduction, and final consonant deletion.

Give one example of each of these processes. Which one of these processes would probably affect intelligibility the most?

The next section introduces more current developments in phonological theories, the so-called nonlinear phonological theories. They represent a radical departure from the conceptual framework that preceded them.

Nonlinear Phonologies: Exemplified by Feature Geometry and Optimality Theory

Phonological theories, theories of generative phonology included, were based on the understanding that all speech segments are arranged in a sequential order. Consequently, underlying phonological representations and surface phonetic realizations, too, consisted of a string of discrete elements. For example:

Wow, what a test. [waʊ wʌt ə tɛst]

The sequence of segments in this phrase begins with [w] and ends with [st]. All segments between follow each other in a specific order to convey a particular message. This assumption that all meaning-distinguishing sound segments are serially arranged characterizes all linear phonologies. Linear phonologies, exemplified by distinctive feature theories and early generative phonology, can be characterized as follows:

1. They emphasize the linear, sequential arrangement of sound segments.
2. Each discrete segment of this string of sound elements consists of a bundle of distinctive features.
3. A common set of distinctive features is attributable to all sound segments according to a binary + and − system.
4. All sound segments have equal value, and all distinctive features are equal; thus, no one sound segment has control over other units.
5. The phonological rules generated apply only to the segmental level (as opposed to the suprasegmental level) and to those changes that occur in the distinctive features (Dinnsen, 1997).

Linear phonologies with sound segments (and their smaller distinguishing, distinctive features) as central analytical units fail to recognize and describe larger linguistic units. Linear phonologies also do not account for the possibility that there could be a hierarchical interaction among segments and other linguistic units (hierarchy refers to any system in which elements are ranked one above another). Nonlinear or nonsegmental phonologies attempt to account for these factors.

Nonlinear phonologies are phonological theories in which segments are governed by more complex linguistic dimensions. The linear representation of phonemes plays a subordinate role. More complex linguistic dimensions—for example, stress, intonation, metrical and rhythmical linguistic factors—may control segmental conditions. These theories explore the relationships among units of various sizes, specifically the influence of larger linguistic entities on sound segments. Therefore, rather than a linear view of equal-valued segments (in a left-to-right horizontal sequence), a hierarchy of factors is hypothesized to affect segmental units. Rather than a static sequence of segments of equal value (as in linear phonology), a dynamic system of features, ranked one above the other, is proposed. For example, syllable structure could affect the segmental level. A child may demonstrate the following pattern:

"man"	[mæn]	"window"	[wɪ doʊ]
"dog"	[dɑg]	"jumping"	[dʒʌ pɪ]
"ball"	[bɑl]	"Christmas tree"	[kɪɪ mə tɹi]

Final consonant deletion does not occur in one-syllable words; however, this child deletes the final consonant of each syllable in a multisyllabic word. In this example, the number of syllables in a word interacts with and affects the segmental level. The number of syllables has priority over the segmental level: It determines segmental features. Nonlinear phonologies rank syllable structure above the level of sound segments. Another factor that may affect the segmental level is stress. Children tend to delete segments in unstressed syllables. The following transcriptions demonstrate this:

ba'nana → ['næ.nə]

po'tato → ['teɪ.toʊ]

'telephone → ['tɛ.foʊn]

In these examples, the syllable stress clearly affects segmental realization; word stress has priority over the segmental level. "Instead of a single, linear representation (one unit followed by another with none having any superiority or

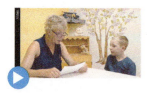

Video Tool Exercise 4.1
Multisyllabic Words and the Impact on Sound Production
Complete the activity based on this video.

control over other units), they [nonlinear phonologies] allow a description of underlying relationships that would permit one level or unit to be governed by another" (Schwartz, 1992, p. 271).

There are many different types of nonlinear phonologies. Several new theories have been advanced, and others have been modified. All nonlinear phonologies are based on a belief in the overriding importance of larger linguistic units influencing, even controlling, the realization of smaller ones. Nonlinear phonologies also attempt to incorporate this hierarchical order of linguistic elements into analytical procedures, using so-called tiered representations of features. Describing the many different nonlinear phonologies is beyond the scope of this book. *Principles of Clinical Phonology: Theoretical Approaches* (Ball, 2016) is an excellent source of more detailed information on many phonological theories. It provides clinical application for most of these theoretical foundations. This section is restricted to an introduction of nonlinear phonologies exemplified by feature geometry and optimality theories. Sonority theory and sonority sequencing principles also are introduced. These theories are in no way superior to other nonlinear phonologies, and clinical application is still rather limited. However, they do seem valuable and offer the reader some insights into current phonological theories.

Feature Geometry

Nonlinear frameworks have been used with a wide variety of populations: children who are developing typically, those with speech sound disorders, those with both speech and morphosyntactic production problems, children and adolescents with hearing loss and speech difficulties, those with autism spectrum disorder, and those with cleft palates, to mention a few (e.g., Ayyad & Bernhardt, 2007; Bernhardt, Bacsfalvi, Gick, Radanov, & Williams, 2005; Bernhardt, Brooke, & Major, 2003; McGee, 2006). Nonlinear assessments have the same general objectives as linear assessments: to determine if the child is communicating effectively, to provide baseline information, to find out if other factors are associated with the speech sound disorder, and to propose a therapeutic plan. However, feature geometry uses independent, hierarchically organized tiers to explain phenomena below the segmental level, a hierarchical arrangement of features. Features are considered autonomous units that are arranged in a hierarchy and can combine and recombine into segments.

There are major organizing features, also called nodes: place, laryngeal, and root (manner). Most accounts show manner features attached to or near the root node, which means that they are ranked higher in this hierarchy. This feature hierarchy uses distinctive features somewhat similar to those used by Chomsky and Halle (1968); however, they are redefined and reorganized in various ways. So, distinctive features play a central role in this feature geometry model. According to Bernhardt and Stemberger (1998), the distinctive elements for feature geometry are based on those of Chomsky and Halle's (1968), except for the features for place of articulation, which follow Sagey (1986). For example, /k/ and /g/ are referred to as + dorsal with this feature system as opposed to + velar with Chomsky and Halle's (1968) system. The reasoning for this is that + dorsal refers to the tongue body, which is the main moving articulator for these sounds (Bernhardt, Bopp, Daudlin, Edwards, & Wastie, 2010).

Across this hierarchy, there is still a distinction between what is unmarked—frequent, less complex—and marked—infrequent, more complex. The term *default* is now used to designate unmarked elements. The features of /t/ are considered the default, consonant features for General American English and many other languages. Therefore, the default setting, so to speak, is – continuant (thus a stop),

– voiced, and coronal [+ anterior] (which refers to the alveolar place of articulation). According to this model, underlying representations are noted by their nondefault features, in other words by those different from this "default" setting of [t]. This relates to another nonlinear theory, the *theory of radical underspecification* (Archangeli, 1988; Archangeli & Pulleyblank, 1994; Bernhardt, 1992; Kiparsky, 1982; Pulleyblank, 1986), which suggests that underlying representations contain only "unpredictable" features. A *predictable feature* is one that is commonly associated with that particular segment or class of sounds. For example, nasals are typically voiced (although there are unvoiced nasals in some African languages). Voicing for nasals is then predictable and would not be contained in the underlying representation. Because all sonorants are voiced, this is also a predictable feature and is not contained in the underlying representation. On the other hand, obstruents can be [+ voice] or [− voice]; therefore, the unpredictable nature of this feature is contained in the underlying representation. As an example, /m/ is considered to be [+ nasal] *and* [labial]. Additional features—[+ consonantal], [+ sonorant], and [+ voiced]—do not need to be added, as they are predictable. With /n/, on the other hand, *only* the feature [+ nasal] needs to be noted since the default (refer to the example with /t/ above) is [coronal].

The tiers of feature geometry interact with one another. Some features are designated as nodes, which means that these nodes may dominate more than one other feature and serve as a link between the dominated feature and higher levels of representation. This can be seen in Figure 4.1, where the place node serves

Figure 4.1 Feature Geometry of the English Consonant System

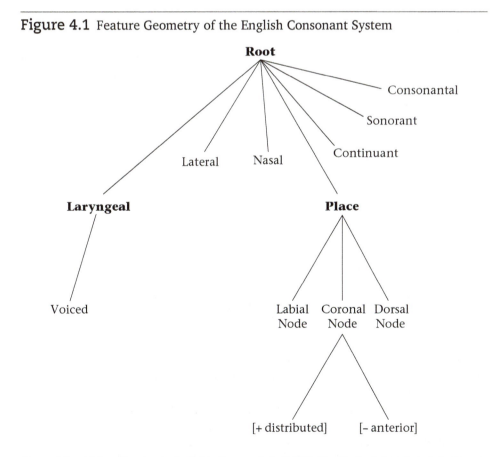

Source: Adapted from Bernhardt, B., & Stemberger, J. P. (1998). *Handbook of phonological development from the perspective of constraint-based nonlinear phonology*. San Diego, CA: Academic Press.

as a link among the labial, coronal, and dorsal nodes and the root node. The place node, for example, dominates the different places of articulation (labial, coronal, and dorsal nodes). The place node must be activated, so to speak, before a specific place of articulation can be chosen. Similarly, the laryngeal node, as a higher level of representation, must be functioning before [+ voice] can be designated. Features that are dominated are considered subordinate or at a lower level of representation.

Feature geometry also attempts to explain why some features are affected by assimilation processes (known as *spreading* or *linking* of features), whereas others are affected by neutralization or deletion processes (known as *delinking*) (Dinnsen, 1997). Figure 4.1 is a feature geometry representation adapted from Bernhardt and Stemberger (1998). These features have been simplified to include only main areas that are pertinent for sounds of General American English.

The following provides a brief explanation of the different nodes and features, summarized from Bernhardt and Stemberger (1998). Note that not all features mentioned by Bernhardt and Stemberger are present in the following list.

Laryngeal Features

1. [+ voiced] sounds produced with vocal fold vibration (e.g., [b, d, g, v, ð, z, ʒ])

Manner Features

1. [+ consonantal] sounds with a narrow constriction in the oral and/or pharyngeal cavities that significantly impede the flow of air (e.g., plosives, affricates, nasals, fricatives, laterals are + consonantal)
2. [+ sonorant] sounds in which the pressure above the larynx allows the vocal cords to vibrate continuously without any rise in pressure above the larynx (e.g., voiced vowels, approximants, and [h] are + sonorant)
3. [+ continuant] sounds in which air continues to move through the oral cavity (e.g., vowels, fricatives and affricates are + continuant)
4. [+ nasal] sounds with the velum lowered so that air moves through the nasal cavity (e.g., nasals are + nasal)
5. [+ lateral] sounds in which central airflow is blocked in the oral cavity but air is directed over at least one side of the tongue (the lateral approximant /l/ is the only + lateral in General American English).

Place Features

Lips. [Labial] sounds made with more involvement of one or both lips (e.g., bilabials [p, b, m], labiodentals [f, v], [w], and possibly [ɹ] are + labial).

The tip of the tongue. [Coronal] sounds made with raising of the tip or blade of the tongue (e.g., [t, d, s, z, ʃ, ʒ, tʃ, dʒ, θ, ð , n, ɹ, l, and j] plus high-front vowels are included). Recall that [Coronal] is a default setting and may not need to be specified.

The tongue body. [Dorsal] sounds made with the back of the tongue (e.g., [k, g, ŋ] (velars and back vowels).

According to these parameters, and allowing for default features, the consonants can be specified accordingly. Refer to Table 4.6. The default features are – continuant, – voiced, and coronal (+ anterior), which were noted for /t/.

Figure 4.2 shows a diagram using the features of "she" [ʃi] becoming "dee" [di].

Table 4.6 Feature Geometry Consonant Specifications

Segment	Root Node	Laryngeal Node	Place Node
/p/	[+ consonantal]		Labial
/b/	[+ cons]	[+ voice]	Labial
/t/	[+ cons]		
/d/	[+ cons]	[+ voice]	
/k/	[+ cons]		Dorsal
/g/	[+ cons]	[+ voice]	Dorsal
/m/	[+ cons] [+ nasal]		Labial
/n/	[+ cons] [+ nasal]		
/ŋ/	[+ cons] [+ nasal]		Dorsal
/f/	[+ cons] [+ continuant]		Labial
/v/	[+ cons] [+ cont]	[+ voice]	Labial
/s/	[+ cons] [+ cont]		
/z/	[+ cons] [+ cont]	[+ voice]	
/ʃ/	[+ cons] [+ cont]		Coronal [– anterior]
/ʒ/	[+ cons] [+ cont]	[+ voice]	Coronal [– anterior]
/θ/ [1]	[+ cons] [+ cont]		Coronal [+ distributed]
/ð/ [1]	[+ cons] [+ cont]	[+ voice]	Coronal [+ distributed]
/tʃ/ [2]	[+ cons] Branching [continuant]		Coronal [– anterior]
/dʒ/ [2]	[+ cons] Branching [continuant]	[+ voice]	Coronal [– anterior]
/w/	[+ sonorant]		Labial [+ round]
/j/	[+ sonorant]		
/ɹ/	[+ cons] [+ sonorant]		Labial + Coronal Place or [– anterior] (used to distinguish /ɹ/ from /l/)
/l/	[+ cons] [+ sonorant]		
/h/	[+ cons] [+ cont]	Laryngeal Node	

[1] + distributed is used for /θ/ and /ð/ according to McCarthy (1988).
[2] The branching structure of the affricates is represented by one branch for the stop portion and one branch for the fricative element, thus [– continuant] (stop portion) and [+ continuant] (fricative portion).

One maps the various features in Table 4.6 onto the diagram in Figure 4.2. Those features that are not a portion of the specific phonemes are not included, and those that are a part of the default /t/ also do not need to be specified. For /t/, the defaults are – continuant, – voiced, and coronal (+ anterior). Vowels are noted as

Figure 4.2 Feature Geometry Tiers with /ʃi/ becoming /di/

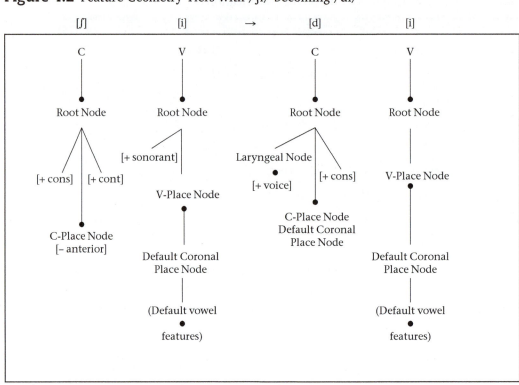

[+ sonorant], front vowels are noted as coronal place node, and back vowels are noted as dorsal place node. Therefore, in Figure 4.2, the [+ cons] and [+ cont] of /ʃ/ changes to just [+ cons] for /d/, whereas the rest of the features are default ones. However, on the laryngeal node, the [+ voice] needs to be added for /d/.

Clinical Exercises Jake substitutes [t] and [d] for [k] and [g] in all word positions. The root node representing + consonantal (with plosives) seems to be present.

At which level is Jake having difficulty according to feature geometry? Examine the places of articulation under the place node.

Rules in nonlinear analysis are restricted to two basic operations: *spreading* (also known as *linking*) and *deletion* (also known as *delinking*) of phonological information from one tier to another. Spreading of features could be exemplified by the production of [gɑg] for *dog*. The coronal place node for /d/ is subject to the linking or assimilation from the dorsal place node feature of /g/. Thus, the dorsal place node of the final [g] in *dog* affects the initial [d]. The result is that the initial [d] is produced as [g]. The place of articulation is moved from coronal [d] to dorsal [g]. Delinking could be exemplified by the production of [dɑ] for *dog*. Under the assumption that the underlying representation is intact, the final consonant slot for that production is delinked from the representation along with the actual features of /g/. Refer to Figure 4.3 for these examples. Linking and delinking result from, and are constrained by, principles of association between tiers. These principles are outlined in Bernhardt and Stemberger (1998). This reference can be used for more detailed analysis procedures.

Figure 4.3 Example of Linking (/dɑg/ → /gɑg/) and Delinking ([dɑg] → [dɑ])

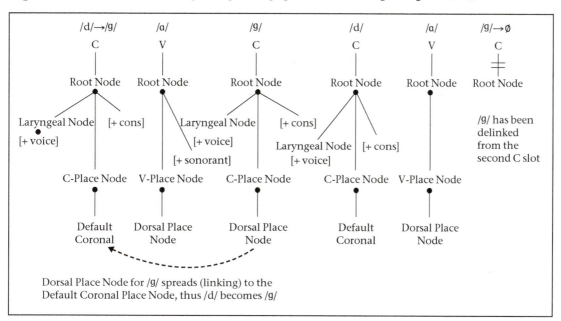

Dorsal Place Node for /g/ spreads (linking) to the
Default Coronal Place Node, thus /d/ becomes /g/

Clinical Application

More Information? Feature Geometry Versus Phonological Processes

Let's look at the difference between how feature geometry versus phonological processes would explain an example of a child who says [gʌ] for *duck* and [dʌ] for *dumb*. If phonological processes are assigned to these substitutions and deletions, the following results are noted:

"duck"	[dʌk]	→	[gʌ]	backing [d] → [g] final consonant deletion [k] → Ø
"dumb"	[dʌm]	→	[dʌ]	final consonant deletion [m] → Ø

Although these phonological processes are easily identifiable, they give no information about a child's underlying representation. Where to begin in therapy would be a relatively arbitrary choice that would be based on the number of times the processes were observed and the age at which they should be suppressed. Feature geometry demonstrates that the underlying representation for this child includes information about the dorsal place node—that is, about /k/ and /g/. This is evidenced by the dorsal production of [g] in [gʌ] for *duck*. Articulatory constraints, however, prevent realization of final consonants. If this was just a case of final consonant deletion, both *duck* and *dumb* should have been realized as [dʌ]. In the underlying representation, the child might be trying to differentiate between *duck* and *dumb*. This suggests that if the articulatory constraints could be eliminated, the child's g/d substitution (backing) might also be eliminated.

Bernhardt and colleagues (2010) also demonstrate how these principles could be used based on the phoneme inventory of a child. One compares the features of the substitutions to the targets, seeing which features are missing. One tries to find a common feature (or features) that when activated would hopefully generalize to other consonants in error with that feature. For example, Ian (age 4 years 6 months) has the following phonemes in his inventory:

/m, n, ŋ, p, b, t, d, k, g, f, v, j, h/

He uses the following substitutions:

/s, ʃ, tʃ/ → /t/, /z, ʒ, ʤ/ → /d/

According to nonlinear geometry, Ian needs the feature of [+ continuant] for all substitutions; this would eliminate the stopping of those fricatives. In addition, the coronal place [– anterior] is necessary for /ʃ, ʒ, tʃ, ʤ/. He has the coronal place [+ anterior] for /t/ but would have to be able to produce [– anterior] The branching [continuant] feature would be needed for /tʃ, ʤ/. Looking for a common set of features, if you taught /ʃ/, for example, the features [+ continuant] and coronal place [– anterior] might be added. This would apply to the fricatives /s, z/ as well.

Other substitutions: /θ/ → /f/, /ð/ → /v/

The only feature distinguishing these substitutions would be the Place node Labial (for /f/ and /v/) versus Coronal for the th-sounds.

/ɹ, l/ → /w/

Here, Ian must add the feature [+ sonorant] to [+ consonantal] for /ɹ, l/. He seems to have the feature [+ sonorant] with /j/ and [+ consonantal] with several other phonemes. It may be necessary to see if Ian can simply combine the two features with /l/ or /ɹ/. In addition, with /ɹ/, either labial + coronal place or [– anterior] is a needed feature.

To summarize, one nonlinear phonology, feature geometry, theorizes that segments are composed of multitiered, hierarchically organized features. Specific nodes that can dominate other features and link various levels of representation are designated. According to this theory, features can link (assimilate) or delink, causing neutralization or deletion. These principles of association are used to explain occurrences between tiers.

> **Clinical Exercises** According to nonlinear analysis, two basic operations may occur: *spreading* (also known as *linking*) and *deletion* (also known as *delinking*). Are the following transcriptions examples of spreading or delinking? Explain why for each: [lɛloʊ] for *yellow*, [kʌ] for *cup*, [fɪndɚ] for *finger*.

Optimality Theory

Optimality theory, first formalized by Prince and Smolensky (1993) and McCarthy and Prince (1995), is considered a constraint-based approach, not a rule-governed one (as is feature geometry). Constraints are limits to what constitutes a possible pronunciation of a word. When constraints are applied linguistically, a set of grammatical universals is said to exist; these universals include the fact that all languages have syllables and that certain syllable patterns seem to be more (or less) common. For example, in General American English, there are words that begin with three consonants, such as *street*, but none that begin with four consonants in a row. Therefore, we could say that General American English has a constraint on how many consonants can occur at the beginning of a word; three consonants are acceptable, but four are not. If languages are compared, they each demonstrate certain constraints. For example, Hawaiian allows no more than one consonant in a row, resulting in words such as *kanaka* for "man." When comparing this to English, which allows several consonants in a row, in such words as *street* and *sixths*, we could say that Hawaiian has a constraint against more than one consonant as an onset (at the beginning of a word or syllable) or as a syllable coda (at the end of a word or syllable). Constraints characterize patterns that are and are not possible within or across languages. Applying this principle generally to children with speech sound disorders, we could state that children who do not produce syllable codas, thus evidencing final-consonant deletion, have a constraint against producing final codas.

Constraints are based on the principles of markedness. Thus, each constraint violation indicates markedness in that respect. Constraints are a means of (1) characterizing universal patterns that occur across languages, (2) demonstrating variations of patterns that occur between languages, and (3) determining markedness indicated by constraint violations (Archangeli & Langendoen, 1997). Markedness is discussed on pages 85–87 of this chapter.

Optimality theory, as a constraint-based approach, was originally developed to explain the differences that occur between and among languages. Optimality theory presupposes a universal grammar and states that constraints characterize universals; however, constraints can be violated. Some constraints are very important (within and across languages) and are rarely violated, whereas others are not as important and can be violated. If we examine constraints in this manner, we find that the following universal trends are considered typical (unmarked) properties of syllables. To the right of each constraint is the name given to it by Archangeli and Langendoen (1997):

Syllables begin with a consonant.	ONSET
Syllables have one vowel.	PEAK
Syllables end with a vowel.	NOCODA
Syllables have at most one consonant at an edge.	*COMPLEX

By examining this list, we can determine whether there are constraint violations in General American English.

1. *Syllables begin with a consonant: ONSET.* Not all syllables begin with a consonant, as demonstrated by words such as *away* and *eat*. Probably, in General American English, most syllables do, however, begin with a consonant. This constraint can be violated (although it is maintained most of the time) in General American English.

2. *Syllables have one vowel: PEAK.* In General American English, this seems to be the case. Some syllables consist of syllabic consonants such as [bi.tl̩] or [fɪʃ.n̩]; however, no syllables contain two separate vowels. In General American English, the constraint of PEAK is *rarely*, if at all, violated.

3. *Syllables end with a vowel: NOCODA.* Not all syllables in General American English end with a vowel. Many syllables end with a consonant in words such as *hat, clock*, and *antique*. This constraint is violated in General American English.

4. *Syllables have at most one consonant at an edge: *COMPLEX.* This is also violated in General American English. Words such as *clocks* and *streets* demonstrate a violation of this constraint.

In summarizing, we could state that some of the previously mentioned constraints can be violated, whereas others typically are not. This could lead to a ranking of constraints from those that are never or rarely violated to those that are sometimes violated to those that are often violated. Constraints that are *rarely* violated are considered higher-order constraints and are separated from others by a double arrow > >. Constraints that are *sometimes* violated are separated from each other by a comma. Based on the previous discussion, the following ranking could be made:

$$PEAK >> ONSET, NOCODA, *COMPLEX$$

Thus, in General American English, the constraint PEAK (syllables have one vowel) is not violated. Therefore, it is separated from the others, ONSET, NOCODA, and *COMPLEX. The other constraints, which can be violated, are separated by commas. Therefore, one important concept within optimality theory is the ranking of constraints.

Optimality theory, like other linguistic theories, proposes an input (an underlying representation), an output (the surface representation), and a relation between the two. The only specification of the input is that it is linguistically well formed; it does not contain variables that are not grammatical. The output is the actual production. Optimality theory does not account for differences between the input and output in terms of rules (as in generative grammar) or processes (as in natural phonology) but in terms of constraints. In optimality theory, the relation between the input and output is mediated by two formal mechanisms: the generator (GEN) and the evaluator (EVAL). The GEN links the input with potential outputs. It can add, delete, or rearrange, for example. The EVAL judges the outputs to determine which one is the *optimal* output. For any given input, such as [pɪg], which is the mental representation of the word "pig," the GEN can generate an infinite number of possible phonetic outputs for that form. All these output forms compete with one another, but one output must be chosen as the optimal one. The EVAL evaluates all these different outputs and chooses the output that is the optimal response for that particular language. These output forms are evaluated through the constraints and their ranking within that language that thus restrict the possible output forms (Ball, 2002; Barlow, 2001).

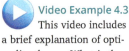 Video Example 4.3

This video includes a brief explanation of optimality theory. What is the difference between rules and constraints? Why are constraints ranked?

https://www.youtube.com/watch?v=xsMea6QhLoA

Two types of constraints function within this mechanism: faithfulness and markedness. Faithfulness constraints require that *input and output forms be identical to one another.* If segments between the input and output are deleted, inserted, or rearranged, the faithfulness constraint is violated. If a child produces the word "skip" as [sɪp], then the faithfulness constraint has been violated. Markedness constraints *require outputs to be unmarked or simplified in structure.* Unmarked features are those that are easier to produce or those that occur frequently across languages. Consonant clusters are considered marked (refer to *COMPLEX mentioned previously). Thus, the child who produces *skip* as [skɪp] violates the markedness constraint. However, a child who says the word "skip" as [sɪp] has not violated this constraint; the output is unmarked or simplified.

As can be seen, faithfulness and markedness constraints are conflicting; there is an antagonistic relationship between the two. The conflict between faithfulness and markedness leads to violation of constraints. Every utterance violates some constraint; if faithfulness is maintained, then markedness is violated. (The most unmarked syllable would be something like [bɑ], so any more complex syllable structure would be some violation of markedness.)

So, how does the EVAL judge which one is the optimal form? At this point, optimality theory postulates that the ranking of the constraints becomes the deciding factor. Lower-ranked constraints can be violated to satisfy higher-ranking constraints. In our previous example, ONSET, NOCODA, or *COMPLEX could be violated to satisfy PEAK.

If optimality theory is applied to phonological development, the hypothesis is that children acquire the correct ranking of the constraints as they develop. Immature patterns demonstrate that this ranking, according to the language in question, has not yet been mastered. In phonological development, the markedness constraint is a higher-ranking one. Children simplify their output until they can apply the faithfulness constraint.

Individual patterns of normal development are seen as products of the individual's idiosyncratic constraint rankings. Application of this to children with phonological disorders indicates that these children also have their own unique constraint rankings. Our job is to determine the rankings that account for the children's error patterns. The next step is to try to re-rank the constraints so that they are more in line with the input. It is assumed that markedness constraints (the typical simplification that occurs in relationship to the production features) must be demoted. *Demotion* is a process in which higher-ranking constraints that do not match the adult rankings become lower, so that the rankings will eventually match the adult ones. Refer to Table 4.7 for a summary of terms and examples within optimality theory.

Table 4.7 Summary of Terms and Examples for Optimality Theory

Constraint Based	Universal, languages differ in the ranking of constraints
Two Types of Constraints	Faithfulness and markedness
Markedness	Output is unmarked or simplified in structure
Faithfulness	Input and output forms are identical
	Conflict results in constraint violability: every output violates some constraint
Types of Markedness Constraints	Complex, Coda, Fricatives, Liquids (Liquid [l], Liquid [ɹ])
COMPLEX	Cluster reduction simplified, "tree" ⇒ [ti], Violation = "tree" ⇒ [tɹi]
CODA	No syllable final consonants, "team" ⇒ [ti], Violation = "team" ⇒ [tim]
FRICATIVES	No fricatives, "sip" ⇒ [tɪp], Violation = "sip" ⇒ [sɪp]
LIQUIDS	No liquids, "lip" ⇒ [wɪp], "rip" ⇒ [wɪp] Violation = "lip" ⇒ [lɪp], "rip" ⇒ [ɹɪp]
LIQUID [l]	No liquid [l], "lose" ⇒ [wuz] Violation = "lose" ⇒ [luz]
LIQUID [ɹ]	No liquid [ɹ], "rock" ⇒ [wɑk] Violation = "rock" ⇒[ɹɑk]
Types of Faithfulness Constraints	Max, Dep, Ident-Feature (Ident-[cons], Ident-[cont])
MAX	Prohibits deletion, "moon" ⇒ [mun] Violation = "moon" ⇒ [mu]
DEP	Prohibits insertion or addition of segments, "sleep" ⇒ [slip] Violation = "sleep" ⇒ [səlip]
IDENT-[feature]	Prohibits changing any feature; input and output forms are the same, "tree" ⇒ [tɹi] Violation = "tree" ⇒ [twi]
IDENT-[cons]	Prohibits changing consonantal features, "led" ⇒ [lɛd] Violation = "led" ⇒ [wɛd]
IDENT-[cont]	Prohibits changing continuant features, "sock" ⇒ [sɑk] Violation = "sock" ⇒ [tɑk]

When using different references for optimality theory, one will find slightly different notations. For example, IDENT[cont] has been labeled IDENT[manner] in Gierut and Morrisette (2005).

Optimality theory offers a new way to view both the acquisition of phonological patterns and the categorization of disordered phonological systems. The concept of constraints and demoting constraints reminds one of phonological process suppression. However, the information gained from the optimality model is far more detailed and gives the clinician valuable information about what the child can do, not just what the child is incapable of doing.

Clinical Exercises The following small sample is from Hector, age 4 years 6 months.

Word Example	Transcription	Hector's Production
grapes	[gɹeɪps]	[deɪ]
feet	[fit]	[fi]
teeth	[tiθ]	[ti]
stove	[stoʊv]	[toʊ]
spoon	[spun]	[un]
bed	[bɛd]	[ɛd]
book	[bʊk]	[ʊt]
nose	[noʊz]	[noʊ]
mop	[mɑp]	[mɑ]
pig	[pɪg]	[ɪd]

Consider the constraints ONSET (syllables begin with a consonant), NOCODA (syllables end with a vowel), and *COMPLEX (syllables have at most one consonant at an edge) for Hector. Which constraints seem to be operating on a regular basis? Look at the four violations of the constraint ONSET. Do you see a pattern? Could this be used to reorganize his constraints?

An analysis using principles of optimality theory is depicted in terms of a *constraint tableau*. The relevant constraints are listed across the top of the tableau. They are ordered from left to right based on their rankings in the child's system. Thus, the highest-ranked constraint is in the left-most column, and the others are listed across the top. Since, theoretically, an infinite number of possibilities could be generated by the GEN, only relevant competitors are listed. The asterisk (*) indicates a constraint violation, and the exclamation point (!) indicates a fatal violation (one of the higher-ranking constraints is violated, and that output will not be selected). The finger (☛) indicates the selected output. Let's look at a sample tableau:

Input	Constraint 1	Constraint 2
Possibility 1	*!	
☛ Possibility 2		*

Possibility 2 is chosen (☛). It does violate a constraint but involves a lower-ranking constraint. In Possibility 1, a higher-ranking constraint is violated; thus, it demonstrates a fatal violation. If an output violates a higher-ranking constraint, this is a fatal violation and will not be the selected output.

Here is a clinical example: Andy demonstrates (1) stopping /s/ → /t/, thus "so" /soʊ/ → /toʊ/. It is also noted that Andy can show (2) stopping and final consonant deletion, "soul" /soʊl/ → /toʊ/, and (3) cluster reduction and final consonant deletion, "stole" /stoʊl/ → /toʊ/. Thus, based on Andy's constraints, the production /toʊ/ will result in three different instances.

The constraint ranking must now be considered for each of these. Recall that in phonological development Markedness features are ranked above Faithfulness.

Constraint Ranking for the Pattern of Stopping: /soʊ/ → /toʊ/.
Markedness constraint
*FRICATIVE: (means that there are no fricatives)
Faithfulness constraint
IDENT[cont]: Input and output must be identical continuants
Constraint ranking *FRICATIVE > > IDENT[cont]

> The constraint ranking of *FRICATIVE is higher than the faithfulness constraint, as Andy uses a simpler sound, a stop, to replace a fricative. Thus, for this example, markedness constraints are ranked higher than faithfulness ones.

Constraint Tableau: Stopping

/soʊ/ → /toʊ/	*FRICATIVE	IDENT[cont]
a. /soʊ/	*!	
☛ b. /toʊ/		*

> A high-ranked constraint is violated (*FRICATIVE); this is a fatal violation. Therefore, the lower-ranking violation (IDENT[cont]) is the selected output.

Constraint Ranking for the Pattern of Final Consonant Deletion
Markedness constraint
*CODA: (means that there is no coda)
Faithfulness constraint
MAX: No deletions
Cumulative constraint ranking (the *FRICATIVE from above must be added)
*CODA, *FRICATIVE > > MAX, IDENT[cont]

> *CODA is ranked above MAX, as MAX says that the input and output correspond in the number of segments. Thus, MAX is violated, whereas *CODA (no coda) is not.
>
> Now *CODA and *FRICATIVE are ranked above MAX and IDENT[cont].

Constraint Tableau: Final Consonant Deletion: /soʊl/ → /toʊ/

/soʊl/ → /toʊ/	*CODA	*FRICATIVE	MAX	IDENT[cont]
a. /soʊl/	*!	*		
b. /toʊl/	*!			*
c. /soʊ/		*!	*	
☛ d. /toʊ/			*	*

> *CODA and *FRICATIVE demonstrate fatal violations, as they are higher-ranking constraints and are violated. Thus, the selected output is /toʊ/.

Constraints and Ranking for the Pattern of Cluster Reduction
Markedness constraint
*COMPLEX: (means that there are no clusters)
Cumulative constraint ranking (now CODA and FRICATIVE are added)
*COMPLEX, *CODA, *FRICATIVE > > MAX, IDENT[cont]

> The only markedness constraint that applies to consonant clusters is *COMPLEX (there are no clusters). This would be a higher-level markedness constraint. For Andy, markedness constraints are higher ranked, as he does use simplifications.

As you work through the various possibilities, you can see that higher-ranking constraints are fatally violated with /stoʊl/; it does have a cluster (*COMPLEX) and a final consonant (*CODA). *CODA is also a fatal violation with /soʊl/ and /toʊl/. A fatal violation occurs with no fricative (*FRICATIVE) with /soʊ/. The MAX is violated several times, but it is a lower-ranking constraint.

Constraint Tableau: Cluster Reduction: /stoʊl/ → /toʊ/					
/stoʊl/ → /toʊ/	*COMPLEX	*CODA	*FRICATIVE	MAX	IDENT [cont]
a. /stoʊl/	*!	*!	*		
b. /soʊl/		*!	*	*	
c. /toʊl/		*!		*	
d. /soʊ/			*!	**	
☞ e. /toʊ/				**	

What does this tell us clinically? First, it demonstrates the *interaction* of the various processes that are occurring with Andy. His errors can be integrated with one another. This gives us more detailed information than simply listing the individual processes. Second, it ranks the relationship among errors. With Andy, we see that both *COMPLEX and *FRICATIVE will be impacted, thus *FRICATIVE will co-occur with *COMPLEX. We also see that markedness constraints for Andy are higher ranked than faithfulness. He simplifies, which is a characteristic of children developing their phonological systems.

For therapy, treating COMPLEX with s-clusters would in turn demote *FRICATIVE and *CODA if the s-clusters, such as /st/, were taught as an onset and a coda ("stop" versus "best," for example). As well, it appears that certain error patterns are predictive. Using optimality theory analyses, Dinnsen and O'Connor (2001) found that children who exhibited stopping also used gliding with liquids. However, this was unidirectional; the presence of liquid gliding did not imply stopping. This seems to reflect certain implicational universals noted earlier in the chapter (pages 86–87).

THE DEVELOPMENT OF NONLINEAR PHONOLOGY. John Firth, professor of general linguistics at the University of London, was a key figure in the development of modern linguistics in the United Kingdom. In a way, nonlinear phonology, too, can be traced back to Firth's (1948) so-called prosodic analysis. For the first time, Firth challenged the one-sided linguistic importance of the phonemic units in their consecutive linearity. He advocated the need for additional nonsegmental analyses, "prosodies," which represent larger linguistic entities, such as syllables, words, and phrases. He postulated that speech is a manifestation of consecutively ordered units *as well as* a manifestation of larger prosodic components that bind phonemes together into linguistically more comprehensive pieces. Firth theorized that different analytical systems may need to be set up to explain the range of contrasts involved. With this approach, known as *polysystemicism*, the concept of nonlinear phonology was born.

Contemporary nonlinear phonologies are seen as an evolution from generative phonology. Chomsky and Halle's (1968) major contribution, *The Sound Pattern of English*, was innovative in its description of two levels of representation: a surface phonetic representation and an underlying phonemic representation. Although the idea of distinctive features was taken from the Prague School of Linguistics, Chomsky and Halle understood the distinctive feature concept in a different way and modified it accordingly. Nonlinear phonologies adopt the generative concepts of distinctive features and surface-level versus underlying representation. However, these new phonologies understand the surface-level representation in a very different way.

Chomsky and Halle's generative phonology described speech components in a linear manner: They were segment based. The components of any utterance were arranged in a sequence, with one discrete segment following the next. A common set of distinctive features is attributed to all segments, and the assignment of a binary value specifies each feature. This limited the possibility of generating phonological rules in several respects. First, only whole segments could be deleted or added. The only other modifications that could occur in the segment were achieved by changing the + or − values of one or more distinctive features. (Thus, this system analyzes only additions, deletions, and substitutions; analysis of nonphonemic distortions is not possible.) Second, because all segments are equally complex and all distinctive features are equal within this system, there is no reason to expect that any one segment or any one distinctive feature might be affected by any given phonological rule. However, many observations and investigations have reported, for example, that certain sounds and sound classes appear to be especially vulnerable to assimilation, whereas others cause assimilation (Dinnsen, 1997). Third, early generative phonology adopted the division between the segmentals and the suprasegmentals that the structural linguists had used to describe and analyze speech events. However, such a division does not allow a vertical, hierarchical understanding of the interaction between segmental units and prosodic features. The nonlinear phonologies represent a challenge to the earlier segment-based approaches. "Nonlinear phonological theory is another step in the evolution of our understanding of phonological systems" (Bernhardt & Stoel-Gammon, 1994, p. 126).

To summarize, many different nonlinear phonologies exist. Some of them have been applied to case studies of children with disordered phonological systems. The results seem to indicate that these phonologies promise new insights into, and a deeper understanding of, these children's phonological systems. Other phonological theories that show promise in their application to disordered speech include, among others, gestural phonology, also known as articulatory phonology (e.g., Browman & Goldstein, 1992, 1995); systemic phonology, which evolved from prosodic analysis (e.g., Halliday & Matthiessen, 2004; Müller, Ball, & Rutter, 2006); and cognitive phonology (e.g., Bybee, 2001). An introduction to these and other phonological models can be found in Martin Ball's (2016) *Principles of Clinical Phonology: Theoretical Approaches.*

The Sonority Theory and Sonority Sequencing Principles

Let's begin with a brief review of phonotactics, as it is an integral part of this discussion. We will be looking at syllable structures, and the phonotactics of syllable structures do play a role. The syllable has been shown to be structured in a hierarchical arrangement, with the onset and rime on one level and the rime further divided into the nucleus and coda (refer to Chapter 2, page 41). The elements of the syllable—onset, nucleus, and coda—can be simple or complex. Their arrangement is language specific and restricted by the phonotactics of that particular language. There are languages in which there are no codas (i.e., no syllable-final sounds), such as Hmong, and those in which complex onsets and codas (i.e., consonant clusters) do not exist, such as Vietnamese. The language-specific phonotactics affects the syllable structure. However, despite all the variation, there are certain commonalities in syllable structure. For example, the nucleus contains a vowel or vowel-like segment. There also seem to be certain patterns in the relationship between the onset and nucleus, and complex onsets and codas have preferred strings of consonants.

The following represents the phonotactic constraints of General American English (Haspelmath & Sims, 2010):

1. All syllables have a nucleus.
2. There is no /h/ as the syllable coda. Although a word may end in the letter "h"—for example, "sigh"—there is no /h/.
3. Complex onsets (those containing more than one element) cannot contain affricates /tʃ/ or /dʒ/.
4. The first consonant in a complex onset must be an obstruent (plosive or fricative).
5. The second consonant in a complex onset cannot be a voiced obstruent (no voiced plosives or fricatives).
6. If the first consonant in a complex onset is not an /s/, the second must be a liquid (/l, ɹ/) or glide (/w, j/)—for example, "flower" or "twin."
7. No glides are in codas of syllables. Words may end with the letter "w"—for example, "cow"—but that is spelling, not pronunciation.
8. If there is a complex coda, the second consonant cannot be /ŋ/, /ʒ/, or /ð/.
9. If the second consonant in a complex coda is voiced, so is the first.
10. Non-alveolar nasals /m, ŋ/ must be homorganic with the next segment (e.g., in "singer" /sɪŋgɚ/, the /ŋ/ and /g/ are homorganic).
11. Two obstruents in the same coda must share voicing (e.g., "bets" /ts/ and "beds" /dz/).

Because phonotactic rules vary in every language, they are an important point when working with individuals who are learning English as a second language. The phonotactics of their native language may influence their pronunciation patterns in English. For example, Cantonese has no consonant combinations (if the labialized /k/, /kʷ/, is counted as one consonant); therefore, no complex onsets or codas exist (except in colloquial Cantonese). This may affect the speaker's production capabilities in General American English.

To discuss sonority, we must consider the syllable specifically as a unit of perception rather than as a unit of production. The sonority theory, according to Ball (2016), is the closest conceptual framework to a phonology of speech perception. Thus, this section represents a wide departure from the nonlinear phonologies discussed in the previous pages. However, sonority theory is a theory and it does have clinical application, most notably with the complexity approaches that have been introduced with implicational universals.

As defined in Chapter 2, the sonority of a sound is its loudness relative to that of other sounds with the same length, stress, and pitch. Different sounds can have various amplitudes, intensities, and amounts of airflow. From these factors, we can arrive at a measure of sonority. However, sonority cannot be correlated directly with instrumental measures. It has to do with the inherent qualities of the sound, the influence of the neighboring sounds, and the overall loudness the speaker uses. In addition, some phonologists equate sonority with an articulatory parameter. Sounds with a relatively open expiratory passageway have more sonority than those with a more constricted airstream during their production. Since each individual sound has a sonority ranking in respect to the other sounds, a sonority scale can be achieved. Figure 4.4 lists the sounds of General American English from most to least sonorous.

The affricates typically do not have a separate category in sonority scales. This list can be further delineated by using numerical values for the various categories. This has been done in various ways. Steriade (1990) used a scale in which the most sonorous sounds, the vowels, were given a sonority ranking of zero. Less sonorous sounds had higher values; thus, voiceless plosives had a value of 7. This seems a bit counterintuitive, with less sonority equating to a higher number and the most sonority equating to zero. Roca (1994) assigned values the other way around. A value of 6 was given to vowels, and a value of 1 was

Figure 4.4 Hierarchy of Sonority Values for Sounds Ranked from Most to Least Sonorous in General American English

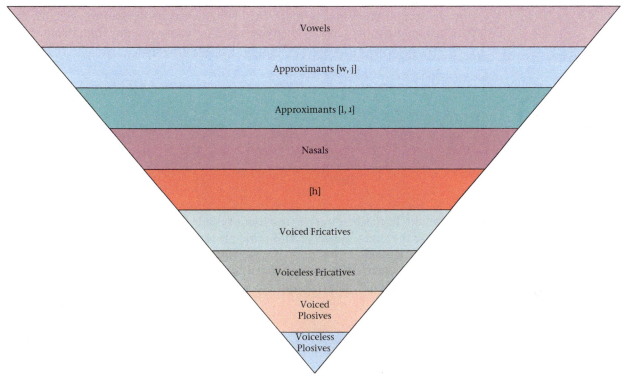

Source: Adapted from O'Grady, W. D., & Archibald, J. (2012). *Contemporary linguistic analysis: An introduction* (7th ed.). Toronto: Pearson Longman.

given to plosives. In Roca's (1994) scale, a differentiation was not made between voiced and voiceless plosives and fricatives. The complexity approach uses the Steriade (1990) model, whereas the Roca (1994) numbering is more practical when mapping sonority to a syllable. Table 4.8 provides both scales. Note that in both scales, /h/ is not assigned a separate number. One assumes that it has been incorporated into the fricatives.

Table 4.8 Numerical Sonority Ranking According to Steriade (1990) and Roca (1994)

Sound Class	Steriade (1990) Values	Roca (1994) Values
Vowels	0	6
Approximants [w, j]	1	5
Approximants [ɹ, l]	2	4
Nasals	3	3
Fricatives		2
Voiced Fricatives	4	
Voiceless Fricatives	5	
Plosives		1
Voiced Plosives	6	
Voiceless Plosives	7	

The sonority scale influences the syllable structure rules. The general rule is that more sonorous elements are closer to the syllable nucleus, and less sonorant elements are farther away. The rules of phonotactics in General American English operate around this sonority hierarchy. The nucleus or peak of the syllable has maximal sonority; the sonority then decreases as you move away from the nucleus.

Let's look at two syllables exemplifying this principle:

Video Example 4.4

In this video, the sonority scale is demonstrated for one- and two-syllable words. If we pick the word "windows," could you map these two syllables according to this scale? Now try the word "stops." Does this word comply to the sonority principles, which have the nucleus as the most sonorous and then sonority falling to the edges?

https://www.youtube.com/watch?v=oKhmBz GzyZ8&t=65s

drift

close

In both of these examples, the sonority falls from the nucleus of the syllable outward to the edges. However, this principle is not an absolute. Certain consonant clusters do not follow this principle exactly. The initial clusters /sp/, /st/, and /sk/ reflect a decrease in sonority from the first to the second element. They are considered "adjunct" clusters and are treated differently when being applied to target selection.

Clinical Application

Sonority Principles and the Complexity Approach

The complexity approach uses sonority principles to select treatment targets. The **sonority value difference** between the consonants of a cluster is used to target specific clusters. To calculate the sonority value difference, the sonority rank of each individual consonant within the consonant cluster is subtracted from the other. In general, the consonant cluster with the least sonority difference, the smallest difference, is selected as a target. Those clusters with the least sonority difference are considered the most complex (more marked), whereas those with greater differences are considered less complex (unmarked). There are some other variables that play a role, but the sonority sequencing principle is a central issue for consonant cluster selection. In this case, the "adjunct" clusters, the ones that do not adhere to the sonority sequencing principle, are not typically targeted.

According to the complexity approach, sonority is used to find the most complex target. There are several other variables for target selection, including the clusters not in the child's inventory and the individual consonants not in the child's inventory. More detail on the complexity approach will be given in Chapter 10.

Summary

This chapter first introduced some of the basic terminology and principles underlying contemporary phonological theories. The relationship between the sound form (as phone) and sound function (as phoneme) was established as a basis for understanding phonological theories. The development of the phoneme concept was traced historically to provide a foundation for understanding how phonological theories could evolve from this concept. Clinical application of these basic principles stressed the interrelationship between sound form and sound function.

The remainder of this chapter summarized several phonological theories that affect the assessment and treatment of phonemic-based disorders. These theories were enumerated in a historical sequence. The linear phonologies were represented by distinctive feature theory, generative phonology, and natural phonology. The nonlinear phonologies included feature geometry and optimality theory. In addition, sonority and the sonority sequencing principle, which play a role in the target selection of the complexity approach, were introduced. Each phonological theory was discussed regarding the conceptual framework of the theory, its development and function, and its clinical implications.

The field of phonology is constantly evolving. Current phonological theories attempt to describe the phonological system, with all its complexity, in a different manner. Although some of the newer models have yet to stand the test of time and research in their use with children with speech disorders, all offer new insights into the intricate nature of normal and impaired phonological systems.

Case Study

The phonological process analysis procedure can be demonstrated using a slightly modified clinical example from Chapter 2, page 43. The following sample is from Tina, age 3 years 8 months.

dig	[dɛg]	boat	[boʊt]
house	[haʊθ]	cup	[tʌp]
knife	[nɑf]	lamp	[wæmp]
duck	[dʌt]	goat	[doʊt]
cat	[tæt]	ring	[wɪŋ]
bath	[bæt]	thumb	[tʌm]
red	[wed]	that	[dæt]
ship	[sɪp]	zip	[ðɪp]
fan	[fɛn]	key	[ti]
yes	[jɛθ]	win	[wɪn]

The following errors are noted:

[s] → [θ]	house, yes
[k] → [t]	duck, cat, cup, key
[θ] → [t]	bath, thumb
[ɹ] → [w]	red, ring

[ʃ] → [s]	ship
[l] → [w]	lamp
[g] → [d]	goat
[ð] → [d]	that
[z] → [ð]	zip

The analysis results are as follows:

	Target → Error	Phonological Process
[s] → [θ]	house, yes	fronting
[k] → [t]	duck, cat, cup, key	velar fronting
[θ] → [t]	bath, thumb	stopping
[ɹ] → [w]	red, ring	gliding
[ʃ] → [s]	ship	palatal fronting
[l] → [w]	lamp	gliding
[g] → [d]	goat	velar fronting
[ð] → [d]	that	stopping
[z] → [ð]	zip	fronting

In summarizing the phonological processes, we see that fronting (including both velar and palatal fronting) affected five sounds (s → θ, k → t, ʃ → s, g → d, and z → ð). Both stopping (θ → t and ð → d) and gliding (l, r → w) were noted on two different sounds.

If this sample is analyzed according to feature geometry, which two place features seem to be problematic for this child, one dominating on certain productions and one dominating on others?

Think Critically

The following are the results of a standardized speech assessment for Ryan, age 6 years 6 months:

horse	[hoʊəθ]	pig	[pɪk]	chair	[ʃɛɚ]
wagon	[wægən]	cup	[kʌp]	watch	[waʃ]
monkey	[mʌŋki]	swinging	[ṣwɪŋɪŋ]	thumb	[fʌm]
comb	[koʊm]	table	[teɪbəl]	mouth	[maʊf]
fork	[foɚk]	cat	[kæt]	shoe	[su]
knife	[naɪf]	ladder	[lærɚ]	fish	[fɪs]
cow	[kaʊ]	ball	[bɑl]	zipper	[ðɪpɚ]
cake	[keɪk]	plane	[pweɪn]	nose	[noʊθ]
baby	[beɪbi]	cold	[koʊd]	sun	[θʌn]

bathtub	[bæftəb]	jumping	[dʌmpən]	house	[haʊθ]
nine	[naɪn]	TV	[tivi]	steps	[stɛp]
train	[tweɪn]	stove	[θtoʊv]	nest	[nɛt]
gum	[gʌm]	ring	[wɪŋ]	books	[bʊkθ]
dog	[dɑg]	tree	[twi]	bird	[bɝd]
yellow	[wɛloʊ]	green	[gwin]	whistle	[wɪθəl]
doll	[dɑl]	this	[dɪθ]	carrots	[kɛɚət]

Summarize the errors according to phonological processes. Which phonological processes occur most frequently?

 Chapter Quiz 4.1 Complete this quiz to check your understanding of chapter concepts.

Chapter 5
Normal Phonological Development

Learning Objectives

When you have finished this chapter, you should be able to:

5.1 Describe early structural and functional developments that are precursors to the child's first words.

5.2 Identify specific early perceptual skills that infants demonstrate prior to their first words.

5.3 Outline the characteristics of the prelinguistic stages.

5.4 Discuss the characteristics of the transition between babbling and the first-50-word stage of language development.

5.5 Trace the consonant, vowel, and prosodic development of preschool-age children.

5.6 Describe the consonant, vowel, and prosodic development of school-age children.

5.7 Explain phonological awareness, its relationship to emerging literacy, and the impact of a phonological disorder.

Chapter Application: Case Study

This is Paula's first semester of graduate school in communication disorders. One of her clinical assignments is Phonology Clinic, where she has been assigned three children. All the children are 4 years old and seem to have no other language, perceptual, cognitive, or motor problems besides their phonological disorders. One of the children, Samantha, has problems with /k/, /g/, /ɹ/, and /s/. She demonstrates velar fronting on /k/ and /g/, gliding on /ɹ/ (which includes vowelization of the rhotic vowels), and a dentalized s-sound. James demonstrates final consonant deletion on many words but specifically if the words are more than one syllable. He also has difficulties with r- and s-sounds. He shows gliding of /ɹ/ at the beginning of words and often deletes the vowels with r-coloring at the end of words. He also exhibits stopping of /s/. Luke uses the plosives /t, d/ to replace all of his fricatives, /s, z, ʃ, ʒ, θ, ð/, as well as the affricates /tʃ, ʤ/. Paula wonders where to begin.

She is aware that these children are still developing their speech sounds, and not all sounds should be accurate. Which sounds and processes are developmentally appropriate at this age?

THIS CHAPTER outlines the prelinguistic behavior and phonological development of children from birth to their school years. **Prelinguistic behavior** refers to all vocalizations prior to the first actual words. **Phonological development** refers to the acquisition of speech sound form and function within the language system. In accordance with current terminology, this sound acquisition process is now referred to as *phonological development* rather than as speech sound development, as it was in the past. **Speech sound development** refers primarily to the gradual articulatory mastery of speech sound forms within a given language. Thus, a child's proficiency in producing typical, adult-like speech sound patterns is measured. Phonological development, on the other hand, implies the acquisition of a functional sound system intricately connected to the child's overall growth in language. Learning to produce a variety of sounds is not the same as learning the contrasts among sounds that convey differences in meaning.

The first goal of this chapter is to explore briefly certain structural and functional developments that must occur prior to speech sound production in the infant. In addition, the chapter discusses the development of specific perceptual skills in infants.

The second goal is to examine some of the available information on speech sound development. Organized according to segmental form as well as prosodic development, this survey ranges from the prelinguistic stages to the near completion of the phonological system during the early school years. In reviewing the literature, an attempt will be made to discuss the various studies so that the reader will become aware of differences in design and purpose that have often resulted in contrasting outcomes. In addition, it should be noted that much of the literature focuses on children's acquisition of speech sounds. Little information is available on children's gradual development of the phonemic function and phonotactic constraints of these segments within a language. When possible, these studies are also included.

Various studies have provided guidelines for determining whether a child demonstrates normal versus impaired phonological development. These "mastery" studies are typically based on the results of (1) testing a large number of children, (2) setting a percentage for each age group for normal articulation of the speech sound in question, and (3) establishing age levels that are considered to be the time frame for acquisition of each sound. In addition, they are cross-sectional studies. As important as these studies are, the role of individual variation, especially in a child's younger years, should not be underestimated. The development of speech sounds and the acquisition of a child's phonological system remains an individual process. Although certain trends can be noted when comparing these studies containing large numbers of children, each child's own differences continue to play a large role in the total acquisition process. Both factors—general trends noted in large-scale studies and a child's individual growth and development—are important to consider when evaluating whether a child has a speech sound disorder.

The third goal of this chapter is to highlight interdependencies among phonological awareness, phonological disorders, and emerging literacy. Phonological awareness is an important topic as clinicians see children, and those with phonological disorders, who struggle with emerging literacy. Definitions and selected activity levels are provided to aid clinicians in their understanding of the various skills that comprise phonological awareness.

Aspects of Structural and Functional Development

As the infant begins its journey from primarily crying behavior to babbling and words, important anatomical structures that are prerequisites for sound production need to be considered. Both the structure and the function of respiratory, phonatory, resonatory, and articulatory mechanisms must change considerably before any regular articulatory activities can occur. These necessary changes, which continue through infancy and early childhood, are directly reflected in the transformation of prelinguistic sound productions to linguistic sound productions. The following summary presents a brief outline of the development of the respiratory, phonatory, resonatory, and articulatory systems during this time span.

The shape, size, and composition of the respiratory system are dramatically modified from infancy to adulthood. Newborns and infants are, of course, perfectly able to accumulate enough air pressure against a closed glottis to "phonate" quite impressively. Although small compared to those of adults, babies' lungs are, relative to their body size, proportionally large. Their subglottal pressure (the pressure that accumulates below the closed glottis) is considerable and continues to be so throughout childhood. For example, when comparable loudness levels are contrasted, children demonstrate higher subglottal pressure values than do adults (Stathopoulos & Sapienza, 1993). In addition, compared to the adult, only approximately one-third to one-half of the alveoli are present in the lungs of the newborn (Hislop, Wigglesworth, & Desai, 1986). It is not until a child is approximately 7 to 8 years old that the number of alveoli approaches the adult value (Hislop et al., 1986; Kent, 1997). It is also around this age that children's respiratory function demonstrates adult patterns. Developmental milestones in the respiratory system are summarized in Table 5.1.

Table 5.1 Milestones in the Development of the Respiratory System of the Child

Age	Typical Patterns
Birth	Rest breathing is approximately 30 to 80 breaths per minute. Frequent paradoxical breathing occurs, exemplified by the rib cage making an expiratory movement as the abdomen performs an inspiratory movement. Compared to the adult, only between one-third and one-half of the number of alveoli are present at birth.
1½ to 3 years	Rest breathing rate decreases to approximately 20 to 30 breaths per minute at age 3. Respiratory control increasingly supports the production of longer utterances during this time frame. The number of alveoli increases rapidly, beginning to approximate adult-like values at the end of this period. Small conducting airways surrounding the alveoli increase their dimensions.
7 to 8 years	Rest breathing is approximately 20 breaths per minute. Adult-like breathing patterns are now beginning to be achieved. The number of alveoli reaches adult values at age 8.

Sources: Data from Hislop, A., Wigglesworth, J., & Desai, R. (1986); Kent, R. D. (1997); Thurlbeck, W. (1982); and Zeltner, T., Caduff, J., Gehr, P., Pfenninger, J., & Burri, P. (1987).

The changes in the phonatory and resonatory systems from infancy to childhood are especially impressive. This anatomical-physiological development leads directly to children's future possibilities to articulate specific speech sounds. However, in newborns, the larynx and vocal tract reflect exclusively **primary functions**, the life-supporting roles of the speech mechanism. At this time, the larynx and vocal tract are unable to fulfill any **secondary functions**, those tasks, including articulation of speech sounds, that occur in addition to the life-supporting ones. For example, the oral cavity (with tongue and lips) and the pharyngeal cavity are used primarily for sucking and swallowing actions. The tongue, which in young infants fills the oral cavity completely, leaves practically no space for the buccal area, the space between the outside of the gums and the inside of the cheeks. In addition, a prenatally acquired "sucking pad" (an encapsulated structure of each cheek that supports the lateral rims of the tongue for more effective sucking action) helps to fill out this space entirely. The production of sounds under these conditions is severely restricted. The ability to produce speech sounds is a highly complex process that depends primarily on many anatomical-physiological changes that occur as a product of growth and maturation. Refer to Figure 5.1 for the tongue displacement and the size of several anatomical structures of the newborn infant.

The larynx, too, has to develop structurally before it can effectively contribute to the speech process. In newborns, for example, the arytenoid cartilages and the posterior portion of the cricoid cartilage are disproportionately large when compared to an adult larynx (refer to Figure 5.2). The vocal processes, where the vocal folds attach, are also large in relationship to the other structures. This means that the vocal processes reach deeply into the vocal folds, thus limiting their vibratory action. In addition, the infant's larynx is close to the angle between neck and chin. This high, restricted position of the larynx does not allow the vocal tract to effectively elongate in a downward direction. This elongation is indispensable for some resonating effects during vowel articulation. Note the movement of the larynx for the vowel [i] versus [u], for example.

Stabilization of the pharyngeal airway (necessary for an upright position) is another significant postnatal development. Anatomical changes include the downward displacement of the hyoid bone and larynx away from the base of the skull and mandible and the loss of the aforementioned sucking pad. All of these changes must occur as prerequisites for the articulation of speech sounds.

Figure 5.1 Sagittal Section of the Head of the Newborn Infant Demonstrating the Forward and Downward Placement of the Tongue

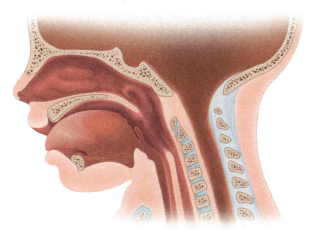

Source: Courtesy of Laura Gallardo.

Figure 5.2 Posterior and Anterior Views of the Laryngeal Structures of an Adult and an Infant

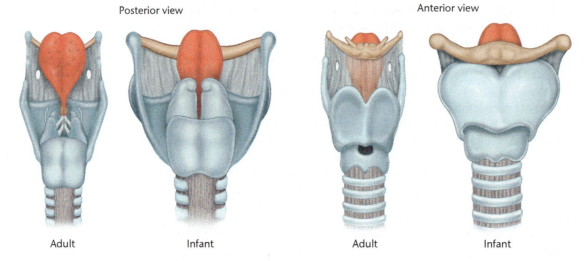

Posterior view Anterior view

Adult Infant Adult Infant

Source: Courtesy of Laura Gallardo.

After a child's first words, which occur around the child's first birthday, the speech mechanism undergoes further enlargement and changes in form. Expansions of the laryngeal and pharyngeal cavities are prominent examples. These expansions co-occur with changes in the form and mobility of the arytenoid cartilages, soft palate, and tongue. The following changes characterize this development:

1. The thyroid cartilage grows more than the cricoid cartilage.
2. The epiglottis becomes larger and firmer.
3. The arytenoid cartilages, which were relatively large in the early stages of this development, now change little in size; they adapt structurally and functionally to the growth of the other laryngeal structures.
4. The vocal and ventricular folds—that is, the "true" and "false" vocal folds—lengthen. This means that more of the vocal folds' muscular portion is now freed for normal vocal cord vibration.

Enlargement of the skull and laryngeal areas during childhood occurs mostly in posterior and vertical directions. This allows the velum more room and thus more mobility. However, the oral area is the site of the greatest changes in available space and resulting mobility. Because of these skeletal changes, the tongue no longer completely fills the mouth. In addition, the tongue and lips change in their dimensions and acquire further flexibility. The fine-tuning and coordination of the lip, mandible, tongue, and velar movements for regular voice and speech production are now increasingly acquired.

To summarize, during infancy, we see enormously complex developmental changes. The infant's larynx, mouth, and pharyngeal areas evolve from a mechanism able to serve only respiratory and feeding purposes to a vocal tract that is structurally and functionally ready to produce speech sounds.

Early Perceptual Development

Although it has often been documented that infants are able to discriminate slight differences in speech sounds within the first months after birth (Best & McRoberts, 2003; Best, McRoberts, & Goodell, 2001; Houston & Jusczyk, 2000; Kuhl et al., 2006), their auditory experiences begin before birth. Human fetuses are able to process auditory stimuli from the external world during the last trimester of pregnancy, with a clear sensitivity to melody contours in language and music (Kisilevsky, Hains, Jacquet, Granier-Deferre, & Lecanuet, 2004; Mampe, Friederici, Christophe, & Wermke, 2009). Newborns prefer their mother's voice over other voices and will actively change their sucking rate to hear her voice more often than another female's voice (Abrams et al., 2016; Augustyn & Zuckerman, 2007). And newborns' cry melodies appear to be shaped by their native language (Mampe et al., 2009).

These results support the notion that infants start to pay attention to and "learn" something about voice and speech prior to birth. However, what evidence do we have about infants' and children's perception and discrimination of speech sounds and phonemic contrasts? The following is a brief overview of these perceptual skills:

- *Categorical perception.* **Categorical perception** refers to the tendency of listeners to perceive speech sounds (which are varied acoustically along a continuum) according to the phonemic categories of their native language. Thus, manipulating variations in voice onset time will produce a clear listener distinction between [ba] and [pa], as if an actual boundary divided the two. Based on changes in measured sucking rates, categorical perception for /b/ and /p/ in the syllables [ba] and [pa] has been demonstrated in infants as young as 1 month of age. Infants under 3 months of age can detect certain differences in place and manner of articulation for consonants. Studies related to the perception of phonemic contrasts in infants are numerous and include those by Cohen and Cashon (2003), Houston and Jusczyk (2000), Jusczyk and Luce (2002), Mareschal and French (2000), Maye and Weiss (2003), and Maye, Werker, and Gerken (2002), for example.

- *Discrimination of non-native sounds in infants.* Since children demonstrate categorical perception between 1 and 3 months of age, it was hypothesized that they might have an inborn ability to make these distinctions. To test this hypothesis, a task was devised in which the discrimination skills of infants were tested with unknown phonemes of non-native languages—that is, languages to which they had not been exposed. Although adult non-native speakers could not differentiate these pairs, results showed that infants up to approximately 6 to 8 months of age could indeed discriminate among non-native sounds that are very similar in their production characteristics. From 6 to 12 months of age, these discrimination abilities decrease, whereas discrimination of native speech sound perception increases (Best & McRoberts, 2003; Kuhl et al., 2006; Rivera-Gaxiola, Silva-Pereyra, & Kuhl, 2005). The conclusion drawn was that language experience may result in the loss of this ability. We do not distinguish between categories that are nonfunctional in our native language. However, there is contrasting evidence to this hypothesis. Polka, Colantonio, and Sundara (2001) found that language experience did not differentiate the group of 10- to 12-month-old English-learning infants when compared to French-learning infants presented with /d/ and /ð/ contrasts. These contrasts do not have phonemic value in French; however, they do in English. It was predicted that the 10- to 12-month-old English learners would be better at this task; however, they were not. This might have to do with the frequency of occurrence of these phonemic contrasts. Refer to the following section on *Perception of Phonemic Contrasts*, Thiessen and Pavlik's (2016) findings.

- *Perceptual constancy.* The ability to identify the same sound across different speakers, pitches, and other changing environmental conditions is known as **perceptual constancy**. Perceptual constancy for vowels and consonants within different contexts has been noted in children from 5½ to 10 months of age (Maye & Gerken, 2000; Werker & Fennell, 2004).

- *Perception of phonemic contrasts.* Shvachkin (1973) and Garnica (1973) examined the ability of toddlers from ages 10 to 22 months to associate minimally paired nonsense syllables to different objects. Could children learn to differentiate phonemes that signal differences in word meaning? These studies found that all children had a developmental progression in the ability to make these distinctions; that is, some distinctions appear to be easier to detect (appear earlier) than others. However, considerable variability was noted among the children as to which features were discriminated earlier and which later. It appears that children still struggle to use phonemic contrasts when confronted with a word-object association task well into the second year of life (e.g., Thiessen, 2007; Thiessen & Yee, 2010). In a series of simulations Thiessen and Pavlik (2016) found that less common phonemes (used in minimal pair contrasts) took longer to be perceived. For example, the very frequent /b/ - /d/ or /d/ - /t/ contrast was established by 18 months of age whereas the less frequent /s/ - /z/ contrast did not emerge until at least 25 months of age. They hypothesize that not all perceptual contrasts are lexical contrasts but are a function of the familiarity with the contrasting phonemes and their frequency of occurrence within the lexicon. It also appears that infants recognize mispronunciations (Aslin, 2014; Swingley & Aslin, 2000). Using eye movements as an indication of recognition/preference, 18- to 23-month-old children recognized both the correctly pronounced and the mispronounced words but recognition was significantly poorer in mispronounced words.

- *Early perceptual abilities related to language development and disorders.* Studies document that early perceptual abilities appear to be related to later language development in children; refer to for example, studies by Kuhl, Conboy, Padden, Nelson, and Pruitt (2005); Tsao, Liu, and Kuhl (2004); and Werker and Tees (2005). Tsao and colleagues (2004) measured speech discrimination in 6-month-old infants using a conditioned head-turn task. At 13, 16, and 24 months of age, language development was assessed in these same children using the MacArthur Communicative Development Inventory. Results demonstrated significant correlations between speech perception at 6 months of age and later language (word understanding, word production, and phrase understanding). The finding that speech perception performance at age 6 months predicts language at age 2 years supports the idea that phonetic perception may play an important role in language acquisition. Early perceptual studies may also show evidence of later difficulties, such as in dyslexia (Bogliotti, 2003; Richardson, Leppaenen, Leiwo, & Lyytinen, 2003). For example, Lyytinen and colleagues (2001) investigated 107 children with a familial risk of dyslexia, comparing them to 93 children without this familial risk. The earliest significant differences between groups were the categorical perception of speech sounds at a few days old (using brain potential responses to speech sounds) and head turning toward the preferred sound at 6 months old. No differences were found between the groups in other measures, such as parental reports of vocalization, motor behavior, or growth of vocabulary (using the MacArthur Communicative Development Scale), before age 2. Similarly, no group differences were found in cognitive and language development assessed by the Bayley Scales of Infant Development and the Reynell Developmental Language Scales before age 2½.

An infant's early perceptual abilities include a wide range of competencies. Many of these abilities develop prior to the actual production of first words. It appears that the infant's early perceptual abilities may also affect later language development, whereas lack of specific skills may be a portion of the symptom complex of disordered language learning.

The next section examines another aspect of the infant's behavior: the prelinguistic stage, which describes vocalizations prior to the first real words. It also shows that specific competencies in this behavior may affect later language development.

Prelinguistic Stages: Before the First Words

Child language development is commonly divided into *prelinguistic behavior*, vocalizations prior to the first true words, and *linguistic development*, which starts with the appearance of the first words. This division is exemplified by the use of early nonmeaningful versus later meaningful sound productions. Jakobson's (1968) *discontinuity hypothesis* clearly emphasized a sharp separation between these two phases. According to his theoretical notion, babbling is a random series of vocalizations in which many different sounds are produced with no apparent order or consistency. Such behavior was seen as clearly separated from the following systematic sound productions evidenced by the first words. The division between prelinguistic and linguistic phases of sound production, according to Jakobson, is often so complete that a child might actually undergo a period of silence between the end of the babbling period and the first real words.

Research since that time (e.g., Boysson-Bardies, 2001; Nathani, Ertmer, & Stark, 2006; Oller, 1980; Oller, Wieman, Doyle, & Ross, 1976; Stark, 1980, 1986) has repeatedly documented that (1) babbling behavior is not random but that children's productions develop in a systematic manner, (2) the consonant-like sounds that are babbled are restricted to a small set of segments, and (3) the transition between babbling and first words is not abrupt but continuous; late babbling behavior and the first words are very similar in respect to the sounds used and the way they are combined. It also appears that children's perceptual abilities are quite developed before the first meaningful utterances. For example, some word comprehension is evident at approximately 7 to 9 months of age (Owens, 2016). The presence of phonemic contrasts in very young children has also been previously documented. Although this acquisition is gradual, more general contrasts begin at approximately 1 year of age. Findings such as these suggest that children's language systems start to develop prior to the first spoken meaningful words during the prelinguistic period.

The following list provides an overview of the *prelinguistic stages* of production described by Stark (1986) and revised slightly by Nathani and colleagues (2006). Although these are referred to as *stages*, there is overlap from one period of development to the next. In addition, individual variations among children necessitate the use of approximate ages.

> *Stage 1: Reflexive crying and vegetative sounds (birth to 2 months).* This stage is characterized by a large proportion of reflexive vocalizations. *Reflexive vocalizations* include cries, coughs, grunts, and burps that seem to be automatic responses reflecting the physical state of the infant. *Vegetative sounds* may be divided into grunts and sighs associated with activity and clicks and other noises associated with feeding.

Stage 2: Cooing and laughter or controlled phonation (1 to 4 months). During this stage, *cooing* or *gooing* sounds are produced during comfortable states. Although these sounds are sometimes referred to as vowel-like, they also contain brief periods of consonantal elements that are produced at the back of the mouth. Early comfort sounds have quasi-resonant nuclei; in other words, they are produced as a syllabic nasal consonant or as a nasalized vowel (Nakazima, 1962; Oller, 1980). From 12 weeks on, a decrease in the frequency of crying is noted, and most infants' primitive vegetative sounds start to disappear. At approximately 16 weeks, sustained laughter emerges.

Stage 3: Vocal play or expansion (3 to 8 months). Although there is some overlap between Stages 2 and 3, the distinguishing characteristics of Stage 3 include longer series of segments and the production of prolonged vowel- or consonant-like steady states. During this stage, the infant often produces extreme variations in loudness and pitch. When compared to those of older children, the transitions between segments in this stage are much slower and incomplete. In contrast to vowels in Stage 2, those in Stage 3 demonstrate more variation in tongue height and position.

Stage 4: Basic canonical babbling (5 to 10 months). Although **canonical babbling**, the collective term for the reduplicated and non-reduplicated babbling stages, usually begins around 5 months of age, most children continue to babble into the time when they say their first words. Stark (1986) describes reduplicated and non-reduplicated, or variegated, babbling as follows: **Reduplicated babbling** is marked by similar strings of consonant-vowel productions. There might be slight quality variations in the vowel sounds of these strings of babbles, but the consonants will stay the same from syllable to syllable. An example of this is [gaga]. **Non-reduplicated** or **variegated babbling** demonstrates variation of *both* consonants and vowels from syllable to syllable. An example of this is [batə]. One major characteristic of this babbling stage is smooth transitions between vowel and consonant productions.

From the previous descriptions, one might conclude that these babbling stages are sequential, with a child first going through reduplicated babbling and later non-reduplicated babbling. This has indeed been documented by Elbers (1982), Oller (1980), and Stark (1986), to mention a few. However, other investigators have questioned this developmental pattern. For example, Mitchell and Kent (1990) assessed the phonetic variation of multisyllabic babbling in eight infants at 7, 9, and 11 months of age. Their findings showed that (1) non-reduplicated babbling was present from the time the infant began to produce multisyllabic babbling (i.e., it did not evolve from an earlier period of reduplicated babbling) and (2) no significant difference existed between the amount of phonetic variation for the vocalizations when the infant was 7, 9, and 11 months old. These and other findings (Holmgren, Lindblom, Aurelius, Jalling, & Zetterstrom, 1986; Smith, Brown-Sweeney, & Stoel-Gammon, 1989) suggest that both reduplicated and variegated forms extend throughout the entire babbling period. A more current study (Geambaşu, Scheel, & Levelt, 2016) using the PhonBank database (Rose & MacWhinney, 2014) analyzed infants' babbling from 7 to 12 months of age for eight different languages. It appears that in certain languages, specific patterns were produced more or less over time. However, in no language did they find the predicted line of development in which reduplicated babbling was most prominent initially and was either gradually or suddenly overtaken by variegated babbling. Instead in most languages, variegated babbling was actually the most prominent pattern from the earliest stages of babbling.

At the beginning of Stage 4, babbling is used in a self-stimulatory manner; it is not used to communicate to adults. Toward the end of this stage, babbling may be used in ritual imitation games with adults (Stark, 1986). This is the beginning of imitative behavior and is an important milestone.

Stage 5: Advanced forms (9 to 18 months). This babbling stage overlaps with the first meaningful words. This is the stage in which jargon as well as diphthongs appear. **Jargon** is characterized by strings of babbled utterances that are modulated primarily by intonation, rhythm, and pausing (Crystal, 1986). It sounds as if a child is actually attempting sentences but without actual words. Because many jargon vocalizations are delivered with eye contact, gestures, and intonation patterns that resemble statements or questions, parents are convinced that the child is indeed trying to communicate something to which they often feel compelled to respond (Stoel-Gammon & Menn, 1997). In this time frame, more complex syllables are also produced, such as CCV (such as [pweɪ] for *play*) or CCVC (such as [bwun] for *balloon*).

The following section examines children's segmental productions toward the end of the canonical babbling stage. Because the productions cannot yet be said to

---

Clinical Exercises Based on the information from the prelinguistic stages, what stage should a child be in before you can hope to verbally stimulate him and possibly expect imitative behavior?

You are working in a birth to 3 years program and are working with a child who you think is beginning to attempt to imitate simple babbling behavior. Based on the information on the most frequently babbled sounds, what type of syllables, vowels, and consonants might you want to attempt to use as stimulation? Refer to pages 124–125.

Clinical Application

Knowledge of Babbling Stages and Diagnostics

Speech-language pathologists, especially those in early intervention services, are often confronted with children beyond 1 year of age who are still within the babbling stages of development. Knowledge of the babbling stages, which includes characteristics and approximate ages of occurrence, can be very helpful in our assessment process. Consider the following information from the parents of Megan, who is 16 months old.

The early intervention program was contacted by Megan's parents, who had been referred by the child's pediatrician. Megan was born 4 weeks premature and had been followed very closely by the parents, the pediatrician, and the early intervention team. She started to walk around 11 months of age, and the parents reported that all developmental milestones up to that point had been within normal limits. The parents were concerned because Megan did not have any real words. All their relatives' children had begun to talk when they were 10 to 12 months old.

The speech-language pathologist visited the family home and noted that Megan was a very active toddler who was busy with her toys and enjoyed attention. Occasionally, Megan produced utterances that consisted of single

(Continued)

vowels, for example, [a], CV structures ([ba], [da], [ma]), and CVCV syllables ([gaga], [babi], [nana], [dati]). According to the parents, repeated attempts to have Megan imitate these babbles had not met with success. It was observed (and the parents verified) that Megan did not use strings of babbles with any intonational patterns; that is, Megan did not produce jargon babbling.

Based on these results, we could deduce that Megan is within the canonical babbling stage. However, she has not reached the point at which she is imitating these babbles in ritualized games with her parents, nor is she using jargon speech. According to the approximate ages presented, jargon babbling begins around 10 months of age. Megan is now 16 months old. This information gives us a general idea of where Megan is within the period of prelinguistic development.

be true vowels and consonants of a particular language system, they are referred to as **vocoids** and **contoids**, respectively. Pike (1943) introduced these terms to indicate *nonphonemic* speech sound productions.

Vocoids: Nonphonemic Vowel-like Productions

Several early investigations with a large number of children were carried out by Irwin and colleagues in the 1940s and 1950s (e.g., Chen & Irwin, 1946; Irwin, 1945, 1946, 1947a, 1947b, 1948, 1951; Irwin & Chen, 1946; Winitz & Irwin, 1958). According to the data on 57 children from 13 to 14 months of age, there was a continued predominance of the [ɛ], [ɪ], and [ʌ] vocoids. Thus, front and central vocoids were found to be favored over high and back vocoids. Later investigations (Davis & MacNeilage, 1990; Kent & Bauer, 1985) generated similar results. However, Selby, Robb, and Gilbert (2000) examined four children between the ages of 15 and 36 months in a longitudinal study. They reported the use of a wide range of vowels by 18 months, with more vowel types being used than had previously been reported. It is interesting to note that the children in their study used a wider variety of back vowels than front vowels, which is in direct contrast to findings in the previous studies.

Contoids: Nonphonemic Consonant-like Productions

Several authors have investigated the contoids, which predominate in the late babbling stage (from 11 to 12 months of age). Locke (1983) provides an excellent overview of the results from three major investigations (refer to Table 5.2). The agreement between these studies is far more striking than the differences. As the data in Table 5.2 indicate, the most frequent contoids were [h], [d], [w], [b], [g], [j] and [m]. The 12 most frequently produced contoids represent about 95% of all the segments transcribed in the three studies (Locke, 1983). In a later study by Robb and Bleile (1994), a slightly different order was established. The most frequent contoids were [h], [m], [d], [b], and [n] (used by at least 50% of the children), and [k], [g], [f], [s], [l] and [w] were used by at least 25% of the children. Both of these results (and many others) stand in contrast to earlier statements that babbling consists of a great multitude of random vocalizations. On the contrary, these and other investigations (Kehoe, 2001; Locke, 1990; Oller, Eilers, Neal, & Schwartz, 1999; Ramsdell, Oller, Buder, Ethington, & Chorna, 2012) suggest that only a rather limited set of phones is babbled.

Table 5.2 English Consonant-like Sounds in the Babbling of 11- and 12-Month-Old American Infants: Percentage of Occurrence[1]

Sound	Frequency	Sound	Frequency
[h]	71%	[l]	3.6%
[d]	64%	[p]	3.2%
[w]	28.8%	[v]	2.0%
[b]	24.8%	[θ]	1.3%
[g]	24.6%	[ð]	1.1%
[j]	22.4%	[f]	.8%
[m]	14.9%	[z]	.6%
[k]	9.4%	[ʃ]	.4%
[n]	8.1%	[ʒ]	.1%
[t]	7.9%	[ɹ]	.1%
[ŋ]	4.5%	[tʃ]	0%
[s]	3.9%	[ʤ]	0%

[1] The percentages are based on a summation of the data found in Irwin (1947a), Fisichelli (1950), and Pierce and Hanna (1974). There are some missing data (2.5%) as certain sounds had no phonemic equivalent in General American English.,

Syllable Shapes

During the later babbling periods, open syllables are still the most frequent type. In the Kent and Bauer (1985) study, for example, V, CV, VCV, and CVCV structures accounted for approximately 94% of all syllables produced. Although closed syllables were present, they were found to be very limited in the repertoires of these infants. However, by 24 months of age, toddlers have expanded their structures considerably. The following syllable structures have been noted: CVC, CVCVC, CCVC, CVCC, CC(C)VCC—for example, by Stoel-Gammon (1987a) and Watson and Scukanec (1997).

Babbling and Its Relationship to Later Language Development

Jakobson's (1968) discontinuity hypothesis denounced any link between babbling and later language development. However, babbling behavior is one aspect of early communication that is emerging as a predictor of later language ability. Several researchers have suggested that both the *quantity* and the *diversity* of vocalizations play a role in later language development.

Attempts have been made to correlate the quantity of vocalizations at a certain babbling age to later language performance (e.g., Brady, Marquis, Fleming, & McLean, 2004; Camp, Burgess, Morgan, & Zerbe, 1987; McCune & Vihman, 2001; Paavola, Kunnari, & Moilanen, 2005; Rothgaenger, 2003). In these studies, *quantity* was defined as the number of vocalizations during a specific time frame. Although somewhat different criteria were used in the various studies, the results showed that the amount of prelinguistic vocalizations was positively related to later language measures.

Diversity of vocalizations was measured in infants by (1) the number of different consonant-like sounds heard in their babbling, (2) the number of structured CV syllables, (3) the proportion of vocalizations containing a true consonant, and (4) the ratio of consonant-like sounds to vowel-like sounds (Boysson-Bardies, 2001; Munson, Edwards, & Beckman, 2005a; Nathani et al., 2006; Oller et al., 1999; Reed, 2018; Rescorla & Ratner, 1996; Whitehurst, Smith, Fischel, Arnold, & Lonigan, 1991). Summarizing the results of these methodologically varying studies, it appears that:

1. Greater language growth is seen in children with more contoid-babble compared to those with more vocoid-babble.
2. Greater language growth is related to greater babble complexity.
3. Greater language growth is related to the increased diversity of contoid productions.

Prosodic Feature Development

Vowels and consonants are combined to produce syllables, words, and sentences. At the same time that we articulate these sound segments, pronunciation varies in other respects. For example, adults use a wide range of pitch and loudness variables that can change the meaning of what is said in a number of ways. Consider the sentence: "You want that. ↘," said with a falling tone at the end, compared to "You want that? ↗," said with a rising tone at the end. (One can even imagine that if *that* is stressed and the vowel prolonged with an excessive rising tone in the second sentence, something incredible is being desired.) The sound segments in these two sentences, [ju wʌnt ðæt], relate to *what* we say; *prosodic features* refer to *how* we say it. **Prosodic features** are larger linguistic units occurring across segments that are used to influence what we say. The linguistically most relevant prosodic features we realize in speech are pitch, loudness, and tempo variations (which include sound duration). They have specific functions and may be analyzed separately. If combined, they constitute the *rhythm* of a particular language or utterance.

The development of prosodic features in infants has gained considerable importance, and research supports the hypothesis positing a close interaction among prosodic features, early child-directed speech (motherese), and early language development (Fernald & Mazzie, 1991; Golinkoff, Can, Soderstrom, & Hirsh-Pasek, 2015; Hsu & Fogel, 2001; Roberts et al., 2013; Song, Demuth, & Morgan, 2010). A better understanding of prosodic features and their development may offer us valuable insights into the transition from babbling to the first words and the close interconnection of segmental and prosodic feature acquisition.

Coinciding with the canonical babbling stage, or starting at approximately 6 months of age, infants use patterns of prosodic behavior. They then consistently use certain features, primarily intonation, rhythm, and pausing (Crystal, 1986). Acoustic analysis shows that falling pitch is the most common intonation contour in the first year of life (e.g., Snow, 1998a, 1998b, 2000). Prosodic patterns continue to diversify toward the end of the babbling period to such a degree that terms such as *expressive jargon* (Stark, 1981) and *prelinguistic jargon* (Crystal, 1986) have been applied to them. These strings of babbles typically sound like adult General American English intonation patterns, giving the impression of sentences without words.

Transition from Babbling to First Words and the First-50-Word Stage

Several studies suggest that babbling and early words have much in common (e.g., Boysson-Bardies & Vihman, 1991; Davis & MacNeilage, 1990; Storkel & Morrisette, 2002; Ttofari, Eecen, Reilly, & Eadie, 2007; Vihman, Ferguson, & Elbert, 1986). In fact, they are often so similar that difficulties arise in differentiating between the two. The main characteristics of the transition from babbling to first words include the following:

1. Primarily monosyllabic utterances
2. Frequent use of stop consonants followed by nasals and fricatives
3. Bilabial and apical productions
4. Rare use of consonant clusters
5. Frequent use of central, mid-front, and low-front vowels ([ʌ, ɛ, æ]).

Despite the similarities, data from Vihman and colleagues (1986) and Davis and MacNeilage (1990) revealed the following distinctions between babbling and first words:

1. A large diversity existed among the children's productions in each of the areas investigated (phonetic tendencies, consonant and vowel inventories, and word selection). The more words the children acquired, the more this diversity seemed to diminish (Vihman et al., 1986).
2. The majority of the children used voiced stops in babbling but not in words; [g] was the most prominent example of this (Vihman et al., 1986).
3. Vowels produced during babbling were used as substitutes for other vowel productions in words. The high-front vowel [i] was a frequent substitute (Davis & MacNeilage, 1990).
4. Productions were context dependent. For example, high-front vowels occurred more frequently following alveolars, high-back vowels following velars, and central vowels following labial consonants (Vihman, 1992). However, Tyler and Langsdale (1996) found little evidence of these context dependencies. The wide range of individual variability could, in part, explain the differences they encountered.

The First-50-Word Stage

Around a child's first birthday, a new developmental era begins: the *linguistic phase*. It starts the moment the first meaningful word is produced. That sounds plain enough, but there are some problems with defining the first meaningful word. Must it be understood and produced by the child in all applicable situations and contexts? Must it have an adult-like meaning to the child? How do we categorize utterances that do not resemble our adult representation but are nevertheless used as words by the child in a consistent manner?

Most define the **first word** as an entity of relatively stable phonetic form that is produced consistently by a child in a particular context and is recognizably related to the adult-like word form of a particular language (Owens, 2016). Thus, if a child says [ba] consistently in the context of being shown a ball, this form would qualify as a word. If, however, the child says [dodo] when being shown the ball, this would not be accepted as a word because it does not approximate the adult form.

Children frequently use "invented words" (Locke, 1983) in a consistent manner, thereby demonstrating that they seem to have meaning for the children. These vocalizations—used consistently but without a recognizable adult model—have historically been called **proto-words** (Menn, 1978), **phonetically consistent forms** (Dore et al., 1976), **vocables** (Ferguson, 1976), and **quasi-words** (Stoel-Gammon & Cooper, 1984).

The time of the initial productions of words is usually called the *first-50-word stage*. This stage encompasses the time from the first meaningful utterance at approximately 1 year of age to when children begin to put two "words" together at approximately 18 to 24 months of age. Whether this stage is actually a separate developmental entity may be questioned. A child's first word may be a plausible starting point, but the strict 50-word cutoff is rather arbitrary. Nevertheless, it appears that children produce approximately 50 meaningful words before the next generally recognized stage of development, the *two-word stage*, begins.

During the first-50-word stage, there seems to be a large gap between the children's productional versus perceptual capabilities. For example, at the end of this stage, when children can produce approximately 50 words, they are typically capable of understanding around 200 words (Ingram, 1989a). This fact must have an effect on the development of semantic meaning as well as on the phonological system. It must be clearly understood that by analyzing children's verbal productions during this stage, we are looking at only one aspect of language development. Their perceptual, motor, and cognitive growth, as well as the influence of the environment, all play indispensable roles in this stage of language acquisition.

In examining the course of phonological development during this period, we see that it is heavily influenced by the individual words children are acquiring. Children are not just learning sounds, which they then use to make up words, but rather seem to learn word units that happen to contain particular sets of sounds. Ingram (2010) called this a *presystematic stage* in which contrastive words rather than contrastive phones (i.e., as phonemes) are acquired. The presystematic stage can be related to Cruttenden's (1981) *item learning* and *system learning* stages of early phonological development. In **item learning**, children first acquire word forms as unanalyzed units, or productional wholes. Only later, characteristically after the first-50-word stage, does **system learning** occur, during which children acquire the phonemic principles of the phonological system in question.

The early portion of the item learning stage is known as the *holophrastic period*, the span of time during which children use one word to indicate a complete idea. In this phase, the link between the object, its meaning, and the discrete sound segments used to represent the object is not yet firmly established. For example, a child might produce [da] to indicate a dog. The next day, the production might change somewhat, perhaps to [do]. This time, the production may not refer to a dog alone but also to a cow or horse. Sounds and meanings drift and change.

Segmental Form Development

Several authors (e.g., Ingram, 1989b; Robb & Bleile, 1994) have noted (1) *phonetic variability*, (2) a *limitation of syllable structures*, and (3) a *limitation of sound segments* during the first-50-word stage. **Phonetic variability** refers to the unstable pronunciations of children's first 50 words. However, it appears that some productions are more stable than others and that some children have a tendency to produce more stable articulations from the beginning of the first-50-word stage. Based on the child's relatively small repertoire of sounds, it would follow that syllable structures and segments might be limited. However, what are the actual limitations during the first-50-word stage?

First, certain syllable types clearly predominate during the first-50-word stage. These are CV, VC, and CVC syllables. Based on the longitudinal investigation of twelve children, Watson and Scukanec (1997) noted the predominance of CV, CVC, and CVCV syllable structures from 2 to 3 years of age. While the CV and CVCV syllable structures decreased during this year time frame, the CVC structures increased. This, of course, does not mean that other syllable types do not occur. For example, the individual longitudinal data from Ferguson and Farwell (1975), French (1989), Ingram (1974), Leopold (1947), Menn (1971), Stoel-Gammon and Cooper (1984), and Velten (1943) indicate that these syllables indeed occur most frequently. However, the children produced other syllables as well. For instance, Menn's Daniel produced CCVC [njaj], Leopold's Hildegard produced CCVCV [pɹti], and Ferguson and Farwell's T produced CVCVVC [wakuak]. Watson and Scukanec (1997) found evidence of both CVCC and CCVC structures in several of the two-year-olds investigated. However, if the 3-year-old children were examined, more CVCC structures (compared to CCVC structures) were noted. This would indicate that consonant clusters in the word-final position are more frequent than word-initially.

If an individual child is examined to see whether patterns emerge, differences can be found. Certain children seem to favor specific types of syllables. For example, some children evidence CVC structures to a moderate degree from the very beginning of the first-50-word stage. With others, CVC syllables appear only later and do not constitute any major part of the children's phonology until after the first-50-word stage (Ingram, 1976).

Although certain phonetic similarities have been verified, several investigations have pointed out the wide range of variability among individual subjects (e.g., Robb & Bleile, 1994; Stoel-Gammon & Cooper, 1984; Vihman, 1992; Vihman et al., 1986). If one wants to generalize, the marked use of voiced labial and dental stops and nasals ([b], [d], [m], [n]) must be underlined. For a summary of findings substantiating these generalizations from five different investigations, refer to Table 5.3. The data in Table 5.3 compare the consonant inventory of 7 children labeled "Stanford" (Vihman et al., 1986) to 19 children from other research studies noted in the table. As can be seen, all the children have words containing [b] and [m]. More than half of the children in the studies produced [p], [t], [d], [k], [g], [ʃ], [n], [w], and [h] consonants as well.

It should be noted that the Vihman and colleagues (1986) data in Table 5.3 reduce the individual variation among children considerably. For example, if child A produces 2 words with word-initial [n] and child B produces 43 words with word-initial [n], both of these children are counted as having [n] use in this table. However, the use of this particular sound in the two children's inventories is hardly comparable.

LONGITUDINAL FINDINGS. Longitudinal research is an important aspect of studying speech sound development. Longitudinal research follows a child or a group of children over a specific time frame. Such research has the advantage of observing the *acquisition* process of individual children. Longitudinal research demonstrates how children actually develop specific skills. This is far better than just the snapshot view of cross-sectional research. In cross-sectional studies, children are typically grouped into age categories. Thus, if the study examines 3-year-old children, one group might consist of children from ages 3 years to 3 years 6 months and the second group would consist of children from ages 3 years 7 months to 4 years. This type of study does not examine how a child develops but rather the general characteristics of a specific age group of children.

Longitudinal research is often limited in that only one child or a small group of subjects is evaluated. Stoel-Gammon (1985) presented a longitudinal investigation that not only used spontaneous speech but also included a sizable number of children. Thirty-four children between 15 and 24 months of age participated in this

Table 5.3 Initial Consonant Productions in the First-50-Word Vocabularies of 7 Stanford Subjects and 19 Other English-Speaking Children

	Stanford	Others[1]		Stanford	Others[1]
p	×	+	ʃ	+	+
b	×	×	ʒ	0	0
t	×	+	tʃ	−	−
d	×	+	dʒ	−	−
k	×	+	m	×	×
g	+	+	n	×	+
f	+	−	ŋ	−	−
v	−	0	l	−	−
θ	+	−	ɹ	+	−
ð	+	−	w	+	+
s	−	−	j	+	−
z	−	−	h	+	+

Note: × = all children in study; + = more than half but not all children in study; − = more than one but less than half the children in study; 0 = none of the children

[1] Data derived from Ferguson and Farwell (1975); Shibamoto and Olmsted (1978); Leonard, Newhoff, and Mesalam (1980); and Stoel-Gammon and Cooper (1984).

Source: Based on M. M. Vihman, C. A. Ferguson, and M. Elbert, *Phonological Development from Babbling to Speech: Common Tendencies and Individual Differences.* Copyright © 1986 by Cambridge University Press.

study. The investigation was constructed to examine meaningful speech only; therefore, the subjects were grouped according to the age at which they began to say at least 10 identifiable words within a recording session. This resulted in three groups of children: Group A, whose children had 10 words at 15 months; Group B, whose children had 10 words at 18 months; and Group C, whose children had 10 words at 21 months. Additional longitudinal investigations by Robb and Bleile (1994) and Watson and Scukanec (1997) in general supported the Stoel-Gammon data. Refer to Table 5.4 for an overview of these three studies. The data from these three longitudinal studies provide information about early consonant development and can be summarized as follows:

1. A larger inventory of sounds was found in the word-initial position than in the word-final position.
2. Word-initial inventories contained voiced stops prior to voiceless ones; the reverse was true for word-final production: In word- or syllable-final positions voiceless stops were used prior to voiced ones.
3. The following phones appeared in at least 50% of the subjects by 24 months of age in all three studies:
   [b, d, t, k, m, n, w, s] word-initial
   [t, k, n, and s] word-final.

Table 5.4 Consonant Inventories of 18- to 30-Month-Old Children According to Three Longitudinal Studies

Age	Research Study	Word- or Syllable-Initial Position Inventories	Word- or Syllable-Final Position Inventories
18 months	Stoel-Gammon (1985)	b, d, m, n, w, h	t
	Robb and Bleile (1994)	b, d, m, n, w, h	t, h, s
21 months	Stoel-Gammon (1985)	b, d, t, k, m, n, h	t, n
	Robb and Bleile (1994)	b, d, g, t, k, m, n, w, s, z	k, n, h, s
24 months	Stoel-Gammon (1985)	b, d, g, t, k, m, n, w, h, f, s	p, t, k, n, s, ɹ
	Robb and Bleile (1994)	b, d, p, t, k, m, n, w, s	t, k, n, s
	Watson and Scukanec (1997)	b, d, p, t, k, m, n, w, j, h, s	p, t, k, m, n, s, z
27 months	Watson and Scukanec (1997)	b, d, g, p, t, k, m, n, w, j, l, h, s, f	p, t, d, m, n, s, z
30 months	Watson and Scukanec (1997)	b, d, g, p, t, k, m, n, w, j, l, h, s, f, ʧ pw, bw	p, t, k, d, m, n, s, z nd, ts

The criteria for inclusion of the phone was somewhat different from study to study. For inclusion in the inventory, Stoel-Gammon (1985) used 50% of the children; Robb and Bleile (1994), 60%; and Watson and Scukanec (1997) stated 7 out of 12 children (58%) must use the phone. For consonant clusters a cut-off of 50% was employed.

Clinical Application

Developmental Research and Therapeutic Implications

It is often stated that speech-language pathologists follow a developmental model in therapy; that is, those sounds or processes that occur earlier developmentally are targeted earlier than those that occur later. The three studies (Robb & Bleile, 1994; Stoel-Gammon, 1985; Watson & Scukanec, 1997) support techniques that are typically used in therapy:

1. *Sounds first appear in the word-initial position.* In therapy, a newly acquired sound is normally placed in the word-initial position. Developmental data give evidence that this is indeed easier for a child.

2. *Anterior stops and nasals are acquired earlier.* In therapy, this is often used as a guiding principle. These sounds occur very early and therefore should be in children's speech. Even most children with phonological disorders have these sounds in their consonant inventories.

Other interesting results from the Stoel-Gammon (1985) study are not often used in therapy:

1. *The vowel -r nearly always appeared in word-final position before the consonantal [ɹ] in word-initial position.* Based on this finding, words such as *more* and *bear* might be easier than *red* and *rope* for children with [ɹ] difficulties (assuming that a specific child has difficulty with the central vowels with r-coloring *and* the approximant [ɹ]).

2. *Word-initial inventories contained voiced stops first; word-final inventories contained voiceless stops first.* According to this finding, children with [k] and [g] problems might benefit from first working on [g] in the word-initial position before addressing [k] in the word-final position. (This is based on the earlier result that sounds appear first in the word-initial position followed by later use in the word-final position.)

(Continued)

3. *Consonant clusters are beginning to emerge at 3 years of age.* The difference between emerging and mastery is a point for clinicians and their work with children. Consonant clusters do appear in the early speech of children and should be seen as emerging, and thus, could be worked on in therapy. Clinicians often feel that consonant clusters are the last phonological units to emerge and avoid them in their therapy practice.

Although individual variability was observed in these investigations, the ability to follow the children in a longitudinal manner seemed to reduce the extreme diversity noted in cross-sectional research. Although these studies did not contain a large number of subjects, it certainly suggests some clinical implications.

A summary of three longitudinal studies is contained in Table 5.4. The Robb and Bleile study had 7 children while the Watson and Scukanec had 12 children. The Watson and Scukanec data began at 24 months so there are no results for the 18- to 24-month-old range. However, consonant clusters are included from that research for 30 months of age.

INDIVIDUAL ACQUISITION PATTERNS. Throughout this discussion, individual variability has been stressed. The next question follows automatically: Do children show individual acquisition patterns or strategies? Do children build their phonological and lexical inventory in a child-centered or adult-centered manner? Thus, is the selection of early words based on children's developing phonological systems, or do children try to match the lexical items noted in adults' speech? After a review of the research, Stoel-Gammon (2011) stated that children from birth to approximately 2 years 6 months of age appear to have some knowledge of their own production abilities. They choose words for their vocabulary that closely match their production preferences or words that can be modified to fit those preferences. Thus, early patterns of word selection are related more to individual production preferences than to the lexicon of the native language.

The following Clinical Application demonstrates two children's variation in their development from 10 to 16 months. Their individual acquisition patterns are very different.

Clinical Application

Comparing Jakobson's Results to the First Words of Two Children

The following are the first words of Joan Velten (Velten, 1943) and Jennika lngram (Ingram, 1974).

	Joan			Jennika	
Age	Words	Actual Production	Age	Words	Actual Production
10 months	up	[ap]	1 year 3 months	blanket	[ba], [babi]
	bottle	[ba]		byebye	[ba], [baba]
11 months	bus	[bas]		daddy	[da], [dada], [dadi]
	put on	[baza]		dot	[dat], [dati]
	that	[za]		hi	[hai]
1 year	down	[da]		mommy	[ma], [mami], [mama]

	Joan			Jennika	
Age	**Words**	**Actual Production**	**Age**	**Words**	**Actual Production**
	out	[at]			
	away	['ba ba]		no	[no]
	pocket	[bat]		see	[si]
				see that	[si æt]
1 year 1 month	fuff	[af], [faf]		that	[da]
	put on	[baɪda]			
1 year 2 months	push	[bus]	1 year 4 months	hot	[hat]
	dog	[uf]		hi	[hai], [haidi]
	pie	[ba]		up	[ap], [api]
3 months	duck	[dat]		no	[nodi], [dodi], [noni]
	lamb	[bap]			
1 year 4 months	M	[am]			
	N	[an]			
	in	[ņ]			

If the month increments are seen as later phases of development, the following order occurs in the first words for Joan and Jennika:

	Joan	Jennika
Vowels	[a] → [u]	[a], [i], [o], [æ], [ai]
Consonants	[p], [b] → [s], [z] → [t], [d] → [f] → [m], [n]	[b], [d], [t], [h], [m], [n], [s] → [p]
Syllable shapes	VC, CV → CVC, CVCV	CV, CVCV, CVC → VC, VCV
	CVCVs are not reduplications	Most CVCVs are reduplications
Phonetic variability	Fairly stable forms	More variability

The difference between the children is remarkable. For example, Jennika has a wide array of sounds before she produces [p], whereas [m] and [n] do not appear until Joan has produced plosives and fricatives.

Prosodic Feature Development

As children move from the end of the babbling period to first words, the previously noted intonational contours continue. The falling intonation contour still predominates, although both a rise–fall and a simple rising contour have also been observed (Kent & Bauer, 1985).

An important aspect of communication during the first-50-word stage is *prosodic variation*. Examples of children's speech during this stage have included pitch variations to indicate differences in meaning. For example, a child realized a falling pitch on the first syllable, [da↓ da], as Daddy entered the room versus a rising pitch on the first syllable, [da↑ da], when a noise was heard outside when Daddy was expected (Crystal, 1986). Prosodic features are also used to indicate differences in syntactical function. A demand or question, for example, is often signaled first by prosody; words are added later. For example, a child 1 year 2 months of age first used the phrase "all gone" after dinner by humming the intonation. Approximately a month passed before the child's segmental productions were somewhat accurate (Crystal, 1986). One widely held view is that these prosodic units fulfill a social function. They are seen as a means of signaling joint participation in an activity shared by the child and the caregiver. Several authors suggest that prosodic features are evidence of developing speech acts (Dore, 1975; Halliday, 1975; Menn, 1976). A word with a specific intonation pattern might indicate requesting, calling, or demanding, for example. The following prosodic features associated with intentional communication have been observed (Marcos, 2001):

10 to 12 Months

First words, naming, labeling

Begin with a falling contour only. A flat or level contour is usually accompanied by variations such as falsettos or variations in duration or loudness.

Example: At 10 and 11 months, Hildegard (Leopold, 1947) lengthened the vowels of words such as [de:] for *there*.

13 to 15 Months

Requesting, attention getting, curiosity, surprise, recognition, insistence, greeting

Rising contour. High falling contour that begins with a high pitch and drops to a lower one.

Example: This is noted in the previous example of [da↑ da].

Prior to 18 Months

Playful anticipation, emphatic stress

High rising and high rising–falling contour.

Example: A child might use a high rising intonation pattern on *ball* to indicate that the game is about to begin.

Around 18 Months

Warnings, playfulness

Falling–rising contour. Rising–falling contour.

Example: A child might use a falling–rising contour on *no* to indicate that she has been warned not to do that—that is, to repeat this warning. The same *no* with a rising–falling contour could be used during a game to indicate that Daddy is not going to get the ball.

As can be noted, intonational changes seem to develop prior to stress. Although various pitch contours appear earlier than the first meaningful words, contrastive stress is first evidenced at the beginning of the two-word stage or at the age of approximately 1 year 6 months. During the first-50-word stage, the observed pitch variations can be said to represent directional sequences (rising versus falling, for example) or range patterns (high versus low within the child's pitch range). For a more detailed analysis of early intonational development, refer to Crystal (1986) and Snow (1998a, 1998b, 2000, 2017).

Consonant, Vowel, and Prosodic Development of the Preschool-Age Child

This section provides information on the developing phonology of children from approximately the end of the first-50-word stage, to the beginning of their sixth year. During this time, the largest growth within the phonological system takes place. However, not only is a child's phonological system expanding but large gains are seen in other language areas. From 18 to 24–30 months of age, a child's expressive vocabulary at least triples from 50 to 150–300 words, and the receptive vocabulary grows from 200 to 1200 words (review by Ingram, 2008). The transition from one-word utterances to two-word sentences, a large linguistic step, typically occurs at this time. With the production of two-word sentences, a child enters the period of expressing specific semantic relationships: the beginning of syntactical development.

By the time children reach kindergarten, they have a vocabulary of approximately 8000 words. Almost all of the basic grammatical forms of the language—such as questions, negative statements, dependent clauses, and compound sentences—are present as well (Berko Gleason & Ratner, 2017; Owens, 2016). More important, the child knows how to use language to communicate in an effective manner. A 5-year-old talks differently to babies than to her friends, for example. The child also knows how to tell jokes and riddles and is able to handle the linguistic subtleties of being polite and rude.

A child's phonological development at 18 to 24 months of age still demonstrates a rather limited inventory of speech sounds and phonotactic possibilities. At this time, perception seems to somewhat precede production. By the end of the preschool period, around the child's fifth birthday, an almost complete phonological system has emerged.

All these changes occur in less than 4 years. Although this section focuses on phonological development, such a discussion must always be seen within the context of the equally large expansions in morphosyntax, semantics, and pragmatics that occur during this time.

Segmental Form Development: Vowels

One area of sound acquisition that has been widely neglected in most discussions of phonological development is the acquisition of vowels. This neglect has been at least partially justified with the statement that children acquire all vowels within the sound inventory of General American English by the age of 3 (Templin, 1957). According to the Irwin and Wong (1983) data, children show the acquisition of [ɑ], [ʊ], [i], [ɪ], and [ʌ] at 18 months of age if the criterion is set at 70% accuracy. For the individual subjects at this age level, the correct production of vowels ranged from 23% to 71%. By 24 months of age, the only vowels that did not reach 70% group accuracy were [ɝ] and [ɚ]. By the age of 3, all the vowels were accounted for, with virtually no production errors. More recently, data from the Memphis Vowel Project (Pollock, 2013; Pollock & Berni, 2003) seem to support Irwin and Wong (1983). Pollock and Berni (2003) noted that between 18 and 35 months of age, the percentage of nonrhotic vowel errors was relatively high. However, after 36 months, nonrhotic vowel errors were minimal (0% to 4%). However, in relationship to rhotic vowels, Pollock (2013) notes that, at 30 to 35 months of age, accuracy was only 61%. It is not until 48 to 53 months of age that accuracy of rhotic vowels is above 90% (at 36 to 41 months of age, accuracy is 80%; at 42 to 53 months of age, accuracy is 78%).

Far more information is needed in the area of vowel acquisition. From the data presently available, it appears that nonrhotic vowels are indeed generally mastered by the age of 3. Whether individual variation plays a large role in this acquisition process still needs to be documented. This is an interesting area of research, especially in light of the deviant vowel systems that can be noted in children with speech sound disorders.

Segmental Form Development: Consonants

CROSS-SECTIONAL RESULTS. It appears that no chapter on phonological development can be complete without looking at the large-sample studies that began in the 1930s (Wellman, Case, Mengert, & Bradbury, 1931) and have continued periodically since that time. However, it seems appropriate to preface such a discussion by highlighting the problems inherent in these studies.

Large-sample studies on phonological development were initiated to examine which sounds were mastered at which age levels. To this end, the studies evaluated most of the speech sounds within a given native language. With a few exceptions (Irwin & Wong, 1983; Olmsted, 1971; Stoel-Gammon, 1985, 1987a), these studies have used methods similar to those used in standardized speech assessments to collect their data; that is, the children were asked to name pictures and certain sounds that were then judged productionally as "correct" or "incorrect."

In this type of procedure, general as well as specific problems arise. First, the fact that a child produces the sound "correctly" as a one-word response does not mean that the sound can also be produced "correctly" in natural speech conditions. Practitioners have always been aware of the often large articulatory discrepancies between one-word responses and the same sounds used in conversation. Second, the choice of pictures and words will certainly affect the production of the individual sounds within the word. Not only does a child's familiarity with the word play a role but factors such as the length of the word, its structure, the stressed or unstressed position of the sound within the word, and the phonetic context in which the sound occurs are also involved. These factors help or hinder production. Therefore, strictly speaking, the only conclusion that can be drawn from cross-sectional studies is that a child could or could not produce a particular sound in a specific word.

The third point is a theoretical issue. As stated repeatedly in this text, certain newer concepts and terminology have been adopted within the field of speech-language pathology. This chapter's title, for example, refers to phonological development, not speech sound development. With the inclusion of the terms *phonology* and *phonological development*, certain conceptual changes have been accepted. These cross-sectional studies are perhaps indicative of the inventory of speech sounds that children typically possess at certain ages, but they do not document a particular child's phonological system.

All large cross-sectional studies have the inherent problem of being just that: cross-sectional. This means that the child says words based on pictures (rather than engaging in conversational speech) for a one-time snapshot of this child's articulation. The end product of these investigations—data for children from 3 to 6 years of age, for example—is simply an artifact of the groupings of the children. Children are put into groups according to their age. This does not demonstrate the development of a particular child's phonology, but rather eliminates individual variations through the process of grouping. Within this chapter, the author has attempted to provide longitudinal data when possible. Longitudinal data follow a child over a period of time. This gives a far more accurate picture of a particular child's development.

Specific methodological differences among various cross-sectional studies, including the criteria used to determine whether a child has "mastered" a particular sound, are also important factors when interpreting the results. Although this has been elaborated on in several articles and books (e.g., Smit, 1986; Vihman, 2004), it is worth mentioning again. Table 5.5 provides a comparison of several of the larger cross-sectional studies.

Table 5.5 Age Levels for Speech Sound Development According to Six Cross-Sectional Studies

	Wellman et al. (1931)	Poole (1934)	Templin (1957)	Prather et al. (1975)	Arlt and Goodban (1976)	Smit (1993b)
m	3	3½	3	2	3	2
n	3	4½	3	2	3	2
ŋ	not tested	4½	3	2	3	4
p	4	3½	3	2	3	2
b	3	3½	4	2 years 8 months	3	2
t	5	4½	6	2 years 8 months	3	2
d	5	4½	4	2 years 4 months	3	3
k	4	4½	4	2 years 4 months	3	2
g	4	4½	4	2 years 4 months	3	2
w	3	3½	3	2 years 8 months	3	2
j	4	4½	3½	2 years 4 months	not tested	3½
l	4	6½	6	3 years 4 months	4	5½
ɹ	5	7½	4	3 years 4 months	5	7
h	3	3½	3	2	3	2
f	3	5½	3	2 years 4 months	3	3
v	5	6½	6	4	3½	4
s	5	7½	4½	3	4	6
z	5	7½	7	4	4	6
ʃ	not mastered by age 6	6½	4½	3 years 8 months	4½	3½
ʒ	6	6½	7	4	4	not tested
θ	not mastered by age 6	7½	6	4	5	5½
ð	not mastered by age 6	6½	7	4	5	4½
tʃ	5	**not tested**	4½	3 years 8 months	4	3½
dʒ	not mastered by age 6	**not tested**	7	4	4	3½

Sources: Data from Wellman, B. L., Case, I. M., Mengert, I. G., & Bradbury, D. E. (1931); Poole, I. (1934); Templin, M. (1957); Prather, E. M., Hedrick, D., & Kern, C. (1975); Arlt, P. B., & Goodban, M. T. (1976); and Smit, A. B. (1993b).

Looking at the age comparisons in Table 5.5, we can observe a difference in reported mastery of 3 or more years for some sounds. For example, note the difference in the ages of mastery for [s] in the Prather, Hedrick, and Kern (1975) and Poole (1934) studies. The Poole investigation has a mastery age of 7½ years, whereas the Prather and colleagues investigation shows a mastery age of 3 years. A 3-year difference can be found for [z] acquisition when the Prather and colleagues data are compared to the Templin (1957) results. Again, Prather and colleagues assign a much earlier age of mastery. Many of these differences result from the way the term *mastery* was defined. Poole, for instance, stated that 100% of the children must use the sound correctly in each of the positions tested. Prather and colleagues and Templin, on the other hand, set the level at 75%. In addition, rather than using a cutoff of 75% for all three positions (initial, medial, and final), as Templin had done, Prather and colleagues used only two positions (initial and final) for their calculations. The Smit (1993b) data noted in Table 5.5 did not report a mastery age. However, these ages have been calculated from the results of the study and set at 75%. The Smit (1993b) study used primarily initial- and final-word positions. Only [l] and [ɹ] were tested in the medial position. This clearly changes the ages at which mastery can be assigned. The shift noted in the Prather and colleagues study could be accounted for by these methodological changes. Also, as Smit (1986) points out, the Prather and colleagues results are based on incomplete data sets, especially for the younger age groupings. Although Prather and colleagues began with 21 subjects in each age group, several of these children did not respond to many of the words. Thus, at times, only 8 to 12 children were used to calculate the norms. The children who did not respond to some words may have been avoiding them because they felt that they could not pronounce them "correctly".

Several investigators (e.g., Irwin & Wong, 1983; Stoel-Gammon, 1985) have attempted to improve the situation by using spontaneous speech and/or longitudinal investigations. Although spontaneous speech samples are in some respects better than the picture-naming tasks, several problems remain. Speech samples can also give us a biased picture. We actually probe only a small portion of a child's conversational abilities and then generalize, assuming that this is representative of the child's overall performance. Also, factors outside our control might determine which words and sounds the child does produce and which ones he does not. As a result, the sample obtained will probably not contain all the sounds in the particular child's phonetic inventory.

Longitudinal data, on the other hand, can give us real insight into the individual acquisition process, an important aspect missing in cross-sectional studies. The following discussion examines data from longitudinal studies on consonant development in children.

LONGITUDINAL RESULTS. Several longitudinal studies of consonant development exist, but they report on either a single child or a small group of children (e.g., Leopold, 1947; Menn, 1971; Vihman, Macken, Miller, Simmons, & Miller, 1985; Watson & Scukanec, 1997). Therefore, the data cannot be readily generalized. Vihman and Greenlee (1987) used a longitudinal methodology to examine the phonological development of ten 3-year-old children, with the following results:

1. Stops and other fricatives were substituted for [ð] and [θ] by all children.

2. More than half of the children also substituted sounds for [ɹ] and [l] (gliding) and used palatal fronting, in which a palatal sound is replaced by an alveolar ([ʃ] becomes [s]).

3. Two of the 10 children demonstrated their own particular "style" of phonological acquisition.

4. On average, 73% of the children's utterances were judged intelligible by three raters unfamiliar with the children. However, the range of intelligibility was broad, extending from 54% to 80%. As expected, children with fewer errors were more intelligible than those with multiple errors. Another factor also played a role: The children who used more complex sentences tended to be more difficult to understand.

This last finding is significant. It documents the complex interaction between phonological development and the acquisition of the language system as a whole. The simultaneous acquisition of complex morphosyntactic and semantic relationships could well have an impact on the growth of the phonological system. In addition, it has been hypothesized that **phonological idioms** (Moskowitz, 1971) or **regression** (Leopold, 1947) occurs as a child attempts to master other complexities of language. Both terms refer to accurate sound productions that are later replaced by inaccurate ones. When trying to deal with more complex morphosyntactic or semantic structures, the child's previously correct articulations appear to be lost, replaced by inaccurate sound productions.

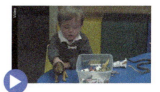

Video Example 5.1
In this video, 2-year-old Ryan plays with toy animals and a farmhouse. Notice the characteristics of his speech productions. The clinician prompts a lot, which helps with understanding his speech. How intelligible would you say his speech is? Could you understand 50% of what he said? How about 75%?

Phonological Processes

According to natural phonology, there seems to be a time frame during which normally developing children do suppress certain processes. This approximate age of suppression is helpful when determining normal versus disordered phonological systems and can be used as a guideline when targeting remediation goals. The following sections address some developmental aspects of syllable structure, substitution, and assimilation processes. Definitions and examples of phonological processes are provided in "Natural Phonology" in Chapter 4.

SYLLABLE STRUCTURE PROCESSES. Syllable structure processes address the general tendency of young children to reduce words to basic CV structures. These processes become evident between the ages of 1 year 6 months and 4 years, when there is a rapid growth in vocabulary and the onset of two-word utterances (Ingram, 1989b).

Reduplication is an early syllable structure process. Ingram (1989b) notes that it is a common process during children's first-50-word stage. There was no evidence of this process, however, in the youngest group of children (ages 1 year 6 months to 1 year 9 months) in the Preisser, Hodson, and Paden (1988) study.

Final consonant deletion is a relatively early process. Preisser and colleagues (1988) state that it was extremely rare in the utterances of the children in the 2 years 2 months to 2 years 5 months age group. Ingram (1989b) and Grunwell (1987) note the disappearance of this process around age 3. However, it seems as if this time frame can extend to a later age. Haelsig and Madison (1986) and James (2001) noted final consonant deletion up to age 4 years 6 months.

Unstressed syllable deletion, sometimes called *weak syllable deletion*, lasts until approximately 4 years of age (Ingram, 1989b). This is also confirmed by Grunwell's (1987)

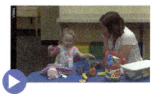

Video Tool Exercise 5.1
Three-Year-Old Carrie Playing with Her Doll
Complete the activity based on this video.

data. However, Preisser and colleagues (1988) noted that most of the children in their sample appeared to have suppressed this process by around their second birthday. (Only 3% of the 20 children over age 2 years 2 months demonstrated unstressed syllable deletion.) Haelsig and Madison (1986) and James (2001) noted this process in children as old as 5 years.

Cluster reduction is a syllable structure process in which a two-consonant cluster is reduced to one element, such as [tɑp] for "stop" or a three-consonant cluster is reduced to one or two consonant elements. Thus, "straw" may become [tɑ] or [twɑ]. Note that a cluster reduction may contain substitutions as well. It appears that consonant cluster reduction is eliminated by approximately 4 years of age (e.g., Bowen, 2011; Grunwell 1987). It appears that consonant cluster reduction is suppressed before consonant cluster substitution. For example, the Smit (1993a) and McLeod, van Doorn, and Reed (2001) data support a general trend of reduction [noʊ] for "snow" followed by consonant cluster substitution [θnoʊ] for "snow".

Epenthesis refers to the insertion of a sound segment into a word, thereby changing its syllable structure. The intrusive sound can be a vowel as well as a consonant, but most often it is restricted to a schwa insertion between two consonants. This schwa insertion—for example, [pəliz] for *please*—is used to simplify the production difficulty of consonant clusters. Smit (1993a) and Smit, Hand, Freilinger, Bernthal, and Bird (1990) report that between the ages of 2 years 6 months and 8 years, schwa insertion in clusters is a common process. Therefore, the suppression of this process can extend to 8 years.

SUBSTITUTION PROCESSES.   *Stopping* refers most frequently to replacing stops for fricatives and affricates. Because fricatives and affricates are acquired at different ages, stopping is not a unified process but should be broken down into the individual sounds for which this process is used. Table 5.6 summarizes the ages at which stopping is suppressed for the different fricative sounds.

Fronting denotes the tendency of young children to replace palatals and velars with alveolar consonants. Frequently occurring fronting processes consist of [ʃ] → [s] palatal fronting and [k] → [t] and [g] → [d] velar fronting. Palatal fronting may also occur in affricate productions, [tʃ] → [ts] and [ʤ] → [dz]. Lowe, Knutson, and Monson (1985) found velar fronting to be more prevalent than palatal fronting. They also found that fronting rarely occurred in normally developing children after the age of 3 years 6 months. Based on the Smit (1993b) data, both velar fronting and palatal fronting were still noted until approximately age 5 years, although the frequency of occurrence was very limited (less than 5% of the 186 children).

Gliding of [ɹ] and [l] seems to extend beyond 5 years of age (Grunwell, 1987; Smit, 1993b) and can be infrequently found even in the speech of children as old as age 7 (Roberts, Burchinal, & Footo, 1990; Smit, 1993b). The suppression of these and other common processes is summarized in Tables 5.6 and 5.7.

Consonant cluster substitution is one of the latest, if not *the* latest, process that is suppressed in normally developing children. Haelsig and Madison (1986) noted cluster substitutions that still occurred in 5-year-old children, whereas Roberts and colleagues (1990) evidenced rare instances of this process in their 8-year-old children. The Smit (1993a) study presented some evidence of cluster substitution in the 8- to 9-year-old children for specific initial consonant clusters (approximately 1% to 4% of the 247 children for primarily three-consonant

Table 5.6 Age of Suppression of Stopping

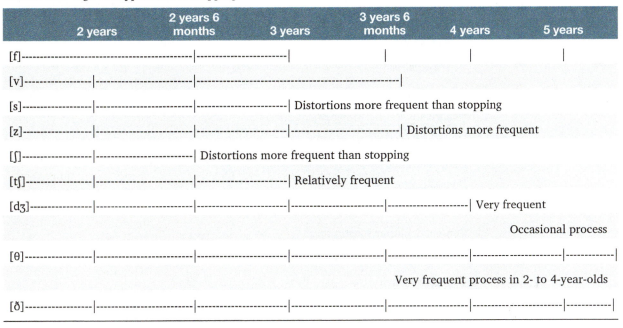

	2 years	2 years 6 months	3 years	3 years 6 months	4 years	5 years
[f]						
[v]						
[s]			Distortions more frequent than stopping			
[z]				Distortions more frequent		
[ʃ]		Distortions more frequent than stopping				
[tʃ]			Relatively frequent			
[dʒ]					Very frequent	
						Occasional process
[θ]						
					Very frequent process in 2- to 4-year-olds	
[ð]						

Source: Data from Smit, A. B. (1993b).

clusters). The suppression of these and other common processes is summarized in Tables 5.6 and 5.7.

ASSIMILATION PROCESSES. Many different assimilation processes occur in the speech of children. At different stages of their speech development, children tend to use assimilation processes in systematic ways. One of the most frequent assimilatory processes is *velar harmony* (Smith, 1973). Prominent examples are as follows:

[gɔk]	for	"dog"
[keɪk]	for	"take"

However, regressive assimilation processes are not limited to velar conso-nants. Smith (1973) reported similar regressive assimilations in which bilabials influenced preceding nonlabial consonants and consonant clusters. Among his examples are the following:

[bebu]	for	"table"
[bɔp]	for	"stop"

Although not all children display these types of assimilation processes, they may be part of the normal speech development in children ages 1 year 6 months to 2 years. If they persist beyond age 3, they begin to constitute a danger sign for a disordered phonological system (Grunwell, 1987).

Table 5.7 Age of Suppression for Several Processes

	2 years	3 years	4 years	5 years	6 years	7 years	8 years	9 years
Labialization[1]	--------	--------	--------	--------				
Alveolarization[1]	--------	--------	--------					
Affrication[1]	--------							
Deaffrication[1]	--------	--------						
Vowelization[1]	--------	--------	--|					
Derhotacization[2]	--------	--------						
Denasalization[3]	--|							
Epenthesis[4]	--------	--------	--------	--------	--------	--------		
Consonant cluster substitution[2]	--------	--------	--------	--------	--------	--------	--------	
Voicing Changes								
Context sensitive[5]	--|							
Initial voicing[6]	--------	--------	--------	--------	--------			
Final devoicing[6]	--------	--------	--------					

[1] Suppression in 75% of the children tested (Lowe, 1996).
[2] Suppression in 90% of the children tested (Smit, 1993b).
[3] The most common error for [m] and [n] but only occasional use (less than 10%) by age 2 years (Smit, 1993a).
[4] From Smit (1993a).
[5] Grunwell (1987).
[6] Suppression in 85% of the children tested (Khan & Lewis, 2015).

Clinical Exercises In Table 5.6, you see that stopping of [s], [z], and [ʃ] seems to be suppressed around age 3 to 3½. After that, distortions become more frequent. Does this suggest anything in the way of a developmental process? In other words, would your assessment results differ if a child is still stopping these sounds at age 4 and beyond?

The data in Table 5.7 suggest that r-problems such as derhotacization and vowelization are suppressed at around age 4 to 4½. Presently, these difficulties are not being treated until children are in first or second grade. What would be your opinion of the relatively late age for treating r-problems?

Prosodic Feature Development

At the time when children begin to use two-word utterances, a further segmental development occurs: *contrastive stress*. This term indicates that one syllable within a two-word utterance becomes prominent. The acquisition process seems to proceed in the following order.

First, within a child's two-word utterance, a single prosodic pattern is maintained; the two words have a pause between them that becomes shorter and shorter. The next step in the acquisition process appears to be the prosodic integration of the two words into one tone-unit. A **tone-unit**, or what is often called a *sense-group*, is an organizational unit imposed on prosodic data (Crystal, 2010). Such a tone-unit conveys meaning beyond that implied by only the verbal production. When the two words become one tone-unit (i.e., without the pause between them and with one intonational contour), one of these words becomes more prominent, usually louder and associated with an identifiable pitch movement (Crystal, 2010). At the end of this process, there exists a unifying rhythmic relationship between the two items; thus, pauses become less likely. The following developmental pattern could be observed:

Daddy (pause) eat

Daddy (pause shortens) eat

'Daddy 'eat (no pause, both stressed)

'Daddy eat (first word stressed)

Contrastive stress in the two-word stage may be used to establish *contrastive meaning* (Brown, 1973). It is assumed that the meaning of the combined one-tone utterance is different from the meaning of the two words in sequence. Later, we see that this contrastive stress is used to signal differences in meaning with similar words. Thus, "Daddy eat" could indicate that Daddy is eating, whereas "Daddy 'eat" could indicate, perhaps, that Daddy should sit down and eat.

The existing studies of prosodic feature development agree that the acquisition of intonation and stress begins at an early age. Adult-like intonational patterns are noted prior to the appearance of the first word, whereas stress patterns seem to occur clearly before the age of 2. However, true mastery of the whole prosodic feature system does not seem to take place until children are in their teens (Crystal, 2010).

Consonants, Consonant Clusters, and Prosodic Development of the School-Age Child

By the time children enter school, their phonological development has progressed considerably. At age 5 years, most of them can converse freely with everyone and make themselves understood clearly to peers and adults alike. However, their pronunciation is still recognizably different from the adult norm. Phonologically, they still have a lot to learn. Although their phonological inventory is nearly complete, this system must now be adapted to many more and different contexts, words, and situations. Other phonological features are obviously not mastered at this time. Certain sounds are still frequently misarticulated, and some aspects of prosodic feature development are only beginning to be incorporated.

Most of the research in child phonology has centered on the development of phonological skills in the first 5 years of life. However, recent interest in later phonological acquisition has evolved in part because of the established relationship between learning to speak and learning to read.

Segmental Form Development

Productionally, children are fine-tuning during the school years. Most of the information on children's production abilities is based on the results of standardized one-word speech assessments (i.e., based on responses to picture naming). If we look at these investigations (e.g., Lowe, 1986, 1996; Templin, 1957), we find that acceptable pronunciation of certain sounds is not achieved until between ages 4 years 6 months and 6 years. The most common later sounds are [θ, ð, ʒ] (Sander, 1972). Other findings (Ingram, Christensen, Veach, & Webster, 1980) include one or more of these consonants: [ɹ, z, v]. Based on single-item pronunciation, most investigators agree that children complete their phonemic inventory by the age of 6 or, at the latest, the age of 7. However, data from the Iowa-Nebraska Articulation Norms (Smit, 1993b) found dentalized [s] productions in 10% of the 9-year-old children tested.

Consonant Cluster Development

As clinicians, we typically do not expect consonant clusters until a later age. A different picture is seen if we separate occurrence and mastery. Many clusters are indeed not mastered until very late. McLeod and Arciuli (2009) state that specific clusters are still being mastered beyond 9 years of age. However, in normally developing children, clusters are present in 2-year-olds, although they may show substitutions such as [pw] for [pl] or [pɹ] (McLeod et al., 2001). It is important to note whether a child uses consonant clusters in the word-initial or word-final position. Although early clusters frequently occur initially, other clusters such as –nt or –nd are noted early in word-final positions.

The mastery of clusters generally takes place anywhere from age 3 years 6 months to age 5 years 6 months. During this time, children may demonstrate consonant cluster reduction, lengthening certain elements of the cluster (e.g., [s:no]), or epenthesis. In epenthesis, children insert a schwa vowel between two consonantal elements of a cluster, as in [səno], for example. The Iowa-Nebraska data (Smit, 1993a) offer interesting insight into 27 different initial clusters. In this study, 1049 children between the ages of 2 and 9 years were screened using an articulation test format. The data can be summarized as follows:

1. On 14 of the 27 initial clusters tested, a small percentage of children in the *8- to 9-year-old group* (N = 247, frequency of occurrence = approximately 2%) reduced two-consonant clusters to a single element. These clusters included [pl], [kl], [gl], [sl], [tw], [kw], [tɹ], [dɹ], [fɹ], [sw], [sm], [sn], [st], and [sk].

2. The consonant clusters [bɹ] and [θɹ] demonstrated a higher frequency of consonant cluster reduction (5% to 15%) for children *ages 5 to 9*.

3. For children *ages 5 years 6 months to 7 years*, the consonant clusters that fell at 75% or below group accuracy included [sl], [bɹ], [θɹ], [skw], [spɹ], [stɹ], and [skɹ].

4. Epenthesis, or schwa insertion in consonant clusters, occurs frequently up to *age 8*. The 9-year-olds rarely exhibited schwa insertion.

These data demonstrate that consonant cluster realizations are not adult-like for all children even at age 9.

The intricate interrelation of normal phonological development with other areas of language growth, which has been emphasized previously, demands attention at this point in children's development as well. The acquisition of vocabulary, for example, is a monumental task that is accomplished in a relatively short time. When children begin kindergarten, they are said to have an expressive vocabulary of approximately 2200 words. New sound sequences occurring in new words require not only increased oral-motor control and improved timing skills but also the internalization of new phonological rules. For instance, the conditions under which voiceless stops in English need to be aspirated might become a new achievement.

The acquisition of morphology is also related to phonological growth. The learning of specific morphological structures implies the learning of phonological rules. Children need to understand under which conditions the plural suffix -s is voiced [z] ("boys") or a voiceless [s] ("hats"), for example. This interconnection between morphology and phonology has been termed **morphophonology**, which refers to the study of the different allomorphs of the morpheme and the rules governing their use. For example, children's production of [əz] to indicate the plural form for *glass* versus [s] as the plural of *boat* falls within the study of morphophonology, as do the rules governing the productional changes from *divide* to *division* and from *explode* to *explosion*. Research findings (e.g., Mealings, Cox, & Demuth, 2013; Mealings & Demuth, 2014; Tomas, Demuth, Smith-Lock, & Petocz, 2015) document that children are acquiring certain morphophonological patterns based on several factors, one of which is their phonological skill. The complex interrelationship among the phonological system and other components of language continues into children's later school years.

Prosodic Feature Development

As prosodic features evolve, they begin to assume grammatical function. For example, specific intonation patterns are used to differentiate between statements and certain questions in English (e.g., "He is coming."↘ versus "He is coming?"↗). Contrasting stress realizations signal different word classes ('construct versus con 'struct). On the sentence level, the combined effects of higher pitch and increased loudness usually convey communicatively important modifications of basic meaning ("This is a 'pen" versus "'This is a pen"). This section examines the grammatical function of prosodic features in school-age children and their relationship to phonological development.

As previously noted, children begin to use intonational patterns toward the end of the first year of life. As these grammatical abilities develop, new uses of intonation emerge. For example, the contrast between rising and falling pitch differentiates the two grammatical functions of a tag question in English ("asking," as in "We're ready, aren't we?"↗, and "telling," as in "We're ready, aren't we!"↘). Differences in intonation patterns such as these appear to be learned during children's third year (Crystal, 2010). However, the learning of intonation goes on for a long time. Studies report that children as old as 11 years were still acquiring some of the fundamental functions of English intonation, especially those for signaling grammatical contrast (Arciuli & Ballard, 2017; Wells, Peppé, & Goulandris, 2004). As Crystal (2010) reported, even teenagers have been shown to have difficulty understanding sentences in which intonation and pausing are used to differentiate meaning. His example was "She *dressed*, and fed the baby" (indicating she dressed herself and then fed the baby) versus "She *dressed* and *fed* the baby" (indicating she dressed as well as fed the baby). Thus, although certain intonational features seem to be among the earliest phonological acquisitions, others may be some of the latest acquired.

Several studies have examined the use of contrastive stress both on the word level (*'record* versus *re'cord*) and on the sentence level (determining whom Mary hit in the following sentences: "John hit Bill and then *Mary* hit him" versus "John hit Bill and then Mary hit *him*") (e.g., Arciuli & Ballard, 2017; Ballard, Djaja, Arciuli, James, & van Doorn, 2012). It appears that the mastery of contrastive stress is not yet at an adult-like level for the majority of the children in the studies even at the age of 11 (Patel & Brayton, 2009; Wells, Peppé, & Goulandris, 2004).

The acquisition of prosodic features is a gradual process that in some respects extends into the teens. It is closely connected to the new phonological, morphosyntactic, semantic, and pragmatic demands placed on developing children. As the complexity of the linguistic environment and the children's interaction with that environment increase, so do the subtle intricacies of each of these language levels.

Phonological Awareness, Emerging Literacy, and Phonological Disorders

Another important aspect that needs to be addressed pertains to the interconnections between learning to speak and learning to read. Early speech abilities and emerging literacy are interactive in a complex manner (McLeod & Baker, 2017). There is also a connection between learning to read and phonological/phonemic awareness. Phonological awareness seems to contribute to word recognition skills and to early spelling, for example. (Refer to Gillon, 2018, for a review.) Research has affirmed the importance of phonological awareness and its relationship to reading acquisition (e.g., Blachman, 2000; Foy & Mann, 2012; Lonigan, Burgess, & Anthony, 2000; Stanovich, 2000). Reviews of the literature have noted that strong phonological awareness skills are characteristics of good readers, whereas children with poor phonological awareness skills in kindergarten and the early school years are far more likely to become poor readers (e.g., Catts, Fey, & Zhang, 2001; Leafstedt, Richards, & Gerber, 2004; Torgesen, 2000). Definitions of the terms that will be used in our discussion of phonological awareness follow.

> **Metaphonology**: A subcategory of metalinguistics, metaphonology involves children's conscious awareness of the sounds within a particular language. It includes how those sounds are combined to form words. Therefore, metaphonological skills pertain to children's ability to discern how many sounds are in a word or which sound constitutes its beginning or end. Phonological awareness abilities are one important metaphonological skill.

> **Phonological processing** refers to the use of sounds in one's language in processing written and oral language (Anthony et al., 2003). The role of phonological processing is to analyze the sound structures of words into smaller units. Thus, one hears the sounds that make up a specific word and can convert them into letters on a page. The use of phonological processing is also inherent in seeing the letters of a word and converting them into something one can read. Phonological processing is a multilevel skill that includes (1) phonological awareness, (2) phonemic awareness, (3) phonological memory (the coding of phonological information in working

memory), and (4) retrieving phonological information from long-term memory (Gillon, 2018). Research provides strong support that phonological processing includes two broad dimensions: coding and awareness (Hurford et al., 1993; Liberman & Shankweiler, 1985). **Coding**, the translation from one form to another—for example, from auditory to written form or from written to auditory form—contains two dimensions, phonetic and phonological, and includes multiple processes that require memory and coding from one form of representation to another. An example of phonetic coding might be that a child learns that the letters *sh* sound a certain way. This knowledge is stored in memory, which the child must access when trying to sound out a new word, *shelf*. The distinction between the two coding dimensions is the type of memory that is accessed. In other words, phonetic coding takes place in working memory for such processes as sounding out unfamiliar words.

In contrast, phonological coding is related to the semantic lexical abilities in long-term memory. This seems to involve a three-step process. First, written symbols are matched to the pronunciation of the written word. Second, the pronunciation of the written word is matched with the pronunciation of words in memory. Third, pronunciations of words in memory are linked with meaning for retrieval of meaning and pronunciation (Wesseling & Reitsma, 2000). At least four types of phonological processing skills demonstrate differences between norm readers and poor readers: memory span (retention of new strings of verbal items), recall of verbal information (in contrast to recall of nonverbal items), articulation rate, and rapid naming (Cornwall, 1992; Torgesen, 2000; Torgesen, Wagner, Simmons, & Laughon, 1990).

Phonological awareness is the ability to pay attention to the sound structure of language separate from the meaning (Hesketh, 2010). It is children's conscious ability to detect and manipulate sound segments, such as moving sounds around in a word, combining certain sounds together, or deleting sounds. Phonological awareness should be examined in the broader scope of phonology because we find that long before children become aware of the phonological structure of words, they have specialized phonological knowledge. This knowledge allows them to make a judgment about whether a word is part of their native language, to self-correct any speech errors or mispronunciations, and to discriminate between acceptable and unacceptable variations of a spoken word.

Phonological awareness uses a single modality—the auditory one. It is the ability to hear sounds in spoken words in contrast to recognizing sounds in written words, which accesses children's coding abilities. Phonological awareness should also be separated from phonemic awareness. *Phonological awareness* is a more general term that refers to all sizes of sound units, such as words (e.g., How many words are in the sentence *He hit the ball*?), syllables (e.g., How many syllables does *banana* have?), onset-rimes (e.g., Which one of these words rhymes with *bed*: *man*, *lock*, or *head*?), and phonemes (e.g., What is the first sound in *dog*?).

Thus, phonological awareness is a subdivision of phonological processing; however, phonological awareness is less complex: Coding puts more demands on memory and processing of information. Phonological awareness is a multilevel skill of breaking down words into smaller units and can be described in terms of syllable awareness, onset-rime awareness, and phoneme awareness (Gillon, 2018). A variety of measures can be used to evaluate a child's knowledge of these three levels.

Phonemic awareness: This skill is a subcategory of phonological awareness. However, it refers only to the phoneme level. It necessitates an understanding that words are composed of individual sounds/phonemes. Phonemic awareness is the understanding that speech is composed of minimal units of sound that can be separated and manipulated (Ukrainetz, 2015). Examples include a child's ability to segment and match sounds (e.g., What is a word that starts with the same sound as *Cathy*?) and the ability to manipulate sounds (e.g., What would *mean* be without the final *n* sound?).

Phonological memory refers to coding information phonologically for temporary storage in working memory. Coding of phonological information into working memory is tested by having the child, based on immediate imitation, recall series of digits or sentence repetition tasks. A deficit in phonological memory does not appear to impair either reading or listening to a large extent, provided the words are already in the child's vocabulary. However, difficulties with phonological memory can limit the ability to learn new written or spoken vocabulary (Wagner, Torgesen, & Rashotte, 1994).

Retrieving phonological information from long-term memory includes the efficiency of retrieving phonological codes associated with individual phonemes, word segments, or entire words. This ability influences the degree to which phonological information is useful in decoding printed words. Rapid naming tasks, such as naming as many animals as fast as you can in a certain time interval, are related to retrieving phonological information from long-term memory.

The following exemplifies some of the phonological awareness tasks that can be implemented with children (Gillon, 2018):

Syllable Awareness. Awareness at the syllable level requires that a child understands that words can be divided into syllables. For example, the word "baby" has two syllables: "ba" and "by." Tasks used to evaluate syllable awareness include (1) syllable segmentation (e.g., How many syllables, or beats, are in *banana*?), (2) syllable completion (e.g., Here is a picture of a rainbow. I'll say the first part of the word and you can complete it. Here is a rain___), (3) syllable identity (e.g., Which part of "rainbow" and "raincoat" sounds the same?), and (4) syllable deletion (e.g., Say "rabbit." Now say it again without the "ra.")

Onset-Rime Awareness. This awareness involves recognition of the onset of the syllable (all sounds prior to the vowel nucleus) and the rime, or the rest of the syllable, that includes the syllable peak and coda. (Refer to Chapter 2 for a review of syllable structure.) Onset-rime awareness is typically measured using some type of rhyming task. To be able to rhyme, children must be able to separate the onset from the rime of the word. Thus, a child knows that *cat, bat,* and *hat* rhyme, as the onset changes in each; however, the rime stays the same: "at." Tasks that measure onset-rime awareness include (1) spoken rhyme recognition (e.g., Do these words rhyme: *hop* and *top*?), (2) recognition of words that do not rhyme (e.g., Which word does not rhyme: *cat, sat, car*?), (3) spoken rhyme production (e.g., Tell me a word that rhymes with *dog*.), and (4) onset-rime blending (e.g., "c" and "at" is blended to "cat").

Phonemic Awareness. This skill can be measured in a number of ways. For each of the tasks, a child's ability to manipulate sounds is tested. Examples include (1) phoneme detection (e.g., Which one of the following words has a different first sound: *rose, red, bike, rabbit*?), (2) phoneme matching (e.g., Which word begins with same sound as "rose"?), (3) phoneme isolation (e.g., Which sound do you hear at the beginning of "road"?), (4) phoneme completion (e.g., Here is a picture of a ball. Can you finish the word for me? "ba____."), (5) phoneme blending (e.g., I am going to say a word in a funny way. Can you tell me what the word is? *b—i—g.*), (6) phoneme deletion (e.g., Can you say "road" without the "d" sound?), (7) phoneme segmentation (e.g., Tell me the sounds in "jeep."), (8) phoneme reversal (e.g., Say "bat." Now say "bat" backwards: "tab."), (9) phoneme manipulation (e.g., Say "meat." Now say it again but this time change the "m" and the "t" around: "team."), and (10) spoonerisms (e.g., *hot dog* becomes *dot hog*).

Clinical Exercises Pick one of the skills noted under each of these categories: syllable, onset-rime, and phonemic awareness. Can you give a different example that you could use with a child?

Explain why the skills under phonemic awareness are considered to be more complex. Think about what a child must do to complete the task. What role would memory play in the tasks listed as (8), (9), and (10)?

There seems to be a developmental progression in the acquisition of phonological awareness skills. First, an awareness of larger units, such as words and syllables, precedes awareness of smaller units, such as individual sounds. In a comprehensive study by Lonigan, Burgess, Anthony, and Barker (1998), which tested several levels of phonological/phonemic awareness in 356 children between the ages of 2 and 5 years, the following results emerged. First, age influenced performance on all tasks. Although accelerated growth was evident between the ages of 3 and 4 years, it was not until around age 5 years that children were able to consistently perform phoneme detection tasks. Second, the linguistic complexity of the task influenced performance. Children across age groups showed stronger performance on blending and deleting at the word level (*dog + house = doghouse*), followed by success at the syllable level (*win + dow = window*), and the weakest performance at the phoneme level (*d + o + g = dog*).

Although stable performance of phonological awareness tasks may not be evident until 4 years of age, some 2- and 3-year-old children can demonstrate phonological awareness knowledge. Maclean, Bryant, and Bradley (1987) appear to be among the earliest investigators who found that a moderate percentage of 3-year-old children can perform competently on a rime detection task. When Lonigan and colleagues (1998) reduced the load on memory by having the children look at three pictures and point to the picture that did not rhyme, nearly 25% of the 2½-year-old children scored above chance on the task.

It must be noted that some researchers have questioned the progressive nature of the development of phonological awareness. In other words, the seemingly noted facts that syllable awareness emerges before rhyme awareness and rhyme awareness emerges before phoneme awareness were not evidenced in all children. For example, individual reports of older poor readers document children who performed better on phoneme manipulation tasks than on rhyme tasks (Duncan & Johnston, 1999). These findings are contrary to the trends noted in most other children.

The next question that arises is whether phonological awareness abilities are predictive of later reading and spelling competencies. In a large number of studies that attempted to control for variables such as memory, intellectual ability, and home and preschool environments (e.g., Frost, Madsbjerg, Niedersøe, Olofsson, & Sørensen, 2005; Gillon, 2018; McLeod & Baker, 2017), the following findings are suggested:

1. There is a positive relationship between phonological awareness and reading. Children with phonological awareness skills learn to read more easily than children who do not have these skills (Goswami & Bryant, 2016).

2. Performance on phonological awareness tasks in kindergarten and first grade is a strong predictor of later reading achievement (e.g., Hecht, Burgess, Torgesen, Wagner, & Rashotte, 2000; Torgesen, Wagner, Rashotte, Burgess, & Hecht, 1997).

3. Direct training on phonological awareness and sound-letter correspondence with children who are not yet reading improves their reading and spelling skills (Schneider, Roth, & Ennemoser, 2000; Walton, Walton, & Felton, 2001).

4. Phonological awareness teaching works best when combined with instruction in sound-letter correspondence (Bradley & Bryant, 1983).

Finally, the relationship among phonological awareness, developing literacy, and speech disorders is relevant to this discussion. Approximately 4% of 6-year-old children will approach reading with a speech sound disorder (Shriberg, Tomblin, & McSweeney, 1999). Are their phonological awareness skills affected by their speech problems? If so, will these children be at greater risk for developing reading and spelling difficulties? It appears that children with articulation-based disorders—and therefore motor-based problems that affect the mechanics of actually producing sound—are not at high risk for literacy problems (e.g., Bishop & Adams, 1990; Catts, 1993; Dodd, 1995). However, those children who have a phonemic-based disorder are potentially at risk for written language difficulties. The extent of this problem is probably determined by their patterns of linguistic strengths and weaknesses (Gillon, 2018). The specific findings from children with expressive phonemic-based difficulties and their phonological awareness skills may be summarized as follows:

1. As a group, children with phonemic-based difficulties show deficits on a variety of phonological awareness tasks (e.g., Bird & Bishop, 1992; Bird, Bishop, & Freeman, 1995; Gillon, 2000; Marion, Sussman, & Marquardt, 1993; Melby-Lervåg, Lyster, & Hulme, 2012; Preston, Hull, & Edwards, 2013; Webster & Plante, 1992).

2. Without intervention, difficulties with phonological awareness persist over time. Difficulties have been especially noted in acquiring phonemic-level skills (e.g., Gillon, 2002; Snowling, Bishop, & Stothard, 2000).

3. Children with other spoken language problems (morphosyntactic or semantic) generally experience poorer long-term outcomes in reading and writing when compared to children with isolated phonemic-based production difficulties (Bishop & Adams, 1990; Catts & Kamhi, 1999; Hodson, 1994; Lewis, Freebairn, & Taylor, 2000; Preston et al., 2013; Snowling, Goulandris, & Stackhouse, 1994; Stackhouse, 1993, 1997; Wells, Stackhouse, & Vance, 1996).

4. In addition to phonological awareness difficulties, children with expressive phonemic-based problems display weaknesses in other areas that appear to be important for literacy development, including letter-name knowledge and verbal working memory (e.g., Webster, Plante, & Couvillion, 1997).

5. The type of phonemic-based disorder is relevant to predicting reading outcomes. Thus, children who show consistent use of unusual or idiosyncratic errors (according to the Dodd [2005] classification system those with a *consistent phonological disorder*) as opposed to normal developmental processes (those classified as having a *phonological delay*) may evidence more severe difficulties in acquiring literacy skills (e.g., Dodd et al., 1995; Leitao, Hogben, & Fletcher, 1997; Preston et al., 2013).

6. The severity of a child's phonemic-based disorder influences literacy outcomes. Children with severe phonemic-based disorders, significant phonological processing difficulties, and other language impairments are very likely to have persistent reading and spelling difficulties (e.g., Bird et al., 1995; Bishop & Robson, 1989; Larrivee & Catts, 1999; Stackhouse, 1982, 1997). However, for the most part, these children respond positively to phonological awareness instruction, which can prevent the negative long-term effects (Gillon, 2000).

To summarize, phonological awareness is a subcategory of phonological processing. It contains many different levels of skills and seems to demonstrate a systematic developmental sequence. It is highly correlated to later reading and spelling abilities. Children with phonemic-based difficulties demonstrate more problems with phonological awareness and, consequently, difficulties with reading acquisition. These reading and spelling deficits may persist, especially in children with idiosyncratic errors and those with severe phonemic-based problems.

Summary

First, this chapter provided an overview of structural and functional development in infancy and early childhood. At birth, the infant's respiratory, phonatory, resonatory, and articulatory systems are not fully developed. Many changes must occur before the systems are ready to support sound and voice production for speech. In addition, children's perceptual abilities are developing. The second portion of this chapter summarized early perceptual skills, including categorical perception and the awareness of phonemic contrasts. The third section of this chapter traced the segmental form and prosodic feature development of children from vocalizations prior to babbling to the time when their speech sound inventory has reached an adult-like form. The prevalence of certain sounds and syllable shapes was traced from babbling to the first words. As the number of words in children's vocabularies increases, inventory and complexity of syllables grow as well. During this early stage of expansion, the prosodic feature intonation begins to be used to signal different intentions.

The linguistic development of preschool-age children is characterized by a large growth in all aspects of language; the acquisition of new phonological features is part of this quickly maturing system. Although cross-sectional studies have attempted to provide so-called mastery ages for sounds, these results cannot be easily generalized. Longitudinal data that document individual variability in sound acquisition as well as the influence of other language areas on phonological skills were then summarized. The suppression of many phonological processes is occurring within this time interval as well. Based on research findings, approximate ages were given for the suppression of several common phonological processes.

Both segmental form and prosodic features continue to mature during children's school years. Although the sound inventory is approaching adult-like form, many aspects of the phonological system are still maturing. Children need to learn morphophonemic variations as well as metaphonological skills. Metaphonological skills were briefly discussed in relation to the emerging literacy of children. During the school years, phonological development often affects children's abilities to learn reading and writing. The close

interdependencies among phonology, language development, and literacy learning point to the importance of normal phonological development in children.

Case Study

Diagnostic Implications of Phonological Process Suppression

Approximate ages of suppression have been provided for several common phonological processes. This information can be helpful during our diagnostic assessment. The following phonological processes were identified in Clint, age 3 years 6 months.

Word	Production	Phonological Process
house	[haʊ]	Final consonant deletion
cup	[kʌ]	Final consonant deletion
gun	[gʌ]	Final consonant deletion
shovel	[ʃʌbəl]	Stopping of [v]
vacuum	[bækju]	Stopping of [v], final consonant deletion
vase	[beɪ]	Stopping of [v], final consonant deletion
scratching	[kɹætʃɪŋ]	Consonant cluster reduction
skunk	[kʌŋk]	Consonant cluster reduction
star	[taɚ]	Consonant cluster reduction
jumping	[dʌmpɪŋ]	Stopping of [dʒ]
jelly	[dɛli]	Stopping of [dʒ]
jeep	[dip]	Stopping of [dʒ]
that	[dæt]	Stopping of [ð]
bath	[bæt]	Stopping of [θ]
feather	[fɛdɚ]	Stopping of [ð]

Similar processes were also noted in Clint's conversational speech.

Which of the noted processes should be suppressed by age 3 years 6 months? Final consonant deletion is usually suppressed by around age 3 years, but research has demonstrated its use until approximately age 4 years. Stopping of [v], [θ], [ð], and [dʒ] extends to age 3 years 6 months or beyond. Consonant cluster reduction is also a process that is suppressed at a relatively late age. Based on these results, the only process that might cause concern at Clint's age would be final consonant deletion.

Think Critically

1. Lori is a 20-month-old toddler who is brought to your clinic by her parents, who are concerned that she has not begun to say real words. Although she babbles strings of sounds, such as [baba], [maba], [toto], and [gaga], she does not evidence true words nor does she impose intonation or rhythmic patterns on the babbles. The parents report that just recently (within the last 2 to 3 weeks), Lori occasionally imitates a babble that she has just produced if the parents have her attention and immediately say her babble back to her. What prelinguistic stage is Lori in? Approximately how delayed is she in respect to the given developmental guidelines?

2. The following results of an articulation test are from Ryan, age 6 years 6 months. We noted his phonological processes in Chapter 4.

horse	[hoʊɚθ]	pig	[pɪk]	chair	[ʃɛɚ]
wagon	[wægən]	cup	[kʌp]	watch	[wɑʃ]
monkey	[mʌŋki]	swinging	[swɪŋɪŋ]	thumb	[fʌm]
comb	[koʊm]	table	[teɪbəl]	mouth	[maʊf]
fork	[foɚk]	cat	[kæt]	shoe	[su]
knife	[naɪf]	ladder	[lærɾ]	fish	[fɪs]
cow	[kaʊ]	ball	[bɑl]	zipper	[ðɪpɚ]
cake	[keɪk]	plane	[pweɪn]	nose	[noʊθ]
baby	[beɪbi]	cold	[koʊd]	sun	[θʌn]
bathtub	[bæftəb]	jumping	[dʌmpən]	house	[haʊθ]
nine	[naɪn]	TV	[tivi]	steps	[stɛp]
train	[tweɪn]	stove	[θtoʊv]	nest	[nɛt]
gum	[gʌm]	ring	[wɪŋ]	books	[bʊkθ]
dog	[dɑg]	tree	[twi]		
yellow	[wɛloʊ]	green	[gwin]		
doll	[dɑl]	this	[dɪθ]		
bird	[bɝd]	whistle	[wɪθəl]		
carrots	[kɛɚət]				

Based on Ryan's age, compare which sounds might be considered in *error* if the ages of speech sound development from the Poole (1934) versus the Templin (1957) investigations are used (page 137). (Actually any two studies could be used for comparison.) Discuss the problems when using these sound mastery age levels.

3. Based on Ryan's age (6 years 6 months), identify which phonological processes are age appropriate, which ones might be considered borderline, and which ones should be suppressed at his age.

> ✓ **Chapter Quiz 5.1** Complete this quiz to check your understanding of chapter concepts.

Chapter 6
Assessment and Appraisal

Collection of Data

Learning Objectives

When you have finished this chapter, you should be able to:

6.1 Summarize the guidelines for the assessment of speech sound disorders, emphasizing specific factors within the child's total communication process.

6.2 Characterize the procedures for a hearing screening and evaluation of the speech mechanism.

6.3 Evaluate standardized speech assessments and note supplemental procedures, including stimulability testing, contextual testing, assessing multisyllabic words (those with three or more syllables), and obtaining a spontaneous speech sample.

6.4 Identify additional screening or testing measures in other areas, including language, prosody, phonological/phonemic awareness, cognitive skills, and assessment of a child's communicative participation.

6.5 Define the special considerations needed in the assessment of a child with emerging phonology.

6.6 Categorize the specific considerations warranted when evaluating an unintelligible child.

Chapter Application: Case Study

Peter has two children who have just come to the clinic and need to be tested. One child, Lillian, is 4 years old. Her parents are very concerned. They state that Lillian is so hard to understand that it causes difficulties in her activities and her participation in everyday communication, such as playing with other children in preschool. They are also worried that she might have language difficulties, as her responses are predominantly one-word expressions. The second child, Collin, who is also 4 years old, talks in

(continued)

multiword sentences, but the words are sometimes "slurred," according to the parents. He also tends to drool when he is very concentrated on an activity and occasionally when he is excited and talking. Peter wonders if there might be some underlying functional or structural deficits that are affecting Collin's speech and contributing to his drooling behavior. Collin's pediatrician has noted no deviancies but, after a preliminary oral structure exam, referred him to a speech-language pathologist for further testing.

Both children present with very different problems, and Peter needs to organize his assessments accordingly. Which basic testing will both children need, and how should Peter individualize his procedures so that the assessments are done in a time-efficient manner? How should he proceed?

ASSESSMENT is one of the most important tasks clinicians perform; it is the basis for treatment decisions. **Assessment** is the clinical evaluation of a client's disorder. It can be divided into two phases: appraisal and diagnosis (Darley, 1991). **Appraisal** refers to the collection of data, whereas **diagnosis** represents the end result of studying and interpreting these data. Appraisal is a very important aspect of our assessment. The collection of too little or unspecific information will not provide enough data for an adequate diagnosis. At the other extreme, collecting too much or unnecessary data wastes the client's and clinician's valuable time. Therefore, professional assessment demands qualified (and verifiable) decisions throughout the appraisal process.

The appraisal process, the collecting of data, continues beyond the initial diagnosis. Collecting data will continue throughout the assessment and, of course, throughout the therapeutic process. Clinicians are professionally obligated to collect data in order to note therapy progress and treatment efficacy. It is vital that, as clinicians, we continue to appraise our clients so that we can realign our goals and procedures if necessary.

This chapter is broad based and is meant to stand at the beginning of our assessment process. It covers basic necessities that are an integral portion of our assessment. For example, information about hearing screening and evaluation of the speech mechanism is included in this chapter, as are other measures typically included, such as language screening or testing. At the core of our initial appraisal is a standardized speech assessment and speech sample. The advantages and disadvantages of standardized procedures are reviewed, and an overview of possible tests is provided. It should be noted that specific analyses of error patterns, phonemic contrasts, and intelligibility are not within the scope of this chapter; they are contained in Chapter 7. Appraisal can also include questions about the child's cognition, prosody, and phonological/phonemic awareness skills, for example. These areas are summarized, and options are discussed. The last portion of this chapter contains information relevant to beginning the collection of data for children with emerging phonology and those who are unintelligible. These children will need specific adaptations to the appraisal process.

The first goal is to identify the different types of data needed for a comprehensive diagnosis. These parts are identified, and procedures are outlined for each method. The second goal is to emphasize clinicians' roles in choosing among available measures—that is, the clinical decision-making process leading to the selection of instruments serving each individual client maximally. Effective assessments are essential for clinical procedures; they lead us through the entire diagnostic and therapeutic process.

Data collection involves at least four different areas: (1) case history, (2) interviews with parents and other professionals, (3) school and medical records, and (4) evaluation by the clinician. Procedures and information important to the

Box 6.1

Interviewing and Obtaining Case History Information: Bibliographical Sources

Flasher, L. V., & Fogle, P. T. (2012). *Counseling skills for speech-language pathologists and audiologists* (2nd ed.). Clifton Park, NJ: Delmar, Cengage Learning.

Luterman, D. M. (2017). *Counseling persons with communication disorders and their families* (5th ed.). Austin, TX: PRO-ED.

Pindzola, R. H., Plexico, L. W., & Haynes, W. O. (2016). *Diagnosis and evaluation in speech pathology* (9th ed.). Boston, MA: Pearson.

Rollin, W. (2000). *Counseling individuals with communication disorders* (2nd ed.). Boston, MA: Butterworth-Heineman.

Ruscello, D. M. (2001). *Tests and measurements in speech language pathology*. Woburn, MA: Butterworth-Heinemann.

Shipley, K. G., & McAfee, J. G. (2016). *Assessment in speech-language pathology: A resource manual* (5th ed.). Boston, MA: Cengage.

Shipley, K. G., & Roseberry-McKibbin, C. (2006). *Interviewing and counseling in communicative disorders: Principles and procedures*. Austin, TX: Pro-Ed.

Tellis, C. M., & Barone, O. R. (2018). *Counseling and interviewing in speech-language pathology and audiology: A therapy resource*. Burlington, MA: Jones & Bartlett Learning.

Tomblin, J. B., Morris, H. L., & Spriestersbach, D. C. (2002). *Diagnosis in speech-language pathology* (2nd ed.). Clifton Park, NJ: Delmar, Cengage Learning.

Westby, C., Burda, A., & Mehta, Z. (2003). Asking the right questions in the right ways: Strategies for ethnographic interviewing. *The ASHA Leader, 8*, 4–17. Retrieved from https://leader.pubs.asha.org/article.aspx?articleid=2292396

first three areas are covered in many texts. This chapter covers only the fourth and most specific task, the evaluation by the clinician. Box 6.1 lists several sources that cover gathering case history information, interviewing, and counselling.

Guidelines for Assessment: Objectives of Appraisal and Diagnosis

The *Scope of Practice in Speech-Language Pathology* (American Speech-Language-Hearing Association [ASHA], 2007a) provides a general framework for the diagnostic process of speech sound disorders (refer to also *Preferred Practice Patterns for the Profession of Speech-Language Pathology*; ASHA, 2004). These generic and universally applicable practice patterns were developed to be consistent with the World Health Organization's *International Classification of Functioning, Disability and Health* (World Health Organization [WHO], 2001). The international classification system in this case addresses the child's (1) health condition, (2) body functions and structures, (3) activities and participation, and (4) environmental and personal factors. These four parameters can be applied to the diagnosis of speech sound disorders, but they could be used as the basis for any speech-language pathologist's diagnosis. Refer to Figure 6.1 for an overview.

Figure 6.1 *International Classification of Functioning, Disability and Health* (WHO, 2001) Applied to the Diagnosis of Speech Sound Disorders

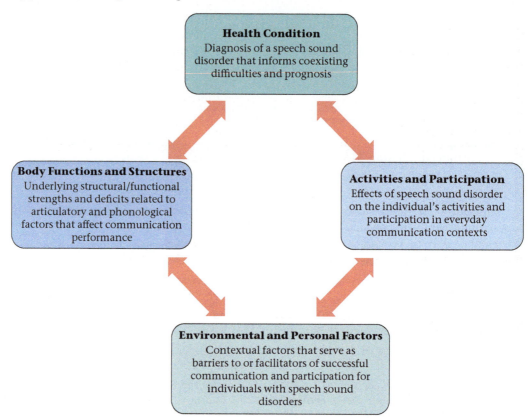

This organization leads to several basic diagnostic questions:

1. How do we determine if a child demonstrates a speech sound disorder?
2. Which coexisting factors seem to be present through either case history information or other evaluations? These could include, for example, a hearing loss, language disorder, or intellectual disability.
3. What is the prognosis of this disorder?
4. Are there any structural or functional deficits or strengths related to communication performance, specific to speech sound production?
5. Are there any factors that serve as barriers to or facilitators of successful verbal communication and participation by this child?
6. What are the effects of this child's speech sound disorder on the child's everyday communication contexts, including at least the school and home environments?

Not all of these questions can be answered easily, and they are not all within the scope of this chapter. Some will need input from family members and those in the community, such as the child's teacher, before answers can be tentatively formulated. However, this chapter will attempt to guide the clinician through some of these questions by offering concrete possibilities.

Initial Procedures: Hearing Evaluation and Speech Mechanism Examination

Clinicians collect data in two different ways: through a procedure known as *screening* or through a more comprehensive evaluation. A **screening** consists of activities or tests that identify individuals who merit further evaluation. A screening procedure does not collect nearly enough data to establish a diagnosis; it only demonstrates the need for further testing. Screening measures can be formal or informal. Formal measures include elicitation procedures and have normative data and cutoff scores. Informal measures are typically devised by the examiner and may be directed toward a specific problem area (such as language or phonemic awareness). Screenings are typically used to give the clinician an initial impression of a certain subset of skills for a particular client.

Screenings are beneficial for those individuals who "fail" the procedure and are later evaluated more comprehensively. Screenings are not always reliable, in that some individuals may "pass" the procedure but still demonstrate impairments. Screenings were not devised to serve as a database for a diagnosis; they are too limited in their scope. In contrast, a **comprehensive evaluation** is a series of activities and tests that allows a more detailed and complete collection of data. A *comprehensive phonetic-phonemic evaluation* includes data from at least the following sources:

- A hearing screening
- A speech mechanism examination
- A standardized speech assessment and stimulability measures
- A conversational speech sample in varying contexts
- Possible additional screening or comprehensive measures such as language testing, phonological/phonemic awareness, contextual testing, and/or cognitive assessment (Bernthal, Bankson, & Flipsen, 2017; Lowe, 1994).

Data from these sources will begin to answer the following questions: (1) Does the child demonstrate a speech sound disorder? (2) Are there any coexisting factors? and (3) Are there are any functional deficits or strengths related to communication performance?

The following sections examine each of the elements of this process, beginning with an initial impression and its usefulness in the collection of data.

Initial Impression

Clinicians can start collecting data even before the formal appraisal begins—for example, by closely observing the conversation between a caregiver and a child, between a teacher and a child in a classroom situation, or between a child and that child's peers. This initial contact will provide an important first impression. The task is to notice certain features of the conversation and document them on a simple form, such as the one in Figure 6.2. Although additional variables must be considered later, this record of the initial impression will aid in planning and organizing the remainder of the assessment.

This type of initial impression also gives us preliminary information about any barriers to or perhaps facilitators of successful communication. If we note that the child, despite the speech sound difficulties, is able to make the intended point (maybe by using gestures, facial expressions, pointing, etc.), this would

Figure 6.2 Sample Form for the Initial Impression

Name _____ Age _____

Conversational partner _____ Date _____

Intelligibility

Good _____ Partly intelligible _____ Unintelligible _____

Single-word responses and continuous speech show comparable intelligibility _____

Single-word responses are more intelligible than continuous speech _____

General overview of misarticulations

Affects consonants _____

Affects consonants and vowels _____

Noted misarticulations _____

_____

Other factors affecting intelligibility (e.g., hypernasality or denasality, vocal loudness or quality, rate of speech)

_____

Caregiver's/teacher's/peer's response to misarticulations

No response _____ Asks for repetition _____ Tries to correct _____

Child's response to parent's/caregiver's intervention _____

_____

Factors the parents and/or teachers think help or hinder this child's communicative efforts

_____

_____

be a positive factor to document. If, on the other hand, the child becomes frustrated easily when not understood, this might prove to be a barrier to communication.

In some states and public schools, observing children in their classroom or school environment is the only "screening" measure allowed by law. Check with your school district to find out the procedure in your school and state.

Procedures for a Hearing Screening

A **hearing screening** is used to identify children who may require a more comprehensive hearing assessment and/or medical management. Hearing screenings during childhood are imperative. Early identification and management of hearing loss is necessary, as "Failure to detect congenital or acquired hearing loss in children may result in lifelong deficits in speech and language acquisition, poor academic performance, personal-social maladjustments, and emotional difficulties" (Harlor & Bower, 2009, p. 1253). The screening of a child's hearing should occur upon initial entry to school, every year in grades K to 3, and in grades 7 and 11 (ASHA, 2006).

Prior to a hearing screening, a visual inspection of the tympanic membrane and the external ear canal should be performed. If you are a screener who is not trained in otoscopy, a general visual inspection of the outer portion of the ear should be done and notes should be made of any abnormalities. In addition, there are four possible protocols for conducting a hearing screening:

1. *Pure tone screening only:* Pure tones are presented in each ear, typically at 20 decibels (dB) for the frequencies 1000, 2000, and 4000 hertz (Hz). Results are Pass (an appropriate response to all stimuli at screening levels in both ears), Fail (a lack of response to any test frequency at screening levels in either ear), or Could Not Screen (lack of cooperation with the task).

2. *Pure tone screening and typanometry:* Typanometry measures the mobility of the tympanic membrane and the status of the middle-ear transmission system. During tympanometry, a small probe is put snugly into the ear canal. Pressure between the probe and the eardrum is varied. Reflected sound from the probe tone is recorded across the pressure range, and a tympanogram is created.

3. *Otoacoustic emissions (OAEs) screening:* A sensitive probe microphone is inserted into the ear canal. OAEs are a direct measure of the hair cells and cochlear function in response to acoustic stimulation. They yield an indirect estimate of peripheral hearing sensitivity, so technically they do not test an individual's hearing. OAEs screening results reflect the performance of the inner ear mechanics.

4. *OAEs and tympanometry:* According to ASHA (2006), these two measures can be used to screen hearing.

If a child fails the hearing screening, rescreening or referral is necessary. ASHA (2006) provides decision trees that represent examples of the decision-making process undertaken during childhood hearing screenings (this information can be found on the ASHA website).

A clinician should also ask about any developmental history that could affect the child's hearing status. This would include a history of episodes of otitis media, "earaches," or the placement of tubes. Shriberg and Kwiatkowski (1982a) verified that one-third of children enrolled in speech or language intervention had histories of recurrent middle ear infections. Although controversy exists surrounding the exact role that chronic otitis media plays in the acquisition of phonology, it may at least interact with other risk factors in some children. This interaction could easily lead to a greater risk of delayed or impaired communication skills.

The next section examines the screening process for the assessment of oral structure and function. This screening is very important because it can identify possible underlying structural and/or functional strengths and deficits related to speech sound production that may affect communication performance.

Evaluation of the Speech Mechanism

An evaluation of both the structure and the function of a client's speech mechanism is a prerequisite for any comprehensive assessment. Its intent is to assess whether the system appears adequate for regular speech sound production. At first glance, the examination of the speech-motor system looks like a relatively simple procedure that has been described often. However, the interpretation of the results is not necessarily as straightforward as it would seem.

It might be beneficial to view the results of the evaluation of the speech mechanism as being along a continuum in which one end indicates normal structure and function and the other end indicates grossly deviant structural and/or functional shortcomings. At the normal end of the continuum, assume that the client has passed all required procedures. This is commonly the case, and no further speech-motor testing appears to be necessary; the client has passed the oral-speech assessment.

At the other end of the continuum, results could show such a pronounced structural or functional aberration that an organic cause of the speech difficulty needs to be considered. If such deviations are noted, further testing and/or referral to a medical expert is warranted.

Between the endpoints of this continuum exists a broad range of structural and functional deviations that may or may not directly affect the adequate production of speech sounds. Often clinicians find minor structural and/or functional inadequacies that do not appear "serious" yet certainly do not qualify as "passing."

Interpreting such results is often difficult. Our evaluation of the speech mechanism is just a screening measure that requires more testing and possible referral when any functional and/or structural inadequacies are found. One possible screening form for the evaluation of the speech-motor system is summarized in Appendix 6.1.

What to Look for When Evaluating the Speech Mechanism

Examining the Head and Facial Structures. A first impression is obtained by sitting opposite the client and evaluating the size and shape of the head. Relative to the body size, the head should appear normal—not too large and not too small. In addition, its shape should be considered. The relationship between the cranium (the upper portion of the skull containing the brain) and the facial skeleton (the lower portion of the skull containing, among other structures, the articulators) should be evaluated. The cranial portion should not appear too large nor the facial area too small, or vice versa. Micrognathia, for example, is marked by an unusually small jaw. Next, the symmetry of the facial features should be inspected. Do the right and left sides of the face appear similar both in proportion and in overall appearance? *Proportion* refers to the structures on both sides being on corresponding planes and their dimensions being similar. For example, right and left eyes are level, and both eyes appear to be about the same size. *Appearance* refers to the overall shape of the structures in question and to the normal state of resting muscle—that is, to the muscular tone. Oddly shaped eyes, nose, or mouth would be a deviancy within this category. In addition, any drooping of the structures or lack of muscle tone on one side of the face should be noted. At rest, the right and left sides of the lips should be even, the red of the lips, or vermilion, forming a smooth curve. Appearance and proportions of the nares (the nostrils), the nasal septum (the structural division of the nose, dividing the nasal cavity into right and left halves), the philtrum (the vertical groove between the upper lip and the nasal septum), and the columella (the vertical ridges on either side of the philtrum) should be evaluated. In short, any striking features of the head and face should be noted. This would include a fairly common syndrome called *adenoid facies*, the result of chronic or repeated infections that lead to enlarged adenoids, mouth breathing, a shortening of the upper lip, and an elongated face (Zemlin, 1998).

Examining Breathing. Respiration can be observed indirectly by examining breathing patterns. The clinician should observe and evaluate the client's breathing patterns at rest (silent breathing) and during speech. During silent breathing, the client's mouth should be closed, with no noticeable clavicular breathing (excursions in the clavicular area that cause the shoulders to move up and down during breathing). In addition, during silent breathing, the amount of time between the inspiratory and expiratory phases should be fairly equal. Therefore, an approximately one-to-one relationship exists between the time for inspiration and the time for expiration. During speech production, the normal time relationship between inspiratory and expiratory phases is somewhere between one and two-plus; that is, depending on the length of the utterance, the expiratory phase should be at least twice as long as the inspiratory phase. Any irregularities in breathing patterns should be noted. This includes muscular jerks or spasms during breathing, forced inhalations or exhalations, or any other (especially recurrent) conspicuous respiratory movements.

Examining the Oral and Pharyngeal Cavity Structures. The structures involved in this area of the speech mechanism examination include the teeth, the tongue, the palate, and the pharyngeal areas.

The Teeth. First, the occlusion of the teeth is important. Normal occlusion (Class I) is characterized by the lower molars being one-half of a tooth ahead of the upper molars. There are different types of malocclusions, including Class II (overbite), Class III (underbite), open bite, and crossbite. (Definitions of these malocclusions are given in Appendix 6.1.) Next, the clinician should check to see whether all teeth are present and their spacing and axial orientation appear adequate. The *axial orientation* of the teeth refers to the positioning of the individual teeth. Abnormalities in this respect would pertain to irregularly "tipped" or rotated teeth. Malocclusions of the teeth and missing teeth may affect the production of specific speech sounds.

The Tongue. First, examine the size of the tongue in its relationship to the size of the oral cavity. Does it appear too large, overfilling the oral cavity (macroglossia), or does it seem too small for the cavity size (microglossia)? Either of these conditions would signal a deviancy. In addition, the tongue's appearance is examined to see whether the color appears normal and the muscular dorsum of the tongue demonstrates a healthy muscle tone. Any "shriveled" tongue appearance might signal a paralytic condition. Next, the surface of the tongue needs to be observed. It should be relatively smooth. Any fissures (grooves or cracks in the dorsum of the tongue), lesions (wounds or abrasions), or fasciculations (visible "bundling" of muscles) would indicate a deviancy. Finally, the tongue needs to be examined in its resting position. It should look symmetrical, without any muscular twitching or movements.

The Hard and Soft Palates. Until this point, the clinician has only observed structures. Examination of the hard and soft palate goes beyond observation. It necessitates feeling the structures with a finger and evaluating the structures within the oral and pharyngeal cavity. Therefore, the clinician must wear examining gloves and be equipped with a small penlight to carry out the task. The hard palate's color; the size and shape of the palatal vault; and the presence or absence of clefts, fissures, and fistulas (openings or holes in the palate) should be determined. The midline of the hard and soft palates is usually a pink and whitish color; a blue tint may suggest a submucous cleft. To exclude this possibility, the clinician should feel along the midline of the hard palate to ensure that the underlying bony structure is intact. The uvula should be examined, and its length and any structural abnormalities noted. A bifid uvula (a uvula that is split into two portions), for example, may indicate a submucous cleft. Finally, the fauces (the passage between the oral and pharyngeal cavities) and the pharyngeal area itself must be assessed. Excessive redness or a swollen appearance of the tonsils and/or adenoids might indicate an inflammation and warrant medical referral.

Functionally Assessing the Speech Mechanism. The functional integrity of the speech mechanism is as important as adequate structures. In this portion of the assessment, the movement patterns of the lips, mandible, tongue, and velum are examined. For the purpose at hand, proper function means not only that the client can move the structures on command but also that the range, smoothness, and speed of the movements are adequate. As the client is performing the various tasks, the clinician should pay attention to the following:

1. Can the client adequately perform the task?
2. Is the range of movements adequate?
3. Are the movements integrated and smooth?
4. Given the age of the client, is the speed of movement within normal limits?

Diadochokinetic rates have often been used to test the speed of movement of the articulators. These rates refer to the maximum repetition rate of the syllables [pʌ], [tʌ], and [kʌ] alone and in various combinations. The rate is measured by either (1) a *count by time* procedure in which the examiner counts the number of syllables spoken in a given interval of time or (2) a *time by count* measurement in which the tester notes the time it takes to perform a specific number of repetitions.

In general, it can be said that diadochokinetic rates increase with age (Fletcher, 1972, 1978; St. Louis & Ruscello, 2000). St. Louis and Ruscello's data show that from about 8 years of age until adulthood the rates remain very similar. According to Kent and colleagues (1987), using diadochokinetic rates for younger children is not suggested due to the variability in the performance of children. In addition, Kent and colleagues (1987) state that, across the lifespan, normative data are limited. The Robbins and Klee (1987) data for children from 2 years 6 months to 6 years 11 months are included in Table 6.1, although the study tested only 10 children in each group. Such tasks and their interpretation should be used with caution. Weismer (1997) questions the role of using these types of procedures in the evaluation of speech disorders. He concludes that these rates may not furnish important diagnostic data because these tasks do not simulate speech production and the rapid repetition of syllables is not consistent with speaking rates or with articulatory movement patterns found in conversational speech. Refer to Table 6.1 for diadochokinetic rates from 2 years 6 months to 8-plus years of age.

> ▶ Video Example 6.1
>
> In this video, 3-year-old Elizabeth is led through a small segment of the functional assessment of the speech mechanism. Note how she reacts to the various tasks; for example, note the lack of smooth movement for licking her lips and moving her lips back and forth. Also note her attempts at the diadochokinetic rates.
>
> https://www.youtube.com/watch?v=TWNWVrcTyEk

Table 6.1 Diadochokinetic Rates (Based on Fletcher [1972, 1978], Kent, Kent, and Rosenbek [1987], Robbins and Klee [1987], and St. Louis and Ruscello [2000]) Based on a Count by Time (Seconds) Procedure

Age	Stimulus	Repetition Rates/Second	Age	Stimulus	Repetition Rates/Second
2 years 6 months to 2 years 11 months	[pʌ] [tʌ] [kʌ] "patticake"	3.7 3.7 3.7 1.3	5 years 0 months to 5 years 5 months	[pʌ] [tʌ] [kʌ] "patticake"	4.8 4.8 4.6 1.6
3 years 0 months to 3 years 5 months	[pʌ] [tʌ] [kʌ] "patticake"	4.7 4.6 3.8 1.4	5 years 6 months to 5 years 11 months	[pʌ] [tʌ] [kʌ] "patticake"	5.1 5.2 4.9 1.7
3 years 6 months to 3 years 11 months	[pʌ] [tʌ] [kʌ] "patticake"	4.8 4.8 4.8 1.8	6 years	[pʌ] [tʌ] [kʌ] [pʌ]-[tʌ]-[kʌ]	4.2 4.1 3.6 1.0
4 years 0 months to 4 years 5 months	[pʌ] [tʌ] [kʌ] "patticake"	4.9 4.8 4.6 1.6	7 years	[pʌ] [tʌ] [kʌ] [pʌ]-[tʌ]-[kʌ]	4.7 4.1 3.8 1
4 years 6 months to 4 years 11 months	[pʌ] [tʌ] [kʌ] "patticake"	4.6 4.5 4.3 1.3	8 years	[pʌ] [tʌ] [kʌ] [pʌ]-[tʌ]-[kʌ]	5.6 5.6 5.6 2

A possible apraxic condition may be questioned if the client cannot move individual structures on command but has movements during involuntary tasks. For example, if the client cannot stick out the tongue when asked to do so but can stick out the tongue to lick ice cream off a spoon, this could indicate an apraxic condition. Further testing is necessary. The sections titled "Childhood Apraxia of Speech: A Disorder of Speech Motor Control" and "Motor Speech Disorders in Adults: Acquired Apraxia of Speech" in Chapter 11 offer further suggestions for diagnostic protocols that could be used for a suspected apraxic condition.

The major goal of this portion of the speech-motor assessment is to determine whether the functional integrity of the articulators appears adequate. Isolated functional deviancies only suggest motor problems but do not necessarily translate to an inability to articulate certain speech sounds. Such functional difficulties should be evaluated considering the client's articulatory performance, articulatory limitations, and intelligibility. Several functional tasks for lips, mandible, tongue, and velum are indicated in Appendix 6.1.

Standardized Speech Assessments and Supplemental Testing

Standardized speech assessments are typically designed to elicit spontaneous naming based on the presentation of pictures. Most consonants of General American English are tested in the initial, medial, and final positions of words.

Advantages and Disadvantages of Standardized Speech Assessments

Using a standardized speech assessment has several advantages. First, these assessments are relatively easy to give and score; the necessary time expenditure is usually minimal. This is an attractive feature for those who feel limited in the time they can spend with appraisal procedures. Second, the results provide the clinician with a quantifiable list of "incorrect" sound productions in different word positions. This is clearly relevant to further assessment and therapy planning. Third, the use of norm-referenced, standardized, single-word tests is typically mandated as a necessary part of an evaluation for a speech sound disorder (ASHA, n.d.-b; Skahan, Watson, & Lof, 2007). Scores from these tests allow the clinician to compare an individual client's performance with the performance of others of a similar age. In addition, these scores could be used to document the client's need for, and progress in, therapy.

However, there are also several problems inherent in standardized speech assessments. They can be summarized as follows:

1. Standardized speech assessments examine sound production in selected, isolated words. Eliciting sounds based on single-word responses can never give adequate information on the client's production realities in connected speech. Sound articulation within selected words may not be representative of a client's ability to produce a particular sound under natural speech conditions.

2. Standardized speech assessments do not typically give enough information about a client's phonological system. These are measures of speech sound

production. As such, they were never meant to provide enough assessment data for a phonological analysis. Although some spontaneous naming measures analyze sounds in error according to phonological processes, the information they provide is typically not enough for a comprehensive phonological analysis.

3. Standardized speech assessments do not test all sounds in all the contexts in which they occur in General American English. Although this would admittedly be a rather large task, some measures do not even test the total inventory of speech sounds of General American English. If scored according to the directions provided, most articulation tests do not test vowels, for example, and very few consonant clusters are sampled.

4. The sounds tested do not occur in comparable phonetic contexts; that is, they are not context controlled. For example, the sounds before and after the tested consonants are different from word to word. The words used also vary in length and complexity. This presents the client with a task that changes the production difficulty from word to word. An analysis by Eisenberg and Hitchcock (2010) found that only 4 of the 11 measures they reviewed demonstrated a controlled environment for a large number of the word-initial consonants. In this same study, none of the tests demonstrated a controlled word environment for a large number of the word-final consonants tested.

5. Standardized speech assessments, like all standardized tests, are selected probes into rather limited aspects of an individual's total articulatory behavior and/or abilities. These measures examine only a very small portion of a person's articulatory behavior; they explore the person's performance with particular test items, on a certain day, in a unique testing situation. It would not be realistic to generalize that such limited results represent a reliable measure of the client's articulatory abilities, let alone the client's phonological system.

Clinical Exercises Pick one standardized speech measure that you have available. Consider that you are testing a child with [s] and [z] problems. How many words does the test contain that would identify these sounds? Count also those words that are not specifically testing [s] or [z] for the articulation score but that do contain these sounds. Do you think you have an adequate number of words?

There are approximately 13 word-initial and 13 word-final [s] clusters in General American English. How many s-clusters does the measure you have chosen include?

Factors to Consider When Selecting a Standardized Speech Measure

In selecting a measure of speech sound competency, several factors are important. In addition to the test's construct and its technical characteristics, the following should be considered: (1) its appropriateness for the client's age or developmental level, (2) its ability to supply a standardized score, (3) its analysis of the sound errors, and (4) its inclusion of an adequate sample of the sounds relevant to the client at hand.

Appropriateness for the Age or Developmental Level of the Client.   Although the age ranges vary, most tests can be administered to children from approximately age 3 years to school age. Selection is troublesome for very young, older adolescent, and adult clients. Younger clients, who may include 2-year-olds or delayed 3- and 4-year-olds, may not respond well to a formal standardized measure. Some younger children might react better to tests that contain large colored pictures or realistic manipulatable objects. For other children, the naming of actual objects or spontaneous speech may be the only way to assess sound production skills. In the evaluation of adolescent and adult clients, two problems exist. First, many of the tests are not standardized for children beyond the ages of 12 or 13 years. In addition, most standardized measures are oriented toward a much younger population. This may prove demeaning for older adolescents and adults and therefore is inappropriate. Certain tests contain printed sentences that can be read by clients. Although the sentence content and the reading level are designed for early school-age children, assessments that provide sentences to be read might prove less of a problem for older clients.

Ability to Provide a Standardized Score.   Some tests are not standardized; that is, standardized scores are not available as outcome measures. Although this is seldom the case in newer tests, some tests—although they are worthwhile probes—do not give standardized measures. Therefore, the results obtained from a client cannot be compared to the performance of other individuals of a similar age. Many sites, especially public school settings, require that the test provide standardized measures for assessment purposes; therefore, tests should be selected accordingly.

Analysis of the Sound Errors.   Many different standardized measures are available. Some are labeled articulation tests, whereas others purport to be tests of phonology. However, these tests do not differ in their examination format (both use the same format: spontaneous picture naming) but in their analysis of the results. Typically, tests of phonology categorize misarticulations according to phonological processes. Although the clinician could go through any measure noting the number and type of phonological processes used, tests that already contain such a procedure will probably allow the clinician a more expedient assessment.

Refer to Table 6.2 for an overview of a few standardized measures that can be used to assess preschool- and school-age children.

Inclusion of an Adequate Sample of the Sounds Relevant for the Client.   Standardized measures typically contain words that sample the sound inventory of General American English. Thus, most of the consonants of General American English are examined within the measure. However, most tests do not sample the most frequently misarticulated sounds in a number of different contexts. For example, the [ʃ] may be tested in only two or three different words. An adequate number of words containing the sound in various word positions is often not available. Supplemental testing with additional words can always be achieved later, but a test that provides adequate goal-directed material for individual clients uses our diagnostic time more efficiently.

Table 6.2 Selected Examples of Standardized Speech Assessments

Name	Age Range	Word Positions Tested	Scores Provided	Comments
Arizona 4: Arizona Articulation Proficiency Scale (4th ed.) (Fudala & Stegall, 2017)	1 year 6 months to 18 years 11 months	Initial- and final-word positions	Standardized; gives standard score, z-score, percentile, speech intelligibility values, and level of articulatory impairment	Gives weighted scores for each consonant. Tests vowels. Offers percentage of occurrence for phonological error patterns.
Assessment Link between Phonology and Articulation—Revised (Lowe, 1996)	3 years to 8 years 11 months	Initial- and final-word positions	Standardized; gives standard scores and percentile ranks	Provides several analyses and gives analysis forms that can be used to document phonological processes, vowel errors, and consonant clusters.
Bankson-Bernthal Test of Phonology (Bankson & Bernthal, 1990)	3 years to 6 years	Initial- and final-word positions	Standardized; gives standard score, percentile rank, and standard error of measurement	Provides various ways to analyze results, phonological processes included.
Clinical Assessment of Articulation and Phonology: CAAP (2nd ed.) (Secord & Donohue, 2002)	2 years 6 months to 11 years 11 months	Pre- and postvocalic consonants	Standardized; gives standard scores, percentile rank scores, and age-equivalent scores	Consonant clusters tested are only words containing [s], [ɹ], and [l] clusters. Vowels are not tested. Sentences are provided and can be used with children who can read.
Diagnostic Evaluation of Articulation and Phonology (DEAP) (Dodd, Hua, Crosbie, Holm, & Ozanne, 2006)	3 years to 8 years 11 months	Initial- and final-word positions	Standardized; gives standard scores and percentile ranks for several measures	Subtests include Sounds in Words, Phonological Process Use, Single Words vs. Connected Speech Agreement Criterion. Contains a diagnostic screen and articulation, phonology, and oral motor screening.
Goldman-Fristoe Test of Articulation (3rd ed.) (Goldman & Fristoe, 2015)	2 years to 16+ years	Initial-, medial-, and final-word positions	Standardized; gives standard score and percentile rank; a confidence interval can be calculated	Can be used with the Khan-Lewis test (Khan & Lewis, 2015) to assess phonological processes.
HAPP-3: Hodson Assessment of Phonological Patterns (Hodson, 2004)	Preschool age	Initial-, medial-, and final-word positions	Standardized; gives percentile rank and severity rating	Assesses phonological processes. Can be used as a direct link to the cycles approach.
Khan-Lewis Phonological Analysis (3rd ed.) (Khan & Lewis, 2015)	2 years to 21 years 11 months	Initial-, medial-, and final-word positions	Ten developmental phonological processes yield standard scores, percentile rank scores, test-age equivalent scores, and percentage of occurrence for individual processes by age	Uses the words from the Goldman-Fristoe Test of Articulation (Goldman & Fristoe, 2015) and translates errors into more common phonological processes. As with the Goldman-Fristoe test, vowels are not tested.
LinguiSystems Articulation Test–Normative Update (LAT-NU) (Bowers & Huisingh, 2018)	3 years to 21 years 11 months	Initial-, medial-, and final-word positions	Standardized; the normative update is more reliable and valid than the last version. However, information about the test does not mention standard scores or percentiles.	A comprehensive Articulation Proficiency Score can be calculated. Provides severity and intelligibility ratings as well as stimulability measures.

Name	Age Range	Word Positions Tested	Scores Provided	Comments
PAT-3: Photo Articulation Test (3rd ed.) (Lippke, Dickey, Selmar, & Soder, 1997)	3 years to 12 years	Initial-, medial-, and final-word positions	Standardized; gives standard scores, age equivalents, and percentiles	Uses actual photographs to test sounds; tests vowels and diphthongs.
Structured Photographic Articulation Test–III (3rd ed.) (Tattersall & Dawson, 2016)	3 years to 9 years	Initial-, medial-, and final-word positions	Standardized; gives standardized scores, including standard scores, percentile score ranks, percentile band scores, and test-age equivalent scores	Uses photographs of Dudsberry, a golden retriever puppy, interacting with various objects. Does not test vowels, although the manual provides a probe for imitation of each vowel in one word. The aim is to test articulation, although seven common phonological processes are provided.

Note: All standardized measures have used the latest U.S. Census reports to determine gender, race/ethnicity, and geographical percentages that are used in direct proportion for their standardization population.

Clinical Application

Many standardized speech measures examine phonological processes. However, phonological processes can be determined from the results of any standardized speech measure. The clinician examines the results and notes the phonological processes used. The following is an example from the PAT-3: Photo Articulation Test (Lippke et al., 1997):

Word	Child's Response	Phonological Process
saw	[tɑ]	stopping [s] → [t]
pencil	[pɛnθəl]	consonant cluster substitution [ns] → [nθ], fronting [s] → [θ]
house	[haʊ]	final consonant deletion [s] → ø
spoon	[pun]	consonant cluster reduction [sp] → [p]
skates	[keɪtθ]	consonant cluster reduction [sk] → [k]
		consonant cluster substitution [ts] → [tθ], fronting
stars	[tɑɚ]	consonant cluster reduction [st] → [t]
		final consonant deletion [z] → ø[1]
zipper	[dɪpɚ]	stopping [z] → [d]

[1] In this example, the production is characterized as a final consonant deletion because [ɑɚ] is considered a centering diphthong.

The phonological processes that are operating and how often they occur could then be analyzed.

Assessment Procedures to Supplement Standardized Speech Measures

The following assessment strategies can be used to minimize the previously mentioned shortcomings of standardized speech assessments:

1. *If a word contains any aberrant vowel or consonant productions, transcribe the entire word.* This gives valuable additional information about the client's sound production skills. For example, assume that the tested word is *yellow*, that the initial [j] is being evaluated, and that the client says [jɛwoʊ]. According to the scoring instructions, the initial [j] would be noted as being "correct," and the clinician would continue to the next item. However, if the entire word has been transcribed, the clinician can later evaluate the [l] production and compare it to the other words on the test that contain [l]. (In addition, some measures test only sounds in the initial and final word positions; however, some clients demonstrate difficulties with medial productions.) Transcribing the entire word complements the test information considerably and also supplies insights into vowels and consonant cluster productions.

2. *Supplement the standardized measure with additional utterances that address the client's noted problems.* The target sounds should be sampled in various vowel contexts and word positions, for example. There are several ways to do this. One method is to develop a list of words containing the needed sounds. This has the advantage of tailoring the supplemental materials to fit the client's needs exactly. One could also use commercially prepared materials. Two examples are McDonald's A Deep Test of Articulation (McDonald, 1964) and Secord's C-PAC: Clinical Probes of Articulation Consistency (Secord, 1981a). McDonald's Deep Test uses pictures to elicit a compound word, such as *hot* + *dog* = *hotdog*. The words formed are not typical compound words of General American English; however, a variety of phonetic contexts can be sampled in this way. Secord's C-PAC assesses the targeted consonant before and after various vowels (in one-syllable words, consonants initiating and terminating the word) in consonant clusters, in sentences, and during storytelling. For children who cannot read, the elicitation mode is imitative. These commercially available protocols have the advantage of assessing a sound in a variety of contexts without any preparation on the part of the clinician.

3. *Always sample and record continuous speech.* Although it has been well documented that production differences exist between single-word tasks (citing) and spontaneous speech (talking) (e.g., Andrews & Fey, 1986; Bernhardt & Holdgrafer, 2001; Morrison & Shriberg, 1992), many practitioners continue to use a standardized speech measure as the sole basis for their analysis procedures. A single-word standardized speech measure alone is not good enough to appraise and diagnose clients with speech sound disorders. See the section titled "Spontaneous Speech Sample" for further information.

4. *Determine the stimulability of the error sounds.* This task can be accomplished easily and relatively quickly at the end of the standardized measure. Refer to the section titled "Stimulability Testing."

Organizing Standardized Speech Assessment Results: Describing the Error

Most standardized measures include a form that can be used to record a client's responses. By completing this form, the clinician obtains information about the accuracy of the sound articulation and the position of this sound within the test word. Each measure gives directions on how to record accurate and inaccurate sound realizations. At least three different scoring systems describe sound errors (Shriberg, Kent, McAllister, & Preston, 2019). The following scoring systems are available:

Two-Way Scoring. A choice is made between a production that is "right" (accurate articulation of the sound in question) or "wrong" (inaccurate articulation). Two-way scoring can be used effectively to give feedback to the client and to document therapy progress. However, because of its limitations and its inability to render any usable information about the type of aberrant articulation taking place, the two-way scoring system is not the best option for scoring standardized speech measures. That said, although most standardized speech measures do give instructions on using phonetic transcription, the scoring for most, if not all, standardized measures is based on a correct–incorrect dichotomy. The clinician counts the number of errors (incorrect responses) and then looks at the standardization tables for a score.

Five-Way Scoring. This system uses a classification based on the type of error. "Correct" productions constitute one category. The other four categories are (1) deletion or omission—a sound is deleted completely, (2) substitution—a sound is replaced by another sound, (3) distortion—the target sound is approximated but not closely enough to be considered a typical realization, and (4) addition—a sound or sounds are added to the intended sound. The five-way scoring system may be suggested in the manuals of standardized speech assessments.

However, this system has several inherent problems. First, standardized measures often do not define, or give examples of, which articulatory patterns are considered within normal limits. The many dialectal and contextual variations could result in a somewhat different but entirely acceptable pronunciation. For example, the alveolar flap [ɾ] is a common pronunciation for [d] in *ladder*. Should this variation be considered "correct" if the medial d-sound is being tested? Clinicians should be aware of these common variations and how they may affect scoring. Second, the category of deletion or omission may include the presence, rather than the absence, of a sound. Normally, deletion implies that a sound segment has been eliminated, as in [mu] for *moon*, for example. However, Van Riper and Irwin (1958) included glottal stops, unvoiced articulatory placements, and short exhalations under omissions. If the production of [wæʔən] for *wagon* is considered, according to these authors, the [g] would be classified as a deletion. However, it would be more accurate to label this as a substitution of a glottal stop for [g]. This ambiguous definition of deletion can detract from the accuracy of the results when sound realizations are analyzed later. Third, the terms *substitution* and *distortion* have a long history of definitional unclarity. Some authors (Van Riper, 1978; Van Riper & Irwin, 1958; Winitz, 1975) state that a more precise way to consider distortions is to regard them as substitutions of non-English sounds. For example, a child produces a [ʃ] in which the articulators are too far back; that is, rather than prepalatal, it has a palatal placement. There is a palatal fricative, transcribed as [ç], that is a phoneme in many languages. Therefore, this palatal [ʃ] production could be designated either as a distortion of [ʃ] or as a substitution of [ç] for [ʃ]. Such vagueness regarding what constitutes a distortion versus a substitution can also affect the scoring of many standardized measures.

Phonetic Transcription. Transcription systems describe speech behavior. The goal of any phonetic transcription is to represent spoken language through written symbols. Of the three scoring systems mentioned, phonetic transcription requires the highest degree of clinical skill. The goal is not to *judge* specific misarticulations but to *describe* them as accurately as possible. Phonetic transcription has several advantages over the other two systems: (1) it is far more precise; (2) it gives more information about the misarticulation, which is helpful for both assessment and intervention; and (3) among professionals, it is the most universally accepted way to communicate information about articulatory features. Phonetic transcription uses broad and narrow transcriptions including diacritics, which are indispensable for a comprehensive evaluation. This system is used for the analyses of citation speech assessments as well as spontaneous speech sampling.

Stimulability Testing

Another assessment procedure often used by clinicians during the assessment process is stimulability testing. **Stimulability testing** refers to testing the client's ability to produce a misarticulated sound in an appropriate manner when "stimulated" by the clinician to do so. Many variations of this procedure exist, but commonly the clinician asks the client to "watch and listen to what I am going to say, and then you say it" (Bernthal et al., 2017). Although there is no standardized procedure for stimulability testing, an isolated sound is usually first attempted. If a normal articulation is achieved, the sound is placed within a consonant-vowel environment and subsequently in a word context. The number of models provided by the clinician typically varies from one to five.

For many clinicians, stimulability testing is a regular procedure that concludes the administration of a standardized speech measure. It determines the consistency of a client's performance on two different tasks: the spontaneous naming of a picture and the imitation of a speech model provided by the clinician. Such information is very helpful in appraising the articulatory capabilities of a client. (Refer to Bleile, 2002; Hodson, Scherz, & Strattman, 2002; Khan, 2002; Lof, 2002; Miccio, 2002; and Tyler & Tolbert, 2002.)

Children's articulatory stimulability has been used to determine therapy goals and to predict which children might benefit more from therapy. It has been suggested that sounds that are more stimulable would be easier to work on in therapy; therefore, highly stimulable sounds are targeted first (Rvachew & Nowak, 2001). When used as a means of predicting which children might benefit from therapy, high stimulability was correlated with more rapid therapeutic success (Miccio, Elbert, & Forrest, 1999). It was also proposed that high stimulability might mean that children are on the verge of acquiring the sounds and would not need therapeutic intervention (Khan, 2002). Although stimulability testing seems to be one type of data collected by most clinicians, its effect on treatment targets is still questionable. In her article on treatment efficacy, Gierut (1998) points out that two studies (Klein, Lederer, & Cortese, 1991; Powell, Elbert, & Dinnsen, 1991) have documented that targeting nonstimulable sounds prompted change in those sounds and other untreated stimulable sounds. In comparison, treatment of a stimulable sound did not necessarily lead to changes in untreated stimulable or nonstimulable sounds. Gierut concludes that treatment of nonstimulable sounds may be more efficient than treatment of stimulable sounds because of the widespread change that seems to occur. However, a second study (Rvachew, Rafaat, & Martin, 1999) noted lack of treatment progress on nonstimulable sounds when compared to stimulable ones. To summarize, stimulability testing provides useful information. However, it should not be the only source when deciding whether a client receives services or which therapy sequence to use.

Contextual Testing

Contextual testing refers to the use of specific phonetic contexts to possibly facilitate correct speech sound production. Commercially prepared materials such as McDonald's A Deep Test of Articulation (McDonald, 1964) and Secord's C-PAC: Clinical Probes of Articulation Consistency (Secord, 1981a) were mentioned previously. Both use different phonetic contexts (i.e., different vowels and consonants) to possibly obtain a correct production or a near-correct approximation. In addition, Secord and Shine (2003) have an articulation measure that supports contextual testing called S-CAT: Secord Contextual Articulation Tests. This measure has three parts: storytelling probes, contextual probes, and target words for contextual training. Another possibility is the Contextual Test of Articulation–CTA (Aase et al., 2000). This measure is designed for prekindergarten to fourth-grade children. The concept of the test is to assist in identifying the phonetic contexts that facilitate correct speech sound production. The CTA examines the following phonemes: / s /, / l /, / k /, / ɹ /, and the schwa. The phonemes are also elicited in 15 consonant clusters: / sm, sn, sl, st, sk, sp, pl, bl, kl, kɹ, tɹ, dɹ, bɹ, mp, nt /. All sounds are embedded in colorful photos that can be elicited spontaneously or prompted with cues.

However, a clinician does not need a commercially prepared instrument to do contextual testing. The basic premise of contextual testing is to present an individual with various phonetic contexts that might facilitate accurate production. Chapter 9 has a section on facilitating contexts for each of the commonly misarticulated sounds. Also, Chapter 9 provides word lists that are ordered from easy to more difficult coarticulatory conditions for each of these sounds.

Testing Multisyllabic (3-Plus Syllable) Words

Assessment of multisyllabic words can reflect many aspects of a child's production possibilities—for example, the child's ability to manipulate phonotactics, prosody (especially word stress), language, and phonological processing skills (James, van Doorn, & McLeod, 2008; Masso, McLeod, Baker, & McCormack, 2016). Multisyllabic words allow clinicians a view into a child's ability to accurately use timing, stress, and the unstressed schwa vowel.

James and colleagues (2008) have criticized single-word speech assessments due to their lack of multisyllabic words. Most measures have two-syllable words but contain very few, if any, words that are three or more syllables in length. Clinicians are well aware of children who stumble and have serious difficulties with 3-plus syllable words but reach a high degree of accuracy with one-syllable words. By not assessing multisyllabic words, James and colleagues (2008) state that a speech sound disorder may be obscured or undiagnosed. James (2006, 2009) provides 10 multisyllabic words that were found clinically useful for revealing speech production difficulties in children: ambulance, hippopotamus, computer, spaghetti, vegetables, helicopter, animals, caravan, caterpillar, and butterfly. There are several informal measures that evaluate multisyllabic words. Table 6.3 contains some examples.

Table 6.3 Examples of Informal Assessments Using Multisyllabic Words

Name	Age Range	Number of Multisyllabic Words	Comments
Assessment of Children's Articulation and Phonology (James, 2001)	2 years to 7 years	199-item test that includes 17 words with 3+ syllables, 77 two-syllable words, and 105 one-syllable words	Research found that words that best differentiated between children with and without speech impairment were monosyllabic words containing word-initial and/or word-final clusters and polysyllabic words (i.e., words with 3+ syllables).
Polysyllable Preschool Test (Baker, 2013)	Preschool-age children	A single-word, picture-naming task that contains a total of 30 words: 20 are 3-syllable words, 8 are 4-syllable words, and 2 are 5-syllable words. The words represent a variety of weak and strong onset stress patterns.	This text's author could not find a copy of this test. One might need to contact the author of the test to get a copy.
Single Word Polysyllable Test (Gozzard, Baker, & McCabe, 2006)	Children from 4 years 0 months to 4 years 11 months were used in the original study. These words would be acceptable for preschool-age and early school-age children.	50 polysyllabic words containing a variety of consonants, vowels, stress patterns, and word shapes were used. The stimuli for the children consisted of a book of 46 colored photographs and clip-art pictures.	The words are contained in the appendix of this article, which is available through Academia's website.

Spontaneous Speech Sample

Over the years, a number of authors have documented the differences that exist in children's speech when single-word citing responses are compared to spontaneous speech (e.g., Andrews & Fey, 1986; Bernhardt & Holdgrafer, 2001; Masterson, Bernhardt, & Hofheinz, 2005; Morrison & Shriberg, 1992; Wolk & Meisler, 1998). However, assessment and treatment protocols continue to be based primarily on the results of standardized speech assessments. Some clinicians may argue that they do not have time to complete the transcription and analysis of a spontaneous speech sample. However, these samples can serve many different functions. For example, conversational speech samples can supply additional information about the language, voice, and prosodic capabilities of the client. Based on the data from the spontaneous speech sample, specific semantic, morphosyntactic, and pragmatic analyses could supplement language testing when required. The conversational speech sample is not optional but rather a basic necessity for every professional assessment.

Although any conversational speech sample is more representative of a client's production capabilities than a one-word assessment, the type of sampling situation also plays a role. Several authors have found an increase or decrease in errors depending on the production task required. First, more complex linguistic contents generally cause an increase in misarticulations (Panagos & Prelock, 1982; Schmauch, Panagos, & Klich, 1978). Second, different communicative needs can influence production accuracy. For example, improvement of speech patterns was noted in five children when they were trying to relate information that was important to them (Menyuk, 1980).

Organization of the Continuous Speech Sample

A continuous speech sample should be planned and executed in a systematic manner to minimize the time investment and maximize the results. Here are some suggestions:

Begin with the Standardized Speech Measure.   One goal of a continuous speech sample in a comprehensive assessment is to compare a client's productions on a single-word task to those in continuous speech. Errors that have been noted in single words can be helpful in planning the continuous speech sample. For example, if a child demonstrates error productions for [s], [ʃ], [tʃ], [dʒ], and [l] on the standardized measure or if your test does not sample particular sounds, these sounds could be targeted.

Provide Objects or Pictures That May Elicit the Targeted Sounds.   Objects and pictures containing the targeted sounds can become a part of the spontaneous speech procedure. Speech-language specialists can increase comparability between naming and talking tasks by attempting to trigger some of the same words that were on the standardized speech measure.

Plan the Length of the Sample.   There has been a lot of discussion about which sample length furnishes adequate information for a comprehensive assessment. Grunwell (1987) states that "100 different words is the minimum size of an adequate sample; 200–250 words is preferable" (p. 55). On the other hand, Crary (1983) found that 50-word samples for process analysis provided as much information as 100-word speech samples. More recently, Heilmann, Nockerts, and Miller (2010) found that the results of a 1-minute sample were as consistent as those of 3- and 7-minute samples.

Keep in mind that, in normal conversation, children articulate between 100 and 200 syllables per minute (Culatta, Page, & Wilson, 1987). Therefore, based on the findings of Heilmann and colleagues (2010), a 1-minute sample of conversational speech should render approximately 100 to 200 words, depending on the length of each word. In most cases, if the sample is organized, this will probably constitute an adequate sample.

It is difficult to transcribe what a child is saying, listen, and respond appropriately to the situation. Therefore, it is a good idea to make a recording of the child's speech sample. To minimize time involvement when listening to the recording, a clinician could simply write out the child's utterances, using phonetic transcription only for errors that may be noted. Assuming that 15 minutes is required to transcribe portions of the sample, the total recording and transcribing time amounts to around 20 minutes. Considering the value this provides in acquiring needed information for goal-directed therapy, this is not a large time investment. Perhaps a lack of the necessary transcription skills deters clinicians more than the actual time involvement. The bottom line for clinicians is that a spontaneous speech sample is not an option but a necessity.

Plan for Diversity in the Sample.   Various communicative situations should be a portion of the recorded speech sample. A variety of situations will ensure that the sample adequately represents the client's phonetic and phonemic skills. This may include several talking situations, such as picture description, storytelling, describing the function of objects, and problem solving. Communicative diversity could also include the client talking with caregivers or siblings. Varying communicative situations also allow for articulatory differences that occur between pragmatically and linguistically diverse samples.

Monitor the Recording and Gloss Any Utterances That Might Later Be Difficult or Impossible to Understand in the Recording.   Diligent monitoring will ensure that the quality of a recording remains constant. This can mean anything from readjusting the device being used to asking the client to repeat an utterance if it is not completely intelligible. It is helpful and often necessary to *gloss* the word or phrase, especially if later transcription difficulties are anticipated. **Glossing** means repeating with normal pronunciation what the client has just said for easier identification later. This can be done quite naturally, so that it does not interfere with the structured situation.

Listen to a Small Portion of the Spontaneous Speech Sample Before Recording. Listening to 1 or 2 minutes of conversation before recording the sample may dramatically increase transcription effectiveness because the clinician can adjust to the client's pronunciation patterns. Later, unintelligible utterances should be clearly marked (language sampling techniques use a series of *X*s to note unintelligibility). It is not necessary to spend time trying to decipher these responses. Instead, it is better to gloss the utterance whenever the intelligibility of the response might be questioned later.

Test the Recording of the Continuous Speech Sample. Be sure to test the sound quality of your recording device *before* you make the recording. Know how to use the sound volume control and where the built-in microphone on the device is located. This text's author missed a complete sample by allowing a child to hold the microphone; unnoticed, the child pushed it into the "off" position. Also, be aware of covers that may fit too closely to the microphone and thus impede its functioning. Children typically like to see and hear the recordings that you have made of them. One idea is to make a short, 10-second segment. Play this back and see whether it is loud enough and the recording can be easily understood. Most clinicians are provided with a computer or a recording device in their workplace. An adequate sound sample can be recorded using that device and a small plug-in external microphone. Microphones are relatively inexpensive and can deliver a good-quality audio signal. Again, be careful when placing the microphone and always test before recording. For portable microphones, the best distance from the child is approximately 6 to 8 inches. The microphone should be slanted slightly toward the client's nose to eliminate distortions because of the expiratory release of certain consonants.

DO NOT use your personal cellphone to videotape or take pictures of your client. This is a violation of the Health Insurance Portability and Accountability Act (HIPAA). Cellphones are insecure devices that should not contain protected health information (PHI), which is defined as all "individually identifiable health information" (Health Insurance Portability and Accountability Act of 1996, Pub. L. No. 104-191, [CFR164.514(b)(2)]). Refer to Box 6.2.

Box 6.2

The Health Insurance Portability and Accountability Act (HIPAA) and Your Cellphone

- The Health Insurance Portability and Accountability Act (HIPAA) was established in 1996 (Public Law Number 104-191).
- The Privacy Rule (2003) pertains to all protected health information (PHI), including paper and electronic. The Security Rule deals specifically with electronic protected health information (EPHI).
- The HIPAA Privacy Rule regulates the use and disclosure of PHI, which is all "individually identifiable health information." If a picture contains any type of health information along with enough detail to identify a specific individual, it is PHI.
- If a photograph can be connected to a client, it is considered PHI.
- THE BOTTOM LINE: Unless your cellphone has been secured and encrypted and is being regulated and monitored, you are in violation of HIPAA if you use your cellphone to record a client.

Selection of Additional Measures in Other Areas

A percentage of our clinical population with "delayed speech" have associated language problems (Keating, Turrell, & Ozanne, 2001; Shriberg, 1991; Shriberg, Kwiatkowski, & Rasmussen, 1990; Toppelberg, Shapiro, & Theodore, 2000). Therefore, at least language screening is recommended for every child who has a speech sound disorder. Selection of additional tests largely depends on an evaluation of the background information, medical and/or school records, and the clinical impression of the individual client.

Language Screening

Because of the high percentage of language problems in children with speech disorders, at least a screening measure for language belongs in the evaluation process. Table 6.4 lists a few of the language screeners available. If the child does not pass the screening measure, a comprehensive, standardized test should be given. There are many standardized language measures. Speech and language treatment sites, including public school settings, hospitals, and private organizations, all have access to standardized measures. Just a few of these standardized tests are the Preschool Language Scale, 5th edition (PLS-5)

Table 6.4 Examples of Language Screening Tools

Name	Age Range Screened	Areas Assessed	Comments
Bankson Language Screening Test (2nd ed.) (Bankson, 1990)	3 years to 6 years 11 months	Tests receptive and expressive language, morphology, syntax, auditory memory, and auditory discrimination	Standardized on 1108 children Administration time: 10–15 minutes
Battelle Developmental Inventory Screening Test (2nd ed.) (Newborg, 2005)	6 months to 8 years	Subtests for fine and gross motor, adaptive, personal-social, receptive and expressive language, and cognitive skills	Standarized on 800 children; gives a range cutoff and age-equivalent scores Administration time: 10–30 minutes
Clinical Evaluation of Language Fundamentals Screening Test (4th ed.) (Semel, Wiig, & Secord, 2004)	5 years to 21 years 11 months	Tests morphology, syntax, semantics, and pragmatics	Standardized on 2000 students; has a cutoff score based on standardization results Administration time: 15 minutes
Early Screening Profiles (ESP) (Harrison et al., 1990)	2 years to 6 years 11 months	Provides a cognitive/language profile, motor profile, self-help/social profile, articulation survey, home survey, health history survey, and behavior survey	Standardized on 1149 children; gives standard scores with confidence intervals, percentile ranks, and age equivalents Administration time: 15–30 minutes. The surveys take an additional 15–20 minutes.
Fluharty Preschool Speech and Language Screening (2nd ed.) (Fluharty, 2000)	3 years to 6 years 11 months	Tests receptive language, expressive language, articulation, and vocabulary	Standardized on 705 children; gives standard scores and age equivalents Administration time: 10 minutes

(Zimmerman, Steiner, & Evatt Pond, 2011); the Clinical Evaluation of Language Fundamentals, 5th edition (CELF-5) (Wiig, Semel, & Secord, 2013); and the Comprehensive Assessment of Spoken Language, 2nd edition (CASL-2) (Carrow-Woolfolk, 2017).

Prosodic Screening and Testing

Prosody or **suprasegmental features** include variations in stress (loudness), pitch (intonation), and duration (rate) that occur across segments. **Rhythm**, another term used within this context, refers to how stressed and unstressed syllables are distributed over time. Occasionally, we notice that children with speech sound difficulties also evidence prosody that is noticeably off or, perhaps, stereotypical. For example, a child may stress words only on the first syllable, or a child may demonstrate equal and even stress on every syllable. Therefore, it is important that we are able to document the prosodic patterns that are noticed. One of the hallmark features of childhood apraxia of speech is aberrant prosody, especially in the realization of word or phrase stress patterns (ASHA, 2007b). Refer to Chapter 11 for more information on childhood apraxia of speech.

There are very few standardized tests available for examining receptive and expressive prosodic abilities in children. Table 6.5 lists those tests that are available for children. Although none of them has robust normative data, if you need to examine a child's prosody in more detail, one of these instruments could be used. Note that there are other tests available that indirectly examine prosody, but these are directed more at examining the emotional aspects of prosody—for example, as conveyed through facial expressions.

Phonological and Phonemic Awareness Screening and Testing

As noted in Chapter 5, early speech abilities and emerging literacy are interactive in a complex manner (McLeod et al., 2017). Phonological awareness is a strong

Table 6.5 Instruments for Assessing or Screening Prosody in Children

Name	Authors, Year	Age Range	Purpose	Normative Data
PEPS-C: Profiling Elements of Prosody in Speech Communication	Peppé & McCann, 2003	4 to 14 years	Assesses receptive and expressive prosodic skills	Normed on 120 children, ages 5 to 14 years
PPAT: Perception of Prosody Assessment	Klieve, 1998	7 to 12 years	Evaluates prosodic perception in children	Normed on 6 children, ages 7 to 12 years
PROP: Prosodic Profile	Crystal, 1982	Children and adults	Obtains information on expressive prosodic patterns	Provides normative data but is not standardized
PVSP: Prosody-Voice Screening Profile	Shriberg, Kwiatkowski, & Rasmussen, 1990	3 to 19 years	Assesses prosody and voice in conversational speech	Normed on 252 individuals, ages 3 to 19 years
Prosody-Voice Profile	Shriberg, 1993	3 to 6 years	A perceptually based assessment of voice and prosody based on a sample of conversational speech	Validated on 62 children with delayed speech and 13 with suspected apraxia of speech

predictor of reading and spelling success in preschool and kindergarten years (e.g., Gillon, 2018; Hesketh, 2010; Kenney, Barac-Cikoja, Finnegan, Jeffries, & Ludlow, 2006). Research has convincingly demonstrated that some children with speech sound disorders have difficulties with phonological awareness. At-risk children, including those with severe speech sound problems, a history of reading problems in the family, or a noticeable delay in phonological and phonemic awareness skills, should receive additional screening or testing in phonological and phonemic awareness. In addition, children with physical, sensory, or intellectual impairment, who frequently struggle with written language acquisition, may present weak phonological awareness skills (Gillon, 2018). Table 6.6 lists selected assessment and screening measures that could be used to further evaluate a child if you suspect the child is having difficulties with phonological awareness.

Table 6.6 Standardized Tools to Assess or Screen Phonological Awareness

Name	Age Range Tested, Administration Time	Areas of Phonological Awareness
Comprehensive Test of Phonological and Print Processing (CTOPP-2) (Wagner, Torgesen, Rashotte, & Pearson, 2013)	Age range: 4 years 0 months to 24 years 11 months Administration time: 40 minutes	Includes the following tasks: elision, blending words, sound matching, phoneme isolation, blending nonwords, segmenting nonwords. The following, which are considered phonological processing tasks involving long-term memory, are also assessed: memory for digits, nonword repetition, rapid digit naming, rapid letter naming, rapid color naming, rapid object naming
HearBuilder® Phonological Awareness Test (H-PAT) (Wiig & Secord, 2011)	Age range: 4 years 6 months to 9 years 11 months Administration time: 15 to 20 minutes	Includes the following tasks: letter-sound identification, rhyming (awareness and production), initial sound identification, blending words (syllables and sounds), segmenting words (syllables and sounds), deleting initial and final sounds, substituting initial and final sounds
Phonological Awareness Test–2 (PAT-2) (Robertson & Salter, 2007)	Age range: 5 years 0 months to 9 years 11 months, grades K–4 Administration time: 40 minutes	Includes the following tasks: rhyming, segmentation, isolation (initial, medial, final sounds), deletion, substitution with manipulatives, blending. Additional subtests for children ages 6 to 9 years: phoneme-grapheme correspondence, phonemic decoding
Phonological Awareness Skills Test (PAST) (Zgonc, 2000)	Age range: pre-K to early elementary grades Administration time: 20 minutes	This test is available online and was originally a portion of Sounds in Action (Zgonc, 2000); it gives a pass/fail score for each grade and includes the following tasks: word in sentence segmenting, rhyme recognition and production, syllable blending and segmentation, syllable deletion, phonemic isolation, initial and final blending and segmentation, deletion of initial, final, and phonemes from consonant blends, phoneme substitutions
Pre-Reading Inventory of Phonological Awareness (PIPA), U.S. version (Dodd, Crosbie, McIntosh, Teitzel, & Ozanne, 2003)	Age range: 4 years 0 months to 6 years 11 months Administration time: 25 to 30 minutes	Includes the following tasks: rhyme awareness, syllable segmentation, alliteration awareness, sound isolation, sound segmentation, letter-sound knowledge
Preschool Comprehensive Test of Phonological and Print Processing (Pre-CTOPP-2) (Lonigan, Wagner, Torgesen, & Rashotte, 2002)	Age range: 3 to 5 years Administration time: 30 minutes	Includes the following tasks: blending, elision, initial sound matching, word span, nonword repetition, rapid naming; the Pre-CTOPPP includes print awareness and reading vocabulary subtests

(Continued)

Table 6.6 Standardized Tools to Assess or Screen Phonological Awareness *(Continued)*

Name	Age Range Tested, Administration Time	Areas of Phonological Awareness
Test of Auditory Analysis Skills (TAAS) (Rosner, 1971)	Age range: grades K–6 Administration time: 3 to 5 minutes	This is a 13-item test that is available online but can be purchased as well; although it is over 40 years old, it could be used as a quick screener Components include: compound word segmenting, deletion of initial and final sounds in words, deletion of a sound in initial consonant blends
Test of Phonological Awareness Skills–Second Edition (TOPAS2+) (Torgesen & Bryant, 2004)	Age range: 5 years 0 months to 8 years 11 months, grades K–3 Administration time: K-version 30 to 45 minutes Early elementary version 15 to 30 minutes	Kindergarten version includes the following tasks: initial sound—same items and initial sound—different items, letter sounds Early elementary version includes the following tasks: ending sound—same items and ending sound—different items, letter sounds
Sutherland Phonological Awareness Test–Revised (Neilson, 2003)	Age range: grades 1–4 Administration time: 15 minutes	Includes the following tasks: syllable counting, rhyme detection, rhyme production, blending CVCs, onset and final phoneme identification, segmentation CVCs and blends, deletion: boundary and internal consonant, nonword reading, nonword spelling

Cognitive Appraisal

Some children who have difficulties communicating in general and specifically those with speech sound disorders may have associated cognitive impairments. The results of a cognitive appraisal may be important when developing further assessment and treatment goals. Testing might then be initiated by referring a client to appropriate professionals. Often such test results can be obtained through medical, school, or client records.

Caution should be exercised, though, when interpreting the results of cognitive measures for children who demonstrate speech sound disorders. First, a large percentage of children with speech sound disorders also demonstrate language difficulties. Some cognitive assessment tools use tasks that are very similar to those used to assess language. Therefore, these scores may be affected by children's language incompetence. For this reason, some authors have suggested using nonverbal cognitive measures (Paul, Norbury, & Gosse, 2018), although tests designed to evaluate nonverbal cognitive skills may appraise only a limited aspect of cognition (Kamhi, Minor, & Mauer, 1990). Second, intelligibility may play a role in the assessment of children with moderate to severe speech sound difficulties, particularly if verbal cognitive measures are used. Nonverbal measures would be helpful with unintelligible children; however, as previously noted, these tests appear restricted. Third, cognitive measures, similar to other standardized tests, do not adequately reflect the abilities of children from culturally and linguistically diverse backgrounds. Although the sample used to norm a particular test typically contains a percentage of children from culturally and linguistically diverse backgrounds (usually the same percentage as represented within the U.S. population), this percentage is typically so small that the inherent test bias for these populations is not eliminated. The presence of language and/or speech sound impairments may further compound the interpretation of scores for children from culturally or linguistically diverse backgrounds.

Although the results of a cognitive appraisal may give helpful guidelines for planning subsequent assessment and remediation strategies, interpretation of the results is not without problems. Clinicians should be aware of the type of cognitive assessment instrument used to appraise the individual (e.g., verbal versus nonverbal) and the limitations of each measure. *Extreme care should be exercised when interpreting the scores of children from linguistically and culturally diverse backgrounds.*

Assessment of a Child's Communicative Participation

At the beginning of this chapter, it was noted that the *Scope of Practice in Speech-Language Pathology* (ASHA, 2007a) provides a general framework for the diagnostic process of speech sound disorders (refer to Preferred Practice Patterns for the Profession of Speech-Language Pathology; ASHA, 2004). These practice patterns were developed to be consistent with the World Health Organization's *International Classification of Functioning, Disability and Health* (WHO, 2001). One of the questions asked was: What are the effects of this child's speech sound disorder on the individual's everyday communication contexts, including at least the school and home environments?

This is an important question and one that is often neglected in our assessment process. However, there are tools that can be used to assess the environment in which the child is functioning (refer to for example, the Index for Inclusion; Booth & Ainscow, 2002) and those that consider the children's own views about their speech and functioning within their environment. Table 6.7 lists a sample of these measures.

Table 6.7 Assessing Children's Views of Their Speech in Educational and Social Contexts

Name	Age Range	Areas Tested	Comments
Communication Attitude Test (CAT) (Brutten & Dunham, 1989)	6 to 15 years (grades 2–8)	This is a 35-item questionnaire that assesses the speech beliefs of children. It was administered to 518 children whose speech was considered normal.	Average CAT score (8.24) indicated the presence of few negative attitudes toward speech. The minimal negative attitudes decreased from second to eighth grade, but this decrease was not statistically significant.
Index for Inclusion: Developing Learning and Participation in Schools (Booth & Ainscow, 2002)	The Index is used to develop inclusion policies and practices within a school setting. It is not specifically directed toward a group of students.	Offers schools a supportive process of self-review and development, which draws on the views of staff, administrators, students, and caregivers, as well as other members of the surrounding communities. It involves a detailed examination of how barriers to learning and participation can be reduced for any student.	Aids in developing policies for a particular school. Examples include: (1) all new students are helped to settle into the school and (2) the school arranges teaching groups so that all students are valued.
Speech Participation and Activity Assessment of Children (SPAA-C) (McLeod, 2004)	No age range given. The 10-item questionnaire is centered on children describing how they feel about talking in different contexts. Children respond by choosing pictures (happy face, sad face, ?, for example).	This measure includes questions for the children themselves, as well as for their siblings, friends, parents, teachers, and others involved in their daily lives. Most questions can be answered in an interview format; however, there is one section in which children indicate their response by drawing.	The SPAA-C is free and downloadable from the Charles Sturt University (Australia) website. The questions for this measure are available in many languages.

Special Considerations: A Child with Emerging Phonology

The period of **emerging phonology** is the time span during childhood in which conventional words begin to appear as a means of communication. Although this level of development usually occurs when children are toddlers, it also may occur in older children who have more severe deficits in language learning. Within the assessment process, special consideration must be given to children with an emerging phonological system. Both the diagnostic procedures themselves and the analysis of the results will be different for this population.

Characteristics of Children with Emerging Phonological Systems. Children with emerging phonology are referred for speech-language services for several reasons. First, some may have been born with known risk factors. Identifiable developmental disorders include Down syndrome and other genetic disorders, known hearing impairments, and cerebral palsy. Second, some children will have early acquired disorders secondary to diseases or trauma such as encephalitis, closed head injury, or abuse. Third, some children will be brought by parents who are concerned about their child's development, as they may have observed differences in the expressive communication abilities and/or intelligibility of their child compared to those of other children of a similar age. Fourth, various sources will refer children because they are "late talkers" and their expressive language is slow to emerge.

Children with developmentally delayed emerging phonology are typically characterized by small expressive vocabularies showing a reduced repertoire of consonants and syllable shapes (Nathani, Ertmer, & Stark, 2006; Paul & Jennings, 1992; Pharr, Ratner, & Rescorla, 2000; Rescorla, Mirak, & Singh, 2000). Often their words are unintelligible. The limited phonological system may also affect further semantic and morphosyntactic development. Therefore, it is important to appraise the phonological system within the broader framework of children's developing language systems. In addition to hearing screening, assessment procedures should always include language screening or testing for this group of children.

Procedural Difficulties with Emerging Phonological Systems. Previously noted assessment procedures encompass several tasks that provide useful and necessary information. However, for children at this level of development, several of these tasks may be difficult to complete.

1. *Standardized speech and stimulability measures.* Depending on the children's developmental level, the administration of standardized speech assessment and stimulability measures might not be possible because these children are not yet skilled at following directions or at imitating. An alternative method might include the naming of objects. However, because of the limited expressive vocabulary of most of these children, this adaptation may have limitations.

   What to Do? With caregivers' help, a clinician can usually procure a fairly complete sample of the words a child is using. Based on the production of these words, the child's consonant and vowel inventory as well as syllable shapes can be established. Such words can be obtained in a number of ways. The following possibilities are given as suggestions:

   a. Have the family record the child saying specific spontaneous and elicited words at home.

   b. Have the caregiver bring a few objects that the child can name from home.

c. Have the caregiver keep a log of the intended words that the child can produce as well as the approximate way in which each word was pronounced.

Although a recording is a good idea, its quality must be ensured so that the child's productions can be evaluated accurately. Based on personal clinical experience, asking a caregiver to bring familiar objects from home and keeping a log of utterances usually provide more diagnostic information than recordings. Bringing in familiar objects from the home environment is especially productive in the initial session. For a young child in an unfamiliar setting, this might provide a small comfort zone that will open communication. Caregiver logs of the child's spoken words become necessary when attempting to assess the shy child who does not communicate at the first or even second meeting. Clinicians need to keep in mind that caregivers are not skilled in phonetic transcription and have limited abilities to write down how the child pronounced a certain word. Explanations and examples should be given to the caregiver on how to proceed with this task.

2. *Spontaneous speech sample.* Children with emerging phonological systems who are being evaluated for a possible communication disorder probably do not talk a lot. When they talk, their utterances may contain only one or two words, and these may be partially unintelligible. Collecting a spontaneous speech sample therefore may be a challenge. However, spontaneous samples not only provide data for establishing sound and syllable inventories but also establish communicative situations that elicit spontaneous utterances. If children are using primarily single words, a one-word utterance analysis such as Bloom's (1973) or Nelson's (1973) will quantify the types of words being used. As mentioned earlier, children's emerging phonological systems should be examined and evaluated within the broader parameters of their emerging language as a whole.

What to Do? Techniques described in the previous section on standardized speech testing can also be used to obtain a conversational speech sample. With shy children who do not respond in an unfamiliar setting, observations of their communicative interaction with the caregivers before or after the session may give valuable information.

3. *Examination of the oral-facial structures and the speech-motor system.* Important diagnostic information will be gained if a relationship between the speech-motor abilities and the slow speech development of these children can be verified. However, the assessment of the structure and function of the speech-motor system is often very difficult to obtain from younger children. This is in part because of their intolerance of the procedures needed to complete an oral examination as well as their limitations in imitating sounds and movements on command.

What to Do? Several fun situations can be initiated to assist in the examination of the speech-motor system. Paul, Norbury, and Gosse (2018) suggest pretending to make clown or fish faces together, letting a child first look inside your mouth with a small flashlight, and then pretending to look for a dinosaur or elephant in the child's mouth. However, even with the best ideas, clinicians often fail to gain the cooperation of a young child. One possibility would be to wait until the child becomes better acquainted with the clinician and then attempt the procedure again. A second possibility is to gather information about the child's babbling behaviors. Babbling history could be used in attempting to establish the quantity and diversity of the child's babbling. Both quantity and diversity of babbling behaviors have been correlated to measures of language. The relationship between babbling and language development is discussed in Chapter 5.

4. *Hearing screening.* A hearing screening is indispensable for children with emerging phonological systems for a number of reasons (the high prevalence of otitis media and its impact on hearing is only one). Speech-language specialists equipped with a portable audiometer typically use a screening procedure that has the client signaling—by raising a hand, for example—when a tone is heard. This type of screening procedure may not be possible with children at this age. However, conditioned response audiometric screening may yield results.

   What to Do? Children who have failed screening attempts need to be referred for a comprehensive audiological evaluation.

5. *Additional measures.* It is well documented that children with phonological disorders often have language problems as well (e.g., Keating et al., 2001; Shriberg, 1991; Webster, Majnemer, Platt, & Shevell, 2005). Therefore, the language abilities of these children need to be assessed. For young children between 2 and 3 years of age, the language assessment instrument must be selected with care. Because of these children's limited attention spans, their difficulties in following directions, and their relatively poor imitation skills, even some standardized language tests normed for these ages might not be successfully administered.

   What to Do? Numerous developmental tests rely partially or totally on the information supplied by the caregiver about a child's level of functioning. The analysis of language in naturalistic contexts can also be used to assess a child's pragmatic, morphological, syntactical, and semantic competencies.

Analysis of Children's Emerging Phonological System.   Several authors suggest that an independent analysis be used with children who are at the emerging level of phonological development (Bernthal, Bankson, & Flipsen, 2017; Paul & Jennings, 1992). An independent analysis considers only a child's productions but

---

Clinical Application

Inventory of Speech Sounds, Syllable Shapes, and Constraints

Ted is age 1 year 8 months and has Down syndrome; he is being followed in the early intervention program. His mother and the speech-language pathologist have recorded these 12 words:

"yes"	[jɛ]	"pig"	[pɪ]
"mom"	[mʌm]	"hug"	[hʌk]
"daddy"	[dædi]	"bike"	[baɪ]
"hello"	[hoʊ]	"duck"	[dʌk]
"grandpa"	[dapa]	"truck"	[tʌk]
"bye"	[bɪ]	"cow"	[daʊ]

Vowel inventory: [i, ɪ, ɛ, æ, a, oʊ, aɪ, aʊ, ʌ]

Consonant inventory: [m, p, b, t, d, k, j, h]

Syllable shapes: CV, CVC, CVCV

Constraints: [k] seems to be used only in a postvocalic position after the central vowel [ʌ].

does not compare them to the adult model. At this stage of children's development, more information can be gained by seeing which sounds and syllable shapes are present. The children's inventory must first be expanded before comparisons to the adult model can be made.

At least three types of data are collected for the independent analysis: the inventory of speech sounds, the syllable shapes a child uses, and any constraints noted on sound sequences. The inventory of speech sounds includes all vowels and consonants found in a child's accumulated word productions. Data on syllable shapes would pertain to sound productions signifying a word (V = vowel, C = consonant) and to the use of both open and closed syllable forms (CV, CVCV, CVC). Sound production constraints would include any sound or sound combinations that are used only in certain word or context positions. Examples of this category would include [p] used only word-initially or [d] in CVCV structures.

Mean Babbling Level and Syllable Structure Level.   For children with emerging language skills, Morris (2010) suggests a procedure used to obtain mean babbling level and syllable structure level. These measures were based on studies by Fasolo, Majorano, and D'Odorico (2008); Paul and Jennings (1992); Pharr and colleagues (2000); Stoel-Gammon (1987b); and Thal, Oroz, and McCaw (1995). The measures provide a metric that summarizes phonetic and syllable shape information for babbles into one score that can be used to show progress over time. The mean babbling level restricts analysis to babbling, whereas the syllable structure level focuses on productive words.

Refer to Table 6.8 for a description of the procedures and subsequent results that can be used to examine the severity of phonological delay.

Table 6.8 Mean Babbling Level and Syllable Structure Level

Mean Babbling Level: Total Number of Consonants		
Procedure	Unstructured parent–child play sample using age-appropriate toys. In the first analysis, the total number of different consonants is counted.	

Results	**Children**	**Age in Months**	**Number of Consonants**
	Norm	18–24	14
	Small expressive vocabulary	18–24	6
	Norm	24–36	18
	Small expressive vocabulary	24–36	10

The child's number of different consonants can be compared to the averages for children in the norm group and for children with small expressive vocabularies to determine which group average is closer. This procedure can also be used to monitor change.

Mean Babbling Level and Syllable Structure Levels		
Procedure:	Unstructured parent–child play sample using age-appropriate toys. Approximately 50 utterances are recorded during a 30-minute session.	

The mean babbling level examines only babbled responses: The vocalization was judged by the parent and the examiner/observer to be nonmeaningful if it contained minimally a voiced vocalic or a voiced syllabic consonant was produced with an expiratory airstream, and was judged to be "speech-like," not a cry, scream, cough, or vegetative sound.

(Continued)

Table 6.8 Mean Babbling Level and Syllable Structure Level *(Continued)*

	Based on the content, each utterance is assigned a certain level.
	A percentage is calculated based on the number of utterances produced at each level.
	The following levels (Levels 1–3) are used to calculate both mean syllable structure level (SSL) and mean babbling level. Mean babbling level examines nonmeaningful utterances, whereas mean SSL examines both meaningful and nonmeaningful utterances.
Levels:	*Level 1*: Vocalization is composed of only a voiced vowel (V syllable shape [ɑ], [u]), a voiced syllabic consonant (C syllable shape [l̩], [m̩]), or a consonant-vowel syllable in which the consonant is a glottal stop, glide, or [h] ([wi], [hɑ]). The following are examples of Level 1 vocalizations: [i], [oʊ], [l̩], [m̩], [n̩], [hɑ], [wa], [ʔa], [ʔa], [ju].
	Level 2: Vocalization is composed of a VC structure ([ʌp], [ɪk]), a CVC with a single consonant ([bab], [mam]), or a CV shape that contains consonants other than those noted at Level 1 ([tu], [mu]). Voicing differences are disregarded; therefore, [bip] or [toʊd] would be considered Level 2. The following are examples of Level 2 vocalizations: [ʌk], [um], [ab], [papa], [baba], [noʊ], [tɛdi], [kaka], [lala].
	Level 3: Vocalization is composed of syllables with two or more different consonant types that differ in place and manner ([dɑli], [kɪti]). Only voicing differences would be considered Level 2. The following are examples of Level 3 vocalizations: [bati], [boʊno], [dʌk], [hɛlo], [jʌki], [hat], [koʊt].
	Count all r-colored vowels and diphthongs as vowels, not consonants.
	Include phonetic variants of the same word if the variation includes a consonant or syllable structure change.
	Include only one instance of each unintelligible word.
Results:	Norm children at 24 months of age SSL = 2.2
	Children with small expressive vocabularies at 24 months of age SSL = 1.7
	The child's SSL average can be compared to the averages for children in the norm group and for children with small expressive vocabularies to determine which group average is closer. This procedure can also be used to monitor change.

Clinical Application

Syllable Structure Levels

Further utterances were gathered from Ted, who was presented in the previous Clinical Application. The syllable structure level is noted for each vocalization.

"yes"	[jɛ]	Level 1	"pig"	[pɪ]	Level 2
"mom"	[mʌm]	Level 2	"hug"	[hʌk]	Level 3
"daddy"	[dædi]	Level 2	"bike"	[baɪ]	Level 2
"hello"	[hoʊ]	Level 1	"duck"	[dʌk]	Level 3
"grandpa"	[dapa]	Level 3	"truck"	[tʌk]	Level 3
"bye"	[baɪ]	Level 2	"cow"	[daʊ]	Level 2

Additional nonconventional vocalizations used to calculate mean babbling level:

[ha]	Level 1	[oʊ]	Level 1
[dɪdɪ]	Level 2	[bubu]	Level 2
[pu]	Level 2	[i]	Level 1
[bæbæ]	Level 2	[pabi]	Level 2
[bʌpi]	Level 2	[ja]	Level 1
[m̩]	Level 1	[ʌ]	Level 1

Total number of consonants: 8

Mean babbling level: 1.5

   Percentage of Level 1: 50%, Level 2: 50%, Level 3: 0%

Syllable structure level: 1.83

   Percentage of Level 1: 33.3%, Level 2: 50%, Level 3: 16.7%

Ted is 20 months old. His total number of consonants is much closer to the average found for children with small expressive vocabularies. Although Ted's syllable structure level is slightly higher than those found with small expressive vocabularies, it is still closer to the average for that group when compared to the norm children at 24 months of age.

Special Considerations: A Child with Unintelligible Speech

The speech of unintelligible children is so disordered that the speaker's message cannot be understood. Unintelligible children are not limited to any specific age group. For example, Hodson and Paden (1981) report children at 8 years of age who were considered unintelligible.

Characteristics of Unintelligible Children. Hodson and Paden (1991) evaluated the speech of 60 unintelligible children ranging in age from 3 to 8 years. All of these highly unintelligible children evidenced varying degrees of difficulty with the production of liquids, stridents, and consonant clusters. Prevalent phonological processes in the speech of these children were cluster reduction, stridency deletion, stopping, gliding and vocalizations of liquids, and labial and nasal assimilations. Hodson (1992) notes that the least intelligible children were those who omitted entire classes of sounds. A few of the children produced no obstruents, either before or after the vowel nucleus (*bed* was realized as [ɛ] or [wɛ]), and a small number of the children did not produce sonorant consonants (*run* was pronounced [ʌ]).

Procedural Difficulties with Unintelligible Children. Children ages 3 years and older usually have no difficulty completing a standardized speech assessment, stimulability testing, or the speech-motor evaluation. Even with reduced intelligibility, a single-word standardized test will probably render transcribable results that can be used for a phonetic-phonemic analysis. The major difficulty for the clinician when evaluating unintelligible children is being able to understand and transcribe a

Video Example 6.2
This video of 3½-year-old Carmen has helpful captions. However, listen to the video without reading the captions. Can you understand Carmen's short sentences? Compare her speech to Toby's in the next video.

https://www.youtube.com/watch?v=szjfC9K190U

Video Example 6.3
In this video, Toby, who is 3 years 10 months old, relies on animal sounds instead of providing the name of the animal. Listen to the prompting that Toby's mom uses. Does just prompting alone—that is, saying the intended word—help Toby with the production?

https://www.youtube.com/watch?v=y0b8Gyumy2E

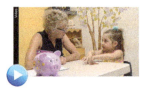

Video Tool Exercise 6.1
A Speech Sample from Kelly, Age 3 Years
Complete the activity based on this video.

spontaneous speech sample. With careful structuring, an understandable spontaneous speech sample may be possible even with unintelligible children.

WHAT TO DO?

1. *Choose the topic and attempt to structure the situation as much as possible.* If the context is unknown—that is, if an unintelligible child is talking about a self-generated topic—the clinician will have even more difficulty understanding the sample. Scripts of action events, scripts of routine events, and scripted events (Lund & Duchan, 1993) will give structure and predictability to the conversation. *Scripts of action events* depict everyday occurrences with predictable elements. Therefore, if a child is asked to explain what one does at McDonald's to get a hamburger, the predictability of the events should aid comprehension. *Routine events* begin, progress, and end in essentially the same way each time they occur. If the topic is baseball and the child is asked to explain what the person coming up to bat must do, the known progression of events will again help the clinician understand the conversation. *Scripted events* are activities that have been performed previously, and therefore all participants have expectations of how they will progress. For example, a child and a clinician could fix the wheel on a broken toy truck. The clinician would then ask the child to explain what they had just done. If the clinician models sentences—for example, "First, we saw that the truck had a missing wheel. Next, we looked for the wheel"—the child might use similar sentence patterns. Again, the predictability of the utterances should increase the clinician's ability to understand what the child is attempting to say.

2. *Gloss the utterances as much as possible.* In other words, say the intended utterance if it is recognized right after the child says it. The clinician should gloss any utterances that may later be difficult to understand on a recording. *Glossing* means repeating the child's utterance according to regular pronunciation. If the child says [aɪ oʊ oʊm] for "I go home," the clinician repeats the utterance in a regular manner so that it is recorded with the sample.

Tables 6.9 and 6.10 can be useful in organizing data for later analysis.

Table 6.9 Considerations When Collecting Data

Hearing screening		
Does not pass screening	→	Referral
Examination of speech mechanism		
Not passing, deviancies	→	Additional testing, referral
Initial impression		
Poor intelligibility	→	Need careful planning of further evaluation, especially spontaneous speech sample; refer to section titled "Special Considerations: A Child with Unintelligible Speech"
Standardized speech measure		
Few errors	→	Stimulability, contextual testing
Many errors	→	Attempt stimulability

Speech sample

   Poor intelligibility   →   Choose topic, structure situation, gloss utterances

Language screening

   Does not pass screening measure   →   Need further evaluation of language skills

Cognitive appraisal

   Necessary   →   Referral, obtain records

Table 6.10 Check Sheet for Data Collection

Hearing screening	Pass _____ Not Passing _____
Examination of speech mechanism	Pass _____ Not passing _____
	Noted deviancies _____ _____
Initial impression	Intelligibility
	Good _____ Fair _____ Poor _____
	Error productions noted _____
Standardized speech assessment	Error productions noted _____
	Stimulability testing
	Sound _____
	Sound level: Yes _____ No _____
	Syllable level: Yes _____ No _____
	Word level: Yes _____ No _____
	Sound _____
	Sound level: Yes _____ No _____
	Syllable level: Yes _____ No _____
	Word level: Yes _____ No _____
	Sound _____
	Sound level: Yes _____ No _____
	Syllable level: Yes _____ No _____
	Word level: Yes _____ No _____
Contextual testing	Sound _____
	Word contexts that elicit norm production _____
	Sound _____
	Word contexts that elicit norm production _____
	Sound _____
	Word contexts that elicit norm production _____ *(Continued)*

Table 6.10 Check Sheet for Data Collection *(Continued)*

Speech sample	Intelligibility
	Good _____ Fair _____ Poor _____
	Error productions noted _____
Language testing	Specific areas of deficiency
	_____
	_____
Information on cognitive appraisal	Necessary _____ Not necessary _____

Summary

First, this chapter summarized the *Scope of Practice* guidelines (ASHA, 2007a), which are based on the World Health Organization's *International Classification of Functioning, Disability and Health* (WHO, 2001). These guiding principles provide a general framework for the diagnostic process of speech sound disorders. The international classification system addresses the child's (1) health condition, (2) body functions and structures, (3) activities and participation, and (4) environmental and personal factors. These four areas were used as general parameters for data collection and included (1) hearing screening, (2) evaluation of the oral mechanism, (3) a standardized speech assessment, and (4) additional measures exemplified by language, prosodic, and phonological and phonemic awareness screening, as well as referral for cognitive appraisal. Methods and examples of screening measures for each of these areas were discussed. In addition, tools that could be used to assess a child's communicative participation were listed. These measures include questionnaires for children, their parents, and school personnel. In the second part of this chapter, special assessment considerations for children with an emerging phonological system and children who are unintelligible speakers were examined. Each of these groups of clients presents the clinician with challenges that will necessitate changes in the assessment process and the evaluation of the results. This chapter serves as a guide to assist the clinician in selecting procedures that will maximize clinical decision making within the diagnostic process.

Case Study

You have just given Ashley, age 4 years 5 months, a standardized speech assessment. Consistent use of the following errors were noted:

[s̪], [z̪] for [s] and [z] on all words

[t], [d] for [θ] and [ð] on all words

[w] for [l]

[w] for [ɹ] for the consonantal [ɹ] and lack of r-coloring on central vowels with r-coloring

[p], [b] for [f] and [v]

Based on the data supplied by Smit (1993b) on page 137, which of these misarticulations would be considered age-appropriate errors?

Which of these difficulties are problems you might want to target in therapy?

How could you structure a spontaneous speech sample to include objects that might stimulate production of these sounds?

Think Critically

The following selected words are from the HAPP-3 (Hodson, 2004).

1. basket	26. candle
2. glasses	27. chair
3. spoon	28. clouds
4. zip	29. fish
5. boats	30. flower
6. cowboy hat	31. glove
7. green	32. gum
8. feather	33. jumping
9. fork	34. horse
10. mask	35. ice cubes
11. star	36. leaf
12. toothbrush	37. page
13. three	38. airplane
14. mouth	39. queen
15. screwdriver	40. yellow
16. truck	41. slide
17. thumb	42. smoke
18. music box	43. snake
19. watch	44. soap
20. rock	45. square
21. shoe	46. nose
22. string	47. swimming
23. crayons	48. television
24. hanger	49. vase
25. yoyo	50. black

The child who you are assessing has [ʃ], [tʃ], [ʤ], and [ɹ] problems.
How many words are tested that contain each of these sounds, and in which word position do they occur?
Make a list that you could use to supplement the results of the articulation testing for these sounds.

 Chapter Quiz 6.1 Complete this quiz to check your understanding of chapter concepts.

Appendix 6.1 Speech-Motor Assessment Screening Form

Each of the following parameters is assessed using the following system:

Pass	Within normal limits
Deviant	Deviant from norm, divided into "slight" or "marked" deviancy
Not passing	Clearly outside of normal limits

Structure Head/Face		Deviant		
Sitting opposite the client, evaluate head and facial structures according to the categories provided.	Pass	Slight	Marked	Not Passing
Size, shape of head				
Symmetry of facial features				
Left half vs. right half				
Absence of drooping or spasticity				
Mandible/maxilla relationship				
Appearance of lips (contact at rest; vermilion)				
Appearance of nose (septum; nares)				
Appearance of philtrum/columella				
Absence of any striking features (e.g., adenoid facies, facial dimensions)				
Comments				

Breathing		Deviant		
Observe and evaluate the client's breathing behavior (as "structural" prerequisite for speaking and voice production) during normal (silent) breathing and during speaking. During silent breathing, the client's mouth should be closed and no clavicular movement should be noticeable.	Pass	Slight	Marked	Not Passing
Silent breathing				
Mouth closed (mouth open would indicate a deviancy)				
Relationship for the time of inspiration versus expiration is about 1:1				
Lack of clavicular breathing				

		Deviant		
	Pass	Slight	Marked	Not Passing
Breathing during speaking				
Breathing through nose (exclusive mouth breathing is a deviancy)				
Relationship for the time of inspiration versus expiration is 1:2 +				
Lack of clavicular breathing				
Comments				

Oral/Pharyngeal Cavity

The head should be bent back slightly for inspection of the palatal areas. A few reminders follow:

Dentition:

Class I (normal) occlusion: lower molars (or canine for children without molars) appear one-half tooth ahead of upper molars.

Class II malocclusion (overbite): Maxilla protruded in relation to mandible, measured by the positions of the first (maxillary and mandibular) molars.

Class III malocclusion (underbite): Mandibular molar more than half a tooth ahead of maxillary molar.

Open bite: Gap between biting surfaces. Especially frontally open bites might influence articulation negatively.

Crossbite: Misalignment of the teeth characterized by a crossing of the rows of teeth.

Missing frontal teeth might have a direct effect on sibilant production.

Macroglossia = tongue appears too large
Microglossia = tongue appears too small
Shrinkage (i.e., a "shriveled" tongue area) might indicate a paralytic condition.
The midline of the hard and soft palates normally appears pink and white; a blue tint suggests a submucous cleft.
Redness of fauces and pharynx might indicate inflammation.

	Pass	Deviant Slight	Deviant Marked	Not Passing
Dentition				
Front teeth present				
Spacing of teeth adequate				
Axial orientation of teeth adequate				
Dentition				
Class I normal occlusion				
If a malocclusion is noted, indicate the type:				

	Pass	Deviant Slight	Deviant Marked	Not Passing
Tongue				
Normal size in relationship to oral cavity				
Normal color				
No shrinkage				
Absence of fissures, lesions, fasciculations				
Normal resting position				
Palate (hard and soft)				
Normal color				

	Pass	Deviant		Not Passing
		Slight	Marked	
Normal width of vault				
Absence of fistulas, fissures				
Absence of clefts				
If cleft, circle one: Repaired Unrepaired				
Normal uvula				
If abnormal, circle one: Bifid Other deviations				
Normal length of uvula				
Appearances of fauces, pharynx				
Comments				

Function				
For older children and adults, these tasks can be elicited by asking the client to complete the task. For younger children (preschool age and below), imitation may be required.				
Head/Face	Pass	Deviant		Not Passing
		Slight	Marked	
Eyes/facial appearance				
Raising of eyebrows is symmetrical				
Can smile, frown on command				
Smiling, frowning symmetrical				
Lips				
Can protrude lips with mouth closed				
Can protrude lips with mouth slightly open				
Can protrude lips to left/right side				

	Pass	Deviant		Not Passing
		Slight	Marked	
Can protrude and spread lips ([u]–[i])				
Demonstrates rapid lip movements				
("pa-pa-pa")				
Mandible				
Can lower mandible on command				
Can move mandible to left/right side				
Comments				

Oral/Pharyngeal Cavity	Pass	Deviant Slight	Deviant Marked	Not Passing
Tongue				
Can stick out tongue				
Can move tongue upward (try to touch nose with tip of tongue)				
Can move tongue downward (try to touch chin with tip of tongue)				
Can move tip of tongue from left to right corner of the mouth				
Can move tongue quickly and smoothly from right to left corner of mouth				
Can move tongue smoothly around vermilion of lips (lick around lips) clockwise and counterclockwise				
Can move tongue from left to right on outside/inside of upper teeth				
Can move tongue from left to right on outside/inside of lower teeth				
Can say "pa-pa-pa" quickly, smoothly				
Can say "ta-ta-ta" quickly, smoothly				
Can say "ka-ka-ka" quickly, smoothly				
Can alternate between quick repetitions of "pa-ta" and "ta-pa"				
Can alternate between quick repetitions of "pa-ta-ka," "ka-ta-pa," and "ta-pa-ka"				
Velopharyngeal function				
During short, repeated "ah" phonation, adequate velar movement is noted				
Can puff up cheeks				
Can maintain intraoral air (puffed cheeks) when slight pressure is applied to cheeks				
Absence of nasal emission				

Breathing	Pass	Deviant Slight	Deviant Marked	Not Passing
Silent breathing				
During quick inspiration breath intake is through nose				
During quick inspiration breath intake is thoracic/abdominal				
Breathing during speaking				
Can sustain "ah" for 5 seconds				
Comments				

Chapter 7
Diagnosis

Summarizing Data and Classifying Speech Sound Disorders

∨ Learning Objectives

When you have finished this chapter, you should be able to:

7.1 Summarize data for the inventory, distribution, and stimulability of speech sounds.

7.2 Evaluate phonemic contrasts and how to establish a phonemic inventory.

7.3 Establish phonemic pattern analysis using phonological processes.

7.4 Classify speech sound disorders according to the following categories: articulation, phonological delay, consistent phonological disorder, and inconsistent phonological disorder.

7.5 Distinguish factors that affect intelligibility and measurements of intelligibility.

7.6 Demonstrate measures of severity, whole-word accuracy, and variability.

Chapter Application: Case Study

Karen had given a standardized speech assessment to Baxter, who was 5½ years old. She had also recorded a spontaneous speech sample for him. The speech sample was a difficult project, and Karen had needed to provide a lot of structure to be able to understand all of what Baxter was saying. Now, everything has been transcribed. The score from the standardized speech assessment demonstrated that Baxter was below average, approximately 2 standard deviations below the norm; therefore, Baxter needed speech therapy. In addition, Karen found that Baxter had an expressive language disorder and his phonological awareness skills were below what was to be expected for his age. Karen felt as if she had a lot of information but somehow needed to organize the data so that she would have a clear overview of Baxter's production skills. She thought that Baxter had a phonological disorder but wanted to know more about what that meant. Karen felt that she should have some type of measure of Baxter's intelligibility, as he was definitely hard to understand if you weren't familiar with him. She has heard that intelligibility measures also might be a good way to document therapy progress. Questions that Karen had included: How should she organize her speech sound data, and how could she know for sure that Baxter had a phonological disorder? Did Baxter's additional language and phonological awareness difficulties present a specific pattern of a phonological disorder? And finally, how could she objectively measure Baxter's intelligibility so that she could use that to note therapy progress?

ONE of the first diagnostic decisions facing clinicians is *how* to organize and analyze the data that they have. There are many possibilities, each of which leads to a somewhat different interpretation. Choosing the organization and analysis that best suits an individual client is important. Above all, a client's type and degree of speech sound difficulties play a major role in this selection process.

The first goal of this chapter is to present some general organizational methods that can be used to give clinicians an overview of the speech sound problems noted on the standardized speech assessment and spontaneous speech sample. This beginning organization is suitable for any dependent or independent analysis, regardless of the age of the client or the type and degree of impairment. The chapter's second goal is to provide analysis procedures that will aid clinicians in possibly determining a specific direction linked to intervention techniques. Variables such as (1) the inventory, distribution, and stimulability of phones; (2) the collapse of phonemic function; (3) phonological process analysis, including idiosyncratic and vowel processes; (4) the differential diagnostic classification system, which provides us with four general subgroups of speech sound disorders; and (5) intelligibility and severity measures, which can be used to document a child's speech are all discussed. Several case studies will be used throughout the chapter to demonstrate the various techniques.

It should be emphasized that the overall aim of this chapter is to provide information that will aid in clinical decision making. There are no prescribed answers. Based on all assessment data collected, each clinician needs to determine for each individual client which analysis procedures must be completed to arrive at a valid diagnosis. This chapter serves as an aid in making those decisions.

Inventory, Distribution, and Stimulability of Speech Sounds

Outcome Measures: Which Sounds the Child Can Produce, Which Sounds the Child Cannot Produce, and Stimulability

One important end product of the standardized speech measure and spontaneous speech sample is the inventory and distribution of speech sounds. The **inventory of speech sounds** includes all speech sounds that a client articulates. However, for many clients, there is not a simple dichotomy between normal and aberrant productions. Some clients show regular production of a speech sound in one context but not in another. This is exemplified by a child who substitutes [t] for [s] within a word and at the end of a word but realizes the target sound correctly when the word begins with [s]. Such inconsistencies should be noted because they provide important clinical information. In addition, some clients produce a sound correctly in contexts in which it does not belong but consistently mispronounce it in contexts in which it should be used. For example, an analysis revealed that a child had no accurate productions of [s] in all words that contained s-sounds. However, in the words "brush" and "wash," [ʃ] was replaced by an accurate [s]. This phenomenon has been reported often and frequently occurs in children with phonemic-based disorders (Fey, 1992). Examples such as these demonstrate that normal articulation of the sound in question is within a client's capabilities; however, the client does not seem to understand the language-specific function and/or organization of specific phonemes. Such information helps considerably when determining which clients show evidence of a phonological disorder.

The **distribution of speech sounds** refers to where within a word the norm and aberrant articulations occur. Standardized speech assessments often categorize according to three word positions: initial, medial, and final. *Word-medial position* is an imprecise term. This lack of precision has bothered many practitioners who were interested in looking more closely at the client's error patterns. Therefore, the analysis procedure offered here is based on where the consonants occur relative to the vowel nuclei. This procedure partially eliminates the necessity of establishing syllable divisions and can be used on words from a standardized speech assessment or from a spontaneous speech sample.

1. *Prevocalic consonants.* Consonants that occur before a vowel. These may be singletons (i.e., single consonants) or consonant clusters primarily at the beginning of a word or utterance.
2. *Postvocalic consonants.* Consonants that occur after a vowel. These may be singletons or consonant clusters primarily at the end of a word or utterance.
3. *Intervocalic consonants.* Consonants that occur between two vowels. These may be singletons or consonant clusters at the juncture of two syllables.

Stimulability measures were discussed in Chapter 6, on page 172. Most standardized speech assessments have a section for stimulability testing. Stimulability for sounds that are in error is an important variable. Some of the specific target selection procedures and resulting intervention methods are based on a child's stimulability for certain sounds. However, a definition of stimulability should be addressed. Does nonstimulable mean that the child has no possibility of imitating a model at all, and thus has 0% stimulability? Several authors state that the child should show 0% accuracy with a model (Gierut, 2001, 2007; Miccio & Elbert, 1996; Powell, Elbert, & Dinnsen, 1991), whereas Barlow, Taps Richard, and Storkel (2010) suggest that nonstimulable means less than 30% accuracy. For the purpose of this chapter's presentation of stimulability, nonstimulable means that the child demonstrates no possibility of providing an accurate model after the clinician's prompts.

What Do the Inventory, Distribution, and Stimulability Results Tell Us as Clinicians?

As a clinician, why is it important to understand the child's inventory, distribution, and stimulability for planning intervention? Let's discuss each of these variables and examine their role in decision making.

Clinical Exercises Divide the following words into prevocalic, intervocalic, or postvocalic consonants: *hats, shoe, today, banana, pajamas, slide.*

Word	Prevocalic	Intervocalic	Postvocalic
hats	[h]		[ts]
shoe	[ʃ]		
today	[t]	[d]	
banana	[b]	[n], [n]	
pajamas	[p]	[ʤ], [m]	[z]
slide	[sl]		[d]

First, the inventory tells us which sounds the child can produce and thus which sounds the child cannot produce. So, we have an idea about the quantity and quality of errors. If a lot of phones are missing from the child's inventory, we would probably choose one of several intervention approaches. For example, we do not want to go sound-by-sound through intervention if the child has many sounds in error. However, we might want to use an approach that causes widespread generalization. If there are so many errors that the child is unintelligible, other options present themselves. Also of note is whether the child has errors on early- *and* later-developing sounds or just on those that are considered to be late sounds. Again, this would steer us in a specific direction. We would also want to note if the inventory demonstrates inconsistency. Inconsistent productions would possibly be exemplified by a child showing many substitutions for several different phones, where a pattern does not seem to be visible. Inconsistent productions are discussed in a later section.

The distribution of phones gives us information necessary for several different intervention directions. If the child can produce prevocalic phones but deletes many postvocalic consonants (final consonant deletion), we might want to work on that pattern initially. If, on the other hand, the child demonstrates prevocalic deletions—that is, initial consonants are deleted—this can be considered for our initial therapy plan. Both initial and final consonant deletion would definitely affect intelligibility. The child who deletes intervocalic phones presents a somewhat different picture. Intervocalic productions are, by definition, two-syllable words. In this case, one- versus two-syllable words might be a factor. The child may exhibit more accuracy with one-syllable words and need help transitioning to two-syllable words.

The stimulability of a phone gives us information about the child's production capabilities. There are treatment methods in which stimulability is a positive factor and other approaches where lack of stimulability is desired. Therefore, a child's stimulability is also significant. Refer to Figure 7.1 for an overview.

Figure 7.2 shows a summary matrix that clinicians could use to organize data from their standardized speech measure. For the purpose at hand, a checkmark (✓) is used to indicate a normal realization, a ø is used to record deletions, and the appropriate phonetic symbols with diacritics are used to document substitutions and distortions. Therefore, this matrix is used to record both standard and aberrant productions of the client. It might not be necessary for clinicians to use this particular form. You might be able to obtain this information from the standardized

Figure 7.1 Analyzing Inventory, Distribution, and Stimulability

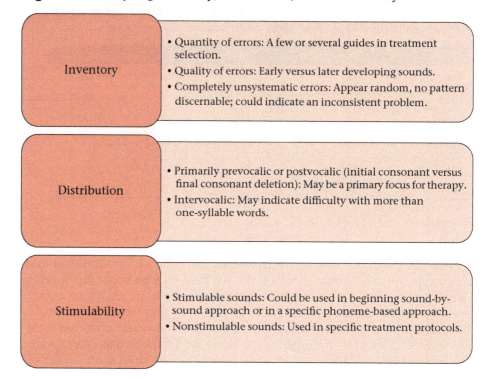

Inventory
- Quantity of errors: A few or several guides in treatment selection.
- Quality of errors: Early versus later developing sounds.
- Completely unsystematic errors: Appear random, no pattern discernable; could indicate an inconsistent problem.

Distribution
- Primarily prevocalic or postvocalic (initial consonant versus final consonant deletion): May be a primary focus for therapy.
- Intervocalic: May indicate difficulty with more than one-syllable words.

Stimulability
- Stimulable sounds: Could be used in beginning sound-by-sound approach or in a specific phoneme-based approach.
- Nonstimulable sounds: Used in specific treatment protocols.

speech measure you are using. However, such a form might be useful when analyzing a speech sample.

Important information for later decision making includes the following:

1. Inventory (Note: For the purpose at hand, if the child demonstrates accurate production of the sound in several instances—but possibly not all of the time—this sound will be considered part of the child's inventory. The inventory would also include consonant clusters produced.)
2. Distribution
3. Stimulability of the child's sounds

Appendix 7.1 presents the transcribed results of the Goldman-Fristoe Test of Articulation (Goldman & Fristoe, 2015) for Jonah, age 7 years 4 months. Spontaneous speech results are also included in the Case Study at the end of this chapter (refer to page 223). The matrix for the Goldman-Fristoe Test of Articulation has been filled out for Jonah and is included as Figure 7.3. Note that consonant clusters are included at the end of the form. The spontaneous speech sample matrix for Jonah is included in Appendix 7.2. As noted, this is filled out somewhat differently. Sounds that are at the beginning of the utterance are marked as prevocalic, those at the end of the utterance are marked as postvocalic, and those in between are marked as intervocalic.

This information can be summarized as follows:

Phones Jonah has in his inventory: [p, b, t, d, m, n, ŋ, w, h], occasionally [f], spontaneous speech sample possibly add [j, l, f , v]

Phones Jonah does not have in his inventory: [k, g, s, z, ʃ, θ, ð, s, tʃ, ʤ]

Prevocalic consonant clusters: All initial clusters are reduced as follows: kw, gɹ, sl, sw, kɹ, tɹ, st → t, dɹ, gl → d, sp, pl, fɹ, pɹ → p, bɹ, bl → b

Figure 7.2 Matrix for Recording Phones According to Prevocalic, Intervocalic, and Postvocalic Word Positions

	Early Sounds	Pre-vocalic	Inter-vocalic	Post-vocalic	Stimulable	Later Sounds	Pre-vocalic	Inter-vocalic	Post-vocalic	Stimulable	
Stops	p					f					Fricatives
Stops	b					v					Fricatives
Stops	t					s					Fricatives
Stops	d					z					Fricatives
Stops	k					ʃ					Fricatives
Stops	g					ʒ					Fricatives
Nasals	m					θ					Fricatives
Nasals	n					ð					Fricatives
Nasals	ŋ					l					Approximants
Approximants	w					ɹ					Approximants
Approximants	j					ʧ					Affricates
Fricative	h					ʤ					Affricates
Fricative											

Note: ✓ indicates a correct production, Ø indicates a deletion, and substitutions are noted with the appropriate phonetic transcription.

Note: Shading indicates a voiced consonant.

Consonant Clusters: Prevocalic:

Intervocalic:

Postvocalic:

Figure 7.3 Recorded Phones for Jonah, Age 7 Years 4 Months

	Early Sounds	Pre-vocalic	Inter-vocalic	Post-vocalic	Stimulable	Later Sounds	Pre-vocalic	Inter-vocalic	Post-vocalic	Stimulable	
Stops	p	✓✓	Ø	✓✓		f	pp✓	✓	pØp	yes	Fricatives
Stops	b	✓	✓p	p		v	bb	bb	p	yes	Fricatives
Stops	t	✓✓✓✓	Ø	✓✓		s	tt	Ø	ttØ	no	Fricatives
Stops	d	✓✓	t	Ø✓		z	dd	t	tØØ	no	Fricatives
Stops	k	tt	t	ttt	no	ʃ	tt	t	t	no	Fricatives
Stops	g	tt	d	Øt	no	ʒ	not tested				Fricatives
Nasals	m	✓	✓✓	✓✓✓		θ	t		f	yes	Fricatives
Nasals	n	✓		✓✓✓✓		ð	d	t		yes	Fricatives
Nasals	ŋ			✓✓✓		l	ww	w	oʊ oʊ oʊ o o	yes	Approximants
Approximants	w	✓✓		----------		ɹ	ww	w	ə ə ə ə ə ə ə ə ə ə	no	Approximants
Approximants	j	d		----------	yes	ʧ	tt	t		no	Affricates
Fricative	h	✓Ø		----------		ʤ	dtd			no	Affricates

Consonant Clusters: Prevocalic: [kw, gɹ, sl, sw, kɹ tɹ, st] → [t]
[dɹ, gl] → [d]
[sp, pl, fɹ, pɹ] → [p]
[bɹ, bl] → [b]

Intervocalic: [ŋk, nt, ŋg] → [n],
[ns] → [nt]
[bɹ] → [b]
[ʤt] → [t]
[kj] → Ø

Postvocalic: [nt] → [n]

Intervocalic consonant clusters: ŋk, nt, ŋg → n, ns → nt, bɹ → b, ʤt → t, kj → Ø

Postvocalic consonant clusters: nt → n

Stimulable phones: [j, l, f, v, θ, ð]

Nonstimulable phones: [k, g, s, z, ʃ, ɹ, ʧ, ʤ]

Note that [ʒ] was not tested. It occurs so infrequently in General American English that most assessment procedures do not include it. This analysis will also not consider [ʒ] as a possibility for further examination.

Comparison of standardized speech assessment and spontaneous speech sample: In the spontaneous speech sample, Jonah shows evidence of an accurate [j] production several times. Therefore, this phone should be added to his inventory. Also, there is an instance of [v] and [f] being produced accurately (in addition, [f] is used as a substitution for [v] three times). Therefore, [v] and [f] could be added to his inventory as well.

Other phone results are very similar to the standardized one-word assessment. Jonah does show one other two-element intervocalic consonant cluster, [nf], on "French fries" [fɛn.faɪθ].

To summarize, Jonah has quite a few phone errors. They are mostly later-developing sounds; however, [k] and [g] are also in error and not stimulable. Consonant clusters are almost always reduced to one element. However, we do see an intervocalic cluster [nt] in "princess" → [pɪn.tət]. This is a cluster that crosses syllable boundaries, as noted by the period. Also noted is a two-element cluster in spontaneous speech, [nf] on "French fries" [fɛn.faɪθ]. Spontaneous speech seems to approximate the standardized one-word assessment.

ERROR PATTERNS: CAN WE FORMULATE PRELIMINARY ERROR ANALYSES?
Examples of initial questions to help us better understand Jonah's results would include the following:

1. Do we see a pattern of substitutions, omissions, or distortions?
2. Are specific sounds often used as substitutions for others?
3. Are the substitutions fairly consistent, or do we see a large degree of inconsistency in productions?
4. Do specific syllable structure phonological process patterns predominate? For example, do we see frequent final consonant deletion, unstressed syllable deletion, or consonant cluster reduction?
5. Do specific substitution phonological process patterns predominate? For example, do we see frequent use of stopping, fronting, or gliding?
6. Based on the 3-plus syllable words that were elicited, do we think the child might be having difficulties with multisyllabic words?

This is meant as a very preliminary analysis to guide us to further possibilities. This is not about going through the entire inventory and doing a phonological analysis, for example. This is just a beginning step, so we get an idea about what should happen next. As clinicians become more experienced, these steps and possibly others become automatic. Let's go through Jonah's results and answer the preceding questions.

1. Do we see a pattern of substitutions, omissions, or distortions?
   Jonah uses a large number of substitutions and relatively few deletions (seven in total).

2. Are specific sounds often used as substitutions for others?

   Jonah uses [t] or [d] as a substitution for 10 different sounds [k, g, j, s, z, ʃ, θ, ð, ʧ, ʤ]

3. Are the substitutions fairly consistent, or do we see a large degree of inconsistency in productions?

   Substitutions are fairly consistent. Jonah used [t] or [d] for the above-mentioned sounds and [w] for [l] and [ɹ],

4. Do specific syllable structure phonological process patterns predominate? For example, do we see frequent final consonant deletion, unstressed syllable deletion, or consonant cluster reduction?

   Jonah uses consonant cluster reduction almost exclusively for two- and three-element clusters.

5. Do specific substitution phonological process patterns predominate? For example, do we see frequent use of stopping, fronting, or gliding?

   Jonah uses stopping very frequently. Gliding is noted with [l] and [ɹ].

6. Based on the 3-plus syllable words that were elicited, do we think that the child might be having difficulties with multisyllabic words?

   Only three multisyllabic words were tested on the standardized speech assessment. Jonah did not delete syllables on those words, and his articulation was comparable to one- and two-syllable words. Jonah does not appear to be having difficulties with multisyllabic words.

The next section addresses those children who show substitutions that relate to phonemic contrasts within their phonological system. It addresses children who demonstrate the use of specific sound substitutions in which one phoneme is used for multiple sounds.

Phonemic Contrasts: Establishing a Phonemic Inventory

Clients with phonemic-based disorders are characterized by impaired phonological systems; they show difficulties using phonemes contrastively to differentiate meaning. Therefore, two or more phonemes represented by the same sound production could indicate that the contrastive phonemic function may not have been realized; *the meaning-differentiating contrast has been neutralized.* The emphasis in this phase of the analysis is on the *contrastive use of phonemes,* not on the accurate production of phones. Loss of phonemic contrast is the central problem of clients with phonological impairments.

Children with a phonological impairment are often difficult to understand because many of their words sound the same. The phonemic contrast between words has been lost. For example, with Jonah one can note in Appendix 7.1 that both "juice" and "zoo" are pronounced as [du]. The contrast between /ʤ/ and /z/ is not there; rather both are now produced as [d]. This is a collapse or neutralization of phonemic contrast.

This neutralization of specific phonemic contrasts can occur on one or many phones. It is inaccurate to think that if a child has only one or two phone errors, that child necessarily has an articulation-based disorder and not a phonemic-based disorder. This is a myth that has been perpetuated for decades. What is true is that the chance of a child having a phonemic-based disorder increases as the number of errors increases. Based on 1100 referrals, Broomfield and Dodd (2010) noted that children with articulation disorders predominantly demonstrated a severity level of mild or moderate. However, children with a phonological disorder also fell into this classification; some of them could also be labelled as mild or moderate in severity. The authors stated that there was an overlap of severity across the groups. That is, "severity alone could not be used to identify subgroups" (Broomfield & Dodd, 2010, p. 87).

The final decision for which speech sounds are indeed used as contrastive phonemes often requires the clinician to check sound oppositions through minimal pairs, for example. The analysis of phonemic contrasts can begin with a matrix such as the one presented in Table 7.1.

Table 7.1 Neutralization of Phonemic Contrasts

First, list the intended target sound. The arrow (→) indicates "becomes." Then list the substitution that is used for that specific target. Only list those sounds that you have determined are *not* in the child's inventory.

Target → Substitution	Target → Substitution

List all sounds that have the same substitution.

Targets	Substitution

List the phonemes that are used correctly (those that are noted as being accurate) and the substitutions from Table 7.1. These are the phonemes in the child's phonemic inventory.

Table 7.2 is a form filled out for Jonah showing his neutralization of phonemic contrasts. Recall that, based on the spontaneous speech sample, the phones [j], [f], [v], and [l] could be added to Jonah's inventory.

For Jonah, several phones have one substitution: [t]. In addition, [d] is used as a substitution for several voiced phones. What does this indicate?

If the child substitutes [t] for [k] in all given situations and never uses [k], we would probably conclude that /t/ is in the child's phonemic inventory but /k/ is not. This is typically how clinicians determine the phonemic inventory of a child. They look specifically at the sound substitutions and use those data to determine a phonemic inventory. For example, Jonah substitutes [t] for [k], [g], [s], [z], [ʃ], [θ], [ð], [tʃ], and [ʤ]. If these target sounds are not noted in other contexts, it could be concluded that Jonah has /t/ in his phonemic inventory, but not /k/,/g/, /s/, /z/, /ʃ/, /θ/, /ð/, tʃ/, or /ʤ/. This would indicate a collapse of phonemic contrasts; that is, specific contrasts that typically occur in the phonemic system of General American English are not realized. The collapse of phonemic contrasts is a central concept for specific types of phonological treatment protocols; for example, multiple oppositions therapy uses this information to establish treatment targets.

Table 7.2 Neutralization of Phonemic Contrasts for Jonah, Age 7 Years 4 Months

Target → Substitution	Target → Substitution
k → t	tʃ → t
g → t, d	ʤ → t, d
s → t	ɹ → w
z → t, d	
ʃ → t	
θ → t, f	
ð → t, d	

List all sounds that have the same substitution.

Targets	Substitution
k, g, s, z, ʃ, θ, ð, tʃ, ʤ	t
g, z, ð, ʤ	d
ɹ	w
θ	f

The following phonemes are in Jonah's phonemic inventory: /p, b, t, d, m, n, ŋ, w, h, f, v, j, and l/.

For the child with a phonological impairment, the phonemic contrast between words is lost. To determine this loss of contrast, minimal pairs might be used to test contrasts. We would want to note that when provided with minimal pair words or pictures, the child is able to produce differences between specific phonemes. Appendix 7.3 lists minimal pair words ordered according to vowels. The words are all CV or CVC words, which the clinician can choose among based on the needs of a specific child. In addition, Chapter 9, pages 336–341, contains minimal word pairs ordered according to frequent substitutions. Several websites can provide pictures for minimal pairs. LessonPix is one in which you input two words with the minimal pair contrast you want and several pictures representing these contrasts are provided. You can then drag and drop them onto a "tray" to create picture materials. Caroline Bowen's speech-language therapy also lets you choose the minimal pair you would like to use and provides pictures. If the child is able to productionally differentiate between the two phonemes pictured in minimal paired words, we can assume that the child contrasts these phonemes and these are a portion of the child's phonemic inventory.

Clinical Application

Jonah and Minimal Pairs

Pictures of minimal pairs were used to assess the targets and substitutions noted for Jonah. The target sound and substitution were placed in the prevocalic position. The results were as follows:

Word Examples	Productions: Same/Different	Word Examples	Productions: Same/Different
cub/tub, kite/tight	Same	than/Dan, then/den	Different
go/doe, got/dot	Same	thin/tin, thick/tick	Different
go/toe, got/tot	Same	than/tan, then/ten	Different
sew/toe, sip/tip	Same	chew/two, chop/top	Same
zip/dip, zoo/do	Same	Jean/teen, joy/toy	Same
ship/tip, shoe/two	Same	Jean/Dean, jeep/deep	Same
rail/whale, red/wed	Same	thought/fought, thin/fin	Different
lake/wake, light/white	Different	fin/pin, fig/pig	Different
vase/base, V/bee	Different	you/do, yacht/dot	Different

The phones [j, f, v, l] can now be safely included in Jonah's phonemic inventory. Also, based on minimal pairs, [θ, ð], which were stimulable, can be included in Jonah's phonemic inventory.
Jonah's phonemic inventory: /p, b, t, d, m, n, ŋ, w, h, f, v, j, l, θ, ð/

Phonemic Pattern Analysis: Phonological Processes

This type of analysis procedure was introduced in Chapter 4. A phonological process analysis is a means of identifying substitutions, syllable structure, and assimilatory changes that occur in clients' speech. Each error is identified and classified as one or more of the phonological processes. Patterns of errors are described according to the frequency of noted phonological processes and/or those that affect a class of sounds. The processes used to identify substitutions are again primarily production based; however, they do account for sound and syllable deletions.

Certain processes seem to occur more frequently in the speech of children who are developing their phonological systems in a normal manner. Others, labeled *idiosyncratic processes*, occur infrequently in the norm population (Stoel-Gammon & Dunn, 1985). On most protocols, substitution processes are limited to consonants, but vowel processes have been identified as well (Ball & Gibbon, 2002; Pollock & Keiser, 1990; Reynolds, 1990; Stoel-Gammon & Herrington, 1990). Refer to Table 7.3 for a list of some of the idiosyncratic processes noted in children. Phonological processes used to identify vowel errors are summarized in Table 7.4.

Table 7.3 Idiosyncratic Processes Found in the Speech of Children with Phonological Disorders

The following are a few examples of the relatively uncommon processes that have been found in the speech of children with phonological disorders.

Process	Example			
Initial consonant deletion	"duck"	[dʌk]	→	[ʌk]
Backing of stops	"tub"	[tʌb]	→	[kʌb]
Backing of fricatives	"fun"	[fʌn]	→	[ʃʌn]
Glottal replacement	"gum"	[gʌm]	→	[ʔʌm]
Denasalization	"knee"	[ni]	→	[di]
Fricatives replacing stops	"toe"	[toʊ]	→	[soʊ]
Stops replacing glides	"yarn"	[jaɚn]	→	[daɚn]
Metathesis (reversal of two sounds)	"step"	[stɛp]	→	[tsɛp]
Affrication (a nonaffricate becomes an affricate)	"top"	[tɑp]	→	[tʃɑp]
Migration (movement of a sound from one position in the word to another position)	"soap"	[soʊp]	→	[oʊps]
Unusual cluster reduction	"plane"	[pleɪn]	→	[leɪn]
Unusual substitution processes	"plane"	[pleɪn]	→	[teɪn]
Vowel processes (e.g., centralization of vowels)	"bed"	[bɛd]	→	[bʌd]

Sources: Data from Bauman-Waengler, J. A., & Waengler, H.-H. (1988), Bauman-Waengler, J. A., & Waengler, H.-H. (1990), Dodd, B., & Iacano, T. (1989), Leonard, L., & McGregor, K. (1991), Roberts, J. E., Burchinal, M., & Footo, M. (1990), Stoel-Gammon, C., & Dunn, C. (1985), and Waengler, H.-H., & Bauman-Waengler, J. A. (1989).

Table 7.4 Phonological Processes Used to Identify Vowel Errors

Several common and idiosyncratic substitution processes that describe changes in consonant productions have been identified. However, children with phonological disorders may also evidence impaired vowel systems. The following processes have been used to describe vowel substitutions in children (Ball & Gibbon, 2002; Bauman-Waengler, 1991; Pollock & Keiser, 1990):

1. *Vowel backing.* A front vowel is replaced by a back vowel of a similar tongue height. Example: [ɪ] → [ʊ]
2. *Vowel fronting.* A back vowel is replaced by a front vowel of a similar tongue height. Example: [u] → [i]
3. *Centralization.* A front or back vowel is replaced by a central vowel. Example: [ɛ] → [ʌ]
4. *Decentralization.* A central vowel is replaced by a front or back vowel. Example: [ʌ] → [ɛ]
5. *Vowel raising.* A front vowel is replaced by a front vowel with a higher tongue position, or a back vowel is replaced by a back vowel with a higher tongue position. Example: [æ] → [ɛ], [ʊ] → [u]
6. *Vowel lowering.* A front vowel is replaced by a front vowel with a lower tongue position, or a back vowel is replaced by a back vowel with a lower tongue position. Example: [u] → [ʊ]
7. *Diphthongization.* A monophthong is realized as a diphthong. Example: [ɛ] → [ɛɪ]
8. *Monophthongization (or diphthong reduction).* A diphthong is realized as a monophthong. Example: [aɪ] → [a]
9. *Complete vowel harmony.* A vowel change occurs within a word and results in both vowels being produced the same. Example: [tɛdi] → [tɛdɛ]
10. *Tenseness harmony.* A lax vowel becomes tense when there is another tense vowel in the same word. Example: [mɛni] → [meni]
11. *Height vowel harmony.* A vowel is replaced with a vowel that is closer in tongue height to another vowel in the same word. Example: [bæskɪt] → [bɛskɪt]

Treatment implications of Stampe's (1979) theory of natural phonology include suppression or decrease of the aberrant phonological processes to increase the complexity of children's phonological patterns. The suppression of these phonological processes occurs naturally in the speech of normally developing children, but for children with phonological disorders, treatment must focus on helping to reduce the use of age-inappropriate processes as well as processes that are not acceptable for the adult language being learned.

Phonological processes provide a means of classifying error patterns noted in disordered speech and suggest a direct and simple way to handle intervention. Although these processes have been labeled phonological, they are based to a large extent on phonetic production features. For example, substitution processes are named after the differences between the production of the target and the error sound. Phonological processes do not give concrete information about the neutralization of specific phonemic contrasts, nor do they account for phonological rules that might be operating.

PLEASE NOTE: The presence of phonological processes in the speech of an individual *does not* necessarily indicate the presence of a phonemic-based disorder. In their contemporary usage, phonological processes are descriptive terms; the existence of a particular process neither explains the problem nor denotes its etiology (e.g., Butcher, 1990; Fey, 1992). Kamhi (1992) has identified the practice of using phonological processes to *imply* a phonemic-based disorder as being the most serious problem associated with this type of analysis.

To summarize, phonological processes, a central aspect of natural phonology, have been extensively used to describe disordered speech patterns and to select treatment goals. The speech of children with disordered phonological systems may show differences in type and use of phonological processes when compared to the speech of children with normally developing systems. However, caution should be exercised when descriptions of phonological processes are used to imply the presence of a phonemic-based disorder. Figure 7.4 is a form that could possibly be used to analyze phonological processes.

Figure 7.4 Phonological Process Analysis Form

Processes	Number of Occurrences
Syllable Structure Changes	
Cluster reduction	_____
Cluster deletion	_____
Reduplication	_____
Weak syllable deletion	_____
Final consonant deletion	_____
Other _____	_____
Substitution Processes	
Fronting	_____
Labialization	_____
Alveolarization	_____
Stopping	_____
Affrication	_____
Deaffrication	_____
Denasalization	_____
Gliding of liquids	_____
Gliding of fricatives	_____
Vowelization	_____
Derhotacization	_____
Voicing	_____
Devoicing	_____
Other _____	_____
Assimilation Processes	
Labial assimilation	_____
Velar assimilation	_____
Nasal assimilation	_____
Liquid assimilation	_____
Other _____	_____
_____	_____

The following section examines the subtypes of one speech sound classification system. The assessment results that have been generated according to this classification system are examined. Where possible, initial directions for intervention are postulated.

Classifying Speech Sound Disorders

In Chapter 1 (pages 10–13), two classification systems were introduced: etiological classification postulated by Shriberg and colleagues (2010) and a descriptive linguistic model, the differential diagnostic system postulated by Dodd (2013). Shriberg and colleagues (2010) noted that the etiological classification system was not intended for clinical practice until more research could validate the initial findings. On the other hand, the differential diagnostic system appears to be useful clinically. Studies have demonstrated that children can consistently be classified according to these parameters (e.g., Broomfield & Dodd, 2004). This section will use the differential diagnostic system proposed by Dodd (2013) to evaluate the results we have obtained in our assessment process.

The differential diagnostic system proposes a classification system consisting of five subgroups of speech sound disorders:

1. Articulation disorder.
2. Phonological delay. These children demonstrate phonological patterns that are evidenced in normal development but typically noted at an earlier chronological age.
3. Consistent phonological disorder. Consistent use of some non-developmental error patterns. These children may demonstrate atypical and idiosyncratic error patterns.
4. Inconsistent phonological disorder. The phonological systems of these children show at least 40% variability of production when the children are asked to name 25 pictures on three separate trials within one session. Thus, multiple errors are demonstrated for the same word.
5. Childhood apraxia of speech. This is seen as a multideficit, motor-speech disorder involving phonological planning and phonetic and motor programming difficulties (Ozanne, 2013).

The last category is not discussed in this chapter. However, it is covered in detail in Chapter 11.

Articulation Disorder

The subgroup articulation disorder involves an inability to pronounce certain phones, typically s- and r-sounds. The child uses a consistent substitution or distortion for the target sound in both spontaneous and imitated productions (Dodd, 2013).

The following factors were noted when using this classification system for 320 children referred to the pediatric Speech and Language Therapy Service in Middlesbrough, UK (Broomfield & Dodd, 2010):

1. The percentage of children diagnosed with an articulation disorder was relatively low (12.5%).
2. The severity was typically in the mild to moderate range. However, within-group variation was large, and severity alone could not be used to identify this subgroup.
3. Children in this group were referred primarily by parents and other health care practitioners, although there was no significant difference between this subgroup and the referral source.

4. An articulation disorder was typically identified in school-age children.

5. In general, there are more boys than girls with communication disorders. However, the gender ratio is much closer for the group of children with an articulation disorder.

6. Children with an articulation disorder were least likely to show comorbidity. When receptive and expressive language and phonological awareness parameters were tested, some children did show evidence of difficulties (a range from 17.5% for comprehension problems to 51.6% for phonological awareness involvement); these were the lowest percentages of any of the other subgroups.

7. Oro-motor difficulties were distributed across the subgroups but were most associated with the articulation group.

WHAT TO DO? Based on this information, the bottom line is that articulation disorders seem to be fairly limited as to the phones in error and the number of children in a clinician's caseload. It is also possible that a child with an articulation disorder might show other language difficulties. This, and specifically phonological awareness, should be tested. Problems with phonological awareness seem to occur in more than half of children with articulation disorders. A detailed oral speech mechanism exam is very important, as children with an articulation disorder might evidence difficulties. These data are consistent with the hypothesis that there may be oro-motor overlays for some children with articulation disorders (e.g., Hewlett, Gibbon, & Cohen-McKenzie, 1998).

The following Clinical Application outlines the factors that help clinicians in the process of decision making when considering a speech sound disorder that is primarily articulation-based versus phonemic-based.

Clinical Application

Speech Sound Disorder Both Articulation- and Phonemic-Based?

It is important to analyze all existing data, possibly supplementing them with additional information, before arriving at the tentative decision that a client does show evidence of a speech sound disorder that is articulation-based. In doing this, speech-language specialists must always keep in mind that articulation- and phonemic-based speech sound disorders can co-occur. "It would be a mistake to adopt an either/or dichotomy" (Elbert, 1992, p. 242). The following example illustrates this point.

Here is a small sample from Sheri, age 6 years 7 months:

fish	[ɪt]	go	[goʊ]	fork	[oʊək]
ball	[bɑl]	spoon	[un]	soap	[oʊp]
up	[ʌp]	red	[wɛd]	thumb	[ʌm]
mouse	[maʊt]	leaf	[lif]	yellow	[jɛ.loʊ]
one	[wʌn]	nose	[noʊd]	house	[aʊt]
wash	[wɑʃ]	chin	[tʃɪn]	cow	[kaʊ]
teeth	[tit]	love	[lʌv]	vacuum	[æ.kum]
wagon	[wæ.ən]	shoes	[ut]	that	[æt]
kiss	[kɪt]	jeep	[ʤip]	swing	[ɪŋ]

Based on this sample, an additional assessment, and a speech sample, the following phones were noted as being in Sheri's inventory: [m, n, ŋ, p, b, t, d, k, g, w, j, h, f, v, l, ʃ, tʃ, ʤ]

Not in Sheri's inventory are: [s, z, θ, ð, ɹ]

Basically, Sheri misarticulates a few later-developing phones. If one examines this small sample, it appears that far more sounds would be in error due to the high number of instances of initial consonant deletion. Placement techniques for [s, z, θ, and ð] were attempted (refer to Chapter 9), and it appeared as if these sounds were good possibilities for this technique. In addition, [ɹ] could be stimulated without the lip rounding.

But what about the initial consonant deletions? It was noted that word pairs with a fricative in the prevocalic position, such as "sew" and "soap," were produced with the initial fricative consonant being deleted. For example, "sew" was produced as [oʊ]. However, if the postvocalic consonant was a fricative, it was produced accurately (refer to the words "love" and "leaf" in the sample above) or with the consistent substitution such as [t] for [s] or [θ]. Words that began with fricatives demonstrated consistent initial consonant deletion. It was tentatively hypothesized that Sheri might have both an articulation-based and a phonemic-based speech sound disorder. She was stimulable for most of the sounds in error but had difficulty with the phonological system (specifically phonotactics). She did not seem to understand that fricatives belonged at the beginning of words, but she was clearly able to produce them at the end of words.

Phonological Delay

According to Dodd (2013), phonological delay is characterized by phonological patterns that one would use to describe a normally developing child at a younger chronological age. These children appear, in the true sense, to have a "delay." Thus, most but not all of the phonological patterns are considered typical. According to Broomfield and Dodd (2010), these children had the following characteristics:

1. More than half of the children (57.5%) diagnosed fell into the group of phonological delay.
2. Children with a phonological delay rarely presented with severe or profound impairments. Since the Broomfield and Dodd (2010) measure for "moderate" allowed for a delay of up to 2½ years, it was rare to have a phonological delay beyond this point.
3. More than half of the children in this group were referred primarily by health visitors (i.e., registered nurses who typically have additional training in community public health nursing).
4. Children with a phonological delay were referred primarily in the 3- to 6-year-old age range.
5. Boys made up 63% of the children with a phonological delay.
6. Comorbidity in the phonological delay group was seemingly comparable to that in other subgroups. Therefore, approximately 50% of the children showed additional difficulties with vocabulary, and almost 75% demonstrated phonological awareness problems.
7. Oro-motor involvement was about the same as in the other subgroups of children with a speech disorder.

Clinical Application

Phonological Delay?

Josie, age 4 years 10 months, was screened by the speech-language pathologist in her prekindergarten class. Her teacher said that Josie was at times hard to understand. The speech-language pathologist summarized her screening results according to phonological processes as follows:

Process	Examples	Total Number of Times Used
Velar fronting	[k] → [t] [kʌp] → [tʌp]	14 times, all words tested
	[g] → [d] [gʌm] → [dʌm]	
Final consonant deletion	[beɪk] → [beɪ] [lɑg] → [lɑ]	5 times, only on words ending with [k] and [g]
Cluster reduction and substitution	[klaʊn] → [taʊn] [gɹæs] → [dæs]	5 times, only on words with [k] and [g] clusters

Josie did show evidence of distortions of later consonants. For example, her s- and r-sounds were distorted. In addition, she was still using the early-process velar fronting. When [k] or [g] was produced in the word-initial position or in consonant clusters, fronting was demonstrated. In the word-final position, the sounds were deleted. More information is needed, but this could be a case of phonological delay.

WHAT TO DO? Phonological delays in children appear to be fairly prevalent. These children typically present in the mild to moderate severity range. Children with a phonological delay are often referred prior to school entry. Language problems, especially vocabulary and phonological awareness, may be present; thus, additional testing may be warranted. Oro-motor skills in these children should be evaluated.

Consistent Phonological Disorder

According to Dodd and colleagues (2013), children with consistent phonological disorder demonstrate consistent use of some non-developmental error patterns. In addition, there may be evidence of some delayed developmental patterns. However, the consistent nature of unusual, non-developmental error patterns marks the impaired acquisition of the child's phonological system. Broomfield and Dodd (2010) list the following qualities of children with a consistent phonological disorder:

1. The group percentage for this type of phonological disorder was relatively high; at 20.6%, it ranked second in the percentage of children diagnosed with a speech sound disorder.
2. Children with a consistent phonological disorder had more severe difficulties. Most of the children were rated in the moderate-severe to severe range.
3. Individuals referring these children for services were consistent with the delayed phonological group (i.e. primarily community health nurses).

4. Approximately 60% of the children in the group with consistent phonological disorder were boys.

5. Additional problems noted in this group included expressive language (46%), vocabulary (60%), and phonological awareness difficulties (82%).

6. Oro-motor deviations were noted in approximately one-quarter of children in the group designated as having a consistent phonological disorder.

WHAT TO DO? The main phonological characteristic of this group appears to be a mixture of delayed phonological error patterns and unusual or idiosyncratic error patterns. Areas of language and phonological awareness should be examined, as should the structure and function of the speech mechanism. The severity of the problem is disconcerting. Treatment for the consistent phonological disorder should focus on system-wide change to increase intelligibility as quickly as possible.

Clinical Application

Jonah

Jonah was recently introduced. Based on the results of a standardized speech assessment, a phonological process analysis for Jonah was completed and is summarized in Figure 7.5.

Figure 7.5 Phonological Process Analysis Summary Sheet for Jonah, Age 7 Years 4 Months

Processes	Number of Occurrences
Syllable Structure Changes	
Cluster reduction	18
Cluster deletion	1
Reduplication	
Weak syllable deletion	3
Final consonant deletion	7
Other: Initial consonant deletion	5
Substitution Processes	
Fronting	15
Labialization	
Alveolarization	1
Stopping	37
Affrication	

(*continued*)

Processes	Number of Occurrences
Deaffrication	_____
Denasalization	_____
Gliding of liquids	5
Gliding of fricatives	_____
Vowelization	6
Derhotacization	9
Voicing	_____
Devoicing	10
Other _____	_____
Assimilation Processes	
Labial assimilation	_____
Velar assimilation	_____
Nasal assimilation	_____
Liquid assimilation	_____
Other _____	
_____	_____
_____	_____

Jonah demonstrates both syllable structure and substitution processes. He is showing consonant cluster reduction as well as some initial and final consonant deletion. Although cluster reduction is a process that may occur later in a child's development, final consonant deletion is a fairly early process, typically suppressed by around 4½ years of age. On the other hand, initial consonant deletion is an idiosyncratic process (refer to Table 7.3). In respect to substitution processes, Jonah demonstrates a very high frequency of stopping, followed by fronting. It appears that Jonah has a phonological disorder that would not be considered just delayed. He shows evidence of both early and later processes (sound substitutions).

Inconsistent Phonological Disorder

An inconsistent phonological disorder, often termed an inconsistent speech disorder, was originally used in reference to a child who was in a research project and did not seem to improve with the strategies that led to improvement in other children's speech (Dodd & Iacano, 1989). It was observed that this child had inconsistent productions of the same lexical items. Thus, for the same object, for example, the child's articulations varied from time to time. Many words demonstrated this pattern, and there were various random changes in their production. In the Dodd and colleagues (2013) differential diagnostic subgroup, an inconsistent phonological disorder was noted when there was at least 40% variability on a given task. This task involved the child identifying the same

25 pictures on three separate occasions within a single therapy session. Each time the articulation varied from instance to instance on the same picture, this was noted as being a variable or inconsistent production. If the child produced 10 or more variations on the 25-picture task (40% or more), the child was considered to have an inconsistent phonological disorder. Other characteristics of this classification include the following:

1. Among the four subgroups, an inconsistent phonological disorder was the least likely to occur (9.4%).
2. Children with an inconsistent phonological disorder had the most severe and the most pervasive speech problems. Some children within this subgroup were classified as having a profound impairment.
3. Both parents and health care practitioners were referral agents for this subgroup. These children were often referred due to their unintelligibility.
4. More than three-quarters of the children in this subgroup were boys.
5. Additional problems included receptive and expressive language, vocabulary and phonological awareness difficulties. When compared to the other three subgroups, these children demonstrated the highest percentage of additional involvement.
6. There seemed to be the least evidence of oro-motor involvement when compared to the other three subgroups.
7. When therapy was considered, these children did not respond to normal phonological treatment methods but first required stabilization of their productions (Crosbie, Holm, & Dodd, 2005).

WHAT TO DO? First, clinicians need to determine the variability shown by a particular child. While some inconsistency in production is normal, these children show a lot of inconstancy. This will initially be evident when looking at the results of their inventories and distribution matrixes. An inconsistent phonological disorder manifests itself in several different phones being used as substitutions for one speech sound. Typically, there is no evident pattern.

A clinician needs to assess this variability. One way to do this is by using the Inconsistency Subtest of the Diagnostic Evaluation of Articulation and Phonology–DEAP (Dodd, Hua, Crosbie, Holm, & Ozanne, 2006). In this assessment, children are asked to name 25 pictures (e.g., girl, elephant, dinosaur) on three trials within one session. Each trial is separated by an activity. A word that is produced identically (but not necessarily accurately) each time is marked by a "0" and is considered consistent. Words that demonstrate variable articulation on at least one of the three trials are marked as "1" and considered inconsistent. Forty percent is the cutoff; therefore, if 10 or more of the productions are inconsistent, a diagnosis of inconsistent phonological disorder is made. Clinicians who do not have a copy of the DEAP can use a set of picture cards representing one-, two-, and three-syllable words to assess variability.

Research has demonstrated that children with an inconsistent phonological disorder do well with the Core Vocabulary Intervention. This technique is used to stabilize the child's productions, which can be done in approximately 2 months of weekly intervention. This therapy targets consistent (although not necessarily accurate) production of highly functional words. Based on research findings, after two months of weekly intervention, consistency and accuracy increased (e.g., Crosbie et al., 2005).

Inconsistent Phonological Disorder

Jared, age 3 years 8 months, was referred to the speech-language specialist due to his lack of intelligibility. Although his rate of speech was a little slow, he did not show evidence of any oral-motor difficulties when given a speech-motor screening test. After giving Jared a standardized speech assessment and listening to his conversation, which centered around summer activities, the clinician noted variable productions of /s/, /z/, /f/, /v/, /l/, /k/, /g/, /ʃ/, /tʃ/, /dʒ/, /θ/, /ð/, and /ɹ/. Sometimes the production was accurate, but in most productions there were several substitutions for one sound. For example, for /s/, Jared produced /t/, /z/, /f/, /ʃ/, and /tʃ/. The /s/ was also deleted in intervocalic and postvocalic positions.

Jared scored below the 1st percentile on the Goldman-Fristoe Test of Articulation (Goldman & Fristoe, 2015), and overall intelligibility was rated as poor. Errors seemed to increase with words of two or more syllables.

Jared was given a consistency probe and demonstrated inconsistent productions on 18 of 25 words—that is, 72% of the time. Due to this high percentage, he could be classified as having an inconsistent phonological disorder.

Examples of Jared's variable production include "kangaroo" [tænhu], [tɑnu], [nəwu]; "thumb" [tʌm], [bʌm], [tɑ]; and "balloon" [bun], [wun], [ədun].

Factors Affecting Intelligibility and Measurements of Intelligibility

Factors Affecting Intelligibility

Intelligibility refers to a judgment made by a clinician based on how much of an utterance can be understood. Measurements of the degree of speech intelligibility are based on a subjective, perceptual judgment that is generally related to the percentage of words that the listener understands. Factors influencing speech sound intelligibility include the number, type, and consistency of speech sound errors (Bernthal, Bankson, & Flipsen, 2017). Clearly, the number of errors is related to the overall intelligibility. However, just adding up the errors does not yield an adequate index of intelligibility.

The intelligibility of an utterance is influenced by several factors. Connolly (1986) lists the following factors:

1. The loss of phonemic contrasts
2. The loss of contrasts in specific linguistic contexts
3. The number of meaning distinctions that are lost because of the lack of phonemic contrasts
4. The difference between the target and its realization
5. The consistency of the target-realization relationship
6. The frequency of abnormality in the client's speech
7. The extent to which the listener is familiar with the client's speech
8. The communicative context in which the message occurs

In addition, Shriberg, Kent, McAllister, and Preston (2019) list several other important factors that may influence scoring and transcription:

1. The age of the child. The younger the child, the more difficult it is for the child to respond to formal testing. Assessment and speech sampling may need to be creative endeavors. In addition, the child's voice quality may demonstrate fluctuations in pitch and loudness, and the child's immature speech development may result in sounds that are ambiguous. This is not to mention the child playing with the microphone and kicking the table, which could result in recordings that are far from optimal.

2. The physical and personality characteristics of the individual. Voice and resonance quality can have an impact on transcription. For example, an individual who is hypernasal or congested with a cold will pose more difficulty when transcribing.

3. Linguistic context and response requirements. Linguistic context refers to the number and type of units (phone, syllable, word, etc.) in which the target is imbedded. For example, if the child has difficulty with [s] and it is produced repeatedly, fluctuations in the production will be difficult to note. Response complexity refers to the number of different units the clinician must note. If the clinician must notice variations in several sounds, this will be more difficult.

4. Successive judgments. If a clinician must judge repeated performance, it becomes difficult to maintain perceptual independence. For example, if a child produces the r-sound accurately in nine successive words, the tenth one will need to be noticeably deviant for our perceptual parameters to change.

Measures of Intelligibility

Even though intelligibility remains essentially a subjective evaluation, many authors have attempted to quantify it and to apply their results to a wide array of children and adults with communication disorders (e.g., Gordon-Brannan & Hodson, 2000; Hodson & Paden, 1981; Kent, Miolo, & Bloedel, 1994; Shriberg & Kwiatkowski, 1982a; Webb & Duckett, 1990; Wilcox, Schooling, & Morris, 1991). Coplan and Gleason (1988) suggest the following guidelines for the percentage of conversation that is intelligible in typical children.

2 years of age	50% intelligible
3 years of age	75% intelligible
4 years of age	100% intelligible; although speech sound errors are possible, speech is intelligible

The following intelligibility measures are based on the frequency of occurrence of misarticulated sounds (Fudala & Stegall, 2017):

Level 6. Sound errors are occasionally noticed in continuous speech.

Level 5. Speech is intelligible, although noticeably in error.

Level 4. Speech is intelligible with careful listening.

Level 3. Speech intelligibility is difficult.

Level 2. Speech is usually unintelligible.

Level 1. Speech is unintelligible.

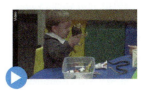

Video Tool Exercise 7.1
Two-Year-Old Ryan
Complete the activity based on this video.

Video Example 7.1

This video provides a short speech sample of 3-year-old Elizabeth telling a story. Mark the words with + if you could understand them and − if you could not. Add all of the + and − marks together, then divide this number by the number of + marks. The result is a percentage of intelligibility. Compare this number to the Coplan and Gleason (1988) guidelines. Is the percentage for Elizabeth higher or lower than the guidelines provided?

https://www.youtube.com/watch?v = PYxM229pAzw

Video Example 7.2

Listen to the first 2 minutes of the following video of Evan, who is 4 years old. According to the Coplan and Gleason (1988) data, a child should be 100% intelligible at age 4. Is Evan 100% intelligible? Would you have been able to understand Evan without many of his father's prompts?

https://www.youtube.com/watch?v = 3jHD-7Bc2rM

Video Example 7.3

Listen to this speech sample of a 3-year-old Star Wars expert. Using the five-point CHIRPA scale (Baker, 2016), how would you rank this child? Compare your results to those of other students. Are they all the same?

https://www.youtube.com/watch?v = EBM854BTGL0

The Children's Independent and Relational Phonological Analysis–CHIRPA (Baker, 2016) can be used for a complete phonological analysis and contains a scale to determine intelligibility. CHIRPA has a five-point rating scale, as follows:

1 = intelligible

2 = mainly intelligible

3 = partially intelligible

4 = mainly unintelligible

5 = completely unintelligible

These types of scales seem to offer a simple solution for rating intelligibility. However, several problems are inherent in this or any type of scale (Flipsen, 2010). First, different listeners will choose different levels, especially in the midrange of the scale; thus, there is a large degree of variability between listeners. A good example is that parents will rank their child more toward the top of the intelligibility scale; they listen to the child every day and have learned how to interpret certain words and phrases. You, as a clinician, will change your scale ratings based on the same principle. As you listen to the child repeatedly, you also will be able to understand more of what the child says, even without treatment changes. With such a scale, how much does it take for the child to move from Level 3: Speech is partially intelligible to Level 2: Speech is mainly intelligible? These scales are not sensitive enough to track change in a child's speech over time (Flipsen, 2010).

Another option is that the clinician can try to calculate the percentage of words understood. However, first the clinician must determine at which linguistic level intelligibility will be analyzed: (1) single words, spontaneous or imitated; (2) sentences, spontaneous or imitated; or (3) conversational speech. The degree of unintelligibility will probably dictate the level. For children who are highly unintelligible, imitated words or sentences may be ideal. However, for less severe speech sound disorders, conversational speech may provide the best measurement. Ideally, different levels should be sampled.

Over the years, many types of intelligibility probes have been developed. Several of these are out of print or unavailable. The sentences from the Beginner's Intelligibility Test (Osberger, Robbins, Todd, & Riley, 1994) are available online. This test, which was originally designed to test the intelligibility of children who are hearing impaired, can be used for any population. There are four sets of sentences that can be used randomly in an imitative task, or if the child can read, they can be read by the child. The sentences are tape recorded and two independent listeners state how many of the words can be understood. According to Osberger and colleagues (1994), a percentage is then calculated based on the number of words the child says (not on the total number of words from the sentences).

A slightly different method, supported by Lagerberg, Åsberg, Hartelius, and Persson (2014) and Martin (2017), can be easily implemented by clinicians. It uses the syllables that can be understood versus the total number of syllables to calculate a percentage. Many clinicians may already be doing this, as it is an easy way to somewhat objectively measure intelligibility. This method uses a 10 × 10 grid in which + is used for an understood syllable and − is used for an unintelligible one. This can be used as the child looks at a picture (if the child is highly unintelligible, some context may be beneficial). When the grid is full, the number of + marks is totaled to determine the percentage of intelligibility. Refer to Appendix 7.4 for a grid and some basic instructions.

Measures of Severity, Whole-Word Accuracy, and Variability

Articulatory competency can also be measured by different severity classifications. Severity measures are attempts to quantify the degree of involvement. Several severity measures are available. Hodson (2004) has developed one that is based on a child's performance on the Hodson Assessment of Phonological Patterns (HAP-3). In addition, Bleile (1996) offers a four-point clinical judgment scale:

1 = no disorder

2 = mild disorder

3 = moderate disorder

4 = severe disorder

BOX 7.1

Determining the Percentage of Consonants Correct (PCC)

What is measured?	A 5- to 10-minute conversational sample is recorded and analyzed.
What is scored?	Only consonants are scored using this metric. The examiner is required to make correct versus incorrect judgments on individual consonant productions. The following sound changes are considered incorrect:

1. Deletion of a target consonant
2. Substitution of a target consonant, including the substitution of a glottal stop or a cognate
3. Partial voicing of a prevocalic consonant
4. Any distortions
5. Addition of a sound to a correct or incorrect target sound
6. Initial [h] deletion and final n/ŋ substitutions in stressed syllables only. For example, [ɪt] for *hit* and [rɪn] for *ring* would be incorrect. However, in unstressed syllables, saying [fɪʃən] for *fishing*, for example, would be considered correct. Acceptable allophonic variations are considered correct. For example, the intervocalic allophonic variation of [t] in *water* [wɑɾɚ] is considered correct.
7. Postvocalic [ɚ], such as in "farm" [fɑɚm], is considered a consonant and is counted as such; [ɝ] and unstressed [ɚ] are classified as vowels and not counted.

What is not scored?	Do not score utterances that are unintelligible or consonants in the second or successive repetitions of a syllable. For example, if the child says [bə bə lun], score only the first [b]. Also, do not score target consonants in the third or successive repetitions of adjacent words unless the articulation changes. For example, if the child says [tɹit], [tɹit], [tɹit], only the consonants in the first two words are counted. However, if the child changes the articulation, saying [tɹit], [twit], [tɹit], then the consonants in all three utterances are counted.
Calculation	The percentage of consonants correct is calculated in the following manner:

$$\frac{\text{Number of correct consonants}}{\text{Number of correct plus incorrect consonants}} \times 100$$

Shriberg and Kwiatkowski (1982a, 1982b) suggest calculating the *percentage of consonants correct (PCC)*, which can then be used with their metric to measure the severity of involvement in children with phonological disorders. Based on research, this type of calculation was found to correlate most closely to listeners' perceptions of severity. This concept was later expanded to other measures (Shriberg, Austin, Lewis, McSweeny, & Wilson, 1997). Quantitative estimates of severity using the PCC give clinicians an objective measure to establish the relative priority of those who might need therapy or to measure progress in therapy, for example. The PCC calculations can be translated into the following severity divisions:

Mild = 85 to 100%

Mild-moderate = 65 to 84.9%

Moderate-severe = 50 to 64.9%

Severe = <50%

Box 7.1 provides the procedure for determining the PCC according to the information from Shriberg and colleagues (1997). It should be noted that the PCC is not intended to score children who evidence primarily sound distortions. If you would like to use a metric that weighs distortion errors, the Articulation Competence Index–ACI (Shriberg et al., 1997) is a possibility.

Jonah's PCC is calculated in the case study at the end of the chapter. It is based on the speech sample collected from Jonah, who was introduced earlier in this chapter.

Shriberg and colleagues (1997) have expanded the original concept of PCC to other measures that examine the percentage of vowels correct (PVC) and a matrix that weighs distortion errors, called the articulation competence index (ACI), to mention just two of their ten indexes. A conversational speech sample is the basis for all calculations. For information on the various metric values, refer to Shriberg and colleagues (1997).

Measures of Whole Words

This section examines two whole-word measures: a measure of accuracy, the Proportion of Whole-Word Correctness (Ingram, 2002), and a measure of variability, the Proportion of Whole-Word Variability (Ingram, 2002; Ingram & Ingram, 2001).

The Proportion of Whole-Word Correctness (PWC; Ingram, 2002) is a simple way to measure the proportion of words that are produced correctly by the child relative to the total number of words in a sample. For example, if the child said 50 words correctly out of a 100-word sample, the PWC would be 50%. The calculation is as follows:

$$\frac{\text{Number of correct words}}{\text{Total number of words (\textit{both correct and incorrect words added together})}}$$

The Proportion of Whole-Word Variability (PWV; Ingram, 2002; Ingram & Ingram, 2001) is a measure of the variability of a child's productions of whole words. This might be a good metric to use with a child who is possibly evidencing an inconsistent phonological disorder. This metric differentiates children who consistently produce words in the same way from those who demonstrate inconsistent productions. The PWV is calculated from a speech sample containing multiple productions of the same word. To calculate the PWV, the following formula is used:

$$\frac{\text{Total number of different forms}}{\text{Total number of productions of that word}}$$

An average of all the words that were produced with variability is then calculated to determine an overall proportion of whole-word variability. Refer to the Case Study at the end of this chapter for an example.

Summary

The goal of this chapter was to show how the data gathered in the appraisal section of our speech sound assessment can be used in different types of analyses. The first portion of this chapter demonstrated how to organize the data according to inventory, distribution, and stimulability of phones. These procedures were illustrated using a case study of Jonah, age 7 years 4 months. The next step in the diagnostic process is to examine the data to determine whether a neutralization of phonemic contrasts exists. A method of analyzing error patterns was illustrated by an analysis of phonological processes. A sample form and analysis using our case study, Jonah, were provided. Next, we returned to one of the classification systems for speech sound disorders discussed in Chapter 1, the Differential Diagnostic System (Dodd, 2013). This system classifies speech sound disorders according to five subgroups: articulation disorder, delayed phonological disorder, consistent phonological disorder, inconsistent phonological disorder, and childhood apraxia of speech. Characteristics of each of the first four subgroups were discussed, as were specific diagnostic parameters.

Finally, measures of intelligibility and severity were described. Several metrics were illustrated along with their calculations. A practical application is included in the Case Study at the end of this chapter. These measures can be used to document the need for, and progress in, therapy as well as to serve as a basis for clinical research.

Case Study

Spontaneous Speech Sample for Jonah, Age 7 Years 4 Months

The following spontaneous speech sample is from Jonah. Using the instructions provided in Box 7.1, determine the PCC.

Looking at Pictures

[dæ ə pɪtə əv ə tɑ]	[oʊ dæt ə tɪti]
That a picture of a dog.	Oh, that a kitty.
[hi ə bɪ dɑ]	[wi hæv ə tɪti]
He a big dog.	We have a kitty.
[hi baʊ ən hæ ə tawə]	[wi dɑt aʊ tɪti ə wɑːŋ taɪm]
He brown an has a collar.	We got our kitty a long time.

Conversation with Mom

[tæn wi do tu mədɑnoʊ]	[hi tʌm tu mədɑnət wɪt ʌt]
Can we go to McDonald?	He come to McDonald with us?
[aɪ wʌ ə ti bɜdə]	[xxxx mɑɪ haʊ]
I want a cheeseburger.	Xxxx my house.
[aɪ wʌ fɛnfɑɪt]	[mɑmi lɛ do]
I want French fries.	Mommy let go.
[wɛ ɪt bɪwi]	[lɛ do naʊ]
Where is Billy?	Let go now.

Talking About Summer Vacation	
[wi doʊf tu dæmɑ]	[ti hæt wɑtə taʊt]
We drove to Grandma.	She has lot'a cows.
[ti wɪf ɪn oʊ + haɪo]	[taʊt ju noʊ mu taʊ]
She live in Ohio.	Cows, you know, moo cow.
[ti hæt ə fɑm]	[deɪ it ə ho wɑt]
She has a farm.	They eat a whole lot.

	Correct Consonants	Incorrect Consonants
That a picture of a dog.	2	5
He a big dog.	3	2
He brown and has a collar.	4	5
Oh, that a kitty.	2	2
We have a kitty.	4	1
We got our kitty a long time.	6	4
Can we go to McDonald?	6	5
I want a cheeseburger.	2	5
I want French fries.	4	6
Where is Billy?	2	3
He come to McDonald with us?	7	6
Xxxx my house.	2	1
Mommy let go.	3	2
Let go now.	2	2
We drove to Grandma.	4	4
She live in Ohio.	2	3
She has a farm.	3	3
She has lot'a cows.	2	5
Cows, you know, moo cow.	3	3
They eat a whole lot.	3	3

Number of correct consonants ≐ 66

Divided by number of correct plus incorrect consonants = 136

66/136 = 0.49 × 100 = 49%

PCC = 49%, which is less than 50% = severe

Proportion of Whole-Word Correctness (PWC)

$$\frac{\text{Number of correct words}}{\text{Total number of words (both correct and incorrect words added together)}}$$

Number of correct words = 33/87 = 37.9% whole-word correctness, which is very low; only slightly more than one-third of the words are produced correctly

Note: "Oh" was not counted, "cheeseburger" counted as two words, and "lot'a" counted as one word.

Proportion of Whole-Word Variability (PWV)

$$\frac{\text{Total number of different forms}}{\text{Total number of productions of that word}}$$

that /ðæt/ → [dæ], [dæt] Total number of different forms = 1 / Total number of productions of that word = 2

PWV = 1/2 = 0.5

dog /dɑg/ → [dɑ], [dɑ] Total number of different forms = 0 / Total number of productions of that word = 2

PWV = 0/2 = 0

want /wʌnt/ → [wʌ], [wʌ] Total number of different forms = 0 / Total number of productions of that word = 2

PWV = 0/2 = 0

kitty /kɪti/ → [tɪti], [tɪti], [tɪti] Total number of different forms = 0 / Total number of productions of that word = 3

PWV = 0/3 = 0

let /lɛt/ → [lɛ], [lɛ] Total number of different forms = 0 / Total number of productions of that word = 2

PWV = 0/2 = 0

she /ʃi/ → [ti], [ti] Total number of different forms = 0 / Total number of productions of that word = 2

PWV = 0/2 = 0

McDonald /mək.dɑ.nəld/ → [mədɑnoʊ], [mədɑnət] Total number of different forms = 1 / Total number of productions of that word = 2

PWV = 1/2 = 0.5

Overall variability = 0.5 + 0 + 0 + 0 + 0 + 0 + 0.5 = 0.14; extremely little variability in productions

Think Critically

The following results are from Brandon, age 5 years 6 months:

house	[haʊs̠]	matches	[mætəs̠]	thumb	[tʌm]
telephone	[tɛfoʊn]	lamp	[wæmp]	finger	[fɪnə]
cup	[tʌp]	shovel	[tʌvoʊ]	ring	[wɪŋ]
gum	[ɣʌm]	car	[tɑə]	jumping	[djʌmpəs̠]
night	[naɪt]	rabbit	[wæbət]	pajamas	[djæməs]
window	[wɪnoʊ]	fishing	[fɪtsʲən]	plane	[pweɪn]
wagon	[ʌæɣən]	church	[tsʲɜtsʲ]	blue	[bwu]
wheel	[ʌiə]	feather	[fɛdə]	brush	[bwʌsʲ]
chicken	[tsʲɪtən]	pencils	[pɪntos̠]	drum	[dwʌm]
zipper	[z̠ɪpə]	this	[dɪs̠]	flag	[fwæɣ]
scissors	[sʲɪtə]	carrot	[tɛwət]	Santa	[s̠ænə]
duck	[dʌ]	orange	[ɔwɪntsʲ]	tree	[twi]
yellow	[jɛwoʊ]	bathtub	[bæftʌb]	squirrel	[twɜwoʊ]
vacuum	[væɣum]	bath	[bæf]	sleeping	[s̠wipən]
bed	[bɛd]	stove	[s̠toʊf]		

1. Which sounds are in the phonetic inventory and which ones are in the phonemic inventory for Brandon?

2. Use Table 7.1 to list the phonemic contrasts for Brandon. Do you notice the collapse of contrasts or any sound that is used frequently as a substitution?

3. Which one of the four classification subgroups (pp. 211–218) do you think fits Brandon the best? What additional information would you need to make that decision?

4. Do you notice any idiosyncratic processes in the results of Brandon's standardized speech assessment?

> ✓ **Chapter Quiz 7.1** Complete this quiz to check your understanding of chapter concepts.

Appendix 7.1 Transcription from Jonah, Age 7 Years 4 Months, from the Goldman-Fristoe Test of Articulation (Goldman & Fristoe, 2015)

1. house [haʊt]
2. door [doə]
3. pig [pɪ]
4. cup [tʌp]
5. boy [bɔɪ]
6. apple [æ.oʊ]
7. go [toʊ]
8. duck [dʌt]
9. quack [tæt]
10. table [teɪ.boʊ]
11. monkey [mʌ.ni]
12. hammer [æ.mə]
13. fish [pɪt]
14. watch [wat]
15. spider [paɪ.tə]
16. web [wɛp]
17. drum [dʌm]
18. plate [peɪt]
19. knife [naɪp]
20. shoe [tu]
21. slide [taɪ]
22. swing [tɪŋ]
23. guitar [ta.ə]
24. lion [waɪ.ən]
25. chair [tɛə]
26. soap [toʊp]
27. glasses [dæ.ə]
28. tiger [taɪ.də]
29. puzzle [pʌ.to]
30. finger [pɪn.ə]
31. ring [wɪŋ]
32. thumb [tʌm]
33. elephant [ɛ.fən]
34. vacuum [bæ.um]
35. shovel [tʌ.boʊ]
36. teacher [ti.tə]
37. zebra [di.bə]
38. giraffe [dɪ.wæ]
39. vegetable [bɛ.tə.po]
40. brushing [bʌ.tɪŋ]
41. blue [bu]
42. yellow [dɛ.doʊ]
43. brother [bʌ.tə]
44. frog [pat]
45. green [tin]
46. that [dæt]
47. leaf [wip]
48. cookie [tʊ.ti]
49. cheese [tit]
50. pajamas [tæ.mə]
51. teeth [tif]
52. princess [pɪn.tət]
53. crown [taʊn]
54. truck [tʌt]
55. red [wɛd]
56. juice [du]
57. zoo [du]
58. star [tɑə]
59. five [faɪp]
60. seven [tɛ.bən]

Appendix 7.2 Matrix for Spontaneous Speech Sample from Jonah, Age 7 Years 4 Months
✓ indicates a correct production, ø indicates a deletion, and substitutions are noted with the appropriate phonetic transcription.

	Early Sounds	Prevocalic	Intervocalic	Post-vocalic	Stimu-lable	Later Sounds	Pre-vocalic	Inter-vocalic	Post-vocalic	Stimu-lable	
Stops	p		✓			f					Fricatives
	b		✓✓✓			v		✓ ✓ f f			
	t		✓✓✓✓✓Ø✓✓✓✓	✓		s			t Ø		
	d		t✓✓			z		ØØ t t	t t		
	k	t t	t t t t Ø t t Ø			ʃ	t t t				
	g		Ø d d d d	ØØ		ʒ					
Nasals	m	✓✓	✓✓✓✓✓	✓✓		θ					
	n		Ø ✓ ✓ ✓✓			ð	d d d				
	ŋ		✓ ✓ ✓			l	✓	w w w w ✓ w w Ø			Approximants
Approximants	w	✓ ✓ ✓ ✓	✓ ✓ ✓ ✓			ɹ					
	j		✓			tʃ		t Ø			Affricates
Fricatives	h	✓ ✓ ✓ ✓	✓ ✓ ✓ ✓ ✓ ✓			ʤ					

Note: Shading indicates a voiced consonant.

Consonant Clusters: Prevocalic:

Intervocalic: ktʃ → t (picture), bɹ → b, nt → Ø, fɹ → f, ntʃfɹ → nf (French fries), dɹ → d, gɹ → d

Postvocalic: ld → oʊ, ət

Also, ɝ → ɜ, ɚ → ə, ɑɚ → ɑ, ɛɚ → ɛ

Note: Phones at the beginning of an utterance have been labeled prevocalic. Phones at the end of an utterance are noted as postvocalic. Phones within the utterance are labeled as intervocalic. Consonant clusters within the utterance have been preserved.

Appendix 7.3 Minimal Word-Pairs Ordered by Vowel

/i/	/ɪ/	/e/	/ɛ/	/æ/	/ɑ, a, ɔ/	/o/
/p/ pea	/p/ pin	/p/ pay	/p/ pen	/p/ pat	/p/ pot	/p/
/b/ bee	/b/ bin	/b/ bay	/b/ Ben	/b/ bat	/b/ bought	/b/ bow
/t/ tea	/t/ tin	/t/	/t/ ten	/t/	/t/ taught	/t/ toe
/d/ Dee	/d/ din	/d/ Dane	/d/ den	/d/	/d/ dot	/d/ doe
/k/ key	/k/ kin	/k/	/k/ Ken	/k/ cat	/k/ caught	/k/ coat
/g/	/g/	/g/ gay	/g/	/g/	/g/ got	/g/ goat
/m/ me	/m/	/m/ may	/m/ men	/m/ mat	/m/	/m/ mow
/n/ knee	/n/	/n/ nee	/n/	/n/ gnat	/n/ knot	/n/ no
/w/ we	/w/ win	/w/ way	/w/ when	/w/	/w/ watt	/w/ whoa
/j/	/j/	/j/ yay	/j/	/j/	/j/ yacht	/j/ yo
/h/ he	/h/	/h/ hay	/h/ hen	/h/ hat	/h/ hot	/h/ hoe
/f/ fee	/f/ fin	/f/ Fay	/f/	/f/ fat	/f/ fought	/f/ foe
/v/ V	/v/	/v/	/v/	/v/ vat	/v/	/v/
/s/ see, sea	/s/ sin	/s/ say	/s/	/s/ sat	/s/ sought	/s/ sew, so
/z/ Z	/z/	/z/	/z/ Zen	/z/	/z/	/z/
/θ/	/θ/ thin	/θ/	/θ/	/θ/	/θ/ thought	/θ/
/ð/ thee	/ð/	/ð/ they	/ð/ then	/ð/ that	/ð/	/ð/ though
/ʃ/ she	/ʃ/ shin	/ʃ/ Shay	/ʃ/	/ʃ/	/ʃ/ shot	/ʃ/ show
/l/ Lee	/l/ Lynn	/l/ lay	/l/	/l/	/l/ lot	/l/ low
/ɹ/	/ɹ/	/ɹ/ ray	/ɹ/ wren	/ɹ/ rat	/ɹ/ rot	/ɹ/ row
/tʃ/	/tʃ/ chin	/tʃ/	/tʃ/	/tʃ/ chat	/tʃ/	/tʃ/
/dʒ/ gee	/dʒ/ gin	/dʒ/ J	/dʒ/ Jen	/dʒ/	/dʒ/ jot	/dʒ/ Joe

/ʊ/	/u/	/ɑɪ/	/ɑʊ/	/ɔɪ/	/ʌ/	/ɝ/
/p/ put	/p/ poo	/p/ pie	/p/ pow	/p/	/p/ putt	/p/ purr
/b/	/b/ boo	/b/ buy	/b/ bow	/b/ boy	/b/ but	/b/ burr
/t/	/t/ two	/t/ tie	/t/	/t/ toy	/t/	/t/
/d/	/d/ do	/d/ dye	/d/	/d/	/d/	/d/
/k/	/k/ coo	/k/	/k/ cow	/k/ coy	/k/ cut	/k/
/g/	/g/ goo	/g/ Guy	/g/	/g/	/g/ gut	/g/ grr
/m/	/m/ moo	/m/ my	/m/	/m/	/m/ mutt	/m/
/n/	/n/ new	/n/ nye	/n/ now	/n/	/n/ nut	/n/
/w/	/w/	/w/ why	/w/ wow	/w/	/w/ what	/w/ were
/j/	/j/ you	/j/	/j/ yow	/j/	/j/	/j/ your
/h/	/h/ who	/h/ hi	/h/ how	/h/	/h/ hut	/h/ her
/f/ foot	/f/ foo	/f/	/f/	/f/	/f/	/f/ fur
/v/	/v/	/v/ Vye	/v/ vow	/v/	/v/	/v/
/s/ soot	/s/ Sue	/s/ sigh	/s/ sow	/s/ soy	/s/	/s/ sir
/z/	/z/ zoo	/z/	/z/	/z/	/z/	/z/
/θ/	/θ/	/θ/ thigh	/θ/	/θ/	/θ/	/θ/
/ð/	/ð/	/ð/ thy	/ð/ thou	/ð/	/ð/	/ð/
/ʃ/	/ʃ/ shoe	/ʃ/ shy	/ʃ/	/ʃ/	/ʃ/ shut	/ʃ/ sure
/l/	/l/ Lu	/l/ lie	/l/	/l/	/l/	/l/
/ɹ/ root	/ɹ/	/ɹ/ rye	/ɹ/ row	/ɹ/ Roy	/ɹ/ rut	/ɹ/
/tʃ/	/tʃ/ chew	/tʃ/ chai	/tʃ/ chow	/tʃ/	/tʃ/	/tʃ/
/dʒ/	/dʒ/	/dʒ/	/dʒ/	/dʒ/ joy	/dʒ/ jut	/dʒ/

Appendix 7.4 Intelligibility Grid

Mark a + for each syllable that is intelligible and a − for each that is unintelligible. The grid contains 100 squares, so when it is full, count the number of + marks. This is your percentage of intelligibility.

The following guideline is from Shriberg and colleagues (1986).

Mild: 85 to 100%

Mild-moderate: 65 to 84.9%

Moderate-severe: 50 to 64.9%

Severe: <50%

Note: For best results, this grid should be filled out by a person who is unfamiliar with the child, especially on repeat measures. For example, a teacher or another speech-language pathologist could help out.

Chapter 8
Dialects and English as a Second Language

	Learning Objectives

When you have finished this chapter, you should be able to:

8.1 Define dialects including formal, informal and regional dialects.

8.2 Describe the characteristics of Appalachian English, Ozark English, and African-American Vernacular English.

8.3 Identify the English as a Second Language Learner noting developmental factors and defining Limited English Proficient students.

8.4 Describe the speech sound and specific prosodic characteristics of Spanish, Vietnamese, Cantonese, Korean, Filipino, Hmong, and Arabic American English.

8.5 Identify cultural competence and recognize general guidelines that could be used when evaluating an English language learner.

Chapter Application: Case Study

Lilly was a darling child who had just moved with her mother to the United States from Vietnam. Both Lilly and her mother did not speak English. However, Lilly's mom did bring a friend to school with her who could speak both Vietnamese and English. According to the friend, Lilly was 7½ years of age, old enough to be in second grade, but she had received limited formal schooling in Vietnam. Lilly's mom said that Lilly had trouble with her speech and "making sentences." Lilly's mom had tried to train her in reading and writing at home, with limited success. Lilly did talk to her mom in Vietnamese. She also tried to imitate simple English words such as "hello," "Lilly," and her brother's name, "Minh."

This was an initial meeting to decide which preliminary steps should be taken to evaluate and help Lilly. The speech-language therapist, Peter, was a new addition to this school, and it seemed that he would play a central role in the process. Peter did not know anything about the Vietnamese language. He was uncertain about the sounds of that language and how they differed from General American English. He was also unsure about how he should evaluate Lilly. It seemed possible that she might have speech and language problems in her native language and would need extra resources to learn English. Would it make a difference for services if Lilly did have speech and language difficulties in Vietnamese? Peter wasn't sure where to start with the evaluation process.

LANGUAGE variations are quite normal in a society composed of a multitude of social groups that have become quite diversified. Most individuals in the United States have ancestors from other countries, and geographical regions have established their own language variations. In addition, immigrants to this country very often do not speak English as their primary language. These and many other factors contribute to a growing diversity in cultural norms, lifestyles, and, of course, speech and language distinctions. The goal of this chapter is to examine a few of these variations that are important as speech-language pathologists work with this diverse population.

The purpose of this chapter is, first, to define *dialect* and to compare technical and professional viewpoints on this term. The second section examines regional dialects, those variations that are primarily related to geographical areas, as well as social and ethnic dialects exemplified by African-American Vernacular English. The last section of this chapter focuses on the phoneme system of several foreign languages. By noting differences between General American English (GAE) and these phonological systems, specific problems can be exemplified. Clinical implications for these speech variations are outlined.

This chapter is positioned between the chapters on diagnostic and treatment principles. Portions of the chapter address diagnostic features, such as noting the differences that can occur between the phonemic system of a speaker's native language and that of General American English or being aware of the features of several common dialects within the United States. Other sections transition into treatment, noting typical error patterns that could be relevant within the treatment process for a non-native speaker. However, because of the importance of this information for speech-language pathologists, it warranted a separate chapter. This chapter is intended as a resource for clinicians who need to be knowledgeable about language variations within the United States.

Dialects

Dialect is a neutral label that refers to any variety of a language that is shared by a group of speakers. Although this section focuses on the speech sound variations within a dialect, readers should keep in mind that dialects also encompass specific use of vocabulary, word forms (such as plural endings), sentence structure, and prosodic patterns.

The technical use of *dialect*, as a neutral term, implies no particular social or attitudinal evaluations; that is, there are no "good" or "bad" dialects. Dialects are simply language variations that typify a group of speakers in a language. The factors that might correlate with the use of a particular dialect can be as simple as geographical locality or as complex as a person's notion of cultural identity. It is important to remember that socially acceptable or so-called standard versions of a language constitute dialects as much as those varieties that are considered socially isolated or stigmatized language differences. General American English also has a dialect referred to as *Standard English*.

There appear to be two sets of representations of Standard English: formal and informal (Wolfram & Schilling-Estes, 2006). **Formal Standard English**, which is applied primarily to written language and most formal spoken language situations, tends to be based on the written language and is exemplified in usage guides and grammar texts. When there is a question as to whether a form is considered Standard English, these texts would be consulted. **Informal Standard English** considers the assessment of members of the American English–speaking community as they judge the "standardness" of other speakers. This notion exists on a continuum ranging from standard to nonstandard speakers of American English and relies far more heavily on grammatical structure than pronunciation patterns (Wolfram & Schilling-Estes, 2006). Listeners accept a range of variations in pronunciation but are not as accepting of specific grammatical structures when evaluating "standardness." For example, a rather pronounced Boston or New York regional dialect would be accepted, but structures such as double negatives would not be considered within the borders of Standard English. **Vernacular dialects** refer to those varieties of spoken American English that are considered outside the continuum of informal Standard English (Wolfram & Schilling-Estes, 2006). Vernacular dialects are signaled by the presence of certain grammatical structures. Therefore, a set of nonstandard English structures marks them as being vernacular. For example, the presence of double negation, lack of subject-verb agreement, and use of variations from standard verb forms would constitute features that could label the speaker as using a vernacular dialect. Although a core of features might exemplify a particular vernacular dialect, not all speakers display the entire set of structures. Therefore, differing patterns of usage exist among speakers of a particular vernacular dialect.

Dialects can vary along several parameters. First, one can describe a dialect according to its hypothesized causative agent. If one examines causation, two main categories are formed: those dialects that (1) correspond to various geographical locations, which are considered **regional dialects**, and (2) are generally related to socioeconomic status and/or ethnic background, labeled **social** or **ethnic dialects**. In addition, dialects are classified according to their linguistic features, including the phonological, morphological, syntactical, semantic, and pragmatic differences that are distinctive when that dialect is compared to Informal Standard English. It appears that regional dialects typically demonstrate at least distinctive phonological and semantic features. On the other hand, social and ethnic dialects can vary along *all* of the previously stated linguistic features.

Regional Dialects

Individuals who study dialects (dialectologists) traditionally have listed three main regional dialect groups in the United States: northern, midland, and southern. More recent scholars prefer a simple north–south distinction, although there are still significant differences in the boundaries of each proposed area. Many researchers believe that there are no discrete dialect boundaries and no clear-cut dialect divisions in American English. However, data from the Telsur Project show clear and distinct dialect boundaries with a high degree of similarity in each dialect. The Telsur Project of the Linguistics Laboratory of the University of Pennsylvania is one of the largest and most extensive ongoing collections of data related to the dialect regions of the United States. The home page for this project is located within the linguistics department at the University of Pennsylvania. The data consist of phonetic transcriptions and acoustic analyses of informants' vowel systems. These data have been compiled in the *Atlas of North American English* (Labov, Ash, & Boberg, 2005) and represent the active processes of change and diversification that the authors have been tracing since 1968 (Labov, 1991, 1994, 1996; Labov, Yaeger, & Steiner, 1972). Their results document four major dialect regions: the North, the South, the West, and the Midland (refer to Figure 8.1). The first three regions demonstrate a relatively uniform development of General American English sound shifts, each moving in somewhat

Figure 8.1 Dialect Areas of the United States Based on Telsur Project Results

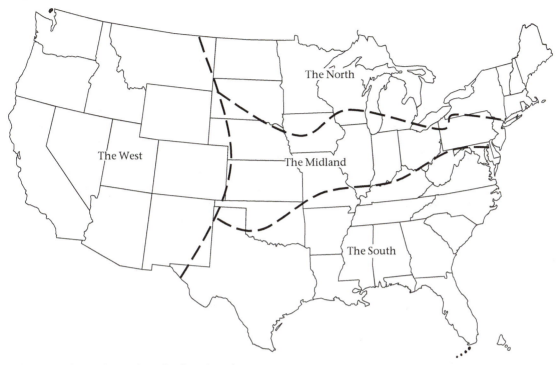

Source: Data from Labov, Ash, and Boberg (2005).

different directions. The fourth region, the Midland, has considerably more diversity, and most of its individual cities have developed dialect patterns of their own.

Three variables seem to have an overall effect on the regional dialects: (1) the Northern cities and South vowel shifts, (2) the merging of specific vowels, and (3) the variations of r-production. The Northern cities and South vowel shifts are examples of chain shifts. These chain shifts are systematic changes in vowel systems in which the vowels shift in respect to their articulatory features. Any feature, such as height, fronting, or backing of the tongue or lip rounding can change. In addition, sets of features can change; for example, vowels can be lengthened or shortened. Chain shifts demonstrate a tendency to maintain specific phonemic distinctions. Therefore, the neighboring vowels will also shift. As one vowel changes—for example, becomes more of a fronted vowel—other vowels change as well, so that distinct articulatory parameters still exist between the vowels. The following is a brief summary of the four major dialect regions as they relate to these three variables.

North. The area referred to as North is divided into the North Central region, the Inland North, Eastern New England, New York City, and Western New England. The short vowels [ɪ], [ɛ], [æ], [ʊ], [ʌ], and [ɑ-a-ɔ] all evidence a specific vowel shift (the Northern Cities Vowel Shift, discussed in Labov, 1991, for example). For the long vowels, which include the diphthongs, the North Central and Inland North regions maintain a long high position, which is typical of the vowel quadrilateral presented in this text. The r-coloring of postvocalic r-productions, such as in *farm* [fɑɚm], is also maintained in these areas.

On the other hand, the Eastern New England area of the North demonstrates r-lessness in which (1) rhotic diphthongs such as those noted in *farm* [fɑɚm] and *porch* [poʊɚtʃ], (2) stressed central vowels with r-coloring such as in *bird* [bɝd] and *shirt* [ʃɝt], and (3) unstressed central vowels with r-coloring such as in *mother* [mʌðɚ] and *over* [oʊvɚ] lose the r-coloring, resulting in possible pronunciations such as [fɑəm] or [fɑm] for *farm*, [poʊətʃ] or [poʊtʃ] for *porch*, [bɜd] for *bird*, [ʃɜt] for *shirt*, [mʌðə] for *mother*, and [oʊvə] for *over*.

In addition, the two vowels [ɑ] and [ɔ] are merged into an intermediate vowel, more frequently [a]. Thus, distinct pronunciations for words such as *caught* [kɔt] and *cot* [kɑt] are not realized. Instead, one similar vowel is used for both words. The exception to this occurs in the city of Providence, Rhode Island, which has the characteristic r-lessness but does not merge the [ɑ] and [ɔ] vowels.

New York City has a distinctive dialect that is not reproduced further west and therefore does not fit neatly into any larger regional group. The long vowels maintain a high position similar to that noted for the North Central and Inland North areas. There is consistent r-lessness of postvocalic "r" except for (1) the central vowel with r-coloring [ɝ] ("bird" is pronounced as [bɝd]) and (2) when a final "r" is followed by a vowel in the next word, such as *The <u>car is</u> gone* [ðə kɑɚ ɪz gɑn]. In addition, the /æ/ vowel splits into lax and tense forms, and the production differences between [ɑ] and [ɔ] are maximal, the [ɔ] vowel being raised to a mid-high position. No clear patterns of sound change seem to occur in Western New England.

South.   The South demonstrates a vowel shift referred to as the Southern Shift (refer to Labov, 1991). However, a small area of the Southeast—the cities of Charleston, South Carolina, and Savannah, Georgia—is distinct from the rest of the South. In these cities, the vowel changes are minimal when compared to the rest of the South. A characteristic of the southern region is the [ɑ]–[ɔ] distinction. With the exceptions of the margins of the South—western Texas, Kentucky, Virginia, and the city of Charleston—this distinction is marked not by a change in the vowel quality but by a back upglide for [ɔ]. Thus, the nuclei of the vowels are acoustically very similar; however, [ɔ] is productionally signaled by a back upgliding movement of the tongue somewhat similar to [ɔo].

Midland.   Speakers in the Midland area do not seem to participate in the vowel shifts that are noted in the South and North. Labov and colleagues (2005) divide the Midland into two sections: South and North. The consistently noted feature of the South Midland is the fronting of [oʊ], resulting in a [ʌ]-like quality. For example, "goes" might be pronounced as [gʌz] or "He goes shopping" [hi gʌz ʃɑpɪŋ]. Exceptions are Louisville, Kentucky, and Savannah, Georgia. Using this criterion, Philadelphia is a member of the South Midland, and Pittsburgh and St. Louis are considered North Midland.

West.   The diversity of dialects declines steadily as one moves westward, resulting in a diffusion of North, Midland, and South characteristics. Although there are exceptions, characteristics of the West are aligned with those of the Midland. The most prominent feature of West phonology is the merger of [ɑ] and [ɔ]; however, as noted previously, this is not restricted to the West. The second feature that emerges is the fronting of the vowel [u], as in *two* or *do*, which is produced with a tongue position that is more anterior than typical, for example. Although these two characteristics are also noted in the South Midland, their occurrence appears to be much higher in the West.

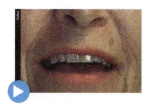

Video Example 8.1
Listen to the two speakers; the first one is from the Northeast (Maine) and the second one is from the South (North Carolina). Listen carefully to the vowels with r-coloring. Do both dialects evidence the same type of changes?

> **Clinical Exercises**   In which regional area were you raised? Do you notice characteristics of your own speech that seem to coincide with that region's particular dialect?
>
> Which regional dialects have some degree of "r-lessness"? Why would this be important to know in your clinical practice?

Characteristics of Appalachian English, Ozark English, and African-American Vernacular English

Appalachian Versus Ozark English

Broadly speaking, *Appalachia* refers to that part of the United States that encompasses the Appalachian Mountain range. However, if the area where Appalachian English is spoken is more narrowly defined, it refers primarily to rural sections of Kentucky, Tennessee, West Virginia, and, to a lesser extent, bordering regions of Virginia and the Carolinas. West Virginia is the only state that is included as a whole in this region. There are differences from one community to another, but many features are shared in these areas.

On the other hand, Ozark English is spoken in a parallelogram-shaped area that includes the Ozark plateaus, Boston Mountains, Arkansas River Valley, and Ouachita Mountains. It includes a portion of northern Arkansas, southern Missouri, southeast Kansas, and southeast Oklahoma and seems to be bounded roughly by the Arkansas, Grand, Missouri, and Black rivers. Again, differences have been noted in communities; however, this area is generally considered the area where Ozark English is spoken.

Appalachian and Ozark English are closely related and share many similarities. It appears, historically, that these two dialects may have descended from a single dialect that was developing in southern Appalachia in the late 1800s and early 1900s. However, as migration to the Ozark area occurred, the dialect developed independently since the 1900s into what is now termed *Ozark English*.

Many phonological and grammatical variations are present in these dialects relative to Standard American English. Table 8.1 provides a summary of

Table 8.1 Differences Noted Between Appalachian English and Ozark English

Feature	Appalachian English	Ozark English
Epenthesis within clusters: Those with [s] + stop are followed by [ɪz].	"across the <u>desks</u>" [dɛskɪz] Relatively infrequent, more common with plurals	"it <u>lasts</u> for three days" [læstɪz] Relatively infrequent
Intrusive [t]: Items ending with [s]; sometimes [f], have a [t] added.	"<u>once</u> a day" [wʌnsət] More extensive in Appalachian English	"<u>twice</u> a month" [twasət]
Fricative stopping: Preceding nasals, voiced fricatives could be stopped. This is particularly prevalent with [z] and can occur with [ð] and [z] as well.	"<u>isn't</u> he?" [ɪdnt] Found in both dialects	They <u>wasn't</u> raising nothing" [wʌdnt] Found in both dialects
Initial [w] reduction: In unstressed position in the sentence, [w] could be deleted.	"a good <u>one</u>" [ən] Fairly prevalent	"<u>they was</u> there" [ðe'əz] Fairly prevalent
Initial unstressed syllables: Initial unstressed syllables are deleted.	"I don't <u>remember</u>" [mɛmbɚ] Prevalent	"<u>between</u> the two" [twin] Prevalent
[h] addition can occur on "it" and "ain't."	"I said I <u>ain't</u> a gonna do that" [haɪnt] Occurs to some extent	"<u>it</u> was bigger" [hɪt] Occurs to some extent
r-lessness (postvocalic "car," intraword vocalic "carry," and following [θ], especially preceding a rounded vowel—for example, "throw").	Following [θ], [ɹ] absence "<u>throw</u>" [θo] Quite prevalent	Following [θ], [ɹ] absence "<u>throwed</u>" [θod] Quite prevalent; other forms present but to a limited degree

(Continued)

Table 8.1 Differences Noted Between Appalachian English and Ozark English *(Continued)*

Feature	Appalachian English	Ozark English
Loss of [l] preceding labial consonants.	"wolf" [wʊf]	"help" [hɛp]
Words with final [oʊ], a vocalic "r" possibly + schwa [ə] replace the [oʊ].	"yellow" [jɛlɚ] More common in Appalachian English	"tomato" [təmetɚə] Occurs
Final unstressed schwa is raised to high front vowel.	"soda" [soʊdi] Occurs	"extra" [ɛkstri] Occurs
"ire" collapse: The sequence "ire" (which is usually two syllables) is reduced to one syllable without the diphthong.	"fire" [fɑr] Stable in Appalachian English	"iron" [ɑrn] Similar to Appalachian English
Lowering of [ɛɚ]: Mid-vowel is lowered so that "bear" sounds similar to "bar."	"bear" [baɚ] Mostly in older speakers, more common in Appalachian English	"there" [ðaɚ] Occurs in older speakers

Source: Adapted from Christian, D., Wolfram, W., & Nube, N. (1988).

▶ **Video Example 8.2**
Listen to the first 2 to 3 minutes of Appalachian English in this video. Which features do you hear that are comparable to Ozark English?
https://www.youtube.com/watch?v=03iwAY4KlIU

phonological features that vary in respect to the two dialects. It is based on the findings of Christian, Wolfram, and Nube (1988).

The data in Table 8.2 include the geographical areas where specific dialects can be heard. Certain phonological changes are associated with each dialect. However, they are not mutually exclusive but rather demonstrate considerable overlap of several features.

Refer to Table 8.3 for some of the productional overlap in the regional dialects as well as those in African-American Vernacular English.

Table 8.2 Regional Dialects with Notable Changes in Pronunciation

Dialect	Geographical Areas
New York	Metropolitan New York
New England	Upper Maine, the Narragansett Bay region, and metropolitan Boston
Southern	Coastal plains from Virginia to eastern Texas, including most of North Carolina, South Carolina, Georgia, Alabama, Mississippi, and Louisiana
Ozark English	Parts of northern Arkansas, southern Missouri, southeast Kansas, and southeast Oklahoma
Appalachian English	Areas of Kentucky, Tennessee, Virginia, North Carolina, and all of West Virginia (urban centers of West Virginia excluded)

Sources: Data from Carver, C. M. (1987) and Christian, D., Wolfram, W., & Nube, N. (1988).

Table 8.3 Specific Phonological Features of Regional and Cultural Dialects

Phonological Feature	Example	Dialects
Changes in r-Sounds		
Loss of r-coloring on central vowels	*bird* = [bɜd] *father* = [fɑðə]	New York, New England, Southern, African-American Vernacular English
Neutralization of [ɹ] in postvocalic clusters	*farm* = [fɑm]	New York, New England, Southern, possibly Ozark English

Phonological Feature	Example	Dialects
Neutralization of [ɹ] in an intervocalic word position	*Carol* = [kɛəl]	African-American Vernacular English, possibly Ozark English
Neutralization of [ɹ] after a consonant	*throw* = [θoʊ]	Appalachian, Ozark, African-American Vernacular English
Changes in Individual Consonants		
Initial [w] reduction	*will* = [ɪl]	Appalachian, Ozark English
Substitution of t/θ and d/ð initiating a word	*that* = [dæt] *think* = [tɪŋk]	African-American Vernacular English
Substitution of f/θ and v/ð intervocalic and in final word position	*bathtub* = [bæftʌb] *mouth* = [maʊf]	African-American Vernacular English
Aspirated vowels initiating a word, sounds like an [h] sound	*it* = [hɪt]	Appalachian, Ozark English
Intrusive [t]	*cliff* = [klɪft]	Appalachian English, can occur in Ozark English
Devoicing of final [b], [d], and [g]	*lid* = [lɪt]	African-American Vernacular English
Changes in Consonant Clusters		
Epenthesis	*ghosts* = [gostəs]	Appalachian, Ozark English
Metathesis	*ask* = [æks]	African-American Vernacular English
Word-final reduction of consonant cluster (especially prominent if one of the consonants is an alveolar)	*test* = [tɛs]	African-American Vernacular English
Deletion of [l] in word-final consonant clusters	*help* = [hɛp]	African-American Vernacular English, also noted in Appalachian and Ozark English before labial consonants
Deletion of word-final consonants with nasalization of preceding vowels	*man* = [mæ̃]	African-American Vernacular English

Sources: Data from Christian, D., Wolfram, W., & Nube, N. (1988); Fasold, R., & Wolfram, W. (1975); Seymour, H., & Miller-Jones, D. (1981), and Wolfram, W. (1994).

Other important variables of dialect have also been recognized in the study of General American English. Among these are ethnicity, race, and cultural dimensions. The next section examines these aspects as they relate to phonological variations in the United States.

Ethnicity, Race, and Culture

Often, the terms *race, culture*, and *ethnicity* are used interchangeably in professional literature and informal conversations. However, there are distinctions between each of these terms. **Race** is a biological label that is defined in terms of observable physical features (such as skin color, hair type and color, and head shape and size) and biological characteristics (such as genetic composition). **Culture** is a way of life developed by a group of individuals to meet psychosocial needs. It consists of values, norms, beliefs, attitudes, behavioral styles, and traditions. **Ethnicity** refers to commonalities such as religion, nationality, and region. Although race is a biological distinction, it can take on ethnic meaning if members of a biological group have evolved specific ways of living as a subculture.

Several types of relationships could exist between ethnicity and language variation. For ethnic groups that maintain a language other than English, language transfer is possible. **Transfer** indicates incorporating language features into a non-native language based on the occurrence of similar features in the native language. In some Hispanic communities in the Southwest, the use of "no" as a generalized tag question ("You go to the movies a lot, no?") could be attributable to the transfer from Spanish, as could phonological features such as the merger of /ʃ/ and /tʃ/ (*shoe* sounds like *chew*), the devoicing of /z/ to /s/ (*lazy* becomes [leɪsi]), and the merger of /i/ and /ɪ/ (*pit* and *peat* sound similar or *rip* and *reap* are pronounced with the same vowel quality).

If one looks through the publications of ethnic dialects, it appears that African-American Vernacular English is one of the most publicized dialects. The next section examines some of the general and phonological characteristics of this dialect.

African-American Vernacular English

Sometimes called *Black English* or *African-American English*, African-American Vernacular English is a systematic, rule-governed dialect spoken by many but not all African American people in the United States. Although it shares many commonalities with Standard American English and Southern English, certain differences distinguish this dialect. These differences affect the phonological, morphological, syntactical, semantic, and pragmatic systems. This section addresses only the phonological variations.

Not all African Americans use African-American Vernacular English, and among those who do, the degree of use differs significantly. Several variables influence the use of this dialect: age, gender, and socioeconomic status being the most noted. Relative to age, evidence suggests that the use of this dialect decreases as the individual ages. Elementary school children use a type of dialect that varies the most from mainstream language, whereas dialect features that appear prominently in adolescence level off in adulthood (Washington, 1998).

Gender differences in the use of African-American Vernacular English have also been reported. Males often exhibit increased use of vernacular, nonstandard forms relative to females. This increase in use in the male population possibly represents differential socialization along gender lines. More positive values of masculinity are associated with more frequent use of vernacular forms, whereas women, particularly middle-class women, use standard forms more frequently (Labov et al., 1972).

Socioeconomic status also seems to contribute to differences in the use of this dialect. Lower- and working-class African Americans reportedly use this dialect more frequently than do middle- or upper-middle-class African Americans. This distinction could also reflect differences in educational background. Terrell and Terrell (1993) suggest that there is a continuum of dialect use from those who do not use the dialect at all to those who use it in almost all communicative contexts. This continuum is significantly influenced by social status variables. African Americans from middle- and upper-middle-class backgrounds appear to be more adept at **code switching,** changing back and forth between African-American Vernacular English and Standard American English, than their lower- and working-class counterparts.

A comparison of the documented phonological features of African-American Vernacular English to other dialects in the United States notes four types of phonological distinctions. First are those features that can occur in all dialects of General

American English but are either more frequent in African-American Vernacular English or appear in a wider range of communicative contexts. The first four items in Table 8.4 belong in this category. Second, some phonological variations are common to African-American Vernacular English and other nonstandard vernacular dialects, but these features are not present in formal or informal standard dialects. Items 5 to 8 in Table 8.4 represent these features. Third, some of the phonological features represent those noted in the phonology of the South. Often these distinctions (items 9 to 12 in Table 8.4) are features of older speakers of southern phonology, and they are rapidly disappearing in present-day speech. Others (items 13 to 17 in Table 8.4) do not or only rarely appear in earlier records of African-American Vernacular English or southern dialect but emerged during the last quarter of the nineteenth century and are expanding rapidly in the speech of both dialects. The final set of features (items 18 to 24 in Table 8.4) seems to be distinctive of African-American Vernacular English.

Table 8.4 Frequently Cited Features of African-American Vernacular English

Feature	Example
Features in Most Dialects of General American English That Appear to Be Most Prevalent in African-American Vernacular English	
1. Final consonant cluster reduction	*first girl* → firs' girl
Loss of second consonant	*cold* → col; *hand* → han
2. Unstressed syllable deletion	*about* → bout
Initial and medial syllables	*government* → gov'ment
3. Deletion of reduplicated syllable	*Mississippi* → miss'ippi
4. Vowelization of postvocalic [l]	*bell* → [bɛə]; *pool* → [puə]
Features in Vernacular Dialects of American English but Not in Standard Dialects	
5. Loss of "r" after consonants and after [θ] and in unstressed syllables	*throw* → [θoʊ] *professor* → [pəfɛsə]
6. Labialization of interdental fricatives	*bath* → [bæf]; *teeth* → [tif]
7. Syllable-initial fricatives replaced by stops	*those* → [doʊz]; *think* → [tɪŋk]
Especially with voiced fricatives	*these* → [diz]
8. Voiceless interdental fricatives replaced by stops	*with* → [wɪt]
Especially when close to nasals	*tenth* → [tɪnt]
Features in Old-Fashioned Southern Dialects	
9. Metathesis of final [s] + stop	*ask* → [æks]; *grasp* → [gɹæps]
10. Loss of r-coloring of stressed central vowel [ɝ]	*bird* → [bɜd]; *word* → [wɜd]
11. Loss of r-coloring of centering diphthongs with [ɚ]	*four* → [foə]; *farm* → [fɑəm]
12. Loss of r-coloring of unstressed central vowel [ɚ]	*father* → [fɑðə]; *never* → [nɛvə]

(Continued)

Table 8.4 Frequently Cited Features of African-American Vernacular English *(Continued)*

Feature	Example
Features Recently Evolving in Southern and African-American Vernacular English Dialects	
13. Reduction of diphthong [aɪ] to [ɑ] before voiced obstruents and in the final syllable position	*tied* → [tɑd]; *lie* → [lɑ]
14. Offglide centering in [ɔɪ] to [ɔə]	*oil* → [ɔəl]; *boil* → [bɔəl]
15. Merger of [ɛ] and [ɪ] before nasals	*pen* → [pɪn]; *Wednesday* → [wɪnzdi]
16. Merger of tense and lax vowels before [l]	*bale* and *bell* → [bɛl]
([i] → [ɪ]; [e] → [ɛ])	*feel* and *fill* → [fɪl]
17. Fricatives become stops before nasals	*isn't* → [ɪdn̩]; *wasn't* → [wʌdn̩]
Features Apparently Restricted to African-American Vernacular English	
18. Stress of initial syllables, shifting the stress from the second syllable	*police* → [ˈpoʊ.lis]; *Detroit* → [ˈdi.tɹɔət]
19. Deletion of final nasal consonant but nasalization of preceding vowel	*man* → [mæ̃]; *thumb* → [θʌ̃]
20. Final consonant deletion (especially affects nasals)	*five* → [fɑː]; *fine* → [fɑː]
21. Final stop devoicing (without shortening preceding consonant)	*bad* → [bæːt]; *dog* → [dɔːk]
22. Coarticulated glottal stop with devoiced final stop	*bad* → [bæːtʔ]; *dog* → [dɔːkʔ]
23. Loss of [j] after specific consonants (loss of palatalization in specific contexts)	*computer* → [kɑmputə]; *Houston* [hustn̩]
24. Substitution of [k] for [t] in [str] clusters	*street* → [skɹit]; *stream* → [skɹim]

Sources: Data from Stockman, I. (1996a) and Wolfram, W. (1994).

Clinical Application

African-American Vernacular English: More Than Phonological Changes

Although several phonological features of African-American Vernacular English have been introduced in this section, semantic, morphological, syntactic, and pragmatic variations are also a part of this dialect (refer to, e.g., Van Keulen, Weddington, & DeBose, 1998, or Terrell & Terrell, 1993). Children could use these dialect features during language assessment; therefore, it is important that clinicians be aware of these variations. The following is a summary of African-American Vernacular English features noted in the grammatical structure of preschool-age children (e.g., Washington & Craig, 1994).

Morphological and Syntactic Form[1]	Examples
Zero Copula or Auxiliary	
Is, are, and modal auxiliaries *will, can*, and *do* not consistently used	"the bridge out" "how you do this"
Subject-Verb Agreement	
Use of a subject and verb that differ in either number or person	"what do this mean"

Morphological and Syntactic Form[1]	Examples
Fitna/Sposeta/Bouta	
Abbreviated forms for "fixing to," "supposed to," and "about to"	*fitna*: "she fitna a backward flip"
Ain't	
Use as a negative auxiliary	"why she ain't comin?"
Undifferentiated Pronoun Case	
Interchange of nominative, objective, and demonstrative cases of pronouns	"him did and him"
Multiple Negation	
Two or more negative markers in one utterance	"I don't got no brothers"
Zero Possessive	
Possession coded by word order that deletes the possessive *-s* marker or uses the nominative or objective case of pronouns rather than the possessive	"he hit the man car" "kids just goin' to walk to they school"

[1] Other morphological and syntactic variations were noted, but the previously noted forms were used by at least one-third of the children in the Washington and Craig (1994) study.

Video Example 8.3

Listen to the first 2½ minutes of this video, which features African-American Vernacular English spoken in North Carolina. Note the variations in phonology, morphosyntax, and semantics of the various individuals. Which of the previously presented phonological features do you hear?

https://www.youtube.com/watch?v=RTt07IVDeww

ASHA's Position on Dialects

It is the position of the American Speech-Language-Hearing Association (ASHA, 2003) that no dialectal variety of American English is a disorder or a pathological form of speech or language. Each dialect is acceptable as a functional and effective variety of American English. Each serves a communicative as well as a social-solidarity function. Each dialect maintains the communication network and the social construct of the community of speakers who use it. Furthermore, each is a symbolic language representation of the geographic, historical, social, and cultural background of its speakers.

A speaker of any language or dialect may exhibit a language disorder unrelated to his or her use of the native dialect. An essential step toward making accurate assessments of communication disorders is to distinguish between those aspects of linguistic variation that represent regular patterns in the speaker's dialect and those that represent true disorders in speech and language.

The speech-language pathologist must have certain competencies in order to distinguish between dialectal differences and communicative disorders. These competencies include the following:

1. Recognizing that all American English dialects are rule-governed linguistic systems
2. Realizing the rules and linguistic features of the American English dialects represented by their clientele
3. Using nondiscriminatory testing and dynamic assessment procedures, such as identifying potential sources of test bias, administering and scoring

standardized tests in alternate ways, using observation and nontraditional interview and language sampling techniques, and analyzing test results in light of existing information regarding dialect use.

IMPLICATIONS FOR APPRAISAL.   For the individual who primarily is speaking a dialect, several issues need to be considered during the assessment process. The most important factor is determining which phonological characteristics constitute dialectal differences. The noted variations in pronunciation, when contrasted to Informal Standard English, could be dialectal differences, rather than signs of a disordered phonological system.

WHAT TO DO?

1. Be sensitive to local dialect patterns and to any regional or cultural dialects that could affect the client's speech. Make an unbiased assessment of an individual's phonology to account for the norms of the particular dialect. In other words, are these phonological variations also represented in individuals with whom this client interacts? In addition, in a society in which the mobility level is high, expect certain regional dialects to appear outside their associated geographical areas.

2. Make a list of assessment instruments that account for dialectal variations, or consider dialect features when scoring any standardized measure. Some articulation tests—the Goldman-Fristoe (Goldman & Fristoe, 2015), for example—have guidelines for scoring certain dialect features. However, some instruments do not. A clinician's knowledge of dialect features (refer to Table 8.3) is helpful in scoring these measures.

3. Evaluate not only the presence of specific dialect features but also their frequency. Research results indicate that a judgment of disordered versus different phonological systems is often influenced by the relative frequency rather than just the categorical presence or absence of certain patterns (Bauman-Waengler, 1993a, 1993b, 1994b, 1995, 1996; Kercher & Bauman-Waengler, 1992; Seymour, Green, & Hundley, 1991; Stockman, 1996b; Wolfram, 1994).

4. Assess a client's communicative effectiveness in the regional or cultural dialect. If the dialect is unfamiliar, ask other professionals or members of the community about the client's communication skills. The client's teachers are often a good source of information.

Clinical Exercises The following is a partial list of words from the Arizona Articulation Proficiency Scale, 4th edition (Fudala & Stegall, 2017):

horse	baby	bathtub	pig	cup	nine	train
monkey	comb	cake	wagon	dog	table	red

Based on the features that are distinctive to African-American Vernacular English (see Table 8.4), describe what dialect variations you might hear in these word productions if you were assessing a child who is speaking African-American Vernacular English.

The Speaker of English as a Second Language

Factors to Consider in the Phonological Development of Children Learning English as a Second Language

There is an increasing number of English language learners within the United States. Within less than 20 years, it is estimated that 40% of the entire school-age population will be English language learners. Certain areas of the United States have already exceeded these estimates. For example, in California, 60% to 70% of school-age children are not native speakers of English (Roseberry-McKibbon & Brice, 2010). In addition, the number of children in the United States who speak a language other than English at home has more than doubled since 1980. It is estimated that 21% of children ages 5 to 17 do not speak English in their home environment (National Center for Children in Poverty, 2010). With these statistics in mind, it is important that we understand the differences in speech development that occur in children who are attempting to learn English as a second language.

First, within the developmental process, there may be **interference** or **transfer** from the children's first language (L1) to English (L2) (Roseberry-McKibbon, 2007). Thus, children may make an error in English because of the direct influence of their first language. This may affect phonological development in several ways. The most direct influence is the phonological inventory. Therefore, if a phoneme does not exist in the first language, children may substitute another phoneme that is somewhat comparable. Both vowels and consonants are typically affected because of the differences in the phonemic systems between L1 and L2. For example, in the Vietnamese phonological system, the [ɪ] and [ʊ] vowels do not exist; however, [i] and [u] are present. Therefore, children may substitute [i] for [ɪ], saying [hit] for "hit" or [u] for [ʊ], as in [luk] for "look." Consonantal inventories are also transferred. Staying with the Vietnamese language, certain dialects do not have "th"-sounds, but [s] and [z] are present. The child learning English may transfer [s] and [z] to English, replacing [θ] and [ð]. Examples of resulting substitutions are "those," which becomes [zoz], and "think," which is pronounced as [sɪŋk].

Not only do the differences between the phonological inventories of L1 and L2 transfer or interfere, but the phonotactic differences will be noticeable within the developmental process. To review, *phonotactics* refers to the arrangement of sounds within a given language; examples include which consonants can be arranged to form consonant clusters and the number and type of consonants that can begin and end a syllable. In Spanish, the [v] at the end of a word is devoiced and transfers to English as [f]—for example, [lʌf] for "love." There are no consonant clusters in Vietnamese or Cantonese (Cheng, 1994; Ruhlen, 1976), and no word-final consonants in Hmong (Matisoff, 1991; Mortensen, 2004). These phonotactic differences may all transfer from L1 to L2. The lack of consonant clusters may affect morphology as well. For example, the plural -s production and the consonant clusters formed by past tense "ed," as in "walked" or "listened," may present difficulties for the learner of English. Of course, syntax, semantics, and pragmatics may also be influenced by the transfer or interference of L1 to L2.

In addition, specific rhythmic patterns (stress, intonation, and duration) exist in a child's first learned language. If these transfer to English, the overall speech pattern may somehow sound different and be more difficult to understand. For a more complete account of the phonology of several languages, refer to later sections of this chapter. The phonological inventories, phonotactic possibilities, and rhythmical differences are provided for several languages.

Although not directly related to the phonological development, many English language learners have been noted to experience a **silent period**. The child may be very quiet, speaking very little as she or he focuses on understanding the new language. Within the classroom, this may be interpreted as the child being extremely "shy" or possibly that the child is not able to meet the demands. The younger a child is, the longer the silent period may last. Older children may stay in this silent period for a few weeks or months, whereas preschool-age children may be relatively silent for a year or more. Again, this is a normal phenomenon and a portion of the developmental process (Roseberry-McKibbon & Brice, 2010).

Clinical Exercises A first-grader, Jessica, is very quiet both in the classroom and in speech-language therapy. Her teacher thinks she is extremely shy. She will often shake her head, which is interpreted as "she doesn't know the answer." She is learning English as a second language; her first language is Spanish. You hypothesize that she might be going through a silent period.

What could you do to help the teacher understand this developmental process?

What could you do as a clinician in speech-language therapy to aid in this transition, remembering that Jessica is trying to understand English as best as she can?

In addition, **code switching** or **code mixing** may occur. In this developmental process, speakers alternate between L1 and L2. This may occur within a phrase or between sentences (Pence Turnbull & Justice, 2017). Zentella (1997) gives the following examples of code switching between Spanish and English: "It's already full, mira" ("It's already full, look") and "Because yo lo dije" ("Because I said it").

As a portion of this developmental process, English language learners may demonstrate a phenomenon referred to as *language loss*. As these children become more proficient in English, they lose skills and fluency in their native language if that language is not reinforced and maintained. This is called *subtractive bilingualism* and can be very detrimental to the children's learning of the native language and family life (Roseberry-McKibbon & Brice, 2010). This may cause difficulties within the family if the parents only speak L1 and no English. As noted earlier, more than 20% of young children do not speak English in their home environment. Clinicians should be sensitive to these issues and reassure the families that this is a normal developmental process. From personal experience, families often voice the opinion that it is harmful to the children to be learning two languages. Families accept the fact that the children's first learned language is not as proficient as before and therefore do not reinforce that language. Bilingualism has many advantages for children both cognitively and linguistically. In our world, which is becoming more and more international, bilingualism is a valuable resource. Families should be encouraged to nurture their children's native language so that loss of L1 does not occur.

Limited English Proficient Students

The term **limited English proficient** is used for any individual between the ages of 3 and 21 who is enrolled or preparing to enroll in an elementary or secondary school, who was not born in the United States, or whose native language is other than English. This term also applies to Native Americans or Alaska Natives and those who come from an environment in which a language other than English has had a significant impact on them. The difficulties in speaking, writing, or understanding the English language compromise the individual's ability to successfully achieve in classrooms where the language of instruction is English or to participate fully in society (PL 107-110, The No Child Left Behind Act [Title III] of 2001). Title III funds are provided to ensure that limited English proficient students (LEPS), including immigrant children and youth, develop English proficiency and meet the same academic content and achievement standards that other children are expected to meet.

The number of immigrants to the United States has increased, averaging more than 1 million a year between 2001 and 2016 (U.S. Department of Commerce, 2017). These individuals come from an array of countries and backgrounds and bring a wealth of different languages to the United States. One way to examine the types and numbers of non-English language backgrounds of a limited English proficient student is by reviewing the statistics contained in the following works:

U.S. Department of Education, Office of English Language Acquisition, Language Enhancement, and Academic Achievement for Limited English Proficient Students (2013), *The Biennial Evaluation Report to Congress on the Implementation of the Title III State Formula Grant Program for School Years 2008–2012*

U.S. Census Bureau (2016), *American Community Survey (ACS), Table B05006, Place of Birth for the Foreign-Born Population*

Migration Policy Institute (2016), State immigration data profiles: Migration Policy Institute tabulations of the U.S. Bureau of the Census' American Community Survey (ACS) and Decennial Census

According to the Migration Policy Institute (2016), more than 460 languages are spoken by limited English proficient students nationwide. The data submitted indicate that Spanish is the native language of the great majority of these students (65.8%), followed by Chinese (6.0%), Vietnamese (3.2%), Korean (2.5%), and Tagalog (2.0%). Languages with more than 10,000 speakers include Hmong, Arabic, Armenian, Chuukese, French, Haitian Creole, Hindi, Japanese, Khmer, Lao, Mandarin, Marshallese, Navajo, Polish, Portuguese, Punjabi, Russian, Serbo-Croatian, and Urdu. It is interesting to note that the total number of LEPS has increased from more than 4 million in 2002 to more than 25 million in 2013.

Spanish is the dominant language among limited English proficient students in 46 states. Tagalog represents the majority of limited English proficient students in Alaska and Hawaii, French is the predominant language of those in Maine, and German is found in North Dakota. Refer to Table 8.5 for the three top languages spoken by limited English proficient students by state (2016 statistics).

The following sections contrast the vowel, consonant, and suprasegmental systems of Spanish, Vietnamese, Korean, Chinese (subdialect Cantonese), Tagalog (Filipino), Hmong, and Arabic to the phonological system of General American English. This contrast is provided as a possible way to predict which features might be difficult for individuals whose native language is one of those listed and who are learning English as a second language. Although other factors play a role in second language acquisition, it appears that a primary cause of difficulty is transfer or interference between the native language and General American English (Yeni-Komshian, Flege, & Liu, 2000).

Table 8.5 Top Three Languages Spoken by Limited English Proficient Students (LEPS) by U.S. State

State	Number of LEPS	1st Language	2nd Language	3rd Language
Alabama	99,600	Spanish	Chinese	Korean
Alaska	32,300	Other Native American Language	Tagalog	Spanish
Arizona	564,700	Spanish	Navajo	Chinese
Arkansas	86,200	Spanish	Vietnamese	Other Pacific Island Language
California	6,763,600	Spanish	Chinese	Vietnamese
Colorado	305,600	Spanish	Vietnamese	Chinese
Connecticut	280,400	Spanish	Portuguese	Polish
Delaware	38,800	Spanish	Chinese	French Creole
District of Columbia	33,200	Spanish	African Languages	French
Florida	2,124,200	Spanish	French Creole	Vietnamese
Georgia	528,300	Spanish	Vietnamese	Korean
Hawaii	172,100	Other Pacific Island Language	Japanese	Chinese
Idaho	61,400	Spanish	Chinese	Other Indic Languages
Illinois	1,116,300	Spanish	Polish	Chinese
Indiana	194,000	Spanish	Chinese	German
Iowa	88,500	Spanish	Vietnamese	Serbo-Croatian
Kansas	114,700	Spanish	Chinese	Vietnamese
Kentucky	83,800	Spanish	Vietnamese	Chinese
Louisiana	121,000	Spanish	French	Vietnamese
Maine	19,500	French	Spanish	African Languages
Maryland	349,000	Spanish	Chinese	Korean
Massachusetts	560,800	Spanish	Portuguese	Korean
Michigan	303,900	Spanish	Arabic	Chinese
Minnesota	211,500	Spanish	African Languages	Hmong
Mississippi	35,800	Spanish	Vietnamese	Chinese
Missouri	119,100	Spanish	Chinese	Vietnamese
Montana	6,400	Spanish	German	Chinese
Nebraska	82,300	Spanish	Vietnamese	African Languages
Nevada	303,800	Spanish	Tagalog	Chinese

State	Number of LEPS	1st Language	2nd Language	3rd Language
New Hampshire	31,200	Spanish	French	Chinese
New Jersey	1,003,400	Spanish	Chinese	Korean
New Mexico	190,600	Spanish	Navajo	Other Native American Language
New York	2,485,400	Spanish	Chinese	Russian
North Carolina	442,000	Spanish	Vietnamese	Chinese
North Dakota	10,500	Spanish	German	African Languages
Ohio	264,400	Spanish	Chinese	German
Oklahoma	142,900	Spanish	Vietnamese	Chinese
Oregon	219,400	Spanish	Vietnamese	Chinese
Pennsylvania	490,100	Spanish	Chinese	Vietnamese
Rhode Island	76,500	Spanish	Portuguese	Chinese
South Carolina	124,700	Spanish	Chinese	Vietnamese
South Dakota	14,600	Spanish	African Languages	German
Tennessee	162,100	Spanish	Arabic	Vietnamese
Texas	3,434,500	Spanish	Vietnamese	Chinese
Utah	126,000	Spanish	Chinese	Vietnamese
Vermont	7,800	French	Spanish	Chinese
Virginia	414,100	Spanish	Korean	Vietnamese
Washington	488,800	Spanish	Chinese	Vietnamese
West Virginia	13,500	Spanish	Chinese	French
Wisconsin	172,300	Spanish	Hmong	Chinese
Wyoming	9,600	Spanish	not given	not given
U.S. Total	25,148,900	Spanish	Vietnamese	

Speech Sound and Selected Prosodic Characteristics of Spanish, Vietnamese, Cantonese, Korean, Filipino, Hmong, and Arabic American English

Spanish American English

Many dialects and language variations of Spanish fall under this one large categorization. Immigrants in the United States who speak Spanish seem to come from (1) Mexico, (2) Central and South America, (3) Puerto Rico, (4) Cuba, (5) the Dominican Republic, and (6) other countries not specifically identified in the 2016 U.S. Census (U.S. Census Bureau, 2016). Refer to Figure 8.2 for an estimate of the distribution of Spanish speakers in the United States according to this census. There seem to be two broad categorizations of Spanish: Hispanic and Latino. According to the Census Bureau, Hispanic and Latino are ethnic, not racial, categories. They include individuals who classified themselves in one of the specific Spanish, Hispanic, or Latino categories ("Mexican, Mexican American, Chicano," "Puerto Rican," or "Cuban") listed on the Census 2000 questionnaire as well as those who indicated that they are "other Spanish/Hispanic/Latino." For the purpose at hand, the author will use the term *Spanish* to include both Hispanic and Latino Spanish speakers.

This discussion first examines some basic qualities of the vowel and consonant system of Spanish and then attempts to note differences that might occur in the various dialects of Spanish, such as Puerto Rican and Nicaraguan.

Spanish has five vowels: [i], [e], [u], [o], and [a]. It has no central vowels with or without r-coloring. In addition, all Spanish vowels are long and tense. Thus, for the Spanish student of English, the contrasts between *beat* and *bit, pool* and *pull, boat* and *bought*, and *cat, cot*, and *cut* are difficult. In addition, the [e] and [o] vowels are monophthongs in Spanish. So, although they are easily recognizable, they sound somewhat different. There is some comparability between the diphthongs of Spanish and English: [aɪ], [aʊ], and [ɔɪ]. However, the gliding action between onglide and offglide in Spanish for each of these vowels is quicker and reaches a higher, more distinct articulatory position than those of General American English (González, 1988).

Spanish consonants show many similarities. The voiced and voiceless stop-plosives are present; however, [t] and [d] are articulated as dentals in Spanish, as opposed to the alveolar production of [t] and [d] in General American English. For the Spanish productions, the tip of the tongue is against the edges of the inner surfaces of the upper front teeth. The production is symbolized as [t̪] and [d̪]. Other shared consonants include [j, w, f, m, l, s, tʃ, and n]; [θ] could occur in some dialects but not in others. The consonants [v, z, h, ð, ʃ, ʤ, ʒ, ŋ] are present in General American English but not in Spanish. Although [ŋ] and [ð] are allophones of other phonemes, they do not form minimal pairs in Spanish. In addition, the letter *r* is pronounced differently in Spanish. Spanish has two *r* phonemes: [ɾ] and [r̄]. The [ɾ], which was introduced in Chapter 3, is a flap, tap, or one-tap trill that is an allophonic variation of [t] or [d] in General American English when they are produced between two vowels. For example, in casual conversation, the word "ladder" or "better" can be pronounced [læɾɚ] or [bɛɾɚ]. The second symbol, [r̄], is an alveolar trill (which, according to the International Phonetic Association Chart [2015], is transcribed [r]; however, to eliminate confusion, it is symbolized here as [r̄]) in which the apex of the tongue flutters rapidly against the alveolar ridge with either two or three vibrations. Therefore, the transference of the Spanish "r" to English produces a somewhat qualitatively different "r" sound. Refer to Table 8.6 for a comparison of the vowel and consonant sounds in General American English to those in Spanish. Based on the inventory and phonotactics of Spanish, Box 8.1 represents possible difficulties a Spanish speaker may have when learning General American English.

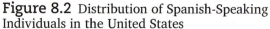

Figure 8.2 Distribution of Spanish-Speaking Individuals in the United States

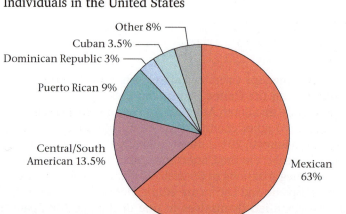

Other 8%

Cuban 3.5%

Dominican Republic 3%

Puerto Rican 9%

Central/South American 13.5%

Mexican 63%

Table 8.6 Phonological Inventory: A Comparison of Spanish to General American English (GAE)

Spanish Vowels	Vowel Differences: Spanish and GAE
[i, e, u, o, a]	• [ɪ, ɛ, æ, ʊ, ʌ, ə, ɝ, ɚ] are not present in Spanish. • Spanish speaker could substitute similar vowels in GAE (e.g., *could* → [kud]). • Spanish speaker could substitute [eɾ̄] for [ɝ], *bird* → [beɾ̄d].
Spanish Consonants	**Consonant Differences: Spanish and GAE**
[p, t, k, b, d, g]	• Because voiceless stops are unaspirated in Spanish, speaker could produce GAE voiceless stops as unaspirated. • In GAE, [t] and [d] are alveolar production; they are dentalized in Spanish.
[f, x, ɣ, s, β] ([x] is a voiceless velar fricative, [ɣ,] is a voiced velar fricative, and [β] is a voiced bilabial fricative)	• The GAE [v, z, ð, θ, ʃ, ʒ] are not present in Spanish.
[tʃ]	• The GAE [dʒ] is not present in Spanish, variable production of [tʃ].
[w, j, l, ɾ, ɾ̄]	• The production of "r" in GAE may be replaced by the [ɾ̄], which is a trilled vibrant production in Spanish.
[m, n, ɲ]	• The GAE [n] is an alveolar production, whereas the [n] in Spanish is a dentalized production. • The GAE production of [ŋ] is not present in Spanish; the [ɲ], which is present in Spanish, is a palatalized nasal.

Shared consonant blends: [pl, pɹ, bl, bɹ, tɹ, dɹ, kl, kɹ, gl, gɹ, fl, and fɹ]. Consonant blends not in Spanish [st, sp, sk, sm, sl, sn, sw, tw, kw, skɹ, spl, spɹ, stɹ, and skw].

Sources: Data from Goldstein (2007), Perez, E. (1994), and Ruhlen, M. (1976).

Box 8.1

Possible Difficulties for Spanish Speakers of American English

According to Goldstein (2007) and Perez (1994), the following vowel, consonant, consonant cluster, syllable structure, and stress difficulties might be problematic for the Spanish speaker learning General American English.

Vowels

Not in Spanish Inventory: [ɪ, ɛ, æ, ʊ, ʌ, ə, ɝ, ɚ]
Leads to:

1. Use of the Spanish [a] vowel for the General American English (GAE) [ʌ] in stressed syllables, thus [dag] for *dug*
2. Tensing of [ɛ] to [e] in GAE, especially preceding nasals, thus [frend] for *friend*
3. Inconsistent realizations of GAE [i] – [ɪ], [e] – [ɛ], [ɛ], [æ], and [u] – [ʊ] oppositions, thus, *sick* could be pronounced [sik]

(Continued)

Consonants

Not in Spanish Inventory: [v, z, ð, θ, ʃ, ʒ, ʤ]
Leads to:

1. Variable production of [ʧ] and [ʃ] in Spanish, thus [tʃoʊ] for *show* and [ʃɛk] for *check* in GAE
2. Possible devoicing of [z] to [s]
3. Devoicing of [v], especially in word-final position, thus [hæf] for *have* or [v] may be realized as [β] (a voiced bilabial fricative) or [b], especially between two vowels, thus [aβan] for *oven*
4. [t] and [d] produced as substitutions for [θ] and [ð]
5. [j] for [ʤ] in word-initial position, thus [jas] for *just*
6. Devoicing of [ʤ] between two vowels and in word-final positions, thus [tineɪtʃɚ] for *teenager* and [læŋwɪtʃ] for *language*
7. Velarization of the GAE [h] to the Spanish [x] (a voiceless velar fricative), thus [xi] for *he*
8. Trilling of the "r" in GAE, which could result in [ɾ] or [r̄] for *r*, thus [əɾaʊnd] or [ər̄aʊnd] for *around*
9. Intrusive [h] in GAE, thus [hændhɪt] for *and it*

Consonant Clusters

Not in Spanish Inventory: [st, sp, sk, sm, sl, sn, sw, tw, kw, skɹ, spl, spɹ, stɹ, skw]
Leads to:

1. Spanish does not allow *s-* in any blend in the initial position; this may become a phonotactic constraint. Spanish speakers learning English may try to maintain that phonological aspect of Spanish (e.g., *snake* becomes *esnake*).
2. Reduction of consonant clusters in GAE in word-final position, thus *gour* for *gourd* or *bar* for *bark*

Syllable Structure and Stress Problems

1. Deletion of intervocalic flaps and occasionally other consonants in GAE, thus [lɪl] for *little*, resulting in syllable reduction
2. Unstressed syllable deletion in GAE, such as [sɛpt] for *accept*
3. Shift of major stress on noun compounds from the first word to the second word in GAE, thus, *mini ˈskirt* instead of *ˈmini-skirt*
4. Shift of major stress on verb particles from the second word to the first word in GAE; for example, *ˈshow up* instead of *show ˈup*
5. Shift of stress on specific GAE words, such as *ˈac cept* for *ac ˈcept*

Sources: Data from Goldstein, B. A. (2007) and Perez, E. (1994).

CUBAN AMERICAN ENGLISH.   Cuban Americans are considered the oldest population of immigrants in the United States. Today, most of them live in New York, New Jersey, California, and Florida. Cuban American Spanish is categorized as a variety of Caribbean Spanish, which includes the three Antilles islands as well as the coastal areas of Mexico, Panama, Colombia, and Venezuela (Otheguy, Garcia, & Roca, 2000).

Clinical Application

Phonological Changes—Cuban American Spanish

According to Hidalgo (1987), the following phonological features are problematic for speakers of Cuban American Spanish.

1. In word-final position, [s] is deleted in Cuban Spanish. This could lead to deletion of the final [s] if a transfer is made between Cuban Spanish and General American English (GAE). Thus, "goose" possibly becomes [gu].
2. The consonants [l] and [r̄] are frequently interchanged before consonants and in word-final position in Cuban Spanish. This could lead to inconsistent realizations of [l] and [ɹ] in GAE.
3. Deletion of intervocalic and word-final [d]-production in Cuban Spanish could lead to a similar deletion pattern for [d] in GAE. Thus, "ladder" could be pronounced as "la-er."
4. The [r̄] in Cuban Spanish can be pronounced like [h] or as a uvular approximate. This could affect the quality of the r-productions in GAE.
5. In Cuban Spanish the labiodental [v] is used as a variant of [b], particularly in words spelled with *v*. This could positively affect the production of GAE, as the previously noted [b] for [v] substitution, often seen in Spanish speakers, would not be present.

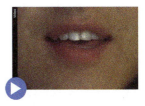

Video Tool Exercise 8.1
Spanish American Speaker
Complete the activity based on this video.

PUERTO RICAN AMERICAN ENGLISH.   Before the invasion of Puerto Rico by the United States in 1898, the island had belonged to Spain for approximately 400 years (Zentella, 2000). Since then, Puerto Rico has experienced intense Americanization. New York presently has the largest population of Puerto Ricans, although a considerable number also live in Massachusetts, Florida, and Pennsylvania (Zentella, 2000). The use of Spanish and English varies according to the situation; however, generation also plays an important role. For example, parents who grew up in Puerto Rico speaking Spanish and moved to the United States tend to use Spanish at home with their children, whereas their children speak both English and Spanish.

Clinical Application

Phonological Changes—Puerto Rican Spanish

Zentella (2000) noted the following pronunciation problems in General American English (GAE) for native Puerto Rican Spanish speakers:

1. The use of [s] for [z] and [tʃ], especially before [i] and [e] in Puerto Rican Spanish, could lead to pronunciation differences such as [sip] for *cheap* or [sen] for *chain*.
2. The consonants [l] and [r̄] are frequently interchanged before consonants and in word-final position in Puerto Rican Spanish. Inconsistent realizations of [l] and [ɹ] could result in GAE.
3. The Spanish [r̄] could be pronounced as a uvular approximant in the middle of words and in the word-initial position. This could affect the quality of r-productions in GAE.

NICARAGUAN AMERICAN ENGLISH.   Most of the immigration from Nicaragua to the United States took place during the Somoza regime in the mid-1970s as a result of the uprising of the Sandinista group (Lipski, 2000). Nicaraguan populations are primarily concentrated in New York City, Los Angeles, New Orleans, and Miami. In the Nicaraguan population, a group of individuals speaks one of two indigenous languages from this area: Miskito or Caribbean Creole English. Because of their English language skills, this second group of Nicaraguans was able to integrate almost immediately into the U.S. job market (Lipski, 2000). Nicaraguan Spanish shares many similarities with the other noted phonemic variations of Spanish speakers in the United States.

Clinical Application

Phonological Changes—Nicaraguan Spanish

According to Lipski (2000), the following phonological features of Nicaraguan Spanish could influence pronunciation of General American English (GAE):

1. Weak production of the intervocalic [j] occurs in Nicaraguan Spanish. In GAE words such as *yoyo* and *oh yes*, the [j] sound could be affected and could be perceived as a sound deletion.
2. Due to the velarization of word-final [n] to [nˠ] or [ŋ] in Nicaraguan Spanish, an inconsistent distinction between [n] and [ŋ] at the end of words in GAE could occur; thus, *sun* could be produced as *sung*.
3. The Nicaraguan Spanish [r̄] may be pronounced as a velar approximant in the middle of words and in the word-initial position. This could affect the quality of r-productions in GAE.

Vietnamese American English

With the end of the Vietnam War in 1975 and the subsequent rule of Vietnam by a communist government, an influx of immigrants came from Indochina to the United States in search of political asylum. Vietnamese is part of the Viet-Muong grouping of the Mon-Khmer branch of the Austroasiatic language family. This family also includes Khmer, which is spoken in Cambodia, and Munda languages spoken in northeastern India and parts of southern China. Vietnamese is a tone language; the variations in tones signify different meanings, and tones have phonemic value. Three dialects of Vietnamese are mutually intelligible: North Vietnamese (Hanoi dialect), Central Vietnamese (Hué dialect), and Southern Vietnamese (Saigon dialect). The tones in each of these dialects vary slightly, although the Hué dialect is more markedly different from the others. Refer to Table 8.7 for a summary of the vowels and consonants of Vietnamese (Hanoi dialect) according to Cheng (1994), Hwa-Froelich (2007), and Tang and Barlow (2006). Box 8.2 notes difficulties for Vietnamese speakers learning General American English.

Table 8.7 Phonological Inventory: A Comparison of Vietnamese to General American English (GAE)

Vietnamese Vowels	Vowel Differences: Vietnamese and GAE
[i, u, e, ɛ, o, ɔ, a, ɯ, ɤ] ([ɯ] is a high-back vowel without lip rounding; [ɤ] is a mid-back vowel without lip rounding)	• [ɪ, ʊ, ɝ, ɚ] and most diphthongs do not exist in Vietnamese; [ie], [ɯɤ], and [uo] are diphthongs in the Southern dialect. • Vowels that do not exist in Vietnamese speakers (such as [ɪ] and [ʊ]) may lead to substitution of similar vowels in GAE (e.g., *hit* → [hit]).

Vietnamese Consonants	Consonant Differences: Vietnamese and GAE
[p, b, t̪, tʰ, ʈ, d, c, k, ʔ] ([ʈ] is a voiceless retroflex stop, whereas [c] is a voiceless palatal stop)	• The [t] consonant is dentalized, and one /t/ has aspiration in Vietnamese. These may replace the alveolar production of [t] in GAE. • There is no [g] in Vietnamese; therefore the voiceless [k], which is present in Vietnamese, may be used to replace [g] in GAE.
[f, s, z (or z̩), x, ɣ, h] ([x] is a voiceless velar fricative, [ɣ] is the voiced velar fricative, and [z̩] is a retroflex fricative)	• [z] seems to be limited to the Northern dialect speakers of Vietnamese; therefore this could create the use of the voiceless [s] in GAE. • [v, ʃ, ʒ] appear only in certain dialects of Vietnamese. Therefore, these consonants may be absent in some Vietnamese natives speaking GAE. • [ð, θ] do not exist in Vietnamese. Substitutions for these sounds, with [s] or possibly [f], may be used by the Vietnamese natives speaking GAE. • [tʃ, dʒ] appear only in certain dialects of Vietnamese. Therefore, production may be variable in GAE, another fricative being used by the Vietnamese speaker of GAE.
[j, w, l, r, ɽ] ([ɽ] is a tap/flap retroflex sound)	• Depending on the dialect, r-sounds are variable in Vietnamese. The tap/flap retroflex [ɽ] is noted in Northern and Southern dialect speakers of Vietnamese, whereas Central dialect speakers produced [r]. This could lead to qualitative differences in GAE pronunciation of "r" by the native Vietnamese speaker.
[m, n, ŋʔ, ɲ] ([ɲ] is a palatal nasal)	• Postdorsal-velar nasals exist in Vietnamese, but they are [ŋʔ] nasals combined with a glottal stop. The palatal nasal of Vietnamese could be substituted for the postdorsal-velar nasal of GAE.
Vietnamese is a tone language	• Vietnamese has no consonant blends. This will present difficulties for the Vietnamese speaker learning GAE, with its many consonant clusters. • Final consonants in Vietnamese are limited to [p, t, k, m, n, ŋ].

Box 8.2

Possible Difficulties for Vietnamese Speakers of American English

According to Cheng (1994) and Hwa-Froelich (2007), the following difficulties may be noted.

Vowels

Not in Vietnamese Inventory: [ɪ, ʊ, ɜ, ɚ] and most diphthongs

1. There are no central vowels with r-coloring in Vietnamese. This sound, especially because of its prevalence in General American English (GAE), might be problematic for Vietnamese speakers of GAE.
2. The long vowel [i] in Vietnamese could be used for the [ɪ] vowel in GAE; thus "pick" sounds like [pik]. Either [e] or [ɛ] could be used as a substitute for [æ]; thus "tap" sounds like [tep] or [tɛp].

Consonants

Not in Vietnamese Inventory: [g, ð, θ]. Only in certain dialects: [z, v, ʃ, ʒ, tʃ, dʒ]

1. [θ] and [ð] are not present in Vietnamese. There is a tendency to substitute the [t] or [s] for [θ] and the [d] or [z] for [ð].
2. The consonants [d, s, z] do not exist in word-final position in Vietnamese; therefore, [t] could be a common substitution.
3. The affricates [tʃ] and [dʒ] do not exist in certain dialects of Vietnamese and could be productionally difficult for a Vietnamese speaker of GAE.
4. Phonotactics: Vietnamese has a limited number of final consonants. The consonants [p, t, k, m, n, ŋ] are the only final consonants used by all three Vietnamese dialects. Therefore, a Vietnamese speaker might have problems realizing other consonants in the word-final position.

Consonant Clusters

Not in Vietnamese: All

1. Vietnamese has no consonant combinations. A Vietnamese speaker could either reduce the combination to a singleton production or insert a schwa sound between the blend. Thus, *stew* might become [sətu].

Syllable Structure and Prosodic Difficulties

Vietnamese is a tone language; specific tones convey phonemic meaning.

1. Vietnamese words are primarily, not exclusively, one-syllable words. The Vietnamese speaker may have problems pronouncing English words of more than one syllable, including using stressed and unstressed syllables correctly.
2. Vietnamese speakers have difficulties learning sentence stress patterns and prosody, including English intonation patterns.

Sources: Data from Cheng, L. L. (1994) and Hwa-Froelich, D. A. (2007).

Korean American English

In 1903, the first Korean immigrants arrived in Honolulu, Hawaii, then a U.S. protectorate. Today, more than 1 million Korean Americans live throughout the United States, representing one of the largest Asian American populations in the country. The largest concentration—about one-quarter of all Korean Americans—is found in the five-county area of Los Angeles, Orange, San Bernardino, Riverside, and Ventura. The next largest area of concentration is in the New York region, including New York City, northern New Jersey, and the Connecticut–Long Island area. This area contains about 16% of the entire Korean American population in the United States. The Baltimore–Washington metro area also has a large number of Korean Americans.

The Korean language belongs to the Altaic language group but contains many words of Chinese origin (Ball & Rahilly, 1999). It has 19 consonants and 8 vowels that occur distinctively long or short. Table 8.8 summarizes the vowels and consonants of Korean (Ladefoged & Maddieson, 1996; Kim & Pae, 2007; Lee, 1999;). Box 8.3 summarizes the possible vowel, consonant, syllable structure, and prosodic difficulties that could be found in the Korean speaker of General American English.

Table 8.8 Phonological Inventory: A Comparison of Korean to General American English (GAE)

Korean Vowels	Vowel Differences: Korean and GAE
[i, e, ø, ɛ, a/ɑ, ɯ, u, o, ʌ] ([ɯ] is a high-back vowel without lip rounding, and [ø] is a close-mid-vowel similar to [e] but with lip rounding)	• Korean has a set of short vowels and long vowels that, according to Lee (1999), demonstrate slightly different tongue positions. • Korean has several diphthongs that begin with [j], ([ja/jɑ, jʌ, jo, ju, jɛ]), [w] ([wa/ɑ, wʌ, wɛ, wi]), and [ɯ] ([ɯi]). • The vowels [ɪ, æ, ʊ] as well as the central vowels with r-coloring are not present in Korean.

Korean Consonants	Consonant Differences: Korean and GAE
[p, pʰ1, t, tʰ, k, kʰ, d][1]	• Voicing is context dependent in Korean; when initiating a syllable, stop-plosives are voiceless; intervocalically, they are voiced. This could cause difficulties with voiced and voiceless stop-plosives in GAE.
[s, z, h]	• [f, v, ʃ, ʒ, θ, ð] are not present in Korean, leading to substitution of another fricative in GAE.
[tʃ, tʰʃ, dʒ, dʰʒ][2] [m, n, ŋ]	• Affricates in Korean appear similar to those of GAE; however, aspiration has phonemic value in Korean and could lead to difficulties understanding specific words in GAE.
[l, ɾ, w]	• The consonants [ɹ, j] are not present in Korean. The [l] in Korean is an allophonic variation of [ɾ], which has certain similarities to [ɹ] but leads to the typical to mix up of these consonants. • The syllable structure of Korean is C, VC, or CVC. • Syllable-final sounds in Korean consist only of [p, t, k, m, n, ŋ, l]. Other final consonants may be difficult for the Korean speaking GAE. • There are no syllable-initial or final consonant clusters in Korean, although intersyllabic clusters are possible. Therefore, consonant clusters may prove problematic for the Korean speaking GAE.

[1] When initiating a word, these sounds are voiceless unaspirated or slightly aspirated, whereas intervocalically, they are voiced.
[2] Lee (1999) describes the affricate dʰʒ as containing palatal stops ([c] and [ɟ]), whereas Ladefoged and Maddieson (1996) use the symbols [tʃ, tʰʃ, dʒ, dʰʒ] noted above. Kim and Pae (2007) transcribe the affricates as [tɕ] and [tʰɕ]—that is, as stops followed by alveolar-palatal fricatives.

Box 8.3

Possible Difficulties for Korean Speakers of American English

Ha, Johnson, and Kuehn (2009) note these characteristic difficulties in Korean speakers speaking American English.

Vowels

Not in Korean Inventory: [ɪ, æ, ʊ] as well as the central vowels with r-coloring

1. The [ɪ] may be pronounced as an [i], so that *ship* sounds like *sheep*.
2. The [æ] vowel may be pronounced as [ɛ], so that *bat* sounds like *bet* or *tan* sounds like *ten*.
3. The central vowels with r-coloring may pose difficulties.

Consonants

Not in Korean Inventory: [f, v, ʃ, ʒ, θ, ð, ɹ, j]

1. Several General American English (GAE) consonant sounds do not exist in the Korean speech sound system. These include the fricatives /f/, /v/, /θ/, and /ð/. These sounds are typically produced as /p/, /b/, /t/, and /d/, respectively, and the /p/ – /f/ and /b/ – /v/ sound distinctions are very often confused.
2. Korean speakers make no distinction between /ɹ/ and /l/ because [l] is an allophonic variation of [ɾ] that may sound somewhat like an r-sound. Combined with the fact that there are no central vowels with r-coloring, this leads to problems with r-sounds and the stereotyped [ɹ] – [l] mix-up.
3. The phonetic realization of word-final stops is different in Korean; word-final stops are always unreleased—that is, produced without audible aspiration—whereas GAE stops can be either released or unreleased. This and the differences in voicing and aspiration initiating a word versus intervocalically can lead to confusion of [p] – [b], [t] – [d], and [k] – [g] pairs of words such as *cap* and *cab*.

Consonant Clusters

Not in Korean Inventory: No syllable-initial or final consonant clusters in Korean, although intersyllabic clusters are possible.

1. Consonant clusters may prove problematic for the Korean speaking GAE.

Syllable Structure and Prosodic Difficulties

1. Korean is a syllable-timed language, and Korean learners of GAE are not accustomed to the patterns of stressed and unstressed syllables in GAE words.
2. The structure of syllables in Korean and English differs. In Korean, word-final consonants are not realized unless they are followed by a vowel in the same syllable. This may cause the insertion of a vowel at the end of GAE words that end with a consonant. For example, *Mark* becomes [maku] and *college* becomes [kalədʒi]. This is a strong characteristic of the speech of Korean speakers who are beginning to learn GAE.
3. Korean learners of English have little or no experience in using GAE in communicative situations in which emphasizing and de-emphasizing words takes on a meaning in context. Korean learners of GAE tend to pronounce each word in a sentence with equal emphasis. They have difficulty producing and perceiving forms with weak stress in GAE and have problems knowing where to speed up, slow down, add stress, or de-emphasize words in their sentences for communicative effect.

Cantonese American English

Standard Chinese (known in China as Putonghua), a form of Mandarin Chinese, is the official spoken language for mainland China. However, most Chinese Americans are from the Canton province in southern China and speak Cantonese. They originally settled in California; according to the *Statistical Abstract of the United States: 2012* (U.S. Census Bureau, 2012), more than 300,000 Chinese Americans live in the San Jose–San Francisco–Oakland–Greater Los Angeles area. More than 500,000 Chinese Americans now reside in New York City.

As one of the Chinese languages, Cantonese belongs to the Sino Tibetan language family, which also includes Tibetan, Lolo Burmese, and Karen (the latter two are also spoken in Burma). The major Chinese languages are Mandarin, Wu, Min, Yue (Cantonese), and Hakka (Li & Thompson, 1987). Because Cantonese has so many dialects, the language is sometimes referred to as a group of *Cantonese dialects*, not just Cantonese. Oral communication is virtually impossible among speakers of some different Cantonese dialects. For instance, there is as much difference between the dialects of Taishan and Nanning as there is between Italian and French. According to its linguistic characteristics and geographical distribution, Cantonese can be divided into four main dialects: Yuehai (including Zhongshan, Chungshan, and Tungkuan), as represented by the Guangzhou city dialect; Siyi (Seiyap), as represented by the Taishan city (Toishan, Hoishan) dialect; Gaoyang, as represented by the Yangjiang city dialect; and Guinan, as represented by the Nanning city dialect, which is widely used in Guangxi province. If not otherwise specified, the term *Cantonese* often refers to the Guangzhou dialect, which is also spoken in Hong Kong and Macao. Refer to Table 8.9 for the vowels and consonants of this dialect. Box 8.4 lists typical problems for Cantonese speakers of General American English.

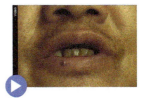

Video Example 8.4
The first section of this video features a Vietnamese American speaker, and the second section features a Korean American speaker. The Vietnamese American speaker says the following words: *cheese, watch, scratch, father, yellow,* whereas the Korean American speaker says the words: *with, thumb, letter, really, first.* They both say the following sentences: "How are you today?" "I am fine, thank you." "It is wonderful weather." "There is sunshine and not rain." "It is simply marvelous." Note the differences in their speech. Which difficulties do you hear in the speech of each speaker?

Table 8.9 Phonological Inventory: A Comparison of Cantonese (Hong Kong) to General American English (GAE)

Cantonese Vowels	Vowel Differences: Cantonese and GAE
[i, y, ɛ, œ, ɔ, u, ɐ, a] + [ɪ, ɵ, ʊ] are allophonic variations of [i, œ, u], respectively ([y] is a high-front vowel with lip rounding, [ɵ] is a central vowel with lip rounding, and [œ] is a vowel similar to [ɛ] but with lip rounding).[1] Diphthongs: [ai, ei, ɐi, ui, ɔi, au, ɐu, ou, ɵy, ɛu]	• Although there are many vowel similarities between Cantonese and GAE, [æ, ɑ, ɝ, ɚ, ʌ, ə] are not present in Cantonese. These may be difficult vowel sounds for the Cantonese speaker of GAE. • Although Cantonese has long and short vowels, they do not differ qualitatively. Therefore, long and short vowels such as [e] and [ɛ] in GAE, which do differ qualitatively, can be difficult for the Cantonese speaker of GAE. • Diphthongs of Cantonese, although not exactly the same, sound fairly close to those represented in GAE.
Cantonese Consonants	**Consonant Differences: Cantonese and GAE**
[p, pʰ,[2] t, tʰ, k, kʰ, kʷ,[3] b, d, g]	• Stop-plosives exist in Cantonese. • In Cantonese, phonemic oppositions are signaled by the presence and absence of aspiration, whereas aspiration in GAE does not have phonemic value. Cantonese speakers can have distributional difficulties with aspirated and unaspirated productions in GAE.
[f, s, h] [m, n, ŋ]	• Voiced fricatives [v, z] as well as [ʃ, ʒ, θ, ð] are not present in Cantonese; therefore, they may be difficult for the Cantonese speaker of GAE.

(Continued)

Table 8.9 Phonological Inventory: A Comparison of Cantonese (Hong Kong) to General American English (GAE) *(Continued)*

Cantonese Consonants	Consonant Differences: Cantonese and GAE
[ts, tʰs, dz, dʰz] [w, j, l]	• Affricates are somewhat different in Cantonese. There is phonemic opposition between aspirated and unaspirated [t, d] in affricate productions. In GAE, aspiration does not have phonemic value and the fricative portion of the affricate is more posteriorly articulated. • [ɹ] is not present in Cantonese but is a fairly frequent consonant in GAE.
Cantonese is a tone language	• In Cantonese, final consonants are limited to [p, t, k, m, n, ŋ]. Therefore, other final consonants may be difficult for Cantonese speakers of GAE. • Consonant clusters do not exist in Cantonese unless [kʷ] and [kʷʰ] are considered. In GAE, consonant clusters are very frequent. • Six possible syllable shapes in Cantonese are C, V, CV, VC, CVV, and CVC. There are many other possible syllable shapes in GAE. • Syllables are equally stressed, and each syllable carries a tone in Cantonese. Stressing is variable in GAE and may prove problematic for the Cantonese speaker learning GAE.

[1] There are long and short variants of many vowels and diphthongs in Cantonese. Officially, Cantonese counts 52 vowels (Cheng, 1994).
[2] The raised [ʰ] indicates that these sounds have aspirated and nonaspirated variations, which is phonemic, and therefore distinguishes meaning between words.
[3] The [kʷ] is a coarticulated consonant; because the [k] and [w] are articulated together, some refer to it as a *consonant cluster*.
Sources: Data from Lee, H. B. (1999) and To, C. K. S., Cheung, P. S. P., & McLeod, S. (2013).

Box 8.4

Possible Difficulties for Cantonese Speakers of American English

According to Chan and Lee (2000), the following difficulties are evidenced:

Vowels

Not in Cantonese Inventory: [æ, ɑ, ɝ, ɚ, ʌ, ə]

1. Long and short vowels are problematic for Cantonese speakers of General American English (GAE). Thus, word pairs with [i] – [ɪ] and [u] – [ʊ] could be difficult.
2. When [i] or [ɪ] occur at the beginning of a word, Cantonese speakers of GAE tend to add a [j] sound; thus, *east* and *yeast* could sound the same. This is a transfer from Cantonese, as the vowel [i] in word-initial position is preceded by [j].

Consonants

Not in Cantonese Inventory: [v, z, ʃ, ʒ, θ, ð, ɹ]

1. Cantonese has no voiced syllable-final plosives; therefore, GAE learners tend to substitute [p, t, k] for [b, d, g] in the word-final position. In addition, Cantonese speakers tend not to release the voiceless plosives, which is transferred to GAE. Thus, *rope* and *robe* or *mate* and *maid* are practically indistinguishable. Cantonese learners of GAE also tend to devoice plosives in syllable-initiating position.
2. Because of the absence of voiced [v] and [z], Cantonese speakers of GAE tend to substitute their voiceless counterparts, [f] and [s].

3. Because [ʃ] and [ʒ] do not exist in Cantonese, [s] is often used in GAE as a substitute for these sounds.

4. Cantonese does not have "th" sounds, and Cantonese GAE speakers often substitute [t] or [f] for [θ] ([tɪn] for *thin*) and [d] or [f] for [ð] ([fe] for *they*).

5. The affricates [tʃ] and [ʤ] do not exist; Cantonese GAE speakers tend to substitute [ts] and [dz] for [tʃ] and [ʤ], which will probably be acceptable substitutions.

6. Cantonese GAE speakers often have trouble distinguishing [l], [n], and [ɹ]. When the [ɹ] is in a word-initial position, these speakers tend to substitute an l-like sound for [ɹ]. There is also a tendency for speakers to substitute [w] for [ɹ]. In word-initial position, [n] could be substituted for [l], whereas in final position, the [l] could be deleted or a [u] sound used, rendering *wheel* as [wiu].

Consonant Clusters

Not in Cantonese Inventory: [kʷ] and [kʷʰ] could be counted as clusters; there are no other consonant clusters in Cantonese.

1. Because Cantonese contains very limited consonant clusters, Cantonese speakers of GAE tend to delete these clusters in words or insert a schwa vowel between the consonant sounds of the cluster.

Prosodic Difficulties

1. Cantonese speakers have a tendency to assign the stress randomly in a word or put equal emphasis on each syllable in a word.

2. These speakers tend to clearly articulate every word separately and put equal stress on each syllable. These fundamental differences make Chinese speakers sound staccato and monotone.

3. The intonation of Chinese speakers of GAE usually falls on the ending words; thus a question may have falling, rather than rising intonation at the end.

Filipino/Tagalog American English

Filipino has been the national language of the Philippines since 1937. It is based on Tagalog, which is a Malayo-Polynesian language. Filipino is primarily Tagalog with borrowed words from several languages, such as Old Javanese, Malay, Sanskrit, Arabic, Spanish, Chinese, and English. Foreign words that have been introduced have affected the Filipino lexicon and phonology, but the morphosyntax has stayed basically the same.

The Philippines has 171 indigenous languages; Filipino is the second language of 70% to 90% of the population. Since 1973, the Philippines has implemented a bilingual Filipino–English educational policy, and the mass media report in both Filipino and GAE. The U.S. Census Bureau's 2011 *American Community Survey* estimated the U.S. population of Filipinos at 4 million. Filipino Americans are the second largest population of Asian Americans and represent the largest population of overseas Filipinos (69% of all Filipinos who are foreign born). Significant numbers of Filipino Americans reside in California, Hawaii, Texas, Illinois, and the New York metropolitan area. Refer to Table 8.10 for the vowels and consonants of Filipino and Box 8.5 for typical problems.

Table 8.10 Phonological Inventory: A Comparison of Filipino (Tagalog) to General American English (GAE)

Filipino/Tagalog Vowels	Vowel Differences: Filipino/Tagalog and GAE
[a, e, i, o, u], all vowels short	• [ɪ, ɛ, æ, ʊ, ʌ, ə, ɝ, ɚ] are not present in Tagalog. Long vowels do not exist in Tagalog, and speakers could have difficulty with the long versus short vowel oppositions.
Diphthongs: [iw, iy/ ey, ɑy, ɑw, uy/oy]	• The diphthongs of Tagalog are close to the articulations of the diphthongs in GAE.
Filipino/Tagalog Consonants	**Consonant Differences: Filipino/Tagalog and GAE**
[p, b, t, d, t̪, d̪, k, g, ʔ]	• In Filipino all stop-plosives that occur in GAE are represented. • The glottal stop is used in Tagalog to differentiate pronunciations that have the same spelling; for example, "bata" [bata] = bathrobe, "bata" [baʔa] = child. Because the glottal stop is not a consonant of GAE, this may be perceived as an intrusive sound.
[s, ʃ, h]	• The fricatives [f, v, z, ʒ, θ, ð] do not exist in Tagalog/Filipino, but are frequent consonants in GAE.
[tʃ, dʒ]	• Affricates in Tagalog/Filipino are the same as in GAE.
[w, j, r̄]	• In Tagalog/Filipino the [ɹ] is similar to the Spanish trilled [r̄], either a flap or a trill. This may be noticeable in "r"-productions of GAE. • In Tagalog/Filipino, [d] and [ɹ] are allophones; therefore, confusion may exist between [d] and [ɹ] in GAE. • There is no [l] in Tagalog/Filipino, but this sound is fairly frequent in GAE.
[m, n, ŋ]	• In Tagalog/Filipino, [ŋg] can occur anywhere in a word, including at the beginning. However, in GAE, [ŋ] occurs only in the word- or syllable-final position. • There are no native root words in Tagalog/Filipino with initial consonant clusters. Words with initial consonant clusters are borrowed words in Tagalog/Filipino. • The most common syllable structures in Tagalog/Filipino are CV and CVC. In syllables where the vowel is in the initial position, a glottal stop acts as the onset. GAE has many more syllable shapes, and glottal stops are not used phonemically in GAE.

Sources: Data from Himmelmann, N. P. (2000) and Malabonga, V., & Marinova-Todd, S. (2007).

Box 8.5
Possible Difficulties for Filipino Speakers of American English

According to Himmelmann (2000) and Malabona and Marinova-Todd (2007), the following problems could occur:

Vowels

Not in Filipino/Tagalog Inventory: [ɪ, ɛ, æ, ʊ, ʌ, ə, ɝ, ɚ]

1. The central vowel [ʌ] does not exist in Filipino/Tagalog. Substitution of [a] for it will occur in General American English (GAE), thus [kap] for "cup." In unstressed syllables, the substitution of [a] for [ə] is probably not noticeable.
2. Inconsistent realizations of [i] – [ɪ], [e] – [ɛ]/[æ], and [u] – [ʊ]. Thus, "ten" in GAE could be pronounced [ten].

Consonants

Not in Filipino/Tagalog Inventory: [f, v, z, ʒ, θ, ð]; the r-sound is similar to the Spanish trilled "r."

1. The "r" is a tap or trill in Filipino/Tagalog and is substituted for GAE central vowels with r-coloring, [ɝ] and [ɚ], and the consonantal-r. This is productionally different but is still perceived as an "r" that is somewhat "off." In Tagalog, the [d] and [ɹ] are allophones; they could be used interchangeably. However, because both [d] and [ɹ] exist in GAE and Tagalog, this may create problems.

2. The th-sounds [ð, θ] do not exist in Tagalog. Substitutions of [d]/[z] (possibly [s] in GAE because [z] does not exist in Filipino) for [ð] and [t]/[s] for [θ] are common. Thus, "thought" becomes [tat] or [sat], and "they" becomes [de] or [ze] or possibly [se].

3. Tagalog has no [f] or [v]. Sound substitutions in GAE are typically [p] and [b]. Thus, the word "Filipino" is typically pronounced [pilopino].

Consonant Clusters

Not in Filipino/Tagalog Inventory: Initial consonant clusters exist, but they are from borrowed words.

1. Initial- and final-word consonant clusters in GAE could be reduced, or a schwa could be inserted; "stop" becomes [sap] or [tap], possibly [sətap].

Hmong American English

Many Hmong people have immigrated to the United States to escape the death and horror of a genocidal war against them. The long campaign of the Laotian and Vietnamese governments to destroy the Hmong is vengeance for Hmong support of the United States in the Vietnam War. According to the *Statistical Abstract of the United States: 2012* (U.S. Census Bureau, 2012), more than 260,000 Hmong people live in the United States and are largely concentrated in California, Wisconsin, and Minnesota. Several million Hmong people remain in China, Thailand, and Laos, speaking a variety of Hmong dialects. The Hmong language group is a monosyllabic, tonal language (7 to 12 tones, depending on the dialect). Hmong appears to have two basic dialects: Mong Leng and Hmong Der. These two dialects are mutually intelligible. In Table 8.11, the consonant and vowel inventories are based on the Mong Leng dialect as identified by Mortensen (2004); the phonology of Hmong Der can be found in Ratliff (1992). Box 8.6 summarizes the noted difficulties of Hmong speakers of GAE.

Video Example 8.5
Listen to this Filipino accent tutorial by Mikey Bustos as he explains a couple of the main difficulties noted in Filipino speakers of American English. What are some of the specific difficulties he notes?

https://www.youtube.com/watch?v=3BBtS1ir4tA

Table 8.11 Phonological Inventory: A Comparison of Mong Leng Hmong to General American English (GAE)

Hmong Vowels	Vowel Differences: Hmong and GAE
[i, ɨ, e, æ, a, u, ɔ] ([ɨ] is a rounded centralized vowel with a high tongue position; the tongue position is moved horizontally so that the maximum elevation of the tongue is mediopalatal rather than prepalatal, as it is with [i])	• In Hmong, [æ] and [a] are variants of one /a/-type vowel; they can be used interchangeably. Hmong speakers might have trouble realizing the distinctions between these two vowels in GAE.
Three nasalized vowels exist: [ĩ], [ũ], and [ã]	• The short vowels [ɪ, ɛ, ʊ, o] and the central vowels of GAE are not part of the Hmong inventory. Hmong speakers of GAE may have difficulty realizing these vowels or may substitute similar vowels.

(Continued)

Table 8.11 Phonological Inventory: A Comparison of Mong Leng Hmong to General American English (GAE) *(Continued)*

Hmong Consonants	Consonant Differences: Hmong and GAE
[p, pʰ, pˡ, pˡ, t, tʰ, t, tʰ, c, cʰ, k, kʰ, q, qʰ, ʔ, d, dʰ] (note: the superscript [ʰ] indicates aspiration, which has phonemic value in Hmong, whereas the superscript elevated [ˡ] or [ˡ] indicates lateral release of the consonant in question)	• The voiced stops [b, g] do not exist in Hmong, but they are consonants in GAE.
[ᵐb, ᵐbʰ, ᵐbˡmbˡ, ⁿd, ⁿdʰ, ⁿɖⁿɖʰ, ⁿɟⁿɟʰ, ᵑgⁿgʰ, ᴺɢᴺɢʰ] ([ɖ] is a retroflexed voiced plosive, [ɢ] a voiced uvular plosive, and [ɟ] a voiced palatal plosive)	• The voiced stops [b, d, g] are prenasalized stops, which is indicated by the [ᵐ, ⁿ, ᵑ, ⁿ, ᴺ] before the sound in question. This indicates that the nasal is produced prior to the stop. This could create qualitative difficulties in GAE, in which the stop-plosives are without nasalization.
[f, v, s, ʂ, ʐ, ç, ʝ, h][1]	• [ʂ, ʐ, ç, ʝ] are retroflexed and palatalized fricatives of Hmong that could be used as substitutions for [ʃ,ʒ]. The GAE consonants [θ, ð] do not exist in Hmong.
[ⁿdz, ⁿdz, ⁿɖ, ⁿɖʐʰ]	• All affricates are prenasalized in Hmong. This is not the case in GAE.
[l, j] [m, mˡ mɬ, n, ɲ, ŋ] Hmong is a tone language	• [ɹ] and [w] are not part of the Hmong inventory but are consonants of GAE. • Hmong has only open syllables, and there are no syllable-final consonants. Although spelling makes a word look like it has a final consonant, those consonants indicate tone, "pab" = "ball" pronounced [pɔ] + high tone. GAE has many different types of syllable shapes and has many words with syllable-final consonants.

[1] For "s," some speakers of Hmong produce an aspirated [s]. The ʝ sound is a voiceless palatal fricative that is similar (but with a narrower opening between the articulators) to a voiceless [j].
Summarized from Matisoff (1991), McCurdy (2010), and Mortenson (2004).

Box 8.6

Possible Difficulties for Hmong Speakers of American English

Matisoff (1991), McCurdy (2010), and Mortensen (2004), summarize the following difficulties.

Vowels

Not in Hmong Inventory: [ɪ, ɛ, ʊ, o, ʌ, ə, ɝ, ɚ]

1. There are no central vowels, including those with r-coloring. These sounds, especially their prevalence in General American English (GAE), might be problematic for Hmong speakers.
2. Short vowels [ɪ, ɛ, ʊ] are not present in Hmong; [i], [e], or [u] may be used as substitutions.

Consonants

Not in Hmong Inventory: [ʃ, ʒ, θ, ð, w, ɹ]

1. Voiced stop-plosives are prenasalized in Hmong. In this context, prenasalized consonants are phonetic sequences of a nasal (one with the same articulators as the voiced stop-plosive) that behave phonologically like single consonants. There is the possibility of transferring these prenasalized stop-plosive productions to GAE.

2. The voiced fricative [z] does not exist in Hmong. Hmong speakers of GAE might substitute the voiceless fricative [s] in words containing [z].

3. The consonant [w] is not in the inventory of Hmong. Hmong learners of GAE may need to learn this sound.

4. An *r*-sound is not present in Hmong. This sound, especially its prevalence in GAE, might be problematic for Hmong speakers of GAE.

5. The affricates in Hmong are prenasalized. Hmong learners of GAE might tend to substitute the prenasalized affricates for [tʃ] and [ʤ]. In addition, the lack of [ʃ] and [ʒ] in Hmong could cause problems.

6. The Hmong language has many stop-plosives with a lateral release, such as [pˡ] and [pˡʰ]. Hmong learners of GAE might substitute these for [pl], as in "play," for example.

Consonant Clusters

Not in Hmong Inventory: Hmong has no consonant clusters.

1. Consonant clusters will prove to be a challenge for Hmong speakers learning GAE.

Syllable Structure and Stress Difficulties

1. Most words are monosyllabic in Hmong. This could pose difficulties when Hmong speakers try to pronounce multisyllabic GAE words and manipulate word stress.

2. Hmong has no word-final consonants.

Arabic American English

In terms of speakers, Arabic is the largest group of the Semitic language family with 206 million speakers. Classified as a Central Semitic language, it is closely related to Hebrew and Aramaic. The Semitic languages are a collection of languages spoken by more than 300 million people across much of the Middle East, North Africa, and the Horn of Africa. Modern Standard Arabic has its historical basis in Classical Arabic, which has documented inscriptions since the sixth century. Classical Arabic has been a literary and liturgical language of Islam since the seventh century. There are several discussion points when proposing a phonological system of Standard Arabic. The following vowel and consonant categorization is based on Huthaily (2003), Newman (2002), and Thelwall and Akram Sa'Adeddin (1999). Refer to Table 8.12 for an overview of the Standard Arabic vowels and consonants. Box 8.7 notes some difficulties which may occur in Arabic speakers of GAE.

Table 8.12 Phonological Inventory: A Comparison of Arabic to General American English (GAE) based on Huthaily (2003), Newman (2002), and Thelwall and AkramSa'Adeddin (1999)

Standard Arabic Vowels	Vowel Differences: Arabic and GAE
[i, a, u]	• Arabic has three vowels, which appear in long and short variations. Tongue position for short vowels is somewhat low, resembling [ɪ] and [ʊ]. The short vowel approaches [ɑ] or [æ]. Arabic has two diphthongs: /aj/ and /aw/. Thus, several GAE vowels are not present in Arabic—for example, [ɪ, e, ɛ, æ, o, ʊ] and the central vowels with and without r-coloring.

(Continued)

Table 8.12 Phonological Inventory: A Comparison of Arabic to General American English (GAE) *(Continued)*

Standard Arabic Consonants	Consonant Differences: Arabic and GAE
[t, tˤ, d, dˤ, k, q, ʔ, ʔˤ]	• [t] is a dentalized production in Arabic; the [ˤ] indicates a pharyngealized production.[1] [b] or [g] productions are inconsistent in Arabic but are a portion of the GAE stop-plosive inventory.
[f, θ, ð, ðˤ, s, sˤ, z, ʃ, x, ɣ, ħ, h]	• [v and ʒ] are inconsistent in Arabic but are a portion of the inventory of GAE. The voiceless and voiced [x, ɣ] have also been labeled as [χ, ʁ], uvular fricatives.
[dʒ]	• The voiceless affricate [tʃ] is not a consistent realization in Arabic but is a portion of the GAE system.
[m, n]	• In Arabic, the [n] is a dentalized production, and [ŋ] is an allophonic variation of [n]. This is not the case in GAE, in which [n] and [ŋ] are two separate phonemes.
[r]	• In Arabic, this r-sound is described as an alveolar trill or as a dental tap or post-velar fricative, depending on the dialect. This is a different type of production than the "r" in GAE.
[l], [lˤ], [j, w]	• The pharyngealized /l/ is noted in Classical Arabic only in the word /alˤlˤah/. • All Arabic consonants can occur syllable-initiating, medially, and in syllable-final positions. Syllables cannot begin with vowels in Arabic. This is not the case in GAE. • Consonant clusters can occur at the beginning and end of words in Arabic. There is some restriction on the types of clusters, and final clusters in Arabic are often simplified with epenthesis—for example, [bint] becomes [binit] ("girl").

[1] *Pharyngealization* involves a secondary approximation of the back and root of the tongue into the pharyngeal area. Based on direct laryngeal observation techniques, Ladefoged and Maddieson (1996) state that there is epiglottal activity.
Sources: Data from Dyson, A. T., & Amayreh, M. M. (2007); Ladefoged, P., & Maddieson, I. (1996); Thelwall, R., & Akram Sa'Adeddin, M. (1999); and Watson, J. (2002).

Box 8.7

Possible Difficulties for Arabic Speakers of American English

The following difficulties are summarized from Altaha (1995), Kharma, and Hajjaj (1989), Power (2003), Val Barros (2003), and Watson (2002).

Consonants

Not in Arabic Inventory: [p], inconsistent productions [b, g, v, ʒ, tʃ]. The Arabic r-sound is described as an alveolar trill or as a dental tap or post-velar fricative, depending on the dialect.

1. The following consonant distinctions seem to be problematic for Arabic speakers learning GAE: /p/ – /b/, /f/ – /v/, /tʃ/ – /dʒ/ – /ʃ/. This results from the absence of these oppositions in Arabic. For example, /p/ does not exist in Arabic, and /v/ and /tʃ/ are inconsistent.

2. Although /n/ and /ŋ/ exist in Arabic, both are allophones of the same phoneme /n/. On the other hand, in GAE they are distinct phonemes. In addition, /ŋ/ never occurs at the end of a word in Arabic; therefore, Arabic speakers tend to add /k/ to the end of GAE words that end in /ŋ/. This results in pronunciations such as [duŋk] for "doing" or [sɪŋk] for "sing."

3. The GAE phonotactics of /l/ are quite different in Arabic; speakers tend to use the light /l/ in all word positions in GAE.

4. In Arabic, the /d/ is always unreleased and voiceless in word-final positions. GAE words such as "bad," "rod," and "mad" are often pronounced as "bat," "rot," and "mat."

5. Although an r-type phoneme exists in Arabic, it is pronounced as a trill. There is a strong tendency to transfer this trilled r-sound to GAE. Although this probably does not cause misinterpretations, it does contribute to the speaker's noted foreign accent.

6. Speakers from Egypt also evidence difficulties with /dʒ/ and /ð/. In modern spoken varieties of Egyptian Arabic, /dʒ/ is replaced by /ʒ/ and /ð/ by /h/.

Vowels

Not in Arabic Inventory: [ɪ, e, ɛ, æ, o, ʊ] and the central vowels with and without r-coloring

1. The central vowels with and without r-coloring do not exist in Arabic. Therefore, a variation of /a/ – /æ/ or /u/ are substituted for /ʌ/ in GAE. The Arabic r-sound could probably replace the central vowels with r-coloring, which will be qualitatively acceptable.

2. The distinctions between specific vowels such as /ɪ/, /ɛ/, and /ʊ/ are problematic for Arabic speakers. As the Arabic speaker learns GAE, the /ɪ/ may become lengthened and lowered to /e/, whereas /ɛ/ could be produced as /i/ or /æ/.

Consonant Clusters

Fewer consonant clusters

1. Arabic has far fewer consonant clusters in both word-initial and word-final positions and has no three-segment consonant clusters. In contrast to GAE, which has 78 three-segment clusters and 14 four-segment clusters occurring at the end of words, Arabic has none. GAE clusters are often pronounced with a short vowel inserted to aid in pronunciation.

Difficulties with Stress and Written–Spoken Correspondence

1. Arabic typically has a one-to-one correspondence between sounds and letters. Therefore, when given written GAE words to pronounce, Arabic speakers could be confused by the lack of sound-letter correspondence in GAE. Also, the influence of the written form can lead to several pronunciation difficulties with both vowels and consonants.

2. In Arabic, word stress is regular and predictable. Arabic speakers often have problems grasping the unpredictable nature of GAE word stress and the concept that stress can alter meaning, as in convict' (a verb) versus con'vict (a noun). Thus, word stress could be a problem for Arabic speakers learning GAE.

Cultural Competence and Implications for Appraisal

As noted in the previous sections, demographic changes in the United States have made cultural competence in service delivery increasingly important. According to ASHA (2017), *cultural competence* requires that audiologists and speech-language pathologists practice in a manner that considers the impact of cultural variables as well as language exposure and acquisition on their clients and their clients' families. It involves understanding and responding appropriately to the unique combination of cultural variables and the complete range of diversity that the professional, client, and family bring to interactions.

> Culture and cultural diversity can incorporate a variety of factors, including but not limited to age, disability, ethnicity, gender identity (encompasses gender expression), national origin (encompasses related aspects e.g., ancestry,

culture, language, dialect, citizenship, and immigration status), race, religion, sex, sexual orientation, and veteran status. Linguistic diversity can accompany cultural diversity. (ASHA, 2017)

Developing cultural competence is a dynamic process that requires ongoing self-assessment and continuous growth of one's cultural knowledge. It evolves over time, beginning with an understanding of one's own culture, continuing through interactions with individuals from various cultures, and extending through one's own lifelong learning.

Clinical approaches—such as interview style, assessment tools, and therapeutic techniques—that are appropriate for one individual may not be appropriate for another. It is important to recognize that the unique influence of an individual's cultural and linguistic background may change over time and according to circumstance (e.g., at home, within the school environment), necessitating adjustments in clinical approaches.

Guidelines

The following are some of the guidelines that can be used by the speech-language pathologist when working with children from different cultural and language backgrounds (summarized and adapted from Peña-Brooks and Hegde, 2000):

1. Understand the phonological characteristics of the child's first language and how these contrast with those of American English.
2. Obtain available information on the child's phonological development in the child's first language. Caregivers are usually aware if their child is developing comparably to other children who have a similar language background.
3. Know the patterns of interference from the child's first language.
4. If possible, choose standardized tests that have been normed on children from that particular cultural background.
5. Obtain the services of a competent interpreter who speaks the child's first language for assessment and treatment completion.
6. Use conversational speech samples, preferably involving the parents, other family members, and/or caregivers, as the primary data for analyzing the child's phonological skills.
7. Appraise the family members' position toward speech disorders, their causes, and treatment possibilities.
8. Carefully collect assessment and treatment data to support or modify the conclusions made in evaluating and beginning therapy.
9. Modify treatment procedures according to the individual child.
10. Be the child's advocate.

Summary

This chapter considered several aspects of General American English dialect and as a second language. The first section defined dialects and differentiated among what is considered Standard English (including Formal and Informal Standard English) and vernacular dialects. It gave examples of each group. The next section defined and summarized regional, ethnic, and social dialects. The dialects outlined were North, South, Midland, West, Appalachian English, and Ozark English. Specific vowel patterns were given for each regional area, and phonological variations that appear to be distinctive to Appalachian English as opposed to Ozark English were summarized. The next sections on ethnic and social dialects included definitions of *race, culture*, and *ethnicity* to provide a background for distinguishing this classification of dialects. The specific phonological characteristics that differentiate African-American Vernacular English from Informal Standard English were listed. The last section of this chapter presented detailed information about speakers of English as a second language. The term *limited English proficient student* was defined, and a discussion of the large number of different languages spoken as a first language in the United States followed. For the most prevalent languages other than English that exist in the United States (Spanish, Vietnamese, Korean, Cantonese, Filipino/Tagalog, Hmong, and Arabic), the phonemic inventories were provided, as were specific pronunciation problems that might occur for each GAE language learner speaking these languages. Cultural competence was discussed, and general guidelines for appraisal were outlined.

Case Study

According to Table 8.4 (pages 239–240), which of the following productions would be indicative of African-American Vernacular English?

house	[haʊs̺]	matches	[mætʃəs]	thumb	[tʌm]
telephone	[tɛfoʊn]	lamp	[wæmp]	finger	[fɪŋgə]
cup	[tʌp]	shovel	[ʃʌvə]	ring	[rĩ]
gum	[gʌ̃]	car	[kɑə]	jumping	[djʌmpən]
knife	[nɑɪt]	rabbit	[wæbət]	pajamas	[djæməs]
window	[wɪnoʊ]	fishing	[fɪʃĩ]	plane	[pweɪn]
wagon	[wædən]	church	[tʃɜtʃ]	blue	[bwu]
wheel	[wiə]	brush	[bwʌʃ]	bath	[bæf]
chicken	[tʃɪkə̃]	pencils	[pɪnsəz]	drum	[dwʌm]
zipper	[zɪpə]	scissors	[sɪzəz]	Santa	[sænə]
duck	[dʌ]	bathtub	[bæftʌb]	street	[skrit]
vacuum	[vækum]				

Answers: thumb (refer to item 7), telephone (item 2), finger (item 12), shovel (item 4), ring (item 19), gum (item 19), car (item 11), fishing (item 19), church (item 10), wheel (item 4), bath (item 6), chicken (item 19), pencils (item 4), zipper (item 12), scissors (item 12), duck (item 20), bathtub (item 6), street (item 24), vacuum (item 23)

Think Critically

1. Based on the data in Table 8.12, which of the words in the preceding case study might be produced differently according to Standard Arabic American English? What might be the characteristic production?

2. Select one of the phonological inventories: Spanish, Vietnamese, Korean, Cantonese, Filipino/Tagalog, Mong Leng Hmong, or Arabic (Tables 8.6 to Table 8.12). Based on these inventories, hypothesize which difficulties children speaking that language might encounter with the GAE words in the preceding case study.

 Chapter Quiz 8.1 Complete this quiz to check your understanding of chapter concepts.

Chapter 9
Therapy for Articulation Disorders

Obtaining an Accurate Production of a Speech Sound

 ## Learning Objectives

When you have finished this chapter, you should be able to:

9.1 Define the traditional motor approach, including guidelines for beginning therapy, and recognizing its applicability to both articulation and phonological disorders.

9.2 Identify the general overview of therapy progression from sensory-perceptual training to establishing sounds in isolation, nonsense syllables, words, structured phrases, and conversational speech emphasizing facilitating and coarticulatory contexts.

9.3 Summarize principles of motor learning and how these affect intervention parameters.

9.4 Differentiate between phonetic placement and sound modification principles and apply this knowledge directly to the most frequently misarticulated sounds: [s] and [z]; [ʃ] and [ʒ]; [k] and [g]; [l]; [ɹ] and the central vowels with r-coloring; [θ] and [ð]; [f] and [v]; affricates; voicing problems; and consonant clusters.

9.5 Understand the structure and dynamics when doing group therapy with the traditional motor approach.

Chapter Application: Case Study

Christine had a new client, Eric, in speech therapy. Eric was in second grade and had just gone through the Individualized Education Program (IEP) to determine his eligibility for services. He had been referred by both his kindergarten and his first-grade teachers for his conspicuous s-sound distortion, but his parents had chosen to wait, thinking that Eric would outgrow his difficulty. Language measures were within normal limits. Eric's s-distortion was conspicuous; he had a lateral s-problem (a unilateral lisp). His mouth deviated to the left side each time he pronounced the s-sound. It was noted that the left lateral edge of his tongue was not elevated, and the resulting sound gave the impression that Eric had too much saliva in his mouth. Using probes, Christine could not find any contexts in which the [s] or [z] was produced correctly or closer to a correct production. Using phonetic placement, Christine started by explaining where the tongue should be and how the edges of the tongue were elevated. After many attempts, Christine decided that she needed a new tactic. Eric was not aware of the deviation of his mouth, so using visual feedback became their first goal. Eric needed to say some sort of s-sound without distorting his mouth to the left. Next, Christine noted that Eric had difficulty elevating the lateral edges of his tongue. Therefore, the next goal became making an "s-sound" (it was clearly distorted) by raising both edges of the tongue with central airflow. It was clear that baby steps were needed to reach a standard s-production. Although Christine had at first not succeeded with her explanation and attempts, this shaping procedure seemed to be getting them closer, step by step, to a typical s-sound.

THIS chapter describes techniques that can be used to treat articulation-based errors in the speech of children and adults. As previously defined, these types of speech sound errors are caused by motor production problems or an inability to produce certain speech sounds. According to the classification noted in Chapter 7, the approach discussed in this chapter traditionally was used for children who demonstrated an articulation disorder (refer to Chapter 7, pages 211–213). However, the techniques discussed, or a portion of them, are relevant for treatment of phonological disorders. As will be noted in Chapter 10, these procedures may precede or be an integral part of various phonological treatment protocols.

This chapter emphasizes a *phonetic approach*, which has also been referred to in the literature as a *traditional motor approach* (e.g., Bernthal, Bankson, & Flipsen, 2017; Klein, 1996; Lowe, 1994; Pena-Brooks & Hegde, 2000; Van Riper, 1978). Using this approach, a clinician instructs a client in how to position the articulators to produce a speech sound that is considered to be within normal limits. Therapy progresses from one error sound to the next. In addition, tasks used to improve auditory discrimination skills (e.g., Van Riper & Emerick, 1984; Weiner, 1979; Winitz, 1989) and principles of motor learning (e.g., Hageman, 2018; Maas et al., 2008; Schmidt & Lee, 2005) have been added to aid clinicians with this process.

The goal of this chapter is to provide an information base that clinicians can use in their efforts to help their clients achieve a standard production of specific speech sounds. This foundation requires an understanding of how the sound is normally produced and knowledge of a client's specific misarticulation. In a continuing attempt to unite articulation- and phonemic-based treatment principles, the linguistic function (exemplified by sound frequency, phonotactics, and examples of minimal pairs) is provided for several of the sounds.

The sounds chosen for inclusion in this chapter represent the most frequently misarticulated sounds noted by McDonald (1964). When applicable, the voiced or voiceless cognates are also treated. Not all possible misarticulations for each individual sound are addressed. Only the most frequent misarticulations referenced in the research or that result from personal clinical experience are included. Therefore, for some sounds—[s], for example—most of the misarticulations treated are distortions. For other sounds, such as [l], most of the errors are sound substitutions.

Defining the Traditional Motor Approach

Phonetic approaches were first described in Europe around the turn of the twentieth century (Gutzmann, 1895; Kussmaul, 1885). Their first documentation in the United States is attributed to Scripture (1902), Scripture and Jackson (1919), and Ward (1923). Through the years, many authors—including Mosher (1929); Mysak (1959); Nemoy (1954); Nemoy and Davis (1937); Van Riper (1939a, 1939b); West and Ansberry (1968); West, Kennedy, and Carr (1937); and Winitz (1969); and Young and Hawk (1955); to mention just a few—have added to and modified the early methods. Van Riper's (1939b) *Speech Correction* is often cited as the text that popularized these techniques, which clinicians have used for decades.

Any contemporary view of treatment needs to stress what is new. Thus, non-contemporary roots might cause clinicians to not take traditional motor approaches seriously. In addition, after so much emphasis has been placed on analyzing our clients' phonemic systems, clinicians wonder whether a traditional phonetic approach should still be used. It should be; there is definitely a place for these methods in our contemporary understanding of speech sound disorders and their remediation. These procedures are certainly used as a part of many phonological treatment procedures. A word of caution: The sound-by-sound treatment approach should not be used for every client who demonstrates a speech sound disorder. There are far more efficient and effective therapy approaches for children with phonological disorders (refer to Chapter 10). However, there might be a time in the course of every treatment, for articulation or phonological disorders, when these principles could be used briefly to obtain a specific sound.

Phonetic or **traditional motor approaches** treat each error sound individually, one after the other. This treatment principle stands in contrast to a **multiple-sound approach**, which attempts to influence several error sounds simultaneously. Traditional motor approaches should not be used automatically with all clients who exhibit a single-sound error. A client with a single-sound error who has problems with the *function* of the sound in the language system—that is, with the underlying system that governs the use of that particular sound—is probably demonstrating a phonemic-based disorder. Omissions and substitutions of an isolated speech sound can be phonological disorders, and other therapy options could be more suitable. The question is never how many sounds are involved but whether the errors, single or multiple, are articulatory or phonological in nature. If they are articulation based, the best treatment option could be a traditional motor, phonetic approach. However, if several sounds are involved, we might want to examine phonological treatment possibilities. They might be more effective and less time consuming than going sound-by-sound through each of the child's errors.

Phonological approaches emphasize the function of sounds in a specific language system. Consequently, the internalization of phonemic rules and contrasts is the main goal of these therapies. However, if the sound is not in a child's repertoire and remains elusive, the phonetic approach could be implemented to establish the speech sound's standard articulation. This does not mean that clinicians need to go through all steps of the phonetic approach but rather that certain ideas and procedures within this approach could prove useful. Thus, one of the treatment goals could be to help a child produce the appropriate articulatory features of the speech sound. This in turn could facilitate the primary goal: increasing the child's ability to understand and use phonemic rules and contrasts with that particular sound.

Guidelines for Beginning Therapy: Articulation Disorders

Data have been gathered, and diagnostic decisions have been made. Any diagnosis should also lead directly to the selection of intervention goals and strategies. Although goals and strategies will change constantly, depending on the client and the noted difficulties, specific diagnostic information should aid in deciding where to begin with therapy. If you do decide to implement a traditional motor approach and your client has more than one sound error, the following guidelines can be used to help you determine where to begin:

Sounds Affecting Intelligibility. Certain sounds affect intelligibility more than others. One main reason is their relatively high frequency of occurrence in conversational contexts. In this chapter, for each of the frequently misarticulated sounds, a frequency of occurrence in General American English is given. Other sounds may affect intelligibility because of their conspicuous aberrant articulation. Therapeutically, high priority should be given to sounds that most affect a client's intelligibility.

Developmentally Earlier Sounds. Under comparable clinical circumstances, sounds that are acquired developmentally earlier should be considered first targets. The term *comparable clinical circumstances* means that both sounds were stimulable to the same degree and that the sounds in question seemed to have a comparable impact on the client's intelligibility.

Stimulability. Although stimulability is not an absolute predictor of which error sounds will improve in therapy and at which level therapy should begin (sound, syllable, word level), stimulability can be used as a probe to find out which sounds might be somewhat easier for a client to realize. If a client is stimulable for a particular sound, the clinician could attempt this sound in therapy for a trial period.

Correct Production of the Sound in a Specific Context. The collected data often give evidence of a typically misarticulated sound produced *accurately* within a specific word context. Such a word might appear on a standardized speech assessment or in the spontaneous speech sample. It is also suggested that test results be supplemented with additional word lists. These probes could yield such a context as well. Standard productions of a word or words containing a usually misarticulated sound verify that, under certain contextual conditions, a client is able to realize its regular articulation. These words, therefore, offer themselves as a therapeutic beginning point.

General Overview of Therapy Progression

This section outlines possibilities for sequencing therapy when working with clients who have articulation disorders. These sequences have been described by numerous authors (e.g., Secord, 1989; Van Riper, 1978; Van Riper & Emerick, 1984; Waengler & Bauman-Waengler, 1984) and have been used by clinicians for many years. Although the following sequencing is presented, clinicians find that certain training items are necessary for some clients but might prove unnecessary for others. A specific client's needs and capabilities cause changes in the sequencing of every therapy program.

Each of the treatment phases assumes that a client enters that particular stage with minimal competency and moves to the next stage when a certain level of accuracy has been achieved. The level of accuracy required before proceeding to the next stage of treatment is usually relatively high. Paul, Norbury, and Gosse (2018) note that correct usage is typically set at 80% to 90% in structured intervention contexts. Therefore, during structured activities in a therapy setting, 80% to 90% accuracy is needed before proceeding to the next stage. However, is this high level of accuracy necessary in spontaneous speech before a client is dismissed from therapy? As dismissal criteria, Lee, Koenigsknecht, and Mulhern (1975) have suggested a much lower level of accuracy in spontaneous, natural contexts. They argue that termination criteria in spontaneous contexts should be set at 50% accuracy. It appears that once children use targeted behaviors in spontaneous speech most of the time, it is probable that they will continue to progress toward more consistent usage. These percentages appear reasonable but, again, can vary according to the clinician's expectations and the client's capabilities.

The therapy progression outlined below first discusses sensory-perceptual training, which, depending on the age and capabilities of a client, may be a necessary first step in therapy. Next, the progression moves from the sound in isolation to nonsense syllables, words, structured contexts, and spontaneous speech. Correct articulation of the sound in question can be attempted in several ways: auditory stimulation or imitation; actual phonetic placement; sound modification (or called shaping); and using sounds in specific contexts, here termed facilitating contexts. Each of these methods is described. Finally, this section ends with an example of how to structure a home program as well as dismissal and re-evaluation criteria. This same general overview (from the sound in isolation to words and structured contexts) is followed for each of the most frequently misarticulated sounds.

Sensory-Perceptual Training

Figure 9.1 shows a schematic of the sensory-perceptual training that Van Riper and Emerick (1984) outlined. Few clinicians implement this type of training with this amount of depth. However, Figure 9.1 can serve as a reference for those clinicians who might think this phase is important or necessary.

As this therapy was originally outlined, sensory-perceptual or ear training was considered the first step in the treatment process. At least two factors should be considered before implementing sensory-perceptual training: the age of the client and whether specific auditory discrimination difficulties are noted for that client. Age is a factor because many of the tasks used to achieve the goals of the training are metalinguistic skills that require the child to think and talk about language, in this case speech sounds. Identifying the position of a sound in a word is a metalinguistic skill, for example. A child must first understand the concept that a "word" is made up of individual "sounds" and their relative relationship to one another. The ability to segment words into sounds begins to develop during the later preschool years. Therefore, for very young children, certain aspects of sensory-perceptual training might not be appropriate. Second, clinicians should carefully evaluate the specific auditory perceptual skills of their clients. The term *specific auditory perceptual skills* refers to clients' abilities to differentiate between their error production and the target sound. If testing reveals no difficulties with specific discrimination tasks, sensory-perceptual training may not be warranted.

The following discussion outlines the general progression of therapy from producing the sound in isolation to finally using it in spontaneous speech. Although sensory-perceptual training might not be used, it is important to remember that

Figure 9.1 Sensory-Perceptual Training Progression

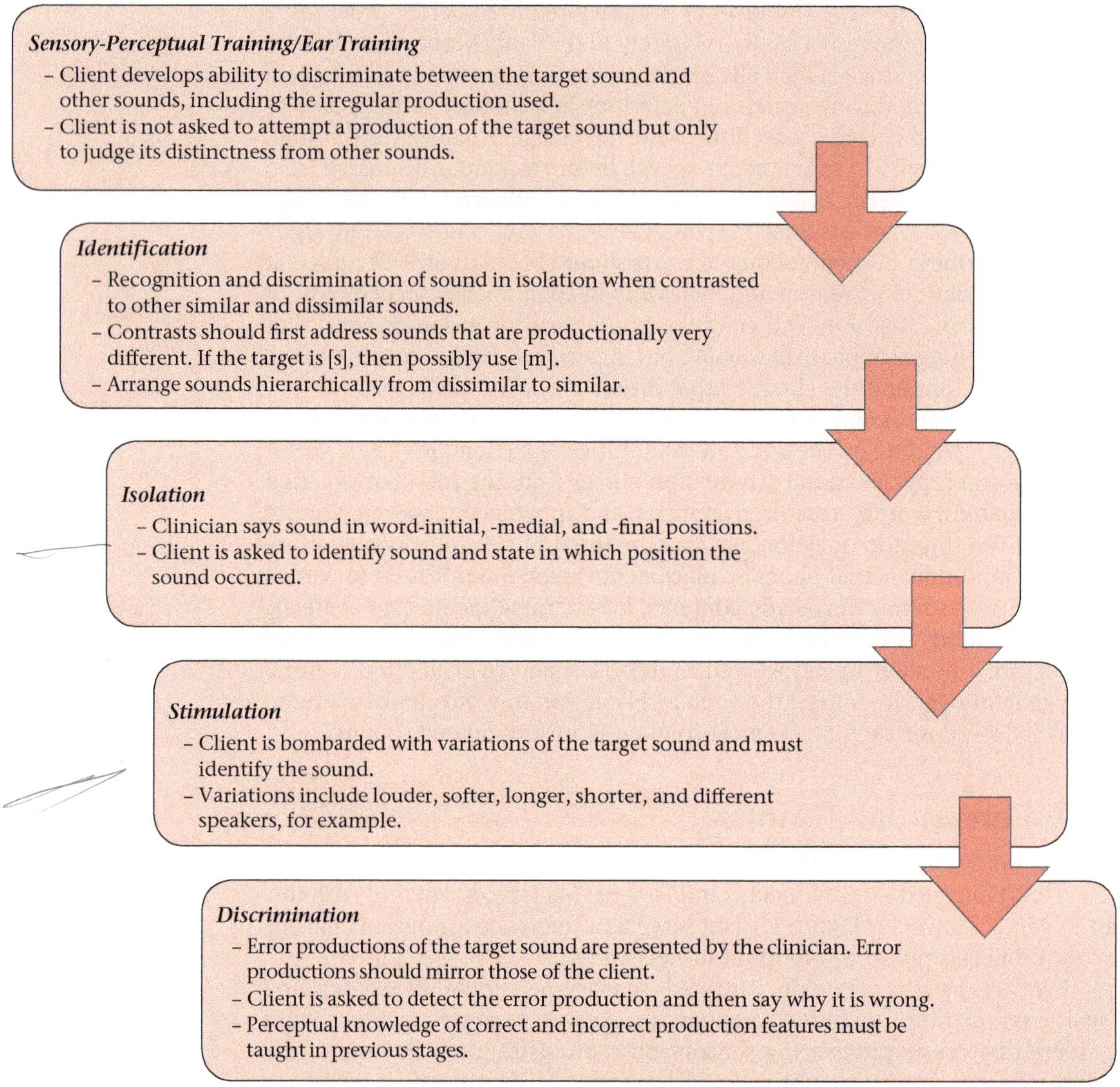

Sensory-Perceptual Training/Ear Training
- Client develops ability to discriminate between the target sound and other sounds, including the irregular production used.
- Client is not asked to attempt a production of the target sound but only to judge its distinctness from other sounds.

Identification
- Recognition and discrimination of sound in isolation when contrasted to other similar and dissimilar sounds.
- Contrasts should first address sounds that are productionally very different. If the target is [s], then possibly use [m].
- Arrange sounds hierarchically from dissimilar to similar.

Isolation
- Clinician says sound in word-initial, -medial, and -final positions.
- Client is asked to identify sound and state in which position the sound occurred.

Stimulation
- Client is bombarded with variations of the target sound and must identify the sound.
- Variations include louder, softer, longer, shorter, and different speakers, for example.

Discrimination
- Error productions of the target sound are presented by the clinician. Error productions should mirror those of the client.
- Client is asked to detect the error production and then say why it is wrong.
- Perceptual knowledge of correct and incorrect production features must be taught in previous stages.

each client must develop specific auditory perceptual abilities in the form of self-monitoring skills. Clinicians constantly need to help their clients develop discrimination of "correct" versus "incorrect" productions. This type of self-monitoring is not an optional portion of therapy.

Production of the Sound in Isolation

The goal of this phase of therapy is to elicit a standard production of the target sound alone, not in combination with other sounds. This can be achieved easily with fricatives and approximants, for example—sounds that are continuants. For stop-plosives, young children might find it easier to articulate the target sound with a central vowel—for example, [kʌ]—or with a noticeable aspiration, [kʰ].

There are several possibilities for eliciting the target sound. Beginning clinicians often think that this task can be achieved in a very short time, and this is indeed often the case. However, if standard or near-standard articulation is not obtained in a reasonable time frame (5 to 10 minutes), persisting with the procedure will probably frustrate both the client and the clinician. In this case, either the technique should be changed or other exercises should be initiated to prepare the client for the correct articulation. The clinician can break the production into stages that approximate the production. For example, if the child has a [w] for [ɹ] substitution, the clinician might first work on simply eliminating the lip rounding of the error production. Once this is achieved, the next step could be changing the high-back tongue positioning of the [w].

WHAT HAPPENS WHEN YOU CANNOT GET A NORM PRODUCTION?   It can often take several therapy sessions to achieve a "correct" production of a specific sound. Which activities can be done to aid this progress? The author offers the following suggestions from clinical experience. First, clinicians should make sure that the client can perceptually distinguish between the error sound and the misarticulations (possibly using a portion of sensory-perceptual training). If the client has a dentalized [s], contrast that to a typical production in words with [s] in various word positions and words of varying lengths and complexities. Second, examine the client's standardized speech assessment and see whether you noted any words or contexts that were closer approximations than others. For example, the word "tree" provided a context in which a correct or near-correct [ɹ] production was obtained. Use these words to determine whether similar words could aid in a norm production. Third, work on stages toward approximating the norm production. For example, have children with a [w] for [l] substitution watch their production in a mirror, noting the characteristic lip rounding on [w] and the visible tongue elevation for [l]. For the Consonant-Vowel (CV) production of "la," the tongue elevation is clearly visible if the [ɑ] is produced with more opening than is usually the case. Fourth, if the sound in question is a sound substitution—for example, a [t] for [k]—use minimal pairs to contrast the target to the substitution.

AUDITORY STIMULATION/IMITATION.   With this procedure, the clinician provides examples of the target sound and asks the client to imitate the sound. A similar procedure is implemented for stimulability testing (refer to Chapter 6). The clinician instructs the client to "watch me and do exactly what I do." If this works, it is perhaps the easiest and quickest way to achieve the target sound. Unfortunately, though, it does not always succeed.

PHONETIC PLACEMENT METHOD.   This method includes instruction by the clinician on how to position the articulators in order to produce a typical sound production. The phonetic production features of the target sound and the error production are analyzed to determine which articulatory changes need to be initiated so that an accurate production results. These methods are described in detail in the sound specific section within "The Traditional Motor Approach and the Most Frequently Misarticulated Speech Sounds."

SOUND MODIFICATION METHOD.   This method is based on deriving the target sound from a phonetically similar sound that the client can accurately produce. This sound is used as a starting point to achieve the target production. The clinician suggests specific adjustments to the articulators that should result in the target sound.

Once the client has produced the target sound acceptably in isolation, the next task is to stabilize it. This is typically achieved by having the client repeat the target sound immediately. At first, this probably needs to be carried out with careful monitoring and feedback by the clinician. When the production is more stable, the client should articulate the sound a number of times successively, with a softer or louder voice, for example, and, when possible, with different durations. This does not need to become a tedious drill for the client and clinician but rather can be achieved in activities that are fun and motivating. For example, the clinician could hide colored cards or favorite objects around the room. Every time the client finds an object, the target sound could be repeated. At first, the clinician constantly provides feedback on the acceptability of the productions, also asking the client to attempt judgments about accuracy.

Sounds in Context

USE OF FACILITATING CONTEXTS. Some clients can produce the target sound quite accurately in some word contexts but not in others. These coarticulatory context conditions seem to aid the client's production of a target sound. Supporting contexts have been called *facilitating contexts* (McDonald, 1964). Van Riper (1978) introduced the term *key words* for words in which the target sound was produced correctly.

Facilitating contexts or key words are often found in the analysis of the client's standardized speech assessment or a conversational speech sample. Additional materials that examine facilitating contexts include McDonald's (1964) deep testing and Secord's (1981a) probes of articulatory consistency. Van Riper (1978) describes how these key words can be used to move directly to the production of the target sound in isolation. In this case, the target sound is isolated by prolonging the sound in the word or by using its natural syllable structure. For example, in one case, the results of an evaluation demonstrated a d/g substitution. However, the word "finger" was found to have a correct production of [g]. The facilitating context of a velar nasal [ŋ] aided the client in producing a velar stop. To take advantage of this situation for the purpose of producing an isolated [g], the client first says *fin-ger*, separating the word between [ŋ] and [g]. The *-ger* is then reduced to [gʌ].

Clinical Exercises Tyler, age 4 years 3 months, can say "blue" with an accurate [l] but says [bwɪŋk] for "blink." Based on Tyler's success with "blue," can you suggest two or three words that might be attempted to facilitate [bl]?

The Goldman-Fristoe Test of Articulation noted that Braydon, age 6 years 4 months, could produce the word "tree" with an acceptable r-sound. All other words with [ɹ] were in error. Based on this context, could you suggest other words that could be practiced to promote a correct [ɹ]?

Facilitating contexts can also be used to begin therapy at the word level. For example, if a small core of words with an acceptable production of the target sound is found, these words can be used to stabilize the production. As Van Riper (1978) pointed out, key words can be used as a model for the client. The clinician should then point out differences between the articulation of these key words and aberrant target sound productions in other words. When the client can feel and hear the target sound, a transition to other words should be attempted. For this transition, it is important that the clinician understand the facilitating contexts in which the sound occurs. For example, is the target sound always preceded or followed by certain vowels or consonants? Are the key words one- or two-syllable words? Does the target sound occur in a stressed or unstressed syllable? If the clinician can predict the facilitating context, words with similar coarticulatory conditions can be added.

Facilitative contexts can be very effective in therapy. If appropriate words can be found, it is relatively easy to isolate the sound in question, which is an excellent start for the isolation phase of production. If the use of meaningful words in a given situation is especially important, facilitative contexts can also be used for work at the word level. As always, the final clinical choice depends on an individual client's circumstances and capabilities.

NONSENSE SYLLABLES. The goal of this therapy phase is to maintain accuracy in producing the target consonant when it is embedded in varying vowel contexts. The therapeutic efficacy of this phase can be greatly increased by ordering the nonsense syllables from those that are easiest for the client to produce to those that are more difficult. The typical sequencing is target sound + vowel (CV), vowel + target sound (VC), and vowel + target sound + vowel (VCV). However, this sequence could change based on the difficulty an individual client demonstrates with each type of nonsense syllable. Vowels can be arranged in a hierarchy from those that provide favorable coarticulatory conditions to those that do not. Suitable vowel sequences are suggested for each of the misarticulations noted in the section titled "The Traditional Motor Approach and the Most Frequently Misarticulated Speech Sounds." However, the individual client's articulatory ease and production accuracy ultimately determine the sequencing of vowels.

Many clinicians skip the nonsense syllable phase of treatment and move directly to the target sound produced in words. One reason is that words are more meaningful and interesting to clients than is drill work with nonsense syllables. However, work with nonsense syllables does not need to be a tedious exercise. Coming up with motivating and enjoyable activities that incorporate nonsense syllables requires only clinical imagination. In addition, although words are more meaningful to children than nonsense syllables, the word material should always be evaluated carefully. Some of the small "articulation cards" with black-and-white line drawings depicting words, for example, are not easily recognizable to the clinician or the client. Such material stretches the concept of meaningfulness. Finally, and probably most importantly, some clients need work with nonsense syllables before they can produce words with any acceptable level of accuracy. If the client produces less than 50% accuracy in two to three practice sessions, the word level is probably still too difficult. The clinician could then work with nonsense syllables or use consonant–vowel words such as *see, sow,* and *saw* until the production has stabilized. In addition, working with nonsense syllables eliminates the interference of the "old" error with the "new" production of the target sound that is inherent in meaningful word material. Years of practice with the old aberrant articulation of the target sound often override the new articulation, especially in familiar words. For example, a child might be quite able to produce the nonsense syllable [ki] accurately in the context of other nonsense syllables. However, when attempting the word "key," the child might suddenly revert back to the "old" substitution and produce [ti].

WORDS. The goal of this therapy phase is to maintain productional accuracy of the target sound in the context of words. A large variation exists in this category, from one-syllable CV structures to multisyllabic words in which the target sound appears several times, often in consonant clusters. Organizing words from relatively easy to more difficult to produce can prove helpful. This should be done in a systematic manner using the articulatory complexity of the word as a guideline. Several factors affect the articulatory complexity of words. These include the length of the word, the target sound's position in the word, the word's syllable structure, where the syllable stress occurs relative to the target sound, coarticulatory factors within the word, and the client's familiarity with the word (refer to Chapter 2, page 42). To summarize, words with fewer syllables, initial-word position, open syllables, and stressed syllables typically are easier to produce.

Coarticulation Factors or Contextual Use. Certain words might be easier to articulate than others because of the influence of neighboring sounds. This relates not only to preceding and following vowels but also to the neighboring consonants in the word. Knowledge of the vowel and consonant articulations can aid in developing a list of words ordered from relatively easy to produce to more difficult. However, the final decision as to ease and difficulty of production depends on the client. Clinicians could find that certain words are "too difficult"—that is, the target sound is consistently misarticulated in that word. These words should then be attempted later, when the regular articulation of the target sound is more stabilized.

Coarticulatory factors also include the number of times the target sound appears in a word and whether it appears as a singleton or as a part of a consonant cluster. Words that contain the target sound only once are normally easier to articulate than those that contain the target sound more than once. Thus, for [k], *cape* is easier than *cake*. Also, words that contain the target sound as a singleton are typically, although not necessarily, easier than those that contain the target sound as a portion of a consonant cluster. Thus, *ray* is usually easier to produce than *tray*.

Familiarity. Familiar words are usually articulated more accurately than unfamiliar words (Secord, 1989). Therefore, clinicians should begin with words that a client knows well or that are high-frequency words. With some clients, however, familiar words might also be more difficult. The impact of years of practicing the misarticulation of a familiar word in a multitude of settings can prove difficult to overcome. These words might need to be targeted later when the client's production and self-monitoring skills have improved.

STRUCTURED CONTEXTS—PHRASES AND SENTENCES. The goal of this therapy phase is to maintain the production accuracy of the target sound as words are placed into short phrases and sentences. However, at this point, phrases and sentences should not yet be spontaneous but rather be structured and elicited. If spontaneous sentences are used, the client could choose words containing combinations with the target sound that are still too difficult. This presupposes that clinicians begin work at this phase while continuing the work at the word level. This is a logical supposition because clinicians typically select a core set of words that can be accurately produced and then put these words into short phrases and sentences.

A *carrier phrase* with a target word at the end is one of the easiest ways to elicit a short phrase. At the beginning of this therapy phase, the carrier phrase should probably not contain any other words with the target sound. Another relatively simple way to elicit an utterance is to embed one target word in the carrier phrase, which can then be modified to create some degree of spontaneity. For example, if a child is working on [s], the carrier phrase could be "I see a ___." The clinician could prepare objects or pictures (at first without any s-sounds) that the client identifies to complete the phrase.

During this therapy phase, the clinician moves from highly structured to less structured tasks and might begin to implement target words with more syllables and consonant clusters.

SPONTANEOUS SPEECH. The goal of this phase is to maintain accuracy of production when the target sound appears spontaneously in conversation. This goal is first addressed in the therapy setting; however, the client needs to transfer this production accuracy to more and more situations outside therapy. This transfer of behavior to conversational speech in various settings is often referred to as *carryover*.

Both inside and outside the therapy setting, this therapy phase should proceed in a systematic manner. One way of accomplishing this is to vary the length of conversation time. Clinicians could start with 1 to 2 minutes of conversation, increasing the time interval as the client's accuracy increases. Initially, before the conversation begins, the client should be aware that the clinician is "listening for our sound." Later, the time interval can be extended and can include specific contexts that trigger the production of the target sound in many different words. For example, pictures containing words with the target sound could serve as the basis for conversation. Also, certain topics might lend themselves to the production of specific sounds. For example, a topic that includes racing, race cars, and race car drivers would probably trigger [ɹ] in a variety of contexts.

After a relatively high level of accuracy is achieved in the therapy setting, the next decisive step is correct production of the sound outside, in the real world. Parents and teachers can serve as valuable assistants during this phase of therapy. When working outside the therapy setting, the amount of time implemented and the specific tasks should be discussed with the assisting helper. This phase can become overwhelming to both the helper and the client if both suddenly think that the sound needs to be produced accurately all the time in every outside setting. (Refer to the following Clinical Application.)

Even when an assistant is employed, the clinician should also monitor a client's level of accuracy in situations outside the immediate therapy setting. This can be accomplished in a variety of ways. For example, to check on the accuracy of sound production outside the therapy setting, the client could bring tape recordings from home. The clinician could also drop by the client's classroom or telephone the client's home.

Dismissal and Re-evaluation Criteria

The last phase of therapy examines dismissal and re-evaluation criteria. Fifty percent accuracy during natural spontaneous speech was mentioned earlier as the criterion for dismissal. This relatively low percentage was suggested under the assumption that the client's competency would continue to increase on its own. Such a supposition needs to be checked by some type of re-evaluation process. It can be as simple as stopping by the child's classroom and listening to conversation, or it can be more structured, such as administering a standardized speech assessment or obtaining a conversational speech sample. Before dismissal, a child who has official school-based documentation for speech-language services (Individualized Family Service Plan or Individualized Education Plan) should be re-evaluated, typically with a standardized test to determine whether the child is within normal limits with those particular speech sound skills. A spontaneous speech sample is again a necessity, as is a consultation with the teacher and parents to ensure that the standard production carries over to other contexts outside the therapy room. Whichever means is employed, *re-evaluation* is a portion of the clinician's clinical responsibility. It is the only way to ensure that therapy was indeed successful and that the client has continued to generalize across situations. The ultimate therapeutic goal is correct production in natural, conversational settings. A re-evaluation is a way of documenting this.

Clinical Application

Structuring a Home Program

When structuring a home program, clinicians need to make sure that a speech assistant (caregiver, teacher, relative, etc.) is informed of several variables:

1. When? Which portion of the day should be set aside for the program?
2. How long? How many minutes should be spent on this program?
3. How often? How many times per week should this program be implemented? Should it be a daily occurrence?
4. What should be done? In detail, what should the assistant do? Does the assistant have written instructions as well as words, phrases, and topics that should be used in the home program?
5. How should accuracy be judged? How should the assistant determine which productions are acceptable and which are not?
6. What should be done if a production is considered unacceptable? How should the assistant react to an aberrant production?
7. How should the assistant motivate and reward the client? What type of reward system should be implemented so that the client stays motivated and continues to work in the home program?

One important question that clinicians need to ask is: How can I be sure that the assistant understands what is to be done? If the assistant does not understand in detail what must be accomplished, this can lead to frustration for both the client and the assistant. (The author had a caregiver assistant who, rather than implement two 5-minute sessions during the day, thought that one 30-minute session twice a week would be better. After two of these long sessions, the child refused to work at home.) Bringing the assistant into therapy can partially solve this problem. The assistant can see and hear which productions are considered accurate and which are not. After a period of observation, the clinician can have the assistant take an active role in the therapy session. The clinician can then give the assistant helpful advice to guide in making decisions about correct and incorrect productions as well as implementation of activities.

Bringing parents into the therapy session is often impractical, especially in a public school setting. If the parents cannot come to therapy, which is often the case, talk to them as their child is dropped off or picked up. The child is present, and a quick demonstration can be implemented. Also, words that a clinician is certain a client can say accurately can be jotted down in a spiral notebook. This notebook can go back and forth between the parents and the clinician. The parents should be instructed to have the child say the word, three to five times per session, possibly putting the word in a short carrier phrase that you have provided. At home, words that are not produced accurately can be crossed off the list by the parents. This method gives you a fairly simple communication link with the parents.

Katie, who was in second grade, was working on [s] in structured conversation. Katie's mother expressed her willingness to work at home with Katie.

1. When? After discussing this with the mother, quiet one-on-one time after dinner was considered the best way to begin.

2. How long? Three to five minutes was determined to be a good time frame.

3. How often? Every weekday.

4. What should be done? Written instructions were put into a small spiral notebook that the mother could transport in her purse between therapy and home. The clinician described in some detail what the topics of conversation should be. These topics had been practiced in therapy, and Katie had been able to reach a fairly high degree of success with them.

5. How should accuracy be judged? After participating in two therapy sessions, the mother knew what to listen for, and she was given written reminders in the notebook. Katie originally had a θ/s substitution. The mother was aware that [s] should have a clear, sharp quality but not sound like [θ].

6. What should be done if a production is considered unacceptable? It was decided that a small stop sign that was constructed in therapy would be used to signal any unacceptable [s]-productions. The mother would simply hold up the sign when she heard [θ]. Katie knew that when the sign went up, she should repeat the whole sentence and try to monitor her [s]-production.

7. How should the assistant motivate and reward the client? It was decided that if Katie participated for the specified minutes of therapy, she could play on the computer, uninterrupted by her two brothers, for 15 minutes. Also, at the end of each week of therapy, Katie could pick one of the movies that the family would watch on the weekend.

Clinical Exercises You are working with a child at the structured sentence level with [ʃ]. Create a simple carrier phrase with [ʃ] that you could use with picture cards. Now try to create a carrier phrase that does not contain sh-sounds that you could use with picture cards or words that begin with [ʃ].

Try to structure a home program with one of your clients. Go through the seven steps that were just outlined and see if you can make suggestions for each.

Principles of Motor Learning and Their Application to Therapy

The principles outlined in this chapter form the basis for the treatment of articulation disorders. As mentioned, this has been called the traditional motor approach. It is a motor approach because the client is instructed to move the articulators in a very specific manner so that an acceptable speech sound will result. It focuses on the motor skills involved in producing a specific target sound. Then drill work to establish this new sound moves through linguistically more complex stages. This type of therapy emphasizes motor repetition and learning a motor task. In this context, it seems appropriate to discuss the principles of motor learning. Although they are imbedded in this chapter, these principles can be used to guide any type of learning of motor tasks. Even if a child is working on minimal pairs in the context of a phonological treatment paradigm, aspects of motor learning are typically involved.

Motor learning is a set of complex processes associated with either experience or practice that leads to permanent changes in the possibilities associated with a specific motor skill (Hageman, 2018; Schmidt & Lee, 2005). We are engaged in motor learning when we learn to play baseball, and a child most certainly uses motor learning to learn a new production of a speech sound. A basic framework for motor learning includes the following: (1) *Performance during acquisition of a specific skill (a child learning to say the s-sound in a word, for example) should be measured separately from performance after the completion of acquisition* (Maas et al., 2008). This determines whether a skill has been learned. For example, if we wanted to measure whether s-sounds have been *learned* in single-syllable words, we could not use the practice words for verification. To say that Sherie scored 100% when practicing her single-syllable [s] words in therapy does not mean that outside of therapy Sherie will say all single-syllable words with 100% accuracy. This should again alert clinicians to the necessity of having probe words, words that are different from those in therapy, so we can see if learning has indeed occurred. (2) There should be a *pre-practice portion of intervention* in which the child is provided with information about the skill to be developed and taught how to produce a correct response. This includes information on what constitutes a correct response. Clinically, this means clear, age-appropriate directions with demonstrations to achieve a correct sound before practice begins. It also presupposes that the child can accurately distinguish between the error sound and a correct response. We often assume that the child can do this perceptual task, but that may not be the case. (3) A *practice phase of intervention* that incorporates conditions of practice and feedback occurs. These should be guided by research on speech and motor learning. The following discussion identifies conditions of practice followed by conditions of feedback.

Conditions of Practice

1. *Practice amount, large or small:* More learning occurs with more practice (Schmidt & Lee, 2005). Children with childhood apraxia of speech were evaluated using Dynamic Temporal and Tactile Cueing (refer to Chapter 11). During a 15-minute period, either 100 to 150 productions (high frequency) or 30 to 40 productions (moderate frequency) were obtained. Children with the higher frequency of practice showed more rapid acquisition of the targets, better performance in the session, and better generalization (Edeal & Gildersleeve-Neumann, 2011). Williams (2012), with multiple oppositions and minimal pair therapy, concluded that a minimum dose of 50 trials in a 30-minute session, 2 times per week, necessitated 30 sessions for intervention to be effective. She also suggested that this frequency be higher for children who have more severe speech sound disorders.

2. *Practice distribution, massed versus distributed:* Practice distribution is how therapy practice is distributed over time. If *x* number of sessions is distributed

with less time between sessions (e.g., three times per week), this is considered massed. If there is more time between sessions (e.g., once per week or once per month), this is distributed practice. Massed practice seems to be the best option, but clinicians are well aware of the child who has been in therapy for the entire school year and becomes bored and unmotivated. One research study that has direct implications for this chapter was conducted by Günther and Hautvast (2010). They examined more than 90 children who were being treated for [s] and [ʃ] difficulties. Those children who regularly completed home practice between sessions (increasing mass distribution) finished intervention in a much shorter time. Caruso and Strand (1999) suggest an increase in massed distribution for more severe speech sound disorders, shifting toward distributed practices as the severity decreases.

3. *Practice variability, constant versus variable:* Practice variability refers to practicing a motor skill in the same way and in the same context (constant) versus practicing the same skill with variations. In this context, *variable* can be defined as practicing a speech sound in varying linguistic contexts. By changing the vowels and the contexts in which we attempt speech sounds, we are using variable practice. Constant practice appears to be more beneficial when first acquiring a new motor skill, whereas variable practice promotes learning or permanent retention of a skill (Preston et al., 2014). Skelton (2004) has taken this a step further with *concurrent treatment* for speech sound disorders. This treatment approach uses randomized variable practice. Randomized variable practice employs various linguistic contexts from (a) word-initial singletons and clusters, (b) word-final singletons and clusters, (c) intervocalic productions in syllables, (d) words, (e) two- to four-word phrases, (f) sentences, and (g) the sound within a conversational topic. All of these variables are randomly practiced for at least 150 productions in each 30-minute session, 2 times per week. For more on concurrent treatment, refer to Skelton (2004).

4. *Practice schedule, blocked versus random:* Blocked practice refers to practicing a skill, a speech target, several times before moving on to the next target ("green" is produced 10 times, then "grow" is produced 10 times, etc.). In the context of speech therapy, random practice refers to different sequences and patterns occurring arbitrarily with no perceptible pattern. The concurrent treatment approach, described above, is an example of random practice. Research results demonstrate a mixed picture. While Skelton (2004) demonstrated progress using a random practice schedule for children with s-problems, Maas and Farinella (2012) found that for children with childhood apraxia of speech, a block approach produced better gains with half of the children they treated. It is suggested that a block practice schedule may be more advantageous at the beginning of therapy, followed by random practice, or that a combination of blocked and random practice may be beneficial (McLeod & Baker, 2017).

5. *Practice task, complex versus simple:* Simple tasks involve the child practicing a specific sound in isolation, whereas more complex tasks could refer to a sound in two- or three-consonant clusters. We typically move through treatment from simple to complex. However, the complexity approach (refer to Chapter 10) is based on selecting targets that are more complex, such as consonant clusters. It has shown to be an effective treatment method for children with phonological disorders (Gierut, 2001).

6. *Practice fraction, whole versus part:* This refers to practicing the motor skill as a whole versus breaking it into its constituent parts. When working with articulation disorders, clinicians use both whole and part practice. We may want the child to practice a whole word or, at times, divide it into its component parts. This is one method discussed in the section on consonant clusters later in this chapter. If the child is having difficulty with the cluster, one possibility is to do part practice. The word "street" is divided into [s] pause [t] pause and [ɹ] + eet.

7. *Practice accuracy, errorless versus learning with errors:* In errorless practice, errors are discouraged. This is used to strengthen accurate acquisition of a motor skill. Learning with errors practice allows the learner to refine and further define a motor skill. Be aware that different treatment methods use these two dichotomies. For example, cycles therapy (Hodson, 2007) discourages errors and places emphasis on choosing very specific targets in which the child has 100% success. On the other hand, minimal pair therapy includes a period of therapy devoted to rule learning (resolving communicative breakdown with the minimal pair).

8. *Attentional focus, external versus internal:* If we ask the child to focus on mouth movements or positioning of the tongue, we are asking the child for internal attention. If, on the other hand, the child is asked to evaluate and judge the perceptual quality of a sound (e.g., Was that a good r-sound? Did it sound like our race car sound?), external focus is being implemented. During pre-practice, internal attention is warranted. After that, as clinicians, we should rely far more on external focus. It appears that reliance on internal focus, such as mouth and tongue movements, hampers the development of unconscious automatic movements such as speech (Lisman & Sadagopan, 2013). Based on this assumption, if a clinician constantly redirects the client to what is being done with the tongue, this is actually detrimental to the end result that we want: automatic movements.

Conditions of Feedback

1. *Feedback type, knowledge of results versus knowledge of performance:* Knowledge of results gives children feedback in a correct or incorrect manner. Knowledge of performance gives feedback on why the responses were correct or incorrect. For example, telling a child, "That wasn't correct, your tongue needs to be further back for an s-sound" is knowledge of performance. Both types of feedback are used during pre-practice, but knowledge of performance should be used primarily during the practice phase of treatment. By using knowledge of performance, you are supporting children's use of their own perceptual and motor feedback.

2. *Feedback frequency, high versus low:* Feedback frequency refers to how often children receive feedback from the clinician based on their productions. Feedback on every production would be considered high, whereas feedback on 50% or fewer productions would be considered low (Maas, Butalla, & Farinella, 2012). As one might anticipate, it appears that high-frequency feedback is more advantageous at the beginning of therapy (pre-practice) and lower-frequency feedback encourages children to rely on their own feedback and self-monitoring somewhat later in the process. Salmoni, Schmidt, and Walter (1984) state that too much feedback does not give children an opportunity to develop their own feedback strategies. A balance between high and

low frequency is probably optimal, with frequency decreasing as the child's production possibilities increase.

3. *Feedback timing, immediate versus delayed:* Immediate feedback follows a response directly, whereas delayed feedback is considered to occur after approximately 3 or more seconds, depending on the situation. While the natural tendency is for clinicians to immediately respond to the child's production, it appears that a short delay is thought to be better for learning (e.g., Murray, McCabe, & Ballard, 2014). The delay encourages the child to possibly self-correct errors or allows the child time to figure out how to revise and improve the next production. If the clinician immediately bombards the child with feedback, these types of reflections by the child become impossible.

New research on motor learning is constantly emerging relative to each of the aforementioned principles. It is important that a clinician stay current on this research, as motor learning is the guiding basis of our work, especially but not only in the area of the traditional motor approach. We have seemingly ignored these principles for too long. An attempt should be made to implement them in every clinician's treatment protocols.

The Traditional Motor Approach and the Most Frequently Misarticulated Speech Sounds

The discussions that follow do not revisit the multitude of traditional motor approaches that have been suggested throughout the years but instead focus on those based on the phonetic features of the target sound in relationship to the error production. Knowledge of the correct phonetic placement and the existing differences between a typical production and the misarticulation is instrumental in facilitating these techniques. Other traditional motor approaches that might not be quite as "phonetically" oriented are referenced in numerous sources. For example, a compilation of phonetic placement, moto-kinesthetic, and sound approximation techniques can be found in Secord's *Eliciting Sounds* (Secord, 1981b).

The following sections contain both phonetic placement and sound modification techniques for s-sounds ([s] and [z]), sh-sounds ([ʃ] and [ʒ]), k-g sounds, l-sounds, r-sounds (including [ɹ] and the central vowels with r-coloring, [ɜ] and [ɚ]), th-sounds ([θ] and [ð]), f-v sounds, affricates, voicing problems (e.g., [p] for [b] substitution), and consonant clusters. The discussions should be considered a reference. They contain a considerable amount of detail that becomes necessary when a clinician is actually working with a client and encountering difficulties in achieving an accurate production. The proposed methods also offer the clinician several possibilities for establishing a standard realization for each of the previously noted sounds. To make reading this chapter less tiresome, several of these techniques have been placed in tables. The word lists with minimal pairs have been placed in Appendix 9.1 at the end of this chapter. The advice and ordering of coarticulatory contexts are based on the author's clinical experience. As noted previously, contexts that might prove advantageous for a specific sound ultimately will depend on the individual client's abilities.

Misarticulations of [s] and [z]

One of the most common speech sound errors is the aberrant production of [s] (Smit, 1993b). Most children have difficulty with [s] realizations at some point in their development. Because [s] and [z] are counted among the latest developing speech sounds, they can pose difficulties into the first school year for some children. This common difficulty can sometimes be heard in the speech of adults. Whether at the grocery store or on television, adults with irregular [s] articulations can be detected.

The productions of [s] and [z] consist of several related physiological factors that make their articulation somewhat complicated: (1) [s] and [z] are both fricatives that are physiologically complex because a rather narrow opening between the articulators must be maintained over a longer period; (2) the fricatives are also the longest sounds in duration (Bauman & Waengler, 1977; Lehiste, 1970), and production requirements necessitate not only a narrow opening between the articulators but also maintaining the right amount of expiratory airflow; (3) there is a precise balance between the articulatory effort required to create the narrow opening and the expiratory air pressure; if this balance is off, even to a small degree, it becomes perceptually noticeable; and (4) aberrant productions can easily cross phonemic boundaries. Thus, if the tongue is too far forward, [s] might sound like [θ]. The same relationship exists between [z] and [ð]. In addition, the voiceless [s] occurs frequently in words in General American English. In summary, [s] and [z] are physiologically difficult, perceptually sensitive, and produced in practically every utterance.

An interesting note: German has no th-sound. The author was surprised by the wide degree of variability that was acceptable for the [s] and [z] sounds in German children. Because there were no distinctive phonemic boundaries between s- and th-sounds, this production variability was generally accepted.

PHONETIC DESCRIPTION. Standard productions of [s] and [z] are articulated in essentially two different ways: as an apico-alveolar or a predorsal-alveolar fricative. These descriptions are somewhat burdensome but necessary for the s-sounds. In this context, *apico* refers to the tip of the tongue, whereas *predorsal* describes the front portion of the body of the tongue. These differences are delineated in Table 9.1. The apico-alveolar variation is produced with the tongue tip up, whereas the predorsal-alveolar [s] is realized with the tongue tip down behind the lower incisors. Sagittal grooving of the tongue, which directs the

Table 9.1 Production Differences: Apico-Alveolar (Tongue Tip Up) Versus Predorsal-Alveolar (Tongue Tip Down) [s] and [z]

	Phonetic Description	
	Apico-Alveolar Fricative	*Predorsal-Alveolar Fricative*
	[s] voiceless [z] voiced	[s] voiceless [z] voiced
Notable differences	Tongue tip up	Tongue tip down behind lower incisors
Articulators	Apex (tip of tongue)	Predorsal (front portion of tongue)
	Alveolar ridge	Alveolar ridge
Productional notes	Narrow opening between tongue tip and alveolar ridge	Tongue arches toward alveolar ridge, narrow opening between the front portion of the tongue and alveolar ridge
	Sagittal grooving of tongue	Sagittal grooving of tongue
	Lateral edges of tongue elevated	Lateral edges of tongue elevated

airstream toward the opening between the articulators, is essential for both types of productions. To achieve this, the lateral edges of the tongue must be elevated and touch the first molars to avoid lateral air escape. Although the tongue-tip-up articulation is probably the most common, many speakers produce the tongue-tip-down [s] and [z]. Each type of s-production has its therapeutic advantages and disadvantages, which are discussed in "Decision Making: Apico or Predorsal Placement" on page 292.

LINGUISTIC FUNCTION

Frequency of Occurrence. [s] ranks among the top five sounds in frequency of occurrence; [z] ranks 11th in the 24 consonants of General American English. The most frequent word-initial clusters include [st], [stɹ], and [sp]; the most frequent word-final clusters are [st], [ns], [nz], [ks], [ts], [ɹz], and [nts] (Dewey, 1923; Roberts, 1965).

Phonotactics. Both /s/ and /z/ can initiate and terminate a syllable. However, in spontaneous speech, the frequency of their occurrence in initial-, medial-, and final-word positions is not comparable. In the speech of first-, second-, and third-grade children, half of the [s]-sounds occurred initiating a word; the other half were divided fairly equally between medial and final positions. In contrast, more than 90% of the [z]-sounds were found in word-final position (Carterette & Jones, 1974).

Refer to Tables 9.2 and 9.3 for the more frequent consonant clusters with [s] and [z] including word examples. All consonant clusters are based on the lists provided by Blockcolsky, Frazer, and Frazer (1987).

Table 9.2 Consonant Clusters with [s]

Word Initiating		Word Terminating			
[sf]	sphere (very infrequent)	[fs]	coughs, roofs		
[sk]	school, skate	[sk]	mask, desk	[ks]	blocks, books
[sl]	sled, sleep	[ls]	false, pulse		
[sm]	small, smile				
[sn]	snow, snack	[ns]	dance, bounce		
[sp]	speed, spin	[sp]	wasp, crisp	[ps]	mops, tips
[st]	stop, stove	[st]	ghost, fast	[ts]	kites, cats
[sw]	sweet, sweater				
[skɹ]	scratch, scrub	[ɹs][1]	horse, nurse		
[skw]	square, squash	[lts]	melts, belts		
[spl]	splash, splurge	[mps]	lamps, jumps		
[spɹ]	spring, spray	[nts]	ants, presents		
[stɹ]	street, string	[ɹst][1]	first, worst	[ɹts][1]	hearts, skirts
		[sks]	desks, masks		
		[sts]	nests, tastes		

[1] These consonant clusters with [ɹ] are considered centering diphthongs (horse, nurse) or centering diphthongs with [st] (first, worst) or [ts] (hearts, skirts) clusters. They are often included in consonant cluster lists and have been included here as well.

Table 9.3 Consonant Clusters with [z]

Word Terminating			
Word- or syllable-initiating clusters with [z] do not exist in General American English.			
[bz]	ribs, tubs	[vz]	gives, waves
[dz]	adds, toads	[zd]	closed, sneezed
[gz]	bags, bugs	[ldz]	builds, folds
[lz]	bells, shells	[lvz]	wolves, elves
[mz]	teams, games	[ɹdz][1]	birds, cards
[nz]	cans, rains	[ɹlz][1]	girls, curls
[ŋz]	wings, rings	[ɹvz][1]	curves, dwarves
[ɹz][1]	bears, ears		
[ðz]	bathes, breathes		

[1] These consonant clusters contain centering diphthongs.

Morphophonemic Function. Word-final clusters ending in [s] or [z] can be used, for example, to signal (1) plurality, as in boo<u>ks</u>, goa<u>ts</u>, nes<u>ts</u>; (2) third-person singular, as in he ju<u>mps</u>, she bui<u>lds</u>; and (3) possessives, as in Mo<u>m's</u>, Da<u>d's</u>. Within phrases, contractible auxiliaries and copulas with the verb *to be* also demonstrate consonant clusters with [s] and [z]. Examples include "the ma<u>n's</u> happy" and "the ca<u>t's</u> running."

Minimal Pairs. Minimal pairs are often used to test the perceptual accuracy of the error production versus the norm production of clients. Several authors (e.g., Grunwell, 1987; Locke, 1980a, b; Winitz, 1984) have devised protocols to test these types of auditory perceptual skills. In addition, minimal pair contrast therapy (discussed in Chapter 10) uses pairs of words that differ by only a single phoneme to re-establish phonemic contrasts that have been lost. Phonemes that are frequently contrasted to /s/ and /z/ include /θ/ and /ð/, /ʃ/ and /ʒ/, and /t/ and /d/. Appendix 9.1 has examples of minimal pair words and sentences incorporating phoneme oppositions with /s/ and /z/.

INITIAL REMARKS. Several important variables must first be considered when a clinician sees a child or adult displaying an [s] problem. First, the disorder could be the result of a hearing loss, specifically a high-frequency hearing loss. Acoustically, both [s] and [z] have high-frequency components (6000 to 11,000 Hz). Because all sound productions are monitored auditorily, even a moderate loss in these frequency areas might impair the perception of intensity relationships between formant regions and therefore lead to a distorted production based on an inability to perceive these fine distinctions. This makes a hearing evaluation prior to conventional diagnostic testing indispensable. If a high-frequency hearing loss is present, a diagnostic evaluation and the subsequent therapy planning need to be organized quite differently.

Second, certain minor structural changes can affect [s] as well. This might include missing teeth in a school-age child or new dentures in an adult. Although circumstances such as these might not cause [s] problems per se, an individual's inability to compensate for such structural deviations can result in unusual production characteristics.

Third, such diagnoses as "**tongue thrust**" or "**tongue thrust swallow**" also need to be considered. The term *tongue thrust* refers to excessive anterior tongue movement during swallowing and a more anterior tongue position during rest (Christensen & Hanson, 1981). Hanson (1988) suggests that a more appropriate term would be **oral muscle pattern disorders**, as it would avoid the misconception that clients forcefully push their tongues forward. Controversy continues to surround these disorders and their impact on articulation, especially the articulation of [s] and [z]. Not everyone with a tongue thrust develops [s] problems. On the other hand, there is a higher incidence of children with [s] distortions who do demonstrate an oral muscle pattern disorder (Fletcher, Casteel, & Bradley, 1961; Hanson, 1988). Although an interdisciplinary approach is strongly urged, it is within the scope of practice of speech-language pathologists to diagnose and treat oral muscle pattern disorders (American Speech-Language-Hearing Association [ASHA], 1991). Prior to ASHA's 1991 position statement, an ad hoc committee report (ASHA, 1989) suggested, as do several clinicians (Hanson, 1988; Hanson & Barrett, 1988; Hilton, 1984), that treatment, often called *oral myofunctional therapy*, might facilitate the correction of [s] difficulties. Knowledge of the diagnostic and treatment procedures of oral muscle pattern disorders is at times necessary to complement work with [s] and [z] misarticulations. Refer to Box 9.1 for literature that refers to tongue thrust.

Box 9.1

Selected Tongue Thrust Literature

Bigenzahn, W., Fischman, L., & Mayrhofer-Krammel, U. (1992). Myofunctional therapy in patients with orofacial dysfunctions affecting speech. *Folia Phoniatrica, 44*(5), 235–242.

Cayley, A., Tindall, A., Sampson, W., & Butcher, A. (2000). Electropalatographic and cephalometric assessment of myofunctional therapy in open-bite subjects. *Australian Orthodontic Journal, 16,* 23–33.

Christensen, M., & Hanson, M. (1981). An investigation of the efficacy of oral myofunctional therapy as a precursor to articulation therapy for pre-first-grade children. *Journal of Speech and Hearing Disorders, 46,* 160–167.

Dworkin, J. P., & Culatta, R. A. (1980). Tongue strength: Its relationship to tongue thrusting, open-bite, and articulatory proficiency. *Journal of Speech and Hearing Disorders, 45,* 277–282.

Forrest, K. (2002). Are oral-motor exercises useful in the treatment of phonological/articulatory disorders? *Seminar in Speech and Language, 23,* 15–26.

Gommerman, S., & Hodge, M. (1995). Effects of oral myofunctional therapy on swallowing and sibilant production. *International Journal of Orofacial Myology, 21,* 9–22.

Hanson, M. L. (1994). Oral myofunctional disorders and articulatory patterns. In J. E. Bernthal & N. W. Bankson (Eds.), *Child phonology: Characteristics, assessment, and intervention with special populations* (pp. 29–53). New York, NY: Thieme.

Hanson, M. L., & Barrett, R. H. (1988). *Fundamentals of orofacial myology*. Springfield, IL: Charles C. Thomas.

Van Dyck, C., Dekeyser, A., Vantricht, E., Manders, E., Goeleven, A., Fieuws, S., & Willems, G. (2016). The effect of orofacial myofunctional treatment in children with anterior open bite and tongue dysfunction: A pilot study. *European Journal of Orthodontics, 38,* 227–234.

TYPES OF MISARTICULATIONS.   As with all treatment plans, a solid diagnostic foundation needs to be established before treating misarticulations of [s] and [z]. It is important to find out exactly how the client produces the error sound. Although the term *distortion* is often used to label abnormal sound changes, this seldom provides enough diagnostic information. Figure 9.2 is presented to help

Figure 9.2 Frequent Misarticulations of [s] and [z]

Interdental [s], [z] θ and ð	• This is a frequent form of distortion. • The tongue tip is too close to posterior surface of upper incisors. • Tongue placement is too far forward, resulting in crossing phonemic boundaries to [θ] and [ð].
Addental [s], [z] s̪ and z̪	• This is the most frequent form of distortion. • The tongue tip is too close to posterior surface of upper incisors. • The tongue placement is too far forward.
Lateral [s], [z] ɬ and ɮ	• Lateral air flow, tip of tongue in direct contact with the alveolar ridge. • No sagittal grooving of tongue. • "Lateral lisp."
Palatal [s], [z] sʲ and zʲ	• More palatal placement of articulators; position is too far back. • The sagittal grooving of the tongue may be more flattened than for [s] and [z]. • Approaches a [ʃ] quality.
Whistled (Strident) [s], [z] s̝ and z̝	• Shrill, irritating auditory impression, a whistle-like component. • Imbalance between air pressure and the opening through which the air must flow. • Too much air pressure or too narrow of an opening between articulators.
[t] for [s] Substitution t and d	• Change in manner of articulation, stopping. • The tongue tip is in direct contact with the alveolar ridge; thus, contact must be eliminated so that a narrow opening occurs.
Nasal [s], [z] s̃ and z̃	• Nasality during [s] production may be organic or functional. • Organic result from physiological anomalies or neuromotor problems—cleft palate, dysarthria. • Functional nasality may be a result of articulatory dyspraxia, faulty learning of sound patterns, or maintenance of a learned pattern that was originally organic.

distinguish between different [s] and [z] "distortions." The last item in Figure 9.2 refers to the production of a nasalized [s] and [z]. As mentioned, there are two types of nasalized productions: organic and functional. Distinguishing functional from organic velopharyngeal competency is the work of a team of professionals. Although an in-depth account of these procedures is not within the scope of this chapter, a few guidelines are given. First, there is a higher probability that a functional problem exists if the nasality is restricted to [s] and [z]. Organic problems usually affect *all* speech sounds, particularly those consonants that require a high degree of intraoral occlusion and the buildup of air pressure (stops, fricatives, affricates). Second, if you are not sure about the nasal quality, nasal airflow and its influence on [s]-productions can be verified by pinching the nostrils closed. The nasal resonance immediately disappears during the occlusion of the nasal passageway and is audible again when the nostrils are released. Third, functional nasal productions are usually accompanied by a normal tongue placement for [s] and [z].

THERAPEUTIC SUGGESTIONS.   Two approaches seem viable when working with a child or an adult who displays an isolated [s] misarticulation: the phonetic placement method and the sound modification (shaping) method. Simply stated, phonetic placement amounts to describing to the client the positioning of the articulators as well as the manner of production of the sound in question. Systematic work toward realizing that goal is then implemented in an attempt to change the aberrant production characteristics. Naturally, with children, this needs to be accomplished in an age-appropriate manner. A mirror might be used to provide visual feedback while the clinician serves as an auditory feedback system. Although this approach is widely used, it is often not easy to describe what exactly needs to be done in a manner that the child can easily understand and follow. The sound modification (shaping) method, on the other hand, uses another sound or sounds that the child can produce in a regular manner as a point of departure for achieving the target sound. Therefore, [t], which the child can produce, might be used to achieve [s], which the child misarticulates. The speech sound chosen should have certain phonetic similarities to the misarticulated sound. In this way, a bridge is built between the similar sound that can be correctly articulated by the child and the target sound that is in error. Both methods are discussed below for problems encountered with [s] and [z].

Clinical Application

A Strident (Whistled) S-Problem

Josh was a bright child who was doing well in first grade. His teacher was satisfied with the skills he was acquiring in reading and writing. However, Josh began to produce a rather conspicuous [s]-production. The teacher referred Josh to the speech-language pathologist.

Assessment revealed that Josh's only speech-language problem appeared to be this [s], which was articulated with a clear and shrill whistle in all contexts. The clinician began to analyze the phonetic characteristics Josh was demonstrating. The placement and the manner of articulation were appropriate. However, it appeared that the more Josh tried to say the sound correctly, the louder the whistle-like component became. Using her phonetic skills, the clinician remembered that there must be a precise balance between the air pressure and the narrow opening between the articulators for [s]-productions. If there is an imbalance between air pressure and the opening through which the air must flow, a whistling component, often referred to as a "strident s," could result. This stridency can be caused by too much air pressure through a slightly narrowed opening or normal air pressure through a very narrow opening (the strident "s" and "z" are transcribed as [s̺] and [z̺], the symbols with a small arrow under each). Thinking about Josh's efforts when attempting to articulate this sound correctly, the clinician was confident that she had found the phonetic reason for Josh's problem. After explanations, some exercises, and some experimenting with openings and air pressure, Josh was able to say [s]-sounds without a whistle.

▶ Video Example 9.1
In this video, Mark is working on s-sounds in speech-language therapy. Note his [s] difficulty. What type of [s] is the clinician trying to achieve: a tongue-tip-up production or a tongue-tip-down production?

https://www.youtube.com/watch?v=nB3D-wi-FSQ

Phonetic Placement. *Decision Making: Apico or Predorsal Placement.* Although most people produce [s] and [z] as apico-alveolar (tongue-tip-up) productions, a predorsal (tongue tip down) articulation is not without merit. For the tongue-tip-up production, the tongue tip is hovering, so to speak, near the alveolar ridge. This precarious position must be precisely maintained over the entire duration of the sound. In contrast, for the tongue-tip-down production, the tongue tip is resting behind the lower incisors. This provides an easily identifiable spot for the tongue tip, which does not waver or fluctuate; it is something definite to "hold on to." For this reason, the predorsal [s] is noted as being a more stable production. Such relative stability is often especially important for children whose motor capabilities are not yet fully developed. In addition, a large percentage of [s] and [z] misarticulations are interdental or addental in nature; that is, the tongue tip is too far forward. To move the tongue tip down for the predorsal-alveolar version provides a solution that is quite different from the child's previous attempts. The natural tendency to return to the previous incorrect [s] is diminished. It is often easier for a child to accomplish a different, new production task than to attempt minor adjustments of a previous one. The final decision on tongue-tip-up or tongue-tip-down [s] production depends on the client's motor abilities or restrictions and on the type and degree of [s] misarticulation. Table 9.4 outlines the procedures for achieving the two different productions based on the various misarticulations.

Sound Modification Methods. Sound modification methods are based on the concept of using a similar, appropriately articulated sound to aid in the production of the misarticulated sound. A similar sound refers to one that is comparable

Table 9.4 Phonetic Placement for Tongue-Tip-Up and Tongue-Tip-Down s-Articulations

Phonetic Placement: Tongue-Tip-Up, Apico-Alveolar [s]

Interdental or Addental Misarticulations

- The tongue tip must be moved back; thus, the client must glide the tongue back to the alveolar ridge.
- Lateral edges of the tongue must be elevated, edges of the tongue must touch the first molars, and the tongue must be grooved.
- Visual and auditory feedback is necessary.

Lateral [s] Misarticulation

- Raise the lateral edges of the tongue so the edges of the tongue touch the first upper molars.
- Direct airstream over the tip of the tongue, thus releasing the contact of the tongue with the alveolar ridge.
- Eliminate the lateral jaw and lip movement using visual feedback. The child can produce an overexaggerated "smile" to help in eliminating these lateral movements.
- If the child has difficulty with tongue grooving, place a straw or small cylindrical object (bamboo stick) lengthwise along the center of the tongue and have the child curl the edges of the tongue around the object, raising the edges of the tongue and creating central airflow.

Palatal [s] Production

- The tongue is too far back.
- The client glides the tongue forward until an acceptable sound is achieved.
- Grooving of tongue must be maintained and possibly increased.

Whistled or Strident [s] Misarticulation

- Balance between expiratory airflow and degree of opening between articulators is crucial.
- The client experiments with reducing the airflow (saying the sound softly) or increasing the opening (slight lowering of the tongue).

Phonetic Placement: Tongue-Tip-Down, Predorsal-Alveolar [s]

- The tongue tip should be behind the lower teeth.
- The front portion of the tongue is directed toward the alveolar ridge.
- Grooving of the tongue is necessary, and the sides of the tongue should touch the first upper molars.
- Visual and auditory feedback is important.

Lateral [s] Misarticulation

- The tongue tip behind the lower teeth eliminates the problem of the contact of the tongue tip and the alveolar ridge.
- The grooving of the tongue is important.
- Eliminate lateral jaw and lip movement using visual feedback.

Palatal [s] Misarticulation

- Predorsal-alveolar production should automatically move the tongue placement forward.
- The grooving of the tongue must be maintained.

---

in some of its phonetic production features. This method is easiest to implement when several direct phonetic similarities exist between the sound to be modified and the target sound. However, some successful techniques have evolved out of very limited articulatory similarities.

1. *[t]-[s] method.*

    a. Begin with a series of rapid [t] repetitions, which typically produce intermittent [s]-like fricatives. This effect is increased if the child is asked to produce [t] with a lot of air pressure. Have the child listen for the sound in between the [t] repetitions; then ask the child to try to prolong this intermittent [s].

b. Begin with a [t]-production in which the stop phase is prolonged, building up air pressure behind the occlusion. The client is then instructed to release the [t] very slowly. The result should approximate [s].

2. *[ʃ]-[s] method.* Three steps are necessary to change [ʃ] to a normal [s]-production:

   a. Eliminate the lip rounding associated with the production of [ʃ]. Have the client smile while saying [ʃ].

   b. Have the client move the tongue slightly forward to change the place where the friction occurs.

   c. Increase the sagittal grooving of the tongue. Have the client raise the lateral edges of the tongue touching the upper molars.

3. *[f]-[s] method.* This method assumes that the tongue tip for [f] is already situated behind the lower incisors; therefore, a tongue tip down [s] is the goal.

   a. Pull the middle of the lower lip away from contact with the upper incisors during the production of [f].

   b. Raise the front portion of the tongue slightly as the upper and lower incisors come closer together.

   For this modification, the client must be aware that a friction sound should be maintained during the entire attempt.

4. *[i]-[s] method.* Phonetic similarities between [i] and [s] consist of the lip spreading and the high, anterior tongue placement for both sounds. For [i], the tongue tip is typically in a lowered position, whereas the anterior portion of the body of the tongue is elevated toward the palate. Thus, this modification normally results in a tongue-tip-down [s].

   a. Instruct the client to bring the teeth slightly closer together during the [i] production.

   b. Elevate the front portion of the tongue (not the tongue tip) until a friction-type sound is heard.

   c. Raise the lateral edges of the tongue touching the upper molars.

The [i] could easily be modified to a voiced [z] if a decision has been made to initiate work with that sound. In addition, the [i]-[z] method has the advantage of maintaining voicing throughout the modification, which is not the case with the [i]-[s] method. Refer to the section titled "Where to Begin: [s] or [z]?"

Functional Nasal [s] and [z] Problems. Therapy for functional nasal [s] and [z] problems does not fit readily into the categorizations of phonetic placement or sound modification methods. The reason for the aberrant nasal [s] is not a deviant tongue placement but rather the inadequate velopharyngeal closure leading to nasal emission. Specific consonants can be used as a bridge to promote sufficient velar closure.

1. *[t]-[s].* If [t] can be produced without hypernasality, instruct the client to hold the stop phase of the [t], building up pressure during the occlusion. [t] is then *slowly* released, producing [s]. Complete velopharyngeal closure is normally necessary when producing [t]. By increasing the air pressure, the occlusion is strengthened because of the higher degree of production effort. This heightened effort might promote more velopharyngeal closure for the following [s]

approximation as well. Visual and auditory feedback should also be implemented to increase the client's awareness of nasal emission versus no nasal emission.

2. *Using consonant clusters [t] + [s] and [s] + [t]*. This method is a slight variation of method #1. It uses the buildup of intraoral air pressure of [t] to facilitate a non-nasal [s] production. The [t] is paired with [s] in a consonant cluster such as "hits" or "bats." If the nasality is eliminated with these phonetic contexts, try [s] + [t], as in "stop" or "stick." At first, do not include any nasal sounds in the word. Therefore, such words as "mats" or "nuts" would be avoided.

Where to Begin: [s] or [z]?   When attempting to achieve an isolated sound production, most clinicians automatically begin with voiceless [s]. The reasoning seems to be that the fricative, although complicated enough for the client, should not be further burdened with the addition of voicing. However, beginning with [z] could be advantageous under certain conditions.

First, voiced consonants normally are produced with less air pressure than voiceless ones. Increased air pressure can at times be counterproductive to establishing typical articulations. Especially with a tongue-tip-up [s], this increased air pressure could lead to the client's "losing" the precariously new approximation between the articulators.

A second factor that supports a choice of [z] is the ability of the voicing component to mask minor productional differences. Listeners seem to be more critical of even slight deviations of the voiceless [s]. The same articulatory features used for the production of [z] are not as noticeable. Naturally, we do not want the client to acquire an [s] that is somehow not acceptable. The following scenario can serve as an example: We have begun work on [s]; however, even with our best efforts and those of the child, the production is still slightly off target. We have tried several times to correct for the minor productional shortcomings, but the articulation is still not quite accurate. We are becoming somewhat frustrated; the child, we feel, is already frustrated. This could be a good time to attempt a voiced [z]. If the articulatory variation is minor enough, the addition of voicing should provide an acceptable sound. It gives the child success (finally) and allows practice time for the new sound. This practice with [z] is often all the child needs to achieve an acceptable [s] articulation.

A third consideration in favor of [z] is a context consideration. If the voiceless [s] is placed in a consonant–vowel (or vowel–consonant) environment, the client must change the voicing halfway through the utterance. This sudden change in voicing could strain an already difficult articulatory-motor task. By using [z], voicing can be maintained throughout the production. To attain [s] once [z] is acceptable is relatively easy. If the child whispers [z], [s] results. The next task is to put the isolated sound production into specific contexts.

COARTICULATORY CONDITIONS.   The phonetic context in which a target sound is placed can have a considerable impact on the production of that sound. Certain contexts can support the production features of the target sound, and others might undermine them. Phonetic contexts that support the production of a target sound can be used effectively by clinicians in certain phases of therapy. On the other hand, ignoring these contexts could lead to endangering a "new" sound production that is still relatively unstable. Facilitative coarticulatory conditions rely on knowledge of, and comparison between, phonetic features.

When analyzing words according to coarticulatory conditions, several factors should be kept in mind:

1. *The vowel following or preceding the target sound.* Consider the comparability of production features of certain vowels relative to the target sound. Some vowels have production features that are phonetically similar to the target sound, whereas others are clearly different. For example, the lip rounding of the high-back vowels and the lip spreading of [s] are dissimilar articulatory conditions.

2. *The syllable structure of the word.* Consider the articulatory gesture as a whole. A word that contains a consonant followed by a vowel (CV) is a less complex articulatory unit than one with a CVC structure. CVCC words are relatively more complex than either CV or CVC structures. Single-syllable words are far simpler to produce than two- or three-syllable words.

3. *The phonetic features of the surrounding consonants.* Consider the movement of the articulators for the production of the overall unit. The target sound's production features can be compared to the other consonants in the word. Again, these similarities can be used to create favorable coarticulatory conditions. For example, the positions of the articulators of [s] and [t] are phonetically similar. This is not the case for [s] and [k].

   Other consonants may provide supportive coarticulatory conditions based on their relative neutral tongue positions. For example, the tongue is not directly involved in the articulation of the bilabials and [h]. Within an articulatory unit, if [s] precedes or follows a sound that does not require tongue activity, the coarticulatory effects on [s] are minimal. Therefore, imbedding [m], [p], [b], and [h] in a word can provide supportive coarticulatory conditions for those consonants in which the tongue is the articulator.

4. *The misarticulation of the client.* Consider the type of misarticulation the client demonstrates. The client is accustomed to this motor pattern and has practiced it, usually for a long time. The unfamiliar motor task, the correct articulation of the target sound, is relatively new. If the new motor task is put into a phonetic environment similar to the misarticulation, the newly established articulation could be jeopardized. For example, if a child's misarticulation of [s] involves a tongue position that is too anterior, an addental or interdental [s] problem, and [s] is in a word together with [θ], this could trigger the original misarticulation. Or, if the child has a lateral [s], it is probably not a good idea to begin with practice words that contain [l], a lateral sound that might trigger the lateral [s] misarticulation.

If the newly acquired [s] is practiced in syllables or words, the vowels that precede or follow it should be considered. Recall that [s] is articulated with the tongue in a relatively anterior position and with some degree of lip spreading; [i] seems phonetically comparable. Both [s] and [i] require unrounding of the lips while the anterior portion of the tongue is elevated toward the palate. This is not the case with [u]. This vowel is produced with the back of the tongue elevated and requires lip rounding. The coarticulatory effects of the lip rounding on [s] can be demonstrated by saying the word "Sue." The lip rounding for [u] is already present as one begins to say the initial [s]. This lip rounding and the additional posterior tongue placement could actually work against a newly acquired [s] articulation.

By examining phonetic comparability, it would seem that the front vowels are better suited for initial context work with [s]. The front vowels [i], [ɪ], [eɪ], [ɛ], and [æ] support the relatively forward tongue placement and the lack of lip rounding. The back vowels have specific features that lack support for [s] and [z]. First, a more posterior tongue placement is associated with all back vowels. In addition, the degree of lip rounding increases from [ɔ] to [oʊ] and from [ʊ] to [u]. The [ɑ] is considered an unrounded vowel. Thus, if lip rounding presents a problem for [s], the low-back vowel [ɑ] should demonstrate more favorable coarticulatory conditions than the mid- and high-back vowels.

The speech-language specialist should keep in mind the phonetic context when moving through every stage of therapy. By contrasting the phonetic features of the target sound and the surrounding consonants and vowels, a hierarchy of contexts can be established that move step by step from more to less supportive coarticulatory conditions. Not every client needs such small steps. However, for those who do, this hierarchy can prove invaluable. On the other hand, some clients might demonstrate "their own" phonetic contexts that could be more facilitating for them than those previously mentioned. The clinician should then use those specific contexts. The suggested sequence should not be seen as part of a "therapy cookbook" approach to be followed with every client but rather as one possibility that incorporates phonetic comparability.

Word Examples.   The following one-syllable words are ordered from relatively easy to more difficult coarticulatory conditions based on comparability of the following vowels:

[s] Words	[z] Words
see - seep - seam - seat - seed - seen	zee - zeal - Zeke
sip - sit - sin - sing	zip - zing - zipped - zinc
say - same - save - sail	Zane
set - said - sell	Zeb - Zed - Zen
sap - sat - Sam - sash - sang	zap - zag - zapped - zagged
sum - sun - suck - sung	
sob - sod - sock - song	czar
sow - soap - sewed - soak	zone - zoned
soot	
Sue - soup - suit - soon	zoo - zoom - zoomed

Clinical Exercises The following words are from a published card set that is available to work on s-sounds.

Word-Initially: Santa, sailboat, cereal, sunflower, soccer player, sock, seal, sand, sandwich, cellphone
Word-Finally: cups, paints, mouse, dice, horse, blocks, jacks, grapes, nurse

How would you rank these words for a child just beginning with s-words? Several of the words should not be used at the beginning of therapy. Which ones should be eliminated until a later date?

Misarticulations of [ʃ] and [ʒ]

This section describes typical and aberrant productions of [ʃ] and [ʒ]. It then addresses specific phonetic placement and sound modification methods. Because [s] and [ʃ] show many similarities in error productions as well as in the diagnostic procedures that would be implemented, the reader is referred to the section on [s] misarticulations at several points.

PHONETIC DESCRIPTION. Phonetically, [s] and [ʃ] are closely related. However, the sagittal groove is considerably wider for [ʃ] than it is for [s]; the tongue is flatter for [ʃ]. This is one reason that the friction noise for [ʃ] is not as "sharp" as that for [s]. In addition, the place of articulation is not the alveolar ridge, as with the [s]; it is located slightly posterior at the anterior part of the palate, the postalveolar area. Finally, [ʃ] has lip rounding rather than the lip spreading common for [s]-productions. Putting this all together, the phonetic description of [ʃ] is a voiceless postalveolar fricative typically with lip rounding. The voiced counterpart of [ʃ] is [ʒ].

LINGUISTIC FUNCTION

Frequency of Occurrence. The voiceless [ʃ] is an infrequent sound, ranking 20th in the 24 consonants of General American English. The voiced [ʒ] is the most infrequent sound in General American English, occurring only in words of foreign origin, such as *beige* or *rouge* (Dewey, 1923; Roberts, 1965).

Phonotactics. Both [ʃ] and [ʒ] can initiate and terminate a syllable. There are very few consonant clusters with [ʃ] and [ʒ]. Refer to the more frequent consonant clusters and word examples in Table 9.5.

Morphophonemic Function. Word-final clusters that end in [ʃ] or [ʒ] can be used to signal past tense in regular verbs that end in these sounds, such as *splashed* and *massaged*.

Minimal Pairs. Frequent sounds that are substituted for [ʃ] and [ʒ] include [s] and [z] and [t] and [d]. Refer to Appendix 9.1 for examples of minimal word pairs and sentences.

INITIAL REMARKS. Preliminary considerations are similar to those presented for [s]. Thus, the client's hearing acuity, minor structural or functional deviations, and auditory discrimination abilities should be assessed before beginning work on the isolated articulation of [ʃ] and [ʒ].

TYPES OF MISARTICULATION. The most common forms of [ʃ] and [ʒ] misarticulations are outlined in Figure 9.3.

Table 9.5 Consonant Clusters with [ʃ] and [ʒ]

Word-Initiating [ʃ]	Word-Terminating [ʃ]	Word-Terminating [ʒ]
[ʃɹ] shrimp, shrub	[ɹʃ] marsh, harsh	[ʒd] rouged, massaged
	[ʃt] washed, wished	

Figure 9.3 Frequent Misarticulations of [ʃ] and [ʒ]

Lateral [ʃ], [ʒ] Typically ɬ and ɮ	• Lateral airflow. • Firm contact of the tongue with prepalatal area. • Lateral edges of tongue are lowered. • Sounds very conspicuous, very similar to lateral [s] and [z].
Addental and [ʃ], [ʒ] ʃ̪ and ʒ̪	• The tongue tip is too far forward; the tongue approximates the alveolar ridge. • Medial grooving may be reduced. • If a child has an addental [s], it is likely that the [ʃ] will be dentalized.
Palatal [ʃ], [ʒ] Voiceless palatal fricative ç and ʝ a voiced palatal fricative	• The tongue is too far back. • Production shifts to the middle of the palate. • Voiceless "sh" sounds like a voiceless [j].
Nasal [ʃ], [ʒ] ʃ̃ and ʒ̃	• It is characterized by nasality during production. • Comparable to nasal [s] or [z], can be organic or functional.
Unrounded [ʃ], [ʒ] ʃ̹ and ʒ̹	• Articulators may be positioned appropriately but there is no lip rounding. • Resulting sound is somewhat "off." • It may occur on the affricates as well.

THERAPEUTIC SUGGESTIONS

Phonetic Placement. Although most [ʃ] and [ʒ] realizations are produced with the tongue tip up, approximating the area directly behind the alveolar ridge, [ʃ] can also be produced with the tongue tip down behind the lower incisors. As with the tongue-tip-down [s], the tongue arches upward, with the front portion of the tongue approximating the postalveolar area. Table 9.6 outlines both productions, the tongue-tip-up and tongue-tip-down [ʃ] and [ʒ].

Sound Modification Methods

1. *[s]-[ʃ] method.* Because [s] and [ʃ] are phonetically similar, clients who have difficulty with [ʃ] often demonstrate [s] problems as well. If that is the case, this method cannot be used. If [s] is intact, the [s]-[ʃ] method would certainly be a good choice. Only lip rounding and a slight retraction of the tongue are initially required. Fortunately, both requirements are often fulfilled simultaneously. If the lips are clearly protruded, the tongue tip has a

Table 9.6 Phonetic Placement for Tongue-Tip-Up and Tongue-Tip-Down [ʃ] and [ʒ]

Placement: Tongue-Tip-Up Production

- Frontal portions of the tongue approximate the anterior area of the palate posterior to the alveolar ridge (postalveolar).
- Sagittal grooving of tongue is present but is wider and flatter than for [s].
- Lips are rounded.

Lateral [ʃ] Misarticulations

- Raise the lateral edges of tongue.
- Release the contact of the tongue with the alveolar ridge.
- Use similar techniques outlined for lateral [s].

Addental [ʃ] Misarticulation

- The tongue must be retracted.
- The client should glide the tongue slowly backward until an acceptable sound is achieved.
- The tongue can be pushed back with a tongue depressor.

Palatal [ʃ] Misarticulation

- The tongue is too far back.
- During production of [ʃ], instruct the client to slowly glide the tongue forward.

Not Enough Lip Rounding

- Lip protrusion is needed.
- The client should place both hands on cheeks and push lips forward; clinician can say to the child, "Look like a fish."

Placement: Tongue-Tip-Down Production

- The tip of the tongue should be down, touching inside of lower incisors.
- The front portion of the tongue arches upward toward the alveolar ridge.
- A narrow opening is created between the front portion of the tongue and the area slightly behind the alveolar ridge.
- A slight medial groove is necessary.
- Lips are slightly protruded and rounded.

tendency to retract a bit (Weinert, 1974). If this natural retraction is still not enough, the client should be instructed to glide the tongue back slightly. If the [ʃ] still sounds somewhat off, slight adjustments might need to be made.

2. *[t]-[ʃ] method.* The main phonetic dissimilarity between [t] and [ʃ] pertains to the manner of articulation, stop versus fricative. The positioning of the articulators is close enough to be usable.

   a. Begin with a prolonged [t] production (prolonging the implosion phase) with lip protrusion.

   b. Maintaining the lip protrusion, instruct the client to slowly release the [t] while gliding the tongue back slightly.

3. *[tʃ]-[ʃ] method.* The goal of this method is to isolate the friction portion of the affricate. This can be done in the following manner:

a. Begin with a very slow production of [tʃ], making sure that lip protrusion is realized.

b. Instruct the client to lengthen the final fricative portion of the affricate.

Functional Nasal [ʃ] Problems. Each of the following methods must first be evaluated to determine whether adequate velopharyngeal closure is achieved. Therefore, no hypernasal resonance should be noted for the sounds coupled with [ʃ].

1. *[t]-[ʃ].* This is similar to the technique described in functional nasal [s] problems. The addition of lip rounding will be necessary for [ʃ] realizations.

2. *[tʃ]-[ʃ].* First, a forceful [tʃ] is produced with an increased buildup of air pressure behind the point of closure. The [t] portion is then slowly released. The client should be instructed that this release should be only minimal. The goal is a slightly narrower opening between the articulators than is normally the case with [ʃ]-productions. This narrow opening with its increased air pressure should help support the velopharyngeal closure necessary for [ʃ].

> **Clinical Exercises** You are seeing Erin, age 7 years 3 months, in speech therapy. She has both lateral [s] and [ʃ] misarticulations, which are also evident in her affricate productions. Which sound would you start with first, or would you work on both simultaneously? Why?
>
> You have chosen to use a sound modification technique for Erin's misarticulations. Which one would you choose for [s] and for [ʃ]? Why?

COARTICULATORY CONDITIONS. When describing context conditions that support regular [ʃ]-productions, two questions must be considered: (1) Is the problem based on difficulties with the tongue placement? and (2) Is the problem primarily the result of not enough lip rounding? The answers to these questions play a role in the selection of coarticulatory conditions.

If the problem is a result of faulty tongue placement—that is, if addental, palatal, or lateral [ʃ]-realizations result—the sequence of supportive vowel coarticulations follows those described for [s]. Thus, the front vowels [i], [ɪ], [eɪ], [ɛ], and [æ], particularly the high-front vowels [i] and [ɪ], support the relatively high anterior position of the tongue during regular [ʃ]-productions.

If the [ʃ] misarticulation is primarily the result of a lack of lip rounding, a different coarticulatory sequence should be considered. The natural lip rounding of the back vowels would support the articulatory necessities for [ʃ]. The high-back vowels [u] and [ʊ] with the most lip rounding would be especially helpful, followed by [oʊ] and [ɔ]. Even the central vowels [ɝ] and [ɚ], which are produced with some degree of lip rounding, could support the lip protrusion necessary for [ʃ]. The unrounded features of the low-back vowel [ɑ] and the front vowels would initially not be indicated.

Word Examples. The following one-syllable words are ordered from relatively easy to more difficult coarticulatory conditions:

[ʃ] Words	
Primary Problem: Tongue Placement	**Primary Problem: Lip Rounding**
she - sheep - sheet - she'd - shield	shoe - shoot
ship - shin - shipped - shift	should - shook
shape - shame - shade - shave - shake	show - showed - shown - shore
shed - chef - shell - shelf	sure - shirt
shack - shag - shaft	shot - shawl - shock - shocked - shop
shut - shove	shack - shag - shaft
shop - shot - shawl - shock - shocked	shed - shell - chef - shelf
show - showed - shown - shore	shade - shave - shake - shape - shame
should - shook	shin - shift - ship - shipped
shoe - shoot	she - sheet - she'd - shield - sheep

Misarticulations of [k] and [g]

Many children go through a phase of substituting [t] for [k] and [d] for [g]. For example, Preisser, Hodson, and Paden (1988) reported that this is the most common deviation involving the [k] and [g] sounds in children from 18 to 29 months of age. Some children seem to "get stuck" in this usually short transient period. Despite a normal progression in other aspects of their speech-language development, they might retain the [t/k] [d/g] substitution into their preschool or even beginning school years. This poses obvious dangers because the child's enormous increase in vocabulary during this time necessitates the understanding and observation of the phoneme oppositions /t/ versus /k/ and /d/ versus /g/. Many minimal pairs exemplify these contrasts in General American English—*tea* versus *key*, for instance.

PHONETIC DESCRIPTION.   [k] and [g] are voiceless or voiced velar stops: The back of the tongue is raised, creating a complete blockage of the expiratory airflow at the anterior portion of the velum. A buildup of air pressure occurs until the tongue suddenly moves away from the velum, releasing the air into the oral cavity. Typically, [k] is produced with higher pressure and more tension than [g]. That makes [k] in most cases aspirated and [g] unaspirated. However, the [k] is not usually aspirated in certain context conditions—for example, in word-medial position and as a component of a consonant cluster.

LINGUISTIC FUNCTION

Frequency of Occurrence.   [k] and [g] occur fairly frequently in General American English. Of 24 consonants, [k] is ranked in the top 10 most frequent, whereas [g] ranks at approximately 15 (Carterette & Jones, 1974; Mines, Hanson, & Shoup, 1978). Frequent word-initiating consonant clusters include [gɹ], [kw], [kl], and [kɹ]. Frequent word-final clusters with these sounds are [ks] and [kt].

Phonotactics.   Both [k] and [g] can initiate and terminate a syllable. Most [g] sounds initiate words, whereas [k] sounds are fairly equally distributed across initial, medial, and final word positions. The more frequent [k] and [g] consonant clusters with word examples are listed in Tables 9.7 and 9.8.

MORPHOPHONEMIC FUNCTION.   Word-final clusters that end in [ks] or [gz] can be used to signal plurality, as in boo<u>ks</u>, le<u>gs</u>, or do<u>gs</u>. In number and tense marking, [k] occurs with [t] or [s] to produce words such as pi<u>cked</u> and pi<u>cks</u>. The [g]

Table 9.7 Consonant Clusters with [k]

Word Initiating		Word Terminating	
[kl]	clown, clean	[kl]	uncle, tickle[1]
[kɹ]	cry, crumb	[ks]	box, six
[sk]	school, sky	[kt]	backed, looked
[skɹ]	scream, scrape	[lk]	milk, silk, elk
[skw]	squeak, squirt	[ɹk]	dark, work[2]
		[ɹkt]	worked, parked[2]
		[sk]	ask, desk
		[sks]	asks, disks

[1] This is not a regular consonant cluster but rather a [k] + a syllabic [l].
[2] These are central vowels with r-coloring (work, worked) or centering diphthongs (dark, parked).

preceding either [d] or [z] can also mark number and tense in verbs such as logged or wags. In phrases, contractible auxiliaries and copulas with the verb *to be* also demonstrate clusters with [k] and [g]. Examples include the duck's waddling and the dog's barking.

MINIMAL PAIRS. The most common substitutions for [k] and [g] are [t] and [d]. Appendix 9.1 contains examples of minimal pairs and sentences that contrast these sounds.

INITIAL REMARKS. Because [k] and [g] misarticulations are often substitutions of one speech sound for another, it is especially important that the client be evaluated for a phonological disorder.

TYPES OF MISARTICULATION. The most frequent forms of [k] and [g] substitutions are noted in Figure 9.4.

THERAPEUTIC SUGGESTIONS.
Phonetic Placement Table 9.9 outlines various ways to establish a correct [k] and [g].

SOUND MODIFICATION METHODS

1. *[ŋ]-[g] method.* These two speech sounds are phonetically very similar: Articulators are directly comparable; however, [ŋ] is a nasal, whereas

Table 9.8 Consonant Clusters with [g]

Word Initiating		Word Terminating	
[gl]	glad, glue	[gz]	pigs, bugs
[gɹ]	grape, grouch	[gd]	wagged, flagged
[gw]	Gwen (very infrequent cluster)		

Figure 9.4 Most Frequent Substitutions for [k] and [g]

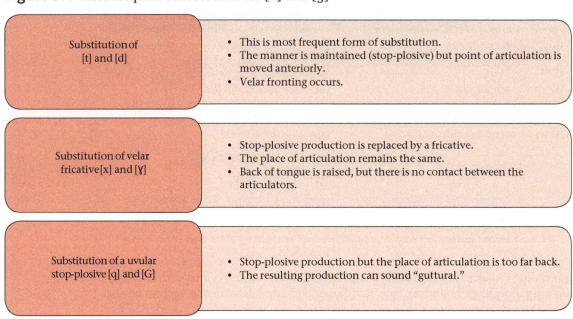

Substitution of [t] and [d]	• This is most frequent form of substitution. • The manner is maintained (stop-plosive) but point of articulation is moved anteriorly. • Velar fronting occurs.
Substitution of velar fricative [x] and [ɣ]	• Stop-plosive production is replaced by a fricative. • The place of articulation remains the same. • Back of tongue is raised, but there is no contact between the articulators.
Substitution of a uvular stop-plosive [q] and [G]	• Stop-plosive production but the place of articulation is too far back. • The resulting production can sound "guttural."

Table 9.9 Phonetic Placement for [k] and [g]

[t] and [d] Substitutions

- Prevent the tip of the tongue from touching the alveolar ridge; the tip of the tongue must remain down behind the lower incisors.
- Place the client's clean finger or clinician's gloved finger (or a tongue depressor can be used if the client can tolerate it) sagittally—front to back—holding down the front half of the tongue (not just the tip). If the entire frontal portion of the tongue cannot be raised, an appropriate [k] can result.
- A similar procedure can be attempted with a tongue depressor placed flat and transversely across the client's tongue, keeping the front portion of the tongue down.
- The client tips his or her head back and tries to "gargle." This demonstrates the posterior positioning of the tongue. The client then attempts [g] maintaining this position.

Velar Fricative Substitution: [x] and [ɣ]

- A fricative is produced instead of a stop; therefore, the tongue needs to be elevated to achieve contact between the articulators.
- Demonstrate with [t] or [d] to emphasize the stop phase and the release aspiration.
- It might be helpful to apply slight pressure under the chin at the throat (do not push too hard, as the client can gag).

Uvular Stop-Plosive Substitution: [q] and [G]

- The place of articulation must be moved more anteriorly.
- The client repeats a rapid sequence of [i] - [k], [i] - [k], [i] - [k], trying to keep the tongue in the [i] position while saying [k]; the front vowel has a tendency to create a more forward positioning of the tongue.

[g] is a stop. The easiest way to use this modification method is to have the client:

    a. Prolong the [ŋ] sound while holding the nostrils closed.

    b. Release the buildup of air pressure into the oral cavity; [g] should result. If [k] is the goal, have the client whisper [ŋ] using the same procedure but with an increase in air pressure.

3. *[u]-[k] method.* This is based on using the high-back vowel [u] to facilitate the tongue positioning for [k]. Have the client:

    a. Prolong [u] and then elevate the back of the tongue.

    b. Try to "stop" the sound by blocking it with the back portion of the tongue. The goal is to obtain complete closure between the posterior portion of the tongue and the soft palate.

    c. Release the sound. If the tongue positioning for [u] is maintained, an acceptable [k] or [g] should result.

COARTICULATORY CONDITIONS. [k] and [g] also demonstrate context-dependent modifications during their productions. In the context of back vowels such as [u] or [ɑ], the articulation is typically made farther back in the mouth. In the context of front vowels, such as in the word "key," the point of contact is more frontally located. These modifications can be used to structure coarticulatory conditions that support specific production goals.

If the goal is to move the positioning of the articulators posteriorly—for example, when a [t] for [k] substitution is realized—combining [k] with the back vowels [u], [ʊ], [oʊ], [ɔ], and [ɑ] is advantageous. During the production of back vowels, the posterior part of the tongue is elevated, supporting the placement necessary for [k]. The front vowels do not provide this coarticulatory support. In fact, the high-front vowels pose an additional danger in this respect. Due to the influence of the high-frontal tongue placement for these vowels, a client might be tempted to revert to the [t] substitution. With a t/k substitution, the phonetically supportive vowel sequence follows the order of high back, mid back, low back, central, low front, mid front, and high front.

If the goal is a more anterior tongue position, as in the substitution of a uvular stop for [k] and [g], the opposite vowel sequence is indicated. In this case, the front vowels aid a more anterior placement with the sequence being high front, mid front, low front, central, low back, and mid back followed by high-back vowels.

It seems advisable to let [g] follow [k] in the sequencing of therapy; the lower degree of the overall muscular effort with the voicing component makes [g] usually more difficult to achieve. According to the author's clinical experience, a coarticulatory condition that seems to support [g] articulation is not a vowel context but an abutting consonant. Often in the context of [ŋ], as in the word "finger," clients have produced a standard [g] that was not evidenced in other g-words. It is always worth a trial period to search for individually based starting points.

Word Examples. The following one-syllable words are ordered from relatively easy to more difficult coarticulatory conditions for a child with a t/k substitution.

[k] Words	[g] Words
coo - coop - cool - cooed[1] - cooled[1]	goof - goose - goofs
could[1]	good[1] - goods[1]
cope - comb - cove - coal - coach - coat[1]	go - goal - goes - ghost[1] - gold[1]
cop - cob - cough - call - caught[1] - cart[1]	gong - gob - gone - gauze - got[1]
cup - cub - come - cuff - cut[1]	gum - gull - Gus - gush - gulp
curb - curve - curl - Kurt[1]	girl
cap - cab - can - calf - cash - cat[1]	gang - gap - gab - gas - gash
Ken - kept[1] - Kent[1]	guess - get[1] - guest[1]
Kay - cape - came - cane - cave - cage	gay - game - gave - gain - gate[1]
king - Kim - kiss - kit[1] - kid[1]	give - gill - gift[1] - guilt[1]
key - keep - keen - keel	geese

[1] These words contain [t] and [d] and probably need to be evaluated to determine whether the coarticulatory influence of [t] and [d] has a negative impact on the newly acquired [k] and [g].

Misarticulations of [l]

Problems with [l]-productions are common in the speech of 3- and 4-year-old children (Prather, Hedrick, & Kern, 1975; Vihman & Greenlee, 1987). By age 4 years 6 months to 5 years, normally developing children demonstrate a decrease in [l] misarticulations (Haelsig & Madison, 1986). Aberrant articulations include substitutions of [w] and [j] for [l]. Because of the relatively high frequency of [l] in General American English, misarticulations are also fairly conspicuous errors.

PHONETIC DESCRIPTION. [l]-sounds are phonetically described as voiced alveolar lateral approximants. During most [l] realizations, the tip of the tongue touches the alveolar ridge. The neighboring coronal areas are relaxed, allowing air to escape laterally. Whereas some articulatory modifications do occur—for example, typical changes take place when [l] is in word-initial versus word-final position—the main feature for [l], which is a laterally free passage for the expiratory airway, remains constant.

Common descriptions of [l] realizations note that the free lateral passage exists on both sides (bilaterally). However, Faircloth and Faircloth (1973) confirm that during spontaneous speech and under certain articulatory conditions, [l] can be realized unilaterally. Heffner (1975) describes the unilateral production as a common [l] realization. Because very little air actually escapes through the lateral openings, a unilaterally free passage usually results in a perfectly acceptable auditory [l] impression. Quite in contrast to the escape of air during lateral [s] misarticulations, the lateral airflow during [l] realizations is very minimal and not actually detectable.

General American English has two [l] varieties: the "light" (or "clear") [l] and the "dark" [l]. Different authors have categorized the production features of the two types in various ways. Some distinguished between them by using the location of the tongue tip (Wise, 1958), whereas others have discussed the qualitative differences (Heffner, 1975). The "light" [l] has an [ɪ] quality that results from a convex shape of the tongue, especially its frontal portion near the palatal or prepalatal area (Heffner, 1975). The "dark" [l] has an [ʊ] or [o] quality caused by the elevation of the tongue's posterior portion. This high-back elevation produces a concave upper surface of the tongue behind the alveolar occlusion. Light l-sounds are transcribed as [l], whereas dark l-sounds are symbolized as [ɫ] or [lˠ].

Although both [l] varieties represent one single phoneme in General American English, /l/, their usage is nevertheless regulated: Light [l] is typically realized in the initial word position when /l/ precedes a vowel or follows an initial consonant—for example, in *like, leap, play,* and *sleep.* Dark [ɫ] is found in word-final positions, as syllabics and when it precedes a consonant—for example, in *full, kettle,* and *cold* (Heffner, 1975). Occasional lack of tongue tip contact has also been noted in [l] following a vowel in word-final position. This becomes important to clinicians when evaluating children. If the tongue tip contact is not established—for example, in the word "wheel"—the final [l] might assume an [o] or [ʊ] quality. It is a good idea to test /l/ production in more than one word position before ascribing the /o/-like sound to an articulatory error.

LINGUISTIC FUNCTION

Frequency of Occurrence. [l] is a frequent sound in General American English; it ranks 8th in children's speech and 5th in adults' speech (Carterette & Jones, 1974). Frequent word-initial clusters include [pl], [kl], and [bl], whereas [ld] and [lz] are common word-final clusters (Dewey, 1923; Roberts, 1965).

Phonotactics. [l] is realized in all word positions, although, as previously noted, allophonic variations that depend on the sound's position in the word exist. It appears that [l] occurs more frequently in medial and final word positions than when initiating a word. Refer to Table 9.10 for lists of the most frequent consonant clusters with [l].

Table 9.10 Consonant Clusters with [l]

Word Initiating		Word Terminating	
[bl]	black, blue	[lb]	bulb
[fl]	flower, flake	[ld]	mild, gold
[gl]	glue, glad	[lf]	Ralph, golf
[kl]	clean, clown	[lk]	milk, elk
[pl]	play, plane	[lm]	film, elm
[sl]	sled, slide	[lp]	help, gulp
[spl]	splash, splinter	[ls]	false, pulse
		[lt]	belt, salt
		[lθ]	health, filth
		[lv]	shelve, twelve
		[lz]	bells, dolls
		[ldz]	folds, worlds
		[lts]	belts, adults
		[lvd]	solved, shelved
		[lvz]	shelves, wolves

Morphophonemic Function. Consonant clusters with [l] are used to signal plurality (do<u>lls</u>, ha<u>lls</u>), possessive (Ji<u>ll's</u>, Bi<u>ll's</u>), third-person singular (he sai<u>ls</u>, she ro<u>lls</u>), and contractible auxiliaries and copulas (the ba<u>ll's</u> rolling, the do<u>ll's</u> little). The consonant clusters [ld] and [lvd] signal past tense, as in sai<u>led</u> or so<u>lved</u>.

Minimal Pairs. Common substitutions for [l] are [ɹ], [w], and [j]. Minimal pair words and sentences exemplifying these substitutions are included in Appendix 9.1.

INITIAL REMARKS. Distortions and substitutions are common [l] errors. Typical substitutions include w/l, j/l, and ɹ/l. Because these substitutions are phonemically relevant, it is important to establish whether they represent phonemic difficulties. This information should be the basis for any therapeutic decision. Also, knowing the articulatory features of the misarticulated [l] is required. Determining these features should include probes into contexts that would promote light and dark [l] realizations. Because their articulations are different, one type could be closer to norm production than the other.

TYPES OF MISARTICULATION. The most common types of [l] misarticulations are outlined in Figure 9.5.

Figure 9.5 Frequent Misarticulations of [l]

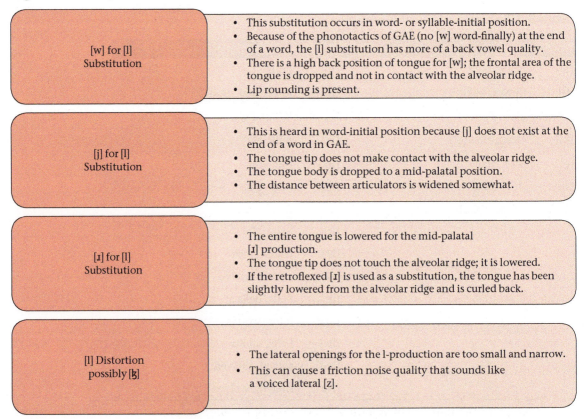

[w] for [l] Substitution	• This substitution occurs in word- or syllable-initial position. • Because of the phonotactics of GAE (no [w] word-finally) at the end of a word, the [l] substitution has more of a back vowel quality. • There is a high back position of tongue for [w]; the frontal area of the tongue is dropped and not in contact with the alveolar ridge. • Lip rounding is present.
[j] for [l] Substitution	• This is heard in word-initial position because [j] does not exist at the end of a word in GAE. • The tongue tip does not make contact with the alveolar ridge. • The tongue body is dropped to a mid-palatal position. • The distance between articulators is widened somewhat.
[ɹ] for [l] Substitution	• The entire tongue is lowered for the mid-palatal [ɹ] production. • The tongue tip does not touch the alveolar ridge; it is lowered. • If the retroflexed [ɹ] is used as a substitution, the tongue has been slightly lowered from the alveolar ridge and is curled back.
[l] Distortion possibly [ɮ]	• The lateral openings for the l-production are too small and narrow. • This can cause a friction noise quality that sounds like a voiced lateral [z].

Table 9.11 Phonetic Placement for [l]

[w] for [l] Substitutions

- The lip protrusion on [w] needs to be eliminated (use [u]-[i] as a contrast of lip protrusion–no lip protrusion).
- The contact with the alveolar ridge needs to be established.
- The edges of the tongue are relaxed; instruct the client to use a "flat tongue" and then raise the tongue to the alveolar ridge.
- If the back of the tongue is still elevated for [w], the result might sound like a dark [l]; put a front vowel after this production and see if it improves qualitatively.

[j] for [l] Substitutions

- The tongue tip must be elevated to the alveolar ridge; this could be the only adjustment necessary.
- If a friction-like sound occurs, the lateral edges of the tongue need to be lowered to allow more airflow.
- A straw or small cylindrical object (bamboo stick) placed along the length of the tongue and pushed down slightly can be used to aid in raising the edges of the tongue if the lateral airflow is too excessive.

[ɹ] for [l] Substitutions

- Contact of the front part of the tongue with the alveolar ridge is needed.
- The body of the tongue needs to be moved forward; refer to "Sound Modification Methods" for using the [i]-[l] sound modification method.

[l] Distortions—[l] Produced as a Lateral Fricative

- If [l] is being produced as a fricative, the opening between the articulators is too narrow. Thus, the edges of the tongue need to be lowered.
- Contrast a flattened tongue versus a rolled tongue, and then place the tongue tip on the alveolar ridge with a more flattened tongue.

Passive Method of Lowering Lateral Edges of the Tongue

- Place a narrow ribbon (½-inch wide) flat across the front of the tongue so that the ends hang down on either side to the client's chin.
- Have the client pull down gently on both sides of the ribbon during [l] production; the tongue tip should be touching the alveolar ridge.

THERAPEUTIC SUGGESTIONS

Phonetic Placement. For accurate productions of [l], the tongue tip is in direct contact with the alveolar ridge. The lateral edges of the tongue are not elevated but rather relaxed, allowing free passage of the air to the right and left of the contact at the alveolar ridge. Visibility of the articulation is often very helpful when establishing the placement of an isolated sound. Because visibility for most [l]-productions is limited, a wide-open mouth posture can enhance it. Under this condition, the tip of the tongue should touch the alveolar ridge in such a way that a good portion of the tongue's underside becomes visible. Table 9.11 outlines the phonetic placement for the various substitutions of [l].

Sound Modification Methods

1. *[d]-[l] method.* Articulators for these two sounds are very similar; the manner of articulation, though, is different.

    a. Use the passive method mentioned in Table 9.11 of pulling the lateral edges of the tongue down with a ribbon during [d]-production.

  b. A second possibility during the stop phase of [d] is to have the client release the air slowly (lowering the lateral edges) without losing the tongue tip–alveolar contact.

2. *[i]-[l] method.* This method is based on similarities between the [i] and the light [l] productions.

  a. Prolong [i] ([ɪ] can also be used) while moving the tongue tip to the alveolar ridge. Although production similarities exist between [i] or [ɪ] and the light [l], this method does not offer much visual feedback for the client. If visibility is important, the [ɑ]-[l] method might be a better choice.

3. *[ɑ]-[l] method.*

  a. Prolong the [ɑ] with a wide-open mouth posture.
  b. Elevate the tongue tip to the alveolar ridge and provide visual feedback. Not only is visibility good with this open-mouth posture but it also helps to lower the lateral edges. Often a child can say la-la-la, which is a slight variation of this method. If the [l] is correct, try [lɑ]—a pause—and then possibly [t] or [d] at the end of the new words ([lɑt], [lɑd]).

COARTICULATORY CONDITIONS. Favorable coarticulatory conditions, specifically the sequence of vowels that support regular [l] articulations, depend on the goal to be achieved. If visibility is important, low vowels might be the choice. Low vowels provide a client with a means of visual control that can be continued until [l] is somewhat stabilized. A desirable sequence of context exercises might begin with the low-back [ɑ] and continue with the low-front [æ]. Mid-front vowels [ɛ] and [eɪ] and mid-back [ɔ] and [oʊ] still offer some visibility if produced with a relatively open-mouth posture. Because of the possible coarticulatory influence of the lip rounding, the mid- and high-back vowels probably should be the last in the sequence for a client who demonstrates a [w/l] substitution.

Clinical Exercises Several published word cards are available for working on many types of misarticulations. The following are presented for [l] in the word-final position:

Word-final position [l] words: seal, pinwheel, whale, pencil, doll, beach ball, squirrel, windmill, apple

How could you rank these words from easiest to most difficult? Are there any words that you might not use or should wait until a much later time to attempt?

In the case of [l] distortions based on an opening that is too narrow creating a lateral fricative sound, the back vowels probably should be the choice. The slightly concave shape of the tongue supports the relaxing of the lateral edges. Here, the dark [l] in word-final position could be easier for a client to achieve.

If a later goal is to produce both light *and* dark /l/-sounds, two coarticulatory conditions need to be considered: first, the position of /l/ in the word, and second, the tendency for certain vowels to promote light versus dark [l]-sounds. Back vowels, especially high-back ones, support the dark [l], whereas front vowels, especially high-front ones, aid the production of light [l]. Depending on the momentary goal—light [l] or dark [ɫ]—the sequence of vowels must vary. For the coarticulatory support of light [l] articulations, the sequence could be [l]: high-front, mid-front, low-front, central, low-back, mid-back, and high-back vowels. The opposite sequence is suggested preceding dark [ɫ] realizations: high-back, mid-back, low-back, central, low-front, mid-front, and high-front vowels.

Several supportive coarticulatory possibilities have been suggested. Based on the momentary goal, different vowel sequences should be considered. However, the order of supporting coarticulatory circumstances for the new sound achievement must be determined by whatever is easiest for a client to attain.

Word Examples   The following one-syllable words are ordered from relatively easy to more difficult coarticulatory conditions for a client with an [l] problem. Word examples are given for both light and dark /l/.

Words with Light l-Sounds	Words with Dark l-Sounds
Lee - leap - leaf - leave - leak - leash	pool - tool - fool - cool - school - spool
limb - lip - lid - lit - lick - live	bull - pull - full - wool[1]
lay - lame - late - laid - lake - lace	bowl - pole - foal - goal - coal
led - let - leg - ledge - left - lend	all - hall - ball - mall - doll - fall - call
lamb - lad - laugh - lag - lamp	hull - dull - gull - skull
lug - luck - love - lump - lunch	bell - tell - fell - sale - shell
law - lot - loss - log - long - lock	mail - bale - pail - Dale - nail - sale - jail
low - load - loan - loaf - loaves	ill - hill - will[1] - Bill - pill - fill - gill
look - looked	eel - heel - meal - deal - kneel - feel
Lou - loom - loop - loon - loot - Luke	

[1] If a client has a [w/l] substitution, these words would need to be evaluated to determine whether the initial [w] might negatively affect [l] articulations.

Misarticulations of [ɹ] and the Central Vowels with r-Coloring

The misarticulations in this section include those occurring with the consonantal r-sound, as in *rabbit* or *red*, and/or the central vowels with r-coloring, [ɝ] and [ɚ], as in *bird* or *father*. A client who has difficulty producing "r-qualities" typically demonstrates problems with both consonantal [ɹ] and central vowels with r-coloring.

Consonantal [ɹ] develops relatively late; it is frequently still in error during the preschool years. Smit (1993b) reported that only by age 7 were 75% of the children in her study able to produce [ɹ] at the word level.

The central vowels with r-coloring appear to be the last vowels to be mastered. Data from the Smit (1993b) study demonstrated that only approximately 80% of the children from 6 to 7 years of age correctly used the vocalic [ɚ] in the middle of a word (as in *earring*).

Although it is expected that r-sounds (both consonantal and central vowels with r-coloring) are "mastered" by school age, some children continue to have difficulties with these sounds. Typical problems include sound substitutions of the consonantal [ɹ] in word- or syllable-initial positions and derhotacization or vowelization of the central vowels with r-coloring.

PHONETIC DESCRIPTION

Consonantal [ɹ]. The articulation of [ɹ] in General American English is extremely variable. In fact, [ɹ] might well be the most inconsistently produced consonant of our language. In different contexts, the same speaker might use various tongue and lip positions when producing this sound. The different types of [ɹ]-productions are usually placed into two broad categories: the bunched and the retroflexed [ɹ] (Shriberg, Kent, McAllister, & Preston, 2019).

The bunched [ɹ] is phonetically classified as a voiced alveolar central approximant. For this production, the corpus of the tongue is elevated toward the palate while the tongue tip points slightly downward. The voiced expiratory air passes sagittally through this fairly wide passageway. The sides of the tongue touch the bicuspids and molars. This tongue position can vary with the vowel context, and lip rounding could be present.

The retroflexed [ɹ] (actually transcribed as [ɻ]) is phonetically classified as a voiced retroflexed central approximant. The tip of the tongue points to the alveolar ridge or its neighboring prepalatal areas. Because the lateral edges of the tongue are raised, preventing lateral air escape, the voiced expiratory air is again channeled sagittally out of the oral cavity. During this action, the dorsum of the tongue is somewhat depressed. This makes the elevation of the tip of the tongue appear even more pronounced. Often the tip of the tongue might even be slightly bent backward or curled up. Such an articulatory position gave these [ɹ] realizations their characteristic name: retroflexed.

Although [ɹ] is extremely variable in its production features, recognizing some frequent allophonic variations that occur in General American English is therapeutically helpful. After [θ], the [ɹ] can be produced as a trill. The term **trill** depicts a sound produced by the vibratory action of the tongue tip against the alveolar ridge. After [t], [ɹ] could have a fricative-like quality caused by the preceding [t], which in its release phase creates a closer approximation between the articulators than is normally the case. This results in a quality approximating [tʃ]. Also, following voiceless consonants, such as in *try, cry*, and *fry*, [ɹ] could be partially devoiced.

Central Vowels with r-Coloring. [ɝ] and [ɚ] have been called *rhotic* or *rhotacized vowels*. The term *r-colored* or *rhotacized vowels* describes their perceptual quality; they appear to contain r-features.

The central vowel [ɝ] is stressed and is usually produced with some degree of lip rounding; [ɚ] is the unstressed counterpart of [ɝ]. Both vowels show similar articulations, although lip rounding could be lacking when [ɚ] is produced. Based on the results of palatography, Fletcher (1992) noted that tongue actions for the rhotic vowels are similar to those for the rhotic approximants. The r-like vowels can be produced in two ways. First, the tongue can be curled upward and backward in a retroflexed position. Second, the tip can be dropped slightly, with the body of the tongue bunched and moved posteriorly in the mouth. These articulations are comparable to the "retroflexed" and "bunched" consonantal [ɹ]-productions previously discussed.

There is some disagreement as to the exact nature of the r-substitutions in children. Very often the misarticulation is simply called a *w/r substitution*. Shriberg and colleagues (2019) argue that most w/r substitutions are actually derhotacized r-productions. Based on extensive clinical experience, Gibbon (2002) states (based on intuition, not clinical data) that most typically developing children acquiring [ɹ] pass through a stage in which they produce [w] substitutions, and some seem to go through another stage in which they progress from [w] to [ʋ], a labiodental approximant, before reaching [ɹ]. Children with speech sound disorders seem to follow the same path, but more slowly, and some continue with [ʊ] into adulthood. However, Gibbon believes that [ɹ] realized as [w] could be more common in children with speech sound disorders.

LINGUISTIC FUNCTION

Frequency of Occurrence. Both consonantal [ɹ] and the central vowels with r-coloring are frequent sounds in General American English. According to Carterette and Jones (1974), these sounds constitute the second most frequently occurring sound category. Many consonant clusters with [ɹ] are also prevalent. These include [pɹ], [tɹ], [fɹ], and [gɹ] in the word-initial position. The central vowels with r-coloring also occur with final consonants exemplified by [ɹd], [ɹt], [ɹn], and [ɹz] (Dewey, 1923; Roberts, 1965). Refer to Table 9.12 for a list of word-initiating and word-terminating consonant clusters with [ɹ]. Word-terminating clusters can be transcribed with the stressed central [ɝ] vowel, thus, "birds" [bɝdz], or with the centering diphthong, "farms" [fɑɚmz] and "forks" [foʊɚks] depending on their sound quality.

Phonotactics. Whereas the consonantal [ɹ] occurs in initiating syllables or in specific clusters, the central vowels with r-coloring function as syllable nuclei. The

Table 9.12 Word-Initiating Consonant Clusters with [ɹ] and Final Consonants and Consonant Clusters Following Rhotic Vowels

Word Initiating		Word Terminating	
[bɹ]	bread, broom	[ɹb]	Herb, curb
[dɹ]	dream, drink	[ɹd]	bird, card
[fɹ]	frog, friend	[ɹg]	iceberg, Pittsburgh
[gɹ]	grass, green	[ɹk]	fork, Mark
[kɹ]	Craig, cry	[ɹl]	Karl, girl
[pɹ]	prune, prince	[ɹm]	arm, worm
[ʃɹ]	shrimp, shrub	[ɹn]	barn, learn
[tɹ]	train, truck	[ɹp]	burp, chirp
		[ɹs]	nurse, horse
[skɹ]	scream, scratch	[ɹʃ]	harsh, marsh
[spɹ]	spring, spred	[ɹt]	dirt, short
[stɹ]	straw, strong	[ɹv]	serve, starve
		[ɹz]	doors, ears
		[ɹdʒ]	large, George
		[ɹkt]	worked, parked
		[ɹlz]	girls, Charles
		[ɹst]	first, pierced
		[ɹts]	shirts, sports
		[ɹtʃ]	March, birch

noted word-final [ɹ] "clusters," such as [ɪn] and [ɪt], contain [ɝ] (e.g., *turn, hurt*) or centering diphthongs preceding a consonant (e.g., *barn, farm*); therefore, they are technically not consonant clusters. They are, however, included in Table 9.11.

Minimal Pairs. The most frequent substitutions for [ɹ] include [w], [j], and [l]. Refer to Appendix 9.1 for examples of minimal pair words and sentences with these phonemic oppositions.

INITIAL REMARKS. Because several misarticulations of the consonantal [ɹ] include substitutions of one phoneme for another, it is important that a client's phonemic system be evaluated. Dialectal variations should also be examined. Dialects that characteristically lose r-coloring on central vowels include Southern, South Midland, Eastern New England, and African-American Vernacular English (e.g., Iglesias & Anderson, 1995; Pollock & Berni, 2001).

TYPES OF MISARTICULATION. Figure 9.6 outlines the most common substitutions for [ɹ] and the central vowels with r-coloring.

THERAPEUTIC SUGGESTIONS
Phonetic Placement: [ɹ]. Two possibilities can be used for phonetic placement therapy with [ɹ]: (1) the apical-alveolar "retroflexed" [ɹ] articulation, and (2) the mediodorsal-mediopalatal "bunched" [ɹ] articulation. The retroflexed [ɹ] is often easier to implement because its features can be explained more easily. The choice of retroflexed or bunched [ɹ] depends on the client and the type of aberrant production presented.

Retroflexed Articulation. The client is instructed to elevate the front of the tongue so that the tongue tip is pointing behind the alveolar ridge. The tongue tip should come close to the area behind the alveolar ridge but should not touch it. The posterior edges of the tongue should be in contact with the upper molars. First, instruct the client to glide the tongue, which is touching the alveolar ridge, forward and backward, "sweeping" the palatal area. Next, instruct the client to execute, with a slightly open-mouth posture, the same action but this time *without* touching the palatal area. If, at the same time, the back edges of the tongue are raised and voicing is added, an r-like quality might be heard. If the [ɹ]-production seems close but is not quite on target, it is important to

Figure 9.6 Common Substitutions for [ɹ], [ɝ], and [ɚ]

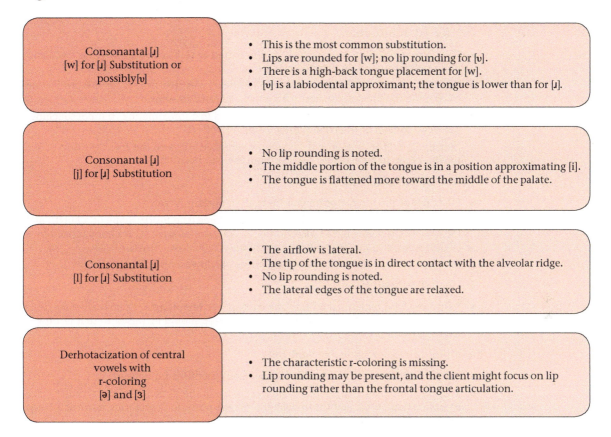

Consonantal [ɹ]
[w] for [ɹ] Substitution or possibly[ʋ]

- This is the most common substitution.
- Lips are rounded for [w]; no lip rounding for [ʋ].
- There is a high-back tongue placement for [w].
- [ʋ] is a labiodental approximant; the tongue is lower than for [ɹ].

Consonantal [ɹ]
[j] for [ɹ] Substitution

- No lip rounding is noted.
- The middle portion of the tongue is in a position approximating [i].
- The tongue is flattened more toward the middle of the palate.

Consonantal [ɹ]
[l] for [ɹ] Substitution

- The airflow is lateral.
- The tip of the tongue is in direct contact with the alveolar ridge.
- No lip rounding is noted.
- The lateral edges of the tongue are relaxed.

Derhotacization of central vowels with r-coloring
[ə] and [ɜ]

- The characteristic r-coloring is missing.
- Lip rounding may be present, and the client might focus on lip rounding rather than the frontal tongue articulation.

remember the tension of the tongue. Clinicians often have a child try to "tense" the tongue by pushing on the desk or pretending that he or she is lifting something heavy. This slight tongue tension could be enough to change the quality to an acceptable-sounding [ɹ].

Mediodorsal-Mediopalatal Bunched Placement. The bunched [ɹ] is produced with the tongue tip down while central portions of the tongue's body are slightly elevated. The characteristic rhotic resonance is created by a sagittal airflow over the relatively broad surface of the tongue. The client should be instructed to lower the tongue tip so that it rests close to the top of the lower incisors. The client must also be aware that the lateral edges of the tongue need to touch the upper molars. A practice progression might start with the client articulating [d], noting how the back portions of the tongue touch the molars. Next, the tongue tip should be lowered, leaving the back of the tongue in the same position. Finally, the whole body of the tongue, including the tongue tip, must be moved posteriorly. The necessary change could be aided by gently pushing back the tip of the tongue with a tongue depressor so that the middle portion of the tongue becomes more elevated. Ehren (2010) suggests that the tongue depressor be placed horizontally in the mouth, pushing the flattened surface back to the corners of the mouth. The child places the tongue against the posterior edge of the tongue depressor inside the mouth and then attempts the [ɹ]-production. Table 9.13 lists the steps that need to be taken for the other substitutions.

Table 9.13 Phonetic Placement for [ɹ], [ɜ˞], and [ɚ]

[w] for [ɹ] Substitutions

- The lip protrusion on [w] needs to be eliminated or reduced (use [u]-[i] as a contrast of lip protrusion–no lip protrusion).
- The back portion of the tongue should not be as elevated as it is for the production of [w]; the tongue body needs to be moved slightly anterior.
- Retroflexed [ɹ]: The tongue tip must be elevated to approximating (but not touching) the front portion of the palatal area for the retroflexed [ɹ].
- Bunched [ɹ]: The lips should be somewhat retracted, and the front portion of the tongue needs to be elevated slightly from the [w] position.

[j] for [ɹ] Substitutions

- Elevation of the tongue or tongue tip is an important factor.
- Retroflexed [ɹ]: This is marked by a concave shape (the inside shape of a bowl), and the tongue tip points in the direction of the prepalatal area; [j] is characterized by a slightly convex shape (the outer shape of an upside-down bowl).
- Bunched [ɹ]: The dorsum of the tongue must be lowered slightly (lower jaw).

[l] for [ɹ] Substitutions

- Retroflexed [ɹ] and bunched [ɹ]: The contact between tongue tip and alveolar ridge should be released; the lateral edges of the tongue should be raised so that airflow is directed medially.

Addition of r-Coloring to [ɜ˞] and [ɚ]

- Only r-coloring needs to be added if the client produces [ɜ] and [ə].
- Two possibilities are (1) to point the tongue tip in the direction of the alveolar ridge or front palatal area, and (2) to push the tongue posteriorly, creating more of a bulge in the middle of the tongue.

Sound Modification Methods: [ɹ] and Central Vowels with r-Coloring. Several of the following modification methods use sounds that were noted as substitutions for [ɹ]. For example, a client could have a [j/ɹ] substitution; [j] is one of the sounds that can be modified to an [ɹ]. The [l]-[ɹ] and [j]-[ɹ] methods are included in Table 9.13. The following methods can also be used:

1. *[d]-[ɹ] method.* With this sound modification method, the goal is a retroflexed r-sound. The client is instructed to:

   a. Produce [d] and note where the tongue placement is.

   b. Attempt to produce [dɹ] by gliding the tongue tip back, pointing into the direction of the frontal area of the palate (past the alveolar ridge). The tongue tip should not touch the palate, but the movement should follow the release of the [d]; that is, the tongue tip should drop and then move back. The [d]-production as a point of departure for [ɹ] also underlines the necessary contact of the posterior edges of the tongue with the molars. This in turn aids the elevation of the lateral edges of the tongue, reinforcing the [ɹ] resonance.

2. *[ɜ˞] or [ɚ]-[ɹ] method.* Clients who have difficulty with [ɹ] usually show problems with the r-colored central vowels as well. However, if a clinician decides to work on the consonantal [ɹ] and the client has acceptable productions of the central vowels with r-coloring, a transfer of this r-coloring would be the method of choice. If the client has [ɜ˞] and [ɚ] but not [ɹ], a word could be specifically

Clinical Application

When to Initiate Therapy with "r" Problems

A clinical decision must be made if the client has either the r-colored central vowels or the consonantal [ɹ] but not both. Should the clinician initiate "r" therapy? The fact that the r-coloring is somehow present should make this an easy sound to remediate. Or, should the clinician wait and watch? The underlying assumption is that if the r-coloring is present in one sound, it probably generalizes to other sounds as well. Do clients in fact generalize r-coloring in such a manner? After reviewing the literature of sound generalization research, Elbert and Gierut (1986) established certain "predictions" that clinicians can use to reduce the number of sounds to be worked on in therapy. The idea is that if a specific sound is taught, certain features of the newly acquired sound might transfer without therapy to other sounds requiring the same features. One prediction is that if one allophone is acquired—[ɝ], for example—norm production of [ɹ] and [ɚ] can probably be achieved without therapy. In this case, a wait-and-watch decision might be best. However, not every child is able to generalize features from one sound to another. In addition, there could be other factors that affect the clinical decision making, such as the age of the child, the intelligibility of the child, parental concerns, and peer pressure, to mention just a few.

divided to elicit the [ɹ] sound. For example, the client could begin with the word "purr." Then the client tries *purring*. Next a pause is made in the word: *pu-rring*. Finally, the last syllable is isolated as *ring*: a consonantal [ɹ] is achieved.

Where to Begin Therapy?   Should therapy begin with the consonantal [ɹ] or with the central vowels with r-coloring? This choice should be based on stimulability probes and the perceptual saliency of the error sound. **Perceptual saliency** refers to the conspicuousness, or noticeability, of the error sound to listeners. If one client has substitutions such as [w/ɹ] or [j/ɹ] and a second client produces derhotacization of central vowels, the substitutions [w/ɹ] and [j/ɹ] are probably more prominent perceptually. Dialect might also play a role in clinicians' decision making. If dialect features include derhotacization of central vowels, the consonantal [ɹ] would be the only therapy choice. Second, which type of [ɹ]-production, the bunched or the retroflexed [ɹ], should be the goal of phonetic placement or sound modification techniques? Again, the client's stimulability plays a role. Placement techniques can be implemented, and the resulting [ɹ] can be evaluated. If an acceptable [ɹ]-production is achieved in isolation, probes can determine which vowels or words promote the accurate use of the newly acquired sound. The therapeutic goal is to appraise the client's individual possibilities and determine the most efficient means of changing aberrant productions to acceptable articulations. Every client presents a different set of challenges.

COARTICULATORY CONDITIONS.   The retroflexed [ɹ] sound offers a challenge when clinicians try to determine which vowel sounds might present coarticulatory conditions that assist its production. There are no vowels in General American English with a tongue placement similar to the retroflexed [ɹ] position. If the retroflexed [ɹ] follows front vowels, especially high-front vowels, at least elevated frontal portions of the tongue are promoted. However, combinations with these vowels would necessitate a quick movement from a concave retroflexed [ɹ] to a rather different tongue shape for the front vowels. On the other hand, the back vowels, with their characteristic posterior elevation of the tongue, do not seem to support a retroflexed articulation. The central vowels without r-coloring, especially those produced with an elevated mandibular position, offer perhaps the best possibility. However, based solely on phonetic production features (and clinical experience), the front vowels might be better than the back vowels in supporting retroflexed [ɹ].

Similar coarticulatory conditions would exist for the central vowels and the bunched r-production with its relative centralized elevation of the body of the tongue. However, the secondary feature of lip rounding, which often characterizes the bunched [ɹ], is also characteristic of the back vowels. Therefore, if the goal is the bunched [ɹ], the sequence of vowels might be central vowels, back vowels, and, finally, front vowels.

As noted previously, the articulatory features of [ɹ] can change with individuals and with the context in which the sound occurs. Because of this, clinicians need to concentrate on the possibilities of each individual client and on the coarticulatory conditions that seem to foster the standard production of these sounds.

Word Examples. Keep in mind that individual and contextual variations often dramatically alter the production of [ɹ]. The following one-syllable words exemplify one possible vowel sequence that could be used for a child with an [ɹ] problem. This order is based on the retroflexed [ɹ] as target. The vowel sequence is the one suggested at the beginning of this section. Word examples are given for both the consonantal [ɹ] and central vowels with r-coloring.

Consonantal [ɹ] Words
rub - rough - run - rut - rush - rug - rung
ram - rap - rat - ran - rag - rack - rang
red - wren - wreck - rent - wrench
Ray - raid - rail - rain - race - rake
rim - rib - rip - ridge - rig - Rick - ring
real - read - reach
raw - rod - rot - Ron - rock - wrong
row - robe - rope - roll - road - wrote
room - roof - rude - root - rule

Central Vowels with r-Coloring	
Words with the central vowel with r-coloring - [ɝ]	**Words with centering diphthongs**
her - burr - purr - fur - sir - spur - stir	air - hair - mare - bear - pear[1]
earn - earth - urge	ear - fear - deer - near - cheer - gear
worm - burn - turn - word - hurt - learn	are - bar - far - jar - car - star
slurp - skirt	oar - more - bore - pour - door
	blur
	lure - tour

[1] Pronunciation of the words with centering diphthongs can vary from speaker to speaker. Thus, the word "hair" might be pronounced [hɛɚ] or [heɪɚ]. These differences could have an influence on the sequencing of the words.

Misarticulations of [θ] and [ð]

[θ] and [ð] are among the latest sounds to develop in the speech of children. Difficulties in articulating them often extend into the beginning school year. Common errors are the substitution of [t/θ] and [d/ð]. Other misarticulations include the substitution of the labiodental fricatives [f] and [v] for [θ] and [ð]. Clinicians should also be aware that variations in [θ] and [ð] productions can be a feature of African-American Vernacular English. The realization of these features is conditioned by the position of [θ] and [ð] in the word. These dialectal features are not considered articulation errors.

PHONETIC DESCRIPTION. [θ] and [ð] are dental fricatives, but they can be produced with the tongue tip slightly between the front teeth or with the tongue tip coming close to the inner surface of the front incisors. The friction that characterizes these sounds as fricatives is created by restricting the breath stream between the tip of the tongue and the backside of the upper front teeth. For both productions, the tongue remains relatively flat.

LINGUISTIC FUNCTION

Frequency of Occurrence. On a frequency of occurrence list for General American English speech sounds, [θ] and [ð] are not neighbors. Whereas [ð] is slightly above the middle, occupying a rank of approximately 10th among 24 consonants, [θ] is among the last on the list, ranking 21st among 24 (Carterette & Jones, 1974). Only word-initial [θɹ] is considered a fairly frequent cluster in General American English.

Phonotactics. Both [θ] and [ð] are found in word-initial and word-final positions. [ð] occurs primarily in word-initial positions, whereas [θ] occurs approximately half the time in word-initial positions; the other half of occurrences are fairly evenly split between word-medial and word-final positions. Refer to Table 9.14 for examples of consonant clusters with [θ] and [ð].

Morphophonemic Function. Word-final clusters that end in [θ] and [ð] can signal (1) plurality, as in mon_ths_ and mou_ths_; (2) third-person singular, as in ba_thes_ and brea_thes_; and (3) past tense, as in ba_thed_ and brea_thed_.

Minimal Pairs. Frequent sounds substituted for [θ] and [ð] include [t]-[d], and [f]-[v]. Refer to Appendix 9.1.

Table 9.14 Consonant Clusters with [θ] and [ð]

Word Initiating		Word Terminating	
[θɹ]	thread, three	[tθ]	width, hundredth
		[lθ]	health, wealth
		[nθ]	ninth, month
		[ŋθ]	length, strength
		[ðd]	bathed, breathed
		[ðz]	bathes, breathes

TYPES OF MISARTICULATIONS. Refer to Figure 9.7 for the most common substitutions for [θ] and [ð].

THERAPEUTIC SUGGESTIONS
Phonetic Placement

Productions with the tongue tip between the front teeth. [θ] and [ð] are articulated as follows:

1. The tongue tip is *slightly* protruded between the upper and lower incisors.
2. The top of the tongue lightly touches the lower edges of the front teeth.
3. The underside of the tongue rests on the top edges of the lower incisors.
4. The body of the tongue is relatively flat.

The expiratory airflow should be directed over the surface of the tongue between the tongue tip and the bottom edge of the front incisors. Specific tongue activities could be implemented before this placement. For example, a client could move the tip of the tongue forward and backward over the bottom edge of the front incisors. Next, with the tip of the tongue placed lightly on the bottom edge of the front incisors, the client lowers the tongue tip minimally during expiration. The goal is to create awareness of the airflow over the surface and tip of the tongue. Because the tip of the tongue is visible during one type of production, visual feedback can be helpful. Care should be taken that this placement is not established with excessive tongue protrusion. The tongue tip should barely be visible between the teeth.

Productions with the tongue tip behind the upper teeth. The tongue tip is placed touching the posterior surface of the front incisors. The body of the tongue should be relatively flat. During expiration, a client should glide the tongue back slightly until a friction noise is heard. The required posterior movement

Figure 9.7 Frequent Misarticulations of [θ] and [ð]

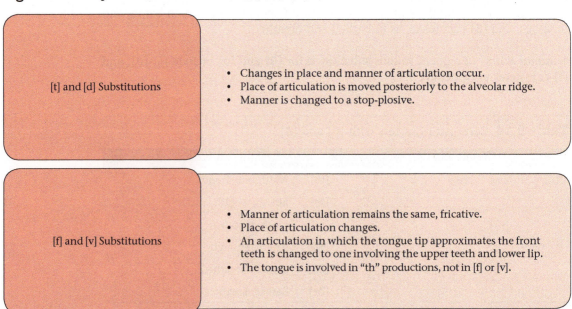

[t] and [d] Substitutions
- Changes in place and manner of articulation occur.
- Place of articulation is moved posteriorly to the alveolar ridge.
- Manner is changed to a stop-plosive.

[f] and [v] Substitutions
- Manner of articulation remains the same, fricative.
- Place of articulation changes.
- An articulation in which the tongue tip approximates the front teeth is changed to one involving the upper teeth and lower lip.
- The tongue is involved in "th" productions, not in [f] or [v].

is minimal. For the client with a [t/θ] substitution, care must be taken that the posterior movement does not result in the tongue tip coming into contact with the alveolar ridge.

Sound Modification Methods. The substitutions [t/θ] and [f/θ] can be effectively influenced by using sound modification methods. The following list describes how to change the articulation from [t] and [f] to [θ] and [ð].

1. *[t]-[θ] method.* These two sounds are distinguished by their place and manner of articulation. To move from [t] to [θ], the place of articulation must be moved anteriorly. Also, the manner of articulation changes from a stop to a fricative. The client should be instructed to:

    a. *Slowly* release [t]. This should result in a friction-like sound.

    b. Maintain this friction-like quality while moving the tongue forward until its tip comes very close to the back of the front incisors. If this constriction is continued, the client should feel the air flowing over the tip of the tongue, forcing its way between the tongue and the back of the upper front teeth.

2. *[f]-[θ] method.* For this method, the place of articulation must be modified; the manner of articulation remains the same. The easiest articulation to achieve when modifying [f] to [θ] is the one with the tongue slightly protruded between the front teeth. Two different methods can be used:

    a. During the production of [f], the client pulls the bottom lip away from the upper incisors.

    b. The friction sound must continue during the placement of the tongue tip between the upper and lower incisors.

Or, during the production of [f], the client is instructed to:

    a. "Split the /f/ in half with his tongue by sticking his tongue between his teeth" (Secord, 1981b, p. 32). The goal is the release of the labiodental placement when the client places the tongue between the incisors.

    b. The friction sound must continue during the placement of the tongue.

3. *[s]-[θ] method.* If the client has an acceptable [s], this could be an easy sound modification method to use because the place of articulation is the only feature distinguishing the two sounds. During the [s]-production, the client should:

    a. Glide the tongue forward until the tip almost touches the back of the upper incisors.

    b. Feel the air flowing between the tongue tip and the back of the upper front teeth.

COARTICULATORY CONDITIONS. Because of the high-front position of the tongue during [θ] and [ð] realizations, high-front vowels offer perhaps the best coarticulatory conditions following these sounds. The back vowels with the positioning of the tongue toward the back of the mouth would not seem to aid the production. Therefore, a possible vowel sequence is high front, mid front, and low front, followed by central vowels and finally the back vowels, moving from the low- to mid- to high-back vowels.

Compared to the voiceless [θ], the voiced [ð] has a much higher frequency of occurrence in General American English. This would suggest that practice with [ð] is an important aspect of therapy.

Word Examples. The following one-syllable words are ordered from relatively easy to more difficult coarticulatory conditions for a child with [θ] and [ð] problems.

[θ] Words	[ð] Words
theme	thee - these
thin - thick - thing - think	this
theft	they
thank - thanks	them - then - their - there
thumb - thud - thug - thump	that - than - that's
third - thirst	the
thaw - thought - thawed - thong	though - those

The remaining sections describe phonetic errors that clinicians encounter less frequently. These errors include difficulties with f- and v-sounds, affricates, voicing problems, and consonant clusters.

Misarticulations of [f] and [v]

One of the earliest fricatives to emerge in the speech of children is [f]; it is usually mastered between 3 and 4 years of age. However, if sound mastery data are examined (refer to Chapter 5), the voiced [v] is consistently noted as being acquired later than its voiceless cognate. When Sander (1972) reinterpreted the data from Wellman, Case, Mengert, and Bradbury (1931) and Templin (1957), he reported that 90% of the children had mastered [f] by age 4 but only 51% had mastered [v] by that age. It was not until age 8 that 90% of the children had mastered the voiced [v]. Therefore, approximately 4 years separate similar levels of competency for [f] versus [v].

What could account for this large difference in the age of acquisition? Although differences between the mastery ages of other consonant cognates exist as well, such large age variations are noted only for [f] and [v]. Perhaps the later acquisition of [v] reflects a much lower frequency of occurrence in General American English when compared to [f]. If it is not a frequent sound, children might simply not be using it, seemingly extending the mastery age. However, frequency of occurrence data for children (Carterette & Jones, 1974) do not support this hypothesis. The frequency of occurrence for [f] and [v] is relatively similar. A second possibility is that it is not the quantity of different words but a limited number of highly frequent words with [v] that raises the frequency count. (A similar case can be made for the voiced [ð]. Its relative high frequency of occurrence can be attributed to a small number of very frequently used words, such as *the*.) Two studies (Denes & Pinson, 1973; Dewey, 1923) might support this hypothesis. These investigators found that *of* [ʌv] was among the 10 most frequently used words in General American English. Such words as *have* and *give* also seem to be fairly common words. If the frequency of occurrence according to the position in the word is examined for first-, second-, and third-grade children, the majority of [v]-sounds occur in word-final positions. These are merely possibilities to explain the differences between the reported ages of acquisition for [f] and [v]. Whatever the reason, the later age of acquisition for [v] could have clinical implications.

The previous therapeutic discussion of phonetic errors has assumed that clinicians would proceed clinically from one consonant cognate to the other. Thus, therapy with [s] would closely coincide with [z] work. The acquisition information might cause clinicians to question the validity of this procedure for [f] and [v]. Acquisition data suggest that therapy for [f] should be initiated prior to therapy for [v]. Depending on the age of the child, it might not be realistic to expect the same level of accuracy for [v]. One of the predictions established by Elbert and Gierut (1986) is that if one member of a cognate pair is achieved in therapy, improvement occurs with the other member. Interpreted with regard to the acquisition data, therapy would most often begin with [f]. However, clinicians might want to wait to see whether [v] will develop on its own. For many children, [v] acquisition appears to take place much later than the mastery of the voiceless [f].

PHONETIC DESCRIPTION.   [f] and [v] are labiodental fricatives. A constriction is created by bringing the inner edge of the lower lip into close contact with the edges of the upper incisors. If this contact is very light, the breath stream can pass between the inner edge of the lower lip and the cutting edge of the upper incisors. Firmer contact between the lower lip and upper teeth might cause the breath stream to flow around the incisors, some of the air being forced out in the region of the canine and premolar teeth. The upper lip remains inactive during [f] and [v] articulation.

TYPES OF MISARTICULATIONS

1. *[p/f] and [b/v] substitutions.* Examples of these substitutions include [pɪŋgɚ] for *finger* or [ʃʌbəl] for *shovel*. Place and manner of articulation have been modified for this substitution. The labiodental articulation is replaced by a bilabial one, and the fricative is changed to a stop-plosive.

   Phonetic transcription of the error: [p] or [b]

2. *Bilabial fricative substitution.* For this substitution, only the place of articulation has been altered from a labiodental to a bilabial production. The symbols [ɸ] and [β] are used to denote voiceless and voiced bilabial fricatives.

   Phonetic transcription of the error: [ɸ] or [β]

THERAPEUTIC SUGGESTIONS

Phonetic Placement.   To develop an awareness of the labiodental articulation, the client should "bite down" on the lower lip with the upper teeth. This probably results in the client's touching the outside edges of the lower lip. However, [f] is produced with the inside of the lower lip approximating the upper incisors. Therefore, the client should then glide the lower lip along the cutting edges of the upper teeth toward the inside of the lip, letting the lip "pop out" of the bite. When the upper incisors are lightly positioned on the inner edge of the lower lip, the client should blow, allowing air to escape between this narrow slit. If the labiodental contact is too firm, the jaw can be lowered *slightly*.

If the client realizes a [p/f] substitution, the presence of airflow should be targeted. Although the airflow for [f] is relatively weak, a light feather or a small piece of tissue placed in front of the mouth should show some movement during the entire [f]-production. This could then be contrasted to the lack of movement during the stop phase of the [p]-articulation. In isolation, producing [p] causes movement of the feather only at the very end during the plosive part of the articulation.

Video Example 9.2
In this video, a speech-language therapist demonstrates one way to achieve an [f]-production with 3-year-old Aiden. As you listen, do you notice any other speech sounds Aiden still has difficulty with?

https://www.youtube.com/watch?v = 9xAoIxsyj38

The labiodental contact is also an important aspect of the phonetic placement for the client who demonstrates a bilabial fricative ([ɸ] or [β]) substitution. Because the substitution and the target sound are both fricatives, if the labiodental positioning can be established, an acceptable [f] results. A passive method might assist in this placement. During the bilabial fricative production, the bottom lip is pushed inward with the tip of the index finger. This should position the bottom lip approximately in the right spot for [f]. When a mirror is used, this passive method offers the client visual feedback regarding the relative positioning of the lower lip and the upper incisors. In addition, auditory feedback is provided when the two different sound qualities are compared.

Sound Modification Methods

[p]-[f] method.   During the stop phase of the [p]-production, the bottom lip is pushed inward with the tip of the index finger so that air can escape. The lower lip should be positioned in such a manner that its inner edge approximates the upper incisors. Initially, maintaining the position of the index finger can serve as an aid until the client is aware of the necessary articulatory placement.

COARTICULATORY CONDITIONS.   Vowels with lip rounding, such as the back vowels (with the exception of [ɑ]), should be avoided when beginning syllable or word practice with a newly acquired [f]. Lip rounding is an unfavorable coarticulatory condition. The central vowels with r-coloring, which are often produced with lip rounding, would not provide a beneficial coarticulatory condition either. When comparing the tongue placement and the relatively closed position of the jaw during normal [f] realizations, the sequence of vowels to be considered might be high front, mid front, and low front followed by the central vowels without r-coloring. The final vowel sequence would start with the low-back vowels followed by the mid- and high-back vowels as well as central vowels with r-coloring.

Word Examples.   The following one-syllable words are ordered from relatively easy to more difficult coarticulatory conditions for a child with [f] difficulties. One-syllable words beginning with [v] are also included. However, keep in mind that a large percentage of [v]-sounds occur in the medial and final word positions.

[f] Words	[v] Words
feet - feed - feel - field	
fit - fill - fin - fig - fish - fist	Vic - Vince
fade - fail - face - fake - faint	veil - vein - vase
fed - fell - fence	vet - vest
fat - fan - fast - fact	van - Val - vamp
fun - fudge	
fought - fall - fog - false	vault
phone - phones - fold	vote
foot - full	
food - fool	
fur - fern	Vern - verb

Affricate Problems

The affricates [ʧ] and [ʤ] develop relatively late in children's speech. The reason for this could be the complexity of their production or their low frequency of occurrence in General American English. Several investigations (e.g., Carterette & Jones, 1974; Shriberg & Kwiatkowski, 1982a) analyzed the utterances of children and adults and consistently ranked both [ʧ] and [ʤ] as two of the least frequently used consonants. This is further exemplified in Olmsted's (1971) study. In spontaneous speech, only 1 of the 48 children ranging from 36 to 54 months of age in the study attempted [ʤ], and that child produced it in an aberrant manner. Although several of the acquisition studies did not test both [ʧ] and [ʤ], others (Arlt & Goodban, 1976; Prather et al., 1975; Smit, 1993b) reported that there is a somewhat later age of acquisition for [ʧ] compared to [ʤ].

PHONETIC DESCRIPTION.   Although some descriptions of affricates give the reader the idea that they are merely the stops [t] and [d] followed by the fricatives [ʃ] and [ʒ], this is not entirely accurate. Based on palatograms, Kantner and West (1960) reported two factors that differentiate isolated consonant sequences from affricate productions: (1) the initial position of the stop portion, and (2) the nature of the movement from the stop to the fricative portion of the affricates. First, the initial stop portion of [ʧ] is articulated closer to the articulatory position for [ʃ]; therefore, it is produced more posteriorly than is normally the case with an isolated [t]. Second, movement from the stop to the fricative portion of the affricate is characterized by the front of the tongue dropping relatively slowly, momentarily creating a constriction that is typical for the [ʃ]-sound. This is different from the release of an isolated [t] in which the tongue drops suddenly to a neutral position. The degree of lip rounding during the production of these affricates depends primarily on the speaker and the phonetic context.

An affricate is not merely a stop followed by a fricative production. Its realization varies in characteristic ways from the articulation of an isolated stop followed by a fricative. However, in order to simplify the directions for children, it often seems that the goal is merely to fuse the stop with the fricative. In addition, the previously reported differences between affricates versus stop plus fricative productions might prove helpful to clinicians if the resulting sound quality is perceptually still not acceptable.

TYPES OF MISARTICULATIONS

1. *[t/ʧ] and [d/ʤ] substitutions.* These misarticulations are characterized by the substitution of a stop for the affricate production. Examples include [tɝt] for *church* or [pədaməz] for *pajamas*. Because the substituted stop and the stop part of the affricate are the same, only the slow release of the stop to [ʃ] distinguishes these two speech sounds.

   Phonetic transcription of the error: [t] or [d]

2. *[ʃ/ʧ] and [ʒ/ʤ] substitutions.* A substitution of a fricative for the affricate is exemplified by [waʃ] for *watch* and [ʒʌmp] for *jump*. The lack of the initial stop portion of the affricate distinguishes this substitution from the affricate production.

   Phonetic transcription of the error: [ʃ] or [ʒ]

3. *[s/tʃ] and [z/dʒ] substitutions.* Examples of these substitutions include [pis] for *peach* and [zæm] for *jam*. This realization does not have any initial stop portion, only a fricative element. In addition, the fricative segment is articulated more anteriorly than the normal fricative portion of the affricates.

Phonetic transcription of the error: [s] or [z]

4. *[ts/tʃ] and [dz/dʒ] substitutions.* Examples for these substitutions include [tsɪp] for *chip* and [dzip] for *jeep*. The fricative element of these substitutions is too far forward.

Phonetic transcription of the error: [ts] or [dz]

THERAPEUTIC SUGGESTIONS

Phonetic Placement.   The tongue tip is placed on the posterior edge of the alveolar ridge in a manner similar to [t]. This [t] realization should be released *slowly*. It is important that the client be aware that during the release, the lateral edges of the tongue need to remain in contact with the premolars and molars, similar to a [ʃ]-production. In addition, the tongue glides slightly back during the release. The posterior movement of the tongue can be aided by pushing the tongue back with a tongue depressor during the slow release of [t].

Sound Modification Method

[t]-[tʃ] method.   The description for using this method is similar to the one explained in "Phonetic Placement" above. To achieve success with this method, it is important that the lateral edges of the tongue remain in contact with the premolars and first molars during the slow release of the [t]. If this is not the case, a [tʰʌ] quality rather than [tʃ] can result.

Secord (1981b) suggests telling "the client to practice saying /t/-/ʃ/ slowly at first, then rapidly until they blend and become one sound" (p. 41).

COARTICULATORY CONDITIONS.   Because of the anterior placement of the tongue for both the stop and the fricative portions of the affricate, the front vowels seem to offer more coarticulatory support than the back vowels. Consequently, a possible vowel sequence would be high-, mid-, and low-front vowels followed by the central vowels and the back vowels. The back vowels, however, offer two advantages: (1) the lip rounding, especially of the high-back vowels, might provide

---

Clinical Exercises The following examples are from word cards that can be purchased for use in therapy. These are the words for "ch":

Initial: chair, chalkboard, chocolate, cherry pie, chicken, Chinese food, cheerleaders, children, cheese, chimpanzee

Medial: high chair, poncho, beach ball, wheelchair, nachos, teacher, enchilada, peaches, pitcher

Final: beach, coach, wrench, ostrich, sandwich, witch, watch, bench, lunch

Which of the words would you want to eliminate at the beginning of therapy work on [tʃ] because the target sound is in a consonant cluster? Rank the remaining words from easiest to more difficult coarticulatory conditions.

coarticulatory support for the lip rounding noted in the [tʃ]-production, and (2) the back positioning of the tongue for the back vowels might enhance the backward gliding movement of the tongue in its transition from stop-plosive to the fricative portion of the affricate. If this proves to aid the production of [tʃ] in a given case, the vowel sequence might be the high-, mid-, and low-back vowels followed by the central vowels and the front vowels. Clinicians should use probes to determine which vowel sequence would be more beneficial for their client.

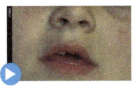

Video Tool Exercise 9.1
Five-Year-Old Hope
Complete the activity
based on this video.

Word Examples. The following one-syllable words are ordered from relatively easy to more difficult coarticulatory conditions for a child with an affricate problem. In this case, affricate-vowel probes demonstrated that the back vowels offer better coarticulatory conditions than the front vowels.

[tʃ] Words	[dʒ] Words
chew - choose	June - juice
choke - chore - chose	Joe - joke - Joan
chalk - chop - chopped - chops	jaw - jog - jar - job - John - jaws
chirp - churn	jerk - germ
Chuck - chug - chum - chunk	jug - junk - jump - jumped
chat - champ - chance	Jack - jam - jab
check - Chet	gem - jet - Jeff
chain - chase	jay - Jane
chick - chin - chill - chips	Jim - Jill
cheek - cheep - cheese - cheat - chief	gee - jeep - Gene - jeans

Voicing Problems

Voicing problems manifest themselves in the substitution of a voiced cognate for a voiceless cognate, such as [du] for *two*, or a voiceless cognate for a voiced cognate, such as when *ball* is pronounced as [pɑl]. Voicing has phonemic value in General American English. Different word meanings are established by the presence or absence of a voicing component. This can be exemplified by the minimal pairs *face* and *vase* and *tot* and *dot*. Because of its phonemic relevance, a voicing problem should trigger evaluation to determine whether a phonological disorder exists.

Several authors (e.g., Grunwell, 1987; Smit & Bernthal, 1983; Smith, 1979) have noted that children at age 4 still show difficulties with certain aspects of voicing. The most common pattern is the voiced production of normally voiceless stops, fricatives, and affricates initiating a syllable or word (prevocalic voicing). Thus, *toe* and *soup* might be pronounced as [doʊ] and [zup]. In addition, voiceless cognates are substituted for their voiced counterparts terminating a word or syllable (postvocalic devoicing); that is, *cub* becomes [kʌp] and *dog* becomes [dɑk]. *Context-sensitive voicing* is a term used to refer to these types of voicing errors. According to Grunwell (1987), context-sensitive voicing, especially postvocalic devoicing, continues in some children beyond 3 years of age.

Specific factors that need to be appraised before implementing therapy for difficulties with consonant voicing–devoicing include the frequency of occurrence in the client's speech and the contexts in which the voicing–devoicing occurs. First, the voicing–devoicing difficulties should occur at a relatively high frequency before therapy is implemented. Second, some specific contextual modifications resulting in devoicing are commonly heard in General American English; these modifications would not be considered misarticulations. For example, devoicing final consonants and assimilations of voicelessness are common (Abercrombie, 1967). Devoicing final consonants can be found most often before a pause. Therefore, devoicing final consonants could be realized during a standardized speech assessment as well as in spontaneous speech samples. The author's clinical experience has shown that final devoicing often occurs on plurals that end in [əz]: *matches* is pronounced as [mætʃəs] and *dishes* as [dɪʃəs]. Assimilations of voicelessness can be either progressive or regressive. During an utterance, these assimilations can often be heard if a voiceless consonant precedes or follows a voiced stop, fricative, or affricate. For example, we pronounce *news* as [nuz]. However, *news* is typically pronounced [nus] in the word *newspaper*. This devoicing of [z] is a regressive assimilation influenced by the following voiceless [p]. Although these types of sound change in context are common, they must be evaluated in relationship to their frequency of occurrence for a particular client. If the frequency is so high that intelligibility is affected, even these "normal" modifications might warrant therapy.

THERAPEUTIC SUGGESTIONS. Probably all children use some voicing distinctions in their speech. The task is to create an awareness of voicing versus lack of voicing for a particular cognate pair. The following guidelines can be supplemented with auditory discrimination exercises to enhance the general awareness of voicing versus devoicing. Minimal pair words that target the particular voicing–devoicing cognate difficulty can also be used.

The following sequencing of auditory discrimination exercises is suggested:

1. Aid a client's general awareness of the presence or absence of voicing by having her or him listen to two sounds—[s] and [z], for example—and identify which one is voiced. This could be combined with the tactile feedback method, which is explained below.

2. Place the cognates in minimally paired words and ask the client to identify voiced versus voiceless sounds at the beginning or end of a word. Word pair discrimination exercises would use the particular consonant cognates and the position of these sounds in words that are problematic for the client. If a client has trouble with devoicing the final stops, word pairs such as *cap* versus *cab* and *lock* versus *log* could be identified.

Tactile Feedback Method. This method develops a client's awareness of the vibratory sensation associated with voicing. This is then contrasted with the lack of vibration present during voiceless sounds. Clients place their fingers on or slightly above the thyroid cartilage during the production of a voiced sound. Attention should be directed to the vibration that is felt. For children, this vibration can be compared to a motor being "on" during voiced consonants versus "off" during unvoiced consonants. This method works well with fricatives and affricates but is difficult to implement with stop-plosives. The natural tendency to add a vowel after the production of stop sounds can trigger the feeling of vibration on unvoiced stop sounds. Actually, the vibration for the vowel *follows* the stop production, but many children will not be able to discern this. A clinician who decides to implement the tactile feedback method for establishing an awareness of voiced versus voiceless stop-plosives should instruct a child to whisper the stop to attain a voiceless realization while saying the voiced cognate with a "big (loud) voice." This should eliminate the voicing influence of the following vowel on the voiceless stop.

Auditory Enhancement Method. This method enhances the humming effect heard during the production of voiced consonants. The client's hands are cupped and placed over the ears. During the production of voiced consonants, the client should hear a humming not present during the production of voiceless consonants. A similar effect can be achieved by plugging each ear with an index finger. Difficulties could arise when using this method to discriminate between voiced and voiceless stops; the instructions noted in the tactile feedback method should be followed here as well.

Whispering Method.   If a child produces a voiced consonant and its voiceless cognate is the goal, the clinician can have the child whisper the sound. As with all previously noted methods, this one is implemented only until the client understands the distinction between voiced and voiceless productions.

Singing Method.   This method is implemented for clients who can produce a voiceless consonant but where the goal is its voiced cognate. Here, the client "sings" the voiceless consonant. A familiar melody such as "Happy Birthday" is sung with the voiceless consonant combined with the [ʌ] vowel replacing the words: [pʌpʌpʌpʌpʌpʌ]. If the client continues to sing—that is, to produce continuous voicing—the voiceless consonant becomes voiced. If this is accomplished, the client is made aware of the voiced production, which can then be isolated from the tune.

Developing Voiced Stop Productions.   This technique is a sound modification method. It modifies the voiced stop-plosives from the nasals [m], [n], and [ŋ]. The author's clinical experience has shown that this technique is often surprisingly effective if one of the previously mentioned methods has failed. During the nasal production, the nostrils are pinched closed. The client releases the air orally. If the voicing of the nasal continues, [b] should result from [m], [d] from [n], and [g] from [ŋ]. The success of this technique depends on the continuation of the voicing component of the nasal sounds.

Consonant Cluster Problems

For some children, the acquisition of consonant clusters can extend into the beginning school years. Smit (1993a) reported that it was not until children were 9 years of age that all consonant clusters were realized in a regular manner. Children also seem to go through certain stages in acquiring consonant clusters (refer to Chapter 5). Consonant cluster reduction and substitution are two processes that describe these stages. One of the earliest stages in a child's attempt to produce consonant clusters is consonant cluster reduction. This is exemplified by the production of [dʌm] for *drum*. Typically, though not always, the marked member of the cluster is the one that is deleted (Ingram, 1989b). The next phase in acquiring clusters is a consonant cluster substitution, which is demonstrated when [dwʌm] is realized for *drum*. The last phase is the regular articulation of the consonant cluster.

According to the phonotactics of General American English, most consonants can be members of a consonant cluster. Consonant clusters at the end of a word are often used to signal certain linguistic functions such as plurality (exemplified by *dogs*), third-person singular tense (as in *kicks*), past tense (as in *kicked*), and possessives (as in *Jack's*). At the spontaneous speech level, any consonant cluster can occur. Therefore, the treatment of consonant clusters often is one stage of a therapy program.

THERAPEUTIC SUGGESTIONS.   In General American English, consonant clusters consist of either two or three consonants in word-initial position and from two to four consonants in word-final position. Consonant clusters with only two consonants are typically easier to produce than those with three or four.

Production of Word-Initial Clusters

Epenthesis. During the acquisition of clusters, children often insert a schwa between the two consonants. This process is referred to as **epenthesis**. Epenthesis can be used to aid a client's production of a cluster. If the cluster is [sk], as in *skate*, the client starts with [səkeɪt]. At first, the word should be pronounced slowly so that the schwa is somewhat prolonged. After a period of practice, the client attempts to shorten the schwa vowel gradually. This can often be achieved by increasing the tempo of the entire word. The end result should be a smooth transition from the first to the second consonant.

Pausing. For this method, a pause is inserted between the first and second members of the consonant cluster. Using the previous example, [sk] becomes [s] (pause) [keɪt]. After a period of practice, the client again shortens the pause between the two consonants. The author's clinical experience has shown that visual feedback in the form of a drawn line or gestures can often aid children in shortening this pause. For example, a long line is drawn and then is successively shortened, or the clinician can start with hands outspread and move them closer and closer together to indicate a shorter pause. Because of the natural pause that occurs between two syllables, this method is especially effective for consonant clusters that could occur across syllable boundaries, such as [ns] in *answer* or *pencil.*

Production of Word-Final Clusters

Prolonging the First Element of the Final Cluster. This method is best suited for clusters whose first element can be prolonged easily, such as the fricatives, affricates, nasals, or approximants [l] and [ɹ]. The first sound is prolonged for about 2 seconds and is then followed by the second element of the cluster, as in *nest*: "sssssssss-t" for [st]. With repeated practice, the prolongation of the first sound is successively shortened.

Pausing. This technique presents itself as a possibility if the first element of the consonant cluster is a stop-plosive. The instructions are similar to those described for initial consonant clusters.

Production of Word-Medial Clusters. Many word-medial clusters, especially two-consonant clusters, occur across syllable boundaries, as in *base-ball* or *an-swer*. Other clusters can be found initiating a syllable, as in *ze-bra* or *A-pril*. Although common pronunciations do not syllabify these clusters between the two elements, for therapeutic purposes they could be artificially divided into *zeb-ra* or *Ap-ril*. The previously mentioned pausing method could be easily implemented by inserting a pause between the two syllables. This pause could first be lengthened and then shortened as the client gains stability of production.

COARTICULATORY CONDITIONS. Three variables should be considered when working on consonant clusters: (1) the length of the cluster, (2) the position of the cluster in the word, and (3) the coarticulation between the specific elements of the cluster.

The *length of the cluster* refers to how many individual consonants form the cluster. Typically, the fewer the consonants, the easier the cluster is for the client. Therefore, consonant clusters with two elements should be attempted prior to those with three elements.

The *position of the cluster in the word* refers to whether the cluster initiates the word, terminates it, or occurs somewhere in the middle. Although most clinicians begin with clusters initiating the word, medial clusters offer some positive features. The "natural" pause between two syllables can be used to separate the cluster into two discrete elements: For example, the [ns] cluster in *pencil* is divided into *pen-cil*. Again, this pause is at first prolonged and later shortened. This procedure gives the client time in a relatively natural word situation to produce the transition between the elements of the cluster. Inserting a pause can also be used for clusters that typically are not syllabified between the two elements. If the consonant cluster [st] is selected, practice could include *Eas-ter, toas-ter*, and *roos-ter*, for example. If the client can produce the cluster without a pause between the syllables, it can then be transferred to the word-initiating position. The client would be instructed to whisper the first part of the word, saying the last *-ster* portion in a louder voice. This necessitates changing the syllable boundary from between the cluster, *s-t*, to initiating the cluster, *st-*. However, if the client can make this transition, the consonant cluster now stands at the beginning of a word, *stir*. A similar technique can be used to gain word-final consonant clusters. In this case, the last *-er* portion of the word is whispered, which results in *east* (from *Easter*), *toast* (from *toaster*), and *roost* (from *rooster*).

A disadvantage of using the clusters medially is that the client must deal with a two-syllable rather than a one-syllable word. If more difficulty is noted when the client has to articulate a two-syllable word, this technique loses its appeal. Both word-initiating and word-terminating consonant clusters should then be practiced in one-syllable word contexts. Words for [st] practice could include *star* and *stone* or *nest* and *lost*. As with all stages of therapy, the clinician needs to establish which sequence offers more favorable effects for each individual client.

The third factor to be considered is the *coarticulation between the specific elements of the cluster*. Given a specific target sound in the cluster, certain sound combinations could be easier to produce than others. For example, if the target sound is [s], consider the consonant cluster [sk], as in *skate*, versus [sp], as in *spot*. For [sk], the tongue must move quickly from a front approximation of the articulators to a stop closure involving the back of the tongue. With [sp], on the other hand, the [p] element can be articulated with very little or no tongue movement from the [s] position. When the coarticulation features are considered, [sp] appears easier to articulate than [sk].

Certain consonant clusters might also need to be carefully evaluated based on the original misarticulation. For a child who originally demonstrated a lateral [s], clusters with [l], a lateral sound, might trigger the old misarticulation, for example. Or, for the child who originally had a [t] for [k] substitution, the word-final cluster [kt], as in *kicked* or *locked*, might prove troublesome.

In addition, specific techniques used to elicit the correct production of a specific sound can be reinforced by selecting certain consonant clusters. If the

Clinical Exercises You have been working with Anna, who had a lateral s-problem. You are now ready to work on consonant clusters. Based on the principles mentioned previously, rank the following clusters from easy to hard: [sp, st, stɹ, sl, sw, sk, skɹ, stɹ, sm, sn].

[k] clusters in both the word-initial and word-final positions are listed in Table 9.7. Rank those clusters from easy to hard.

[t]-[s] method was used to establish [s], the cluster [ts] used at the beginning of therapy might reinforce the [s]-production. Similarly, a clinician who has established an acceptable [ɹ] realization by means of the [d]-[ɹ] method might use the consonant cluster [dɹ] to aid in stabilizing [ɹ] during the initial stages of therapy.

The preceding guidelines have been provided to suggest, not dictate, clinical decision making. The choice of the cluster and the sequencing of clusters in the therapy program depend on the needs and the articulatory possibilities of an individual client. However, one task of a clinician is to understand and consider the factors that could have a positive or negative influence on the production of a specific target sound. This understanding increases the efficacy of therapy.

Group Therapy with the Traditional Motor Approach

In many speech-language therapy positions, the clinician has the opportunity to work one-on-one with a client. University clinics, hospitals, and private practice, for example, usually offer these opportunities. However, for clinicians working in public schools—and more than 50% of speech-language therapists do (ASHA, 2013)—group therapy must be incorporated into their sessions. The following are a few suggestions for clinicians working with speech sound disorders in a group setting.

First, it is a good idea to group the clients according to grade levels. Even if a child in kindergarten and one in first grade have similar goals, the differences at this young age are large. With older children (e.g., fifth grade and middle school), it might be possible to group them according to similar grades. For example, a group of sixth- and seventh-graders would probably be functional, whereas a group of sixth- and eighth-graders would be problematic. Occasionally, you will have a student who is mature or immature for the particular grade level, and the grouping could be adjusted accordingly. However, students enjoy being with other members of their grade, and activities can be at the same level when these students are grouped together.

Second, limit the number of children in each group. Groups of two students are best; a group of three is still feasible. When four or more students are in one group, the author has found that, even with middle school students, problems occur. When you have larger groups, it is very easy for the students to be unruly. Remember that the reason students typically enjoy speech therapy is that it is fun. They get to interact and do interesting activities. When discipline becomes a continual issue, the fun is gone, and students withdraw from therapy. They make up excuses for not going to therapy, they sit in therapy and don't talk, and they complain. This is not a conducive atmosphere for speech services. Also, keep in mind that from about fifth grade on, speech therapy becomes a chore. Students are often teased about going to "speech" (although bullying is supposed to be totally unacceptable), or they feel "different," singled out. At fifth-grade age, being part of the group is very important. This is another reason why it is essential to address speech sound disorders as early as possible and dismiss the child from services. As a last note, most speech-language therapy sessions in public schools last 25 to 30 minutes. If you have four students in a group and alternate between them, this means that each student has a total of 6 to 7 minutes of individual time per session. That is certainly not much time for changing speech behavior.

Third, if possible, put students with similar speech sound disorders in one group. If you have two or three second-graders who are still working on r-sounds, they would make a great group. Again, that might not be possible. However, a group can function if all members have different speech sound disorders. It is important that students know what sound they are working on. A therapy session can begin by all students stating the sound that is their goal. It is often surprising that, after months in therapy, some children still might not know why they are in speech services. If they do not know "their" sound, a clinician cannot expect that there will be any conscious carryover to the classroom. You can have a group with one student working on some language goals; this just takes a bit more planning. However, it is difficult to put students with fluency problems and children who are autistic in a group of students with speech sound disorders. Children who are autistic should be put in a group of students who are not autistic, if possible. Social interaction with other nonautistic children is often very beneficial.

During a school year, a clinician will continually be evaluating new students, and some children, especially those in kindergarten and first grade, will come to speech services with articulation-based speech sound disorders. It is perhaps a good idea to see a child who cannot produce a target sound individually until the goal sound can at least be produced in some type of syllable, either a nonsense syllable or simple CV words such as "see" for [s] or "ray" for [ɹ]. There are two reasons for this. First, the child who is trying to acquire a new sound needs a clinician's constant and undivided attention to try to position the articulators, and the clinician is possibly trying to find facilitating contexts and give feedback on the correct and incorrect sound productions. This is very hard to do in a group. Second, a child might be very self-conscious about the speech sound error, and therapy is difficult to complete in front of a group of fellow students. If the clinician's time is restricted due to a very large caseload, the clinician might say, "I really don't have time for individual therapy." One possible approach to dealing with a child individually would be to take the child out of class, sit somewhere close to the classroom (speech therapy rooms are often on the outskirts of the campus, and the walk back and forth could take more than 5 minutes), and try to get the sound in isolation for 5 minutes. If a clinician attempts this procedure for even a very limited amount of time every day for a week, often enough progress can be made to move the student into a group after that week. Clinicians should continue to look for facilitating contexts. Those contexts are true shortcuts to word production with a particular sound.

It is the clinician's task to know the exact level at which each child in each group is working. Is the child at the CV, CVC level, or has the child progressed to short carrier sentences or even short spontaneous sentences? *It is critically important to keep notes on every therapy session.* You could have a list of words that seem to be good possibilities and then jot down the word with a + or − depending on the student's production accuracy. From the author's experience, the best approach is to have a sheet for each child. The date can be written at the margin and the words written in with a + or − for each therapy session. This log can be used later to document progress when speech "report cards" are needed. In public schools, these are usually prepared at the same time that classroom report cards or progress reports are given to the parents. If you have no notes, these progress reports become guesswork and therefore meaningless.

What type of activities lend themselves to group work? One possibility is a set of games from which one child in the group picks each therapy session. (Some favorites for even second-graders are Chutes and Ladders, Candyland, and Monkeying Around.) These must be games that do not require a lot of time to set up or take turns. The students enjoy choosing a game and often keep very close track of whose turn it is to pick. Turns move from one child to the next. The goal is to get as many productions from a student as possible in one 30-minute session. One possibility is to have the student repeat each word at least 10 times before taking a turn, make up 4 sentences with a specific word, or use his or her sound in spontaneous sentences for 30 seconds. The possibilities for activities are only as limited as your imagination. Although tempting, clinicians should use published packs of word cards with care. They are boring, and students tire quickly of just looking at a picture and saying the word. As noted earlier, these word cards range from coarticulatory conditions that are easy to very difficult. This is also true for workbooks for particular sounds, which have pages and pages that can be copied and distributed. These also are boring and do not have the words ordered according to any type of phonetic principles.

Again, clinicians should try to keep speech therapy services fun. Students should be praised and rewarded when they are doing a good job. One idea is to give each child a small, colorful sheet of paper with his or her name on it. Staple it to the bulletin board and stamp it at the end of every therapy session (stickers take too much time). A child who accumulates a certain number of stamps can choose a prize from a treasure chest. This has proven to be a real incentive for children up to fourth grade.

Summary

This chapter first defined the phonetic (traditional motor) approach to the treatment of articulation disorders, which focuses on placement of the articulators in such a manner as to achieve an acceptable articulation of the sound in question. A sequence for therapy was outlined, including sensory-perceptual training and beginning at the sound level, systematically moving to more complex articulatory conditions. Dismissal criteria were also suggested in the first portion of this chapter.

An overview of principles of motor learning was also included. These principles are important to guide the clinician through any type of treatment process. They provide a framework for conditions of practice and feedback that have documented efficacy.

Misarticulations of several consonants were discussed in detail in the second part of this chapter. These consonants represent the most frequently misarticulated speech sounds: [s] and [z], [ʃ] and [ʒ], [k] and [g], [l], [ɹ] and the central vowels with r-coloring, and [θ] and [ð]. Other sound problems included misarticulations of [f] and [v], the affricates [tʃ] and [ʤ], voiced and voiceless substitutions, and consonant clusters. When applicable, phonetic placement as well as sound modification techniques were described. In addition, effects of coarticulation were examined for each noted problem.

Therapy with a group of students is often necessary. The final section of this chapter examined some possibilities for group therapy. Suggestions of how to structure the groups were given, and examples of activities were provided.

Any successful application of the traditional motor approach to articulation therapy presupposes a firm knowledge base not only of the phonetic characteristics of the sound's typical realization but also of the misarticulated sound. An attempt has been made to provide both in this chapter.

Case Study

The following are results from the Arizona Articulatory Proficiency Scale for Lori, age 7 years 6 months.

1. horse	[hoɚθ]	18. pig	[pɪg]	35. this	[ðɪθ]
2. wagon	[wægən]	19. cup	[kʌp]	36. whistle	[wɪθəl]
3. red	[ɹɛd]	20. car	[kɑɚ]	37. chair	[tɛɚ]
4. comb	[koʊm]	21. ear	[ɪɚ]	38. watch	[wat]
5. fork	[foɚk]	22. swing	[θwɪŋ]	39. thumb	[θʌm]
6. knife	[naɪf]	23. table	[teɪbəl]	40. mouth	[maʊθ]
7. cow	[kaʊ]	24. cat	[kæt]	41. shoe	[ʃu]
8. cake	[keɪk]	25. ladder	[lærɚ]	42. fish	[fɪʃ]
9. baby	[beɪbi]	26. ball	[bɑl]	43. zipper	[ðɪpɚ]
10. bathtub	[bæθtəb]	27. airplane	[ɛɚpleɪn]	44. nose	[noʊð]
11. nine	[naɪn]	28. cold	[koʊld]	45. sun	[θʌn]
12. train	[tɹeɪn]	29. jumping	[dʌmpɪŋ]	46. house	[haʊθ]
13. gum	[gʌm]	30. television	[tɛləvɪzən]	47. steps	[s̪tɛpθ]
14. dog	[dɑg]	31. stove	[s̪toʊv]	48. nest	[nɛst]
15. yellow	[jɛloʊ]	32. ring	[ɹɪŋ]	49. carrots	[kɛɚəts]
16. doll	[dɑl]	33. tree	[tɹi]	50. books	[bʊkθ]
17. bird	[bɝd]	34. green	[gɹin]		

Lori demonstrates difficulties with [s], [tʃ], and [dʒ]. If you analyze the patterns for [s]-production, you find that she substitutes [θ] for [s] and [ð] for [z] in most words. However, she dentalizes [s] when it occurs at the beginning of a word with [t] (refer to *steps* and *stove*). Facilitating contexts can be noted at the end of a word in which [s] is produced correctly in [s] + [t] or [t] + [s] blends (refer to *nest* and *carrots*). It seems as if the combination with [t] produces coarticulatory conditions that are favorable for [s]. Although [s] is a sound that develops later than [tʃ] or [dʒ], these facilitating contexts could be used initially to begin work on [s]. In addition, [s] is a sound that occurs frequently in General American English.

Think Critically

1. You are working with a 7-year-old child, Larry, who has a [θ] for [s] substitution (as well as a [ð] for [z] substitution). He seems unable to distinguish between /s/ and /z/ when used in minimal pairs with voiced and voiceless "th." Based on his errors and his lack of discrimination abilities, construct a sensory-perceptual training program using identification, isolation, stimulation, and discrimination. Try to be as specific as possible about the targets you would use for each of the phases.

2. Maureen, age 7 years 6 months, shows evidence of consistent dentalized [s̪] and [z̪] productions for [s] and [z] in all contexts. You cannot find facilitating contexts and have decided to do phonetic placement with the child. Describe

the advantages and disadvantages of using a tongue-tip-up versus a tongue-tip-down production. Select one of the phonetic placement techniques and describe step-by-step how you would explain the tongue placement and what the child would need to do to achieve a correct [s]-production.

3. Molly has a [w] for [ɹ] substitution. Describe in detail the steps you would complete to achieve an [ɹ]-production using the phonetic placement technique for the retroflexed [ɹ].

✅ **Chapter Quiz 9.1** Complete this quiz to check your understanding of chapter concepts.

Appendix 9.1 Minimal Word-Pairs with Frequently Misarticulated Sounds

Minimal Pair Words and Sentences Contrasting /s/ and /z/ to /θ/ and /ð/

/s/ and /z/

/s/ versus /θ/		/z/ versus /ð/		/s/ versus /θ/		/z/ versus /ð/	
sank	thank	Zen	then	bass	bath	breeze	breathe
sick	thick			Bess	Beth	close	clothe
sink	think			face	faith	seize	seethe
sing	thing			mass	math	she's	sheathe
saw	thaw			miss	myth	Sue's	soothe
sigh	thigh			moss	moth	tease	teethe
sin	thin			mouse	mouth		
song	thong			pass	path		
sought	thought						
sum	thumb						

He was *sicker* after dinner.
He was *thicker* after dinner.

He had to *saw* the pipes.
He had to *thaw* the pipes.

The captain was *sinking*.
The captain was *thinking*.

Something was wrong with his *sum*.
Something was wrong with his *thumb*.

Did he *breeze* close by her?
Did he *breathe* close by her?

They walked by the *closing* store.
They walked by the *clothing* store.

There's a strange-looking *moss* on the tree.
There's a strange-looking *moth* on the tree.

The boy had a big *mouse*.
The boy had a big *mouth*.

Minimal Pair Words and Sentences Contrasting /s/ and /z/ to /t/ and /d/

/s/ versus /t/		/s/ versus /t/		/z/ versus /d/		/z/ versus /d/	
sell	tell	ace	ate	Z	D	as	add
cent	tent	base	bait	zing	ding	bees	bead
sack	tack	brass	brat	zip	dip	buzz	bud
sag	tag	case	Kate	zoo	do	cries	cried

sail	tail	kiss	kit	zoom	doom	dries	dried
sank	tank	hiss	hit	zipper	dipper	knees	need
sea	tea	lice	light			rose	rode
seam	team	mice	might			size	side
sew	toe	nice	night			toes	towed
sip	tip	peace	Pete			ways	wade
sock	talk	rice	write			trays	trade

He wanted to *sell* his story.
He wanted to *tell* his story.

The *seam* was split.
The *team* was split.

He thought it was *nice*.
He thought it was *night*.

She gave him a large *kiss*.
She gave him a large *kit*.

He looked at the big *zipper*.
He looked at the big *dipper*.

The airplane *zipped* through the clouds.
The airplane *dipped* through the clouds.

It wasn't the right *size*.
It wasn't the right *side*.

The *bees* can't be lost.
The *bead* can't be lost.

/ʃ/ and /ʒ/

Minimal Pair Words and Sentences Contrasting /ʃ/ and /ʒ/ to /s/ and /z/

/ʃ/ versus /s/		/ʒ/ versus /z/	/ʃ/ versus /s/		/ʒ/ versus /z/
shack	sack	No words found	bash	bass	No words found
shag	sag		clash	class	
shame	same		gash	gas	
shave	save		leash	lease	
she	see		mesh	mess	
shed	said		plush	plus	
sheep	seep				
sheet	seat				
shell	cell				
shine	sign				
ship	sip				
shock	sock				
shoe	Sue				
shoot	suit				
show	sew				
shy	sigh				

What a *shine*!
What a *sign*!

The *shell* was very small.
The *cell* was very small.

It was a large *shock*.
It was a large *sock*.

It was a big *bash*.
It was a big *bass*.

He broke the *leash*.
He broke the *lease*.

The *clash* was over.
The *class* was over.

Minimal Pair Words and Sentences Contrasting /ʃ/ and /ʒ/ to /t/ and /d/

/ʃ/ versus /t/		/ʒ/ versus /d/	/ʃ/ versus /t/		/ʒ/ versus /d/	
shack	tack	No words found	bash	bat	rouge	rude
shag	tag		cash	cat	beige	bade
shake	take		fish	fit		
shape	tape		flash	flat		
sharp	tarp		hash	hat		
she	tea		mash	mat		
shed	ted		rash	rat		
shell	tell		rush	rut		
ship	tip		wish	wit		
shop	top					
shoe	two					
shoot	toot					

He found a large *shack* in the woods.
He found a large *tack* in the woods.

The *ship* was broken.
The *tip* was broken.

He tried to *shake* it.
He tried to *take* it.

It was a long *shape*.
It was a long *tape*.

She had a funny *wish*.
She had a funny *wit*.

He couldn't find his *cash*.
He couldn't find his *cat*.

What a *fish* he had!
What a *fit* he had!

It was a large *flash*.
It was a large *flat*.

/k/ and /g/

Minimal Pair Words and Sentences Contrasting /k/ and /g/ to /t/ and /d/

/k/ versus /t/		/k/ versus /t/		/g/ versus /d/		/g/ versus /d/	
cake	take	ache	ate	gate	date	bag	bad
cop	top	back	bat	gown	down	beg	bed
cape	tape	bake	bait	go	doe	bug	bud
cub	tub	beak	beat	got	dot	leg	led
key	tea	bike	bite	gull	dull	sag	sad
kite	tight	knock	knot				
cool	tool	lake	late				
car	tar	like	light				
corn	torn	neck	net				

They didn't like the cold *coast*. They didn't like the cold *toast*.	The *cub* was small. The *tub* was small.	They had a *bake* sale. They had a *bait* sale.
The teacher *caught* the boy. The teacher *taught* the boy.	The *gate* was fixed. The *date* was fixed.	He twisted his *neck*. He twisted his *net*.
He was stuck in the *car*. He was stuck in the *tar*.	There is a scratch on her *back*. There is a scratch on her *bat*.	He *likes* it. He *lights* it.
Hand me the *key*. Hand me the *tea*.	The *lock* was big. The *lot* was big.	Her big brother made her *beg*. Her big brother made her *bed*.

Minimal Pair Words and Sentences Contrasting /l/ to /ɹ/, /ɚ/, /w/, and /j/

/l/

/l/ versus /ɹ/		/l/ versus /ɚ/		/l/ versus /w/		/l/ versus /j/	
lace	race	bowl	boar	lag	wag	lung	young
lane	rain	Dale	dare	life	wife	loose	use
led	red	feel	fear	lake	wake	lard	yard
lick	Rick	male	mare	leave	weave	Lou	you
long	wrong	mole	more	leap	weep	less	yes
lie	rye	owl	our	leak	weak	let	yet
light	right	tile	tire	light	white		
lead	read			let	wet		
lock	rock						

She knew it was the *long* way home. She knew it was the *wrong* way home.	She didn't want to *leave*. She didn't want to *weave*.
He stumbled on the *lock*. He stumbled on the *rock*.	*Lou* cannot come to the party. *You* cannot come to the party.
What a *deal*! What a *dear*!	It was a *light* coat. It was a *white* coat.
The *tile* needed to be replaced. The *tire* needed to be replaced.	The *lung* fish swam in the aquarium. The *young* fish swam in the aquarium.

Minimal Pair Words and Sentences Contrasting /ɹ/ and /ɝ/ with /l/, /w/, and /j/

/ɹ/, /ɝ/, and /ɚ/

/ɹ/ versus /l/		/ɚ/ versus /l/		/ɹ/ versus /w/		/ɹ/ versus /j/	
race	lace	boar	bowl	rag	wag	rung	young
rain	lane	dare	Dale	rail	whale	ram	yam
red	led	fear	feel	rake	wake	rank	yank

Rick	lick	mare	male	rate	wait	rot	yacht
wrong	long	more	mole	red	wed	rear	year
rye	lie	our	owl	ray	way	roar	you're
right	light	tire	tile	right	white		
read	lead			rent	went		
rock	lock			ring	wing		
				ripe	wipe		
				ride	wide		
				raced	waste		
				rest	west		
				round	wound		
				rake	wake		
				run	won		

It was a long *rain*.
It was a long *lane*.

She won the *race* at the county fair.
She won the *lace* at the county fair.

He walked to the *right*.
He walked to the *light*.

He *feels* the earthquake.
He *fears* the earthquake.

Across the field ran a large *mare*.
Across the field ran a large *male*.

The *ring* was broken.
The *wing* was broken.

The athletes always *run*.
The athletes always *won*.

She didn't want to *rake* it up.
She didn't want to *wake* it up.

The *rot* was moldy and damp.
The *yacht* was moldy and damp.

Roar loud, he said.
You're loud, he said.

Minimal Pair Words and Sentences Contrasting /θ/ and /ð/ to /s/ and /z/, /t/ and /d/, and /f / and /v/

/θ/and /ð/

/θ/ versus /s/		/θ/ versus /s/		/ð/ versus /z/		/ð/ versus /z/	
thank	sank	Beth	Bess	then	Zen	clothe	close
thick	sick	faith	face			teethe	tease
thin	sin	path	pass			breathe	breeze
think	sink	mouth	mouse				
thinner	sinner	myth	miss				

/θ/ versus /t/		/θ/ versus /t/		/ð/ versus /d/		/θ/ versus /d/	
thank	tank	bath	bat	than	Dan	breathe	breed
thick	tick	Beth	bet	then	den	loathe	load
thin	tin	math	mat	though	dough		
thought	taught	tooth	toot	thine	dine		
		path	pat				

/θ/ versus /f/		/ð/ versus /v/		
thin	fin	than	van	
		that	vat	
		thine	vine	

The fog was *thickening*.
The fog was *sickening*.

They walked by the *clothing* store.
They walked by the *closing* store.

It hurts when children *teethe*.
It hurts when children *tease*.

She couldn't *breathe* through the testing, so she left.
She couldn't *breeze* through the testing, so she left.

Chapter 10
Treatment of Phonological Disorders

⌄ Learning Objectives

When you have finished this chapter, you should be able to:

10.1 Define minimal pair therapy exemplified by minimal opposition contrast therapy and multiple oppositions, noting target selection and intervention.

10.2 Explain minimal pair target selection represented by maximal oppositions and the complexity approach.

10.3 Characterize the cycles phonological remediation approach, its goals, and therapeutic progression.

10.4 Understand evaluation procedures to determine an inconsistent speech disorder and how to implement the resulting core vocabulary approach.

10.5 Describe metaphon therapy as a phonological awareness approach to treating phonological disorders in preschool children.

10.6 Identify speech sound disorders with concurrent language problems, specifically the treatment of morphosyntax, vocabulary, and the child with emerging phonology.

10.7 Analyze vowel errors and prepare an intervention program.

Chapter Application: Case Study

Oscar, age 4 years 5 months, had just been evaluated at the clinic. Now he was going to be part of John's caseload. Oscar had been diagnosed as having a moderate to severe consistent phonological disorder. That diagnosis and the multitude of speech sound errors he demonstrated made the sound-by-sound approach out of the question. Oscar's intelligibility was poor, and several phonological processes were noted in his speech. Most of the fricative sounds were articulated as stops, a considerable number of final consonants were deleted, syllable reductions were present on two- and three-syllable words, and he did not seem able to produce any consonant clusters. In addition, Oscar had expressive language difficulties. John was overwhelmed. Which type of therapy should John use and where should he begin?

This is a question that many clinicians face. There are many possibilities for phonological treatment, but each option is intended for specific children with various degrees of severity. In addition, all of the treatment approaches are structured differently and have distinctive ways to select targets for intervention. This chapter attempts to guide a clinician through this process with different treatment protocols (including combining phonology with language problems) for phonological intervention.

THIS CHAPTER focuses on phonological approaches to treatment. Fey (1992) lists the following three basic principles underlying most of these approaches:

1. *Groups of sounds with similar patterns of errors are targeted.* In direct contrast to treating individual sounds in a sequential order, patterns of errors are noted, and selected targets are chosen for therapy.
2. *Phonemic contrasts that were previously neutralized are established.* Many of the phonemic-based treatment methods use minimal pairs to contrast phonemic oppositions. If these distinctions can be made, the assumption is that the child will generalize this knowledge to other contrasts.
3. *A naturalistic communicative context is emphasized.* Work on individual sounds or nonsense syllables is, strictly speaking, not a part of phonemic-based therapy techniques.

Several treatment approaches are described in this chapter. Although each uses a somewhat different analysis system to describe the patterns of errors, most use minimal pairs in their remediation program. These *minimal pair contrast therapies* have been grouped together; however, their differences are discussed. Other treatment techniques, such as *cycles training, metaphon therapy,* and *core vocabulary,* incorporate different concepts into their methodology. The final portion of this chapter contains some guidelines for combining phonemic-based approaches with language therapy, with an emerging phonological system, and with *vowel therapy* in children who have multiple vowel errors.

The production of speech sounds—the phonetic form—and the contrastive use of phonemes within the phonological system—the phoneme function—are closely related. In addition, the phonological system interacts with other language areas. Although phonological approaches emphasize the function of phonemes, both the production of speech sounds and the relationship of phonology to other language areas should not be overlooked. This chapter attempts to integrate these factors with a discussion of intervention techniques for phonological disorders.

Several principles underlie the treatment of phonemic errors in most of the following approaches. First, the phoneme as a basic unit differentiating between word meanings is at the core of these phonemic-based therapies. Consequently, intervention begins at the word level. This differs considerably from the traditional or motor approach, which typically begins with the production of the respective sounds in isolation. In addition, in most of the following therapy discussions, word materials are structured in a very specific manner. Phonemes are usually arranged contrastively between words, resulting in "minimal pairs"—two distinct words that differ by only one phoneme value.

Second, treatment focuses on a child's phonological system. An analysis of the child's phonology as an integrated system results in knowledge of (1) the inventory and distribution of speech sounds, (2) the syllable shapes and phonemic contrasts used, and (3) the error patterns displayed. All of these factors become important when the child's phonological system, not the individual speech sound, is at the center of the remediation process.

Third, very often groups of sounds or sound classes rather than only individual speech sounds are targeted. Children with these speech sound disorders often have difficulties with several phonemes. Their aberrant realizations might extend to whole classes of sounds, making it impossible for the children to establish phonemic contrasts; thus, neutralization of phonemic oppositions occurs. Phoneme-based remediation focuses on more than one sound or perhaps on an entire class of sounds at the same time. Several sounds can be targeted in a specific sequence, as in the cycles training approach (Hodson & Paden, 1991), or several sounds can be used to demonstrate phonemic contrasts, as in multiple oppositions therapy (e.g., Williams, 2010). With phonologically based therapies, generalization is assumed to occur to other sounds or sound classes.

Important differences exist between the traditional motor approach (which is often used to treat articulation errors) and phonemic-based remediation methods (which target phonological disorders). Traditional motor approaches represent therapy for *speech form*, the production of speech sounds. In contrast, phonemic-based remediation methods target *phonemic function*, the contrastive use of phonemes to establish meaning differences. However, in the actual therapy situation, separating these two different approaches entirely is often impossible. Form and function constitute an interactive unity in our treatment of children with phonological difficulties.

Minimal Pair Therapy: Minimal Oppositions Contrast Therapy and the Multiple Oppositions Approach

Minimal Opposition Contrast Therapy

The term **minimal opposition contrast therapy** refers to the therapeutic use of pairs of words that differ by only one phoneme. This type of therapy has a long history within the field of speech-language pathology and has been referred to by a variety of labels, including minimal pairs therapy (Velleman, 2016), method of meaningful minimal contrast (Weiner, 1981), conventional minimal pair therapy (Barlow & Gierut, 2002), and minimal opposition contrast therapy (Gierut, 1990). The author has chosen one of these classifications, which seems just as descriptive as any of the other labels.

OVERVIEW OF MINIMAL OPPOSITION CONTRAST THERAPY. Minimal opposition contrast therapy is a method in which minimal pairs are used as the beginning unit of therapy. Target sounds for this therapy can be selected according to a number of parameters, but for the purpose at hand phonological processes will be used. The clinician chooses a phonological process based on the developmental order of suppression, the frequency of occurrence of the process, how many sounds are affected, and how the process affects intelligibility. A sound pair is then selected based on this specific phonological process.

For the sound pair, a phone that the child can produce is typically paired with one that is not produced correctly. For example, let's use stopping as the phonological process that is selected. We find that our child stops most of the fricatives (/s, z, ʃ, ʒ, θ, ð/). This child produces either [t] or [d] for all these phonemes. We would choose the sound that the child uses for a substitution (in this case, either [t] or [d]) and pair it with one of the sounds the child cannot produce. Based on the high frequency of occurrence and the impact on the child's intelligibility, /s/ might be a good choice. In this case, our minimal pairs would be structured with /t/ versus /s/. Further information is provided in the section titled "How to Select Target Sounds for Minimal Opposition Contrast Therapy."

WHICH CHILDREN MIGHT BENEFIT FROM MINIMAL OPPOSITION CONTRAST THERAPY?   Which clients seem to be good candidates for this type of remediation? Beginning with Weiner's (1981) study, more than 40 peer-reviewed published investigations of the minimal pair approach have documented its use with children (refer to Baker, 2010, for a summary). First, all children had normal hearing, age-appropriate receptive language skills, and no evidence of oral-motor difficulties. Second, children participating in these studies evidenced a wide range of age and severity levels. Across the literature, age ranged from 2 years 10 months to over 10 years of age, with 4 to 5 years being the most common age. Severity ranged from mild to severe phonological impairments. However, Baker (2010, 2016) and Williams (2000b) conclude that, based on research findings (e.g., Tyler, Edwards, & Saxman, 1987), minimal opposition contrast therapy is best suited to children who experience a mild to moderate phonological disorder. According to Dodd's (2013) diagnostic system, this would probably be children who were diagnosed with a phonological delay. Children with moderate to severe or severe phonological difficulties may be better suited to another approach, such as multiple oppositions or the complexity approach. Regarding the age of the child, it appears that most children were from 3 to approximately 7 years of age. Thus, minimal opposition contrast therapy is suitable for even younger children.

In addition, Lowe (1994) states that "the minimal opposition procedure is most appropriate for clients who are stimulable for the target sound" (p. 190). Hodson (1992) supports this view and adds that it appears inappropriate to set up a potentially frustrating situation by requiring differential productions of word pairs until a child can spontaneously and effortlessly say the target sounds in the pairs. Saben and Costello-Ingham (1991) found that therapy based on minimal opposition contrasts alone produced little progress in two clients. However, these clients improved when a traditional motor approach was implemented, to first establish the contrasting phones, and then using minimal opposition contrasts.

HOW TO SELECT TARGET SOUNDS FOR MINIMAL OPPOSITION CONTRAST THERAPY.   Phonological processes are frequently used to assess patterns of phonemic errors. They can easily be used for target selection for minimal opposition contrast therapy. A specific phonological process should be chosen based on:

1. *Its relative frequency of occurrence:* Processes that occur most often in the child's speech will probably affect intelligibility to a higher degree.
2. *The consequence this process has on a client's intelligibility, which includes how many sounds are affected:* Certain processes will have more impact on intelligibility than others. For example, final consonant deletion could affect many different sounds, whereas velar fronting is limited to /k/ and /g/. In most cases, the more sounds that are affected, the more intelligibility will be undermined.

3. *A child's age and phonological development:* Some phonological processes, such as final consonant deletion, are suppressed at a relatively early age, whereas others, such as consonant cluster reduction, can persist until beginning school grades. The child's age and level of phonological competence must be considered when selecting phonological processes.

Consider an example: A child who is 4 years 6 months old demonstrates a high frequency of final consonant deletion, consonant cluster reduction, gliding (/ɹ/ → /w/), and stopping of /θ/ and /ð/. Based on the child's age and the impact on intelligibility, final consonant deletion would possibly be a good choice for beginning therapy. The others are "later" processes that would probably not affect the intelligibility of a 4-year-old as much as deletion of many final consonants would.

After an appropriate phonological process is selected, word pairs must be found for the beginning phase of minimal opposition contrast training. The child's phonetic inventory and the stimulability of specific sounds often guide the selection. Refer to Table 10.1 for examples of numerous phonological processes and target selection.

SELECTION OF TREATMENT TARGETS: CASE STUDY.   Jonah, 7 years 4 months old, was introduced in Chapter 7. The results of his phonological analysis will be used to demonstrate the selection of a phonological process and a minimal word pair. *Note*: Because of the severity of Jonah's phonological disorder, minimal opposition contrast therapy would not be a good choice for him. However, his data are used to exemplify the process. A phonological process analysis form is completed for Jonah (refer to Figure 7.5, pages 215–216) and shows the following:

1. *Frequency of occurrence of phonological processes:* Fronting (15 times), stopping (37 times), and consonant cluster reduction (18 times) are very frequent phonological processes for Jonah.
2. *Consequence on intelligibility, including how many sounds are affected:* Jonah uses stopping for seven different sounds: /s/, /z/, /ʃ/, /θ/, /ð/, /tʃ/, and /ʤ/. Since specifically /s/ and /z/ are high-frequency sounds in General American English, intelligibility would be affected.
3. *Age and phonological development:* Jonah is age 7 years 4 months. At his age, stopping should be suppressed. Fronting is also suppressed at an early age, but for Jonah this process involves primarily velar fronting of only two phonemes, /k/ and /g/.

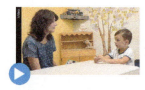

Video Tool Exercise 10.1
**Conversational Speech
with Patrick**
Complete the activity
based on this video.

Based on this information, the phonological process of stopping was selected. If we look for stimulability within the group of sounds that are replaced by [t] and [d], we find that the th-sounds are stimulable but, based on minimal pair production, have been included in Jonah's inventory. The /s/ and /z/ would affect intelligibility the most. However, before beginning with the minimal pairs, we would probably need to attempt some phonetic placement so that Jonah could possibly articulate a correct or near-correct [s].

OVERVIEW OF MINIMAL OPPOSITION CONTRAST THERAPY.   The two target sounds selected are placed in minimal pair words with the chosen sounds typically at the beginning: *toe-sew, talk-sock,* or *tick-sick*, for example. This would not

Table 10.1 Examples for Constructing Minimal Pairs Using Phonological Processes

Substitution Processes	
Underlying principle	Construct word pairs with the target sound and the substitution. If the target sound is not stimulable, a traditional approach might be necessary to achieve correct production of the sound in a specific word context.
Velar fronting	For t/k and d/g substitutions, find word pairs contrasting /t/ and /k/ or /d/ and /g/. Examples: *tea* versus *key*, *tape* versus *cape*. *Dumb* versus *gum*, *dull* versus *gull*.
Palatal fronting	For s/ʃ substitution, find word pairs contrasting /s/ and /ʃ/. Examples: *sip* versus *ship*, *sell* versus *shell*.
Stopping of /s/ and /z/	For t/s and d/z substitutions, find word pairs contrasting /t/ and /s/ or /d/ and /z/. Examples: *toe* versus *sew*, *T* versus *sea*, *D* versus *Z*, *do* versus *zoo*.
Gliding /ɹ/ → /w/	For w/ɹ substitution, find word pairs contrasting /w/ and /ɹ/. Examples: *wed* versus *red*, *weed* versus *read*.

More Uncommon Processes

Stops replacing glides /j/ → /d/	For d/j substitution, find word pairs contrasting /d/ and /j/. Examples: *dot* versus *yacht*, *darn* versus *yarn*.
Denasalization of /n/ → /d/	For d/n substitution, find word pairs contrasting /n/ and /d/. Examples: *knot* versus *dot*, *near* versus *deer*.

Processes Affecting Groups or Classes of Phonemes	
Underlying principle	Select contrast pairs containing sounds that the child can produce or that are stimulable.
Final consonant deletion	Start with word pairs with and without final consonants, such as *bow* versus *boat*. If generalization does not occur, present word pairs contrasting another final consonant against no final consonant. Example: Child can produce [m, n, t, d, l, f, v, p, b] but not in word-final position. First, present contrasts such as *toe* versus *toad*, *low* versus *load*.
Consonant cluster reduction	Use singletons in the child's inventory to structure reduced consonant clusters contrasted to standard consonant clusters. Example: Cluster reductions are noted on several consonant blends. Child can produce [b], [p], [k], and [l] but says [kaʊn] for *clown*, [peɪ] for *play*, [bu] for *blue*. If you begin with [pl], word pairs such as *plan* versus *pan*, *please* versus *peas* could be used.
Stopping of fricatives	Select a stimulable fricative, which is then contrasted with the homorganic stop. Example: Child is stimulable for [f] but uses p/f substitution in most contexts. Use word pairs such as *pig* versus *fig*, *pin* versus *fin*.
Initial consonant deletion	Start with word pairs contrasting one initial consonant versus no initial consonant. If generalization does not occur, present word pairs with another initial consonant. Example: Child can produce [p, b, t, d, h, w, m, n] but inconsistently deletes these sounds at the beginning of a word. Use word pairs such as *beet* versus *eat*, *bee* versus *E*.

be the case, however, if you were working on final consonant deletion. Often pictures of these words that are appropriate for children are very limited. Therefore, it has been suggested that if meaningful minimal pairs cannot be found for contrastive phonemes, near-minimal pairs should be used (Elbert & Gierut, 1986). **Near-minimal pairs** are pairs of words that differ by more than one phoneme;

however, the vowel following (or preceding, in the case of final consonant deletion) remains constant in both words. For example, *sir-third* or *sore-thorn* would be considered near-minimal pairs. These near-minimal pair words can be very helpful in establishing more practice material for the client. In addition, nonsense words can be used quite effectively. The nonsense word can be the name of a character or an action that is given meaning. For example, "Thote" could be a dog's name, or "thup" could be an action (I had to "thup" the ball).

After minimal pairs are chosen, the following steps are suggested (Blache, 1989):

STEP 1: *Discussion of words.* The therapist must be certain that the child knows the concepts portrayed. To confirm this, the child can be asked to point to the picture named, and the clinician could ask questions about it. For example, for the chosen word pair *fig-pig*, ask, "Which one is a fruit?" or "Which one is an animal?"

STEP 2: *Discrimination testing and training.* In this phase, the client's discrimination between the two sounds is tested. The therapist repeats the two words in random order and the child is instructed to point to the respective picture. If the response is correct seven consecutive times, the therapist can be reasonably certain that the client is differentiating between the two sounds. If the criterion of seven correct discriminations in a row cannot be reached, poor auditory discrimination or memory skills may be the cause (Blache, 1989). These skills need to be addressed before continuing the program.

STEP 3: *Production training.* This phase is directed toward elicitation of the minimal pair words. The child is instructed to be the teacher, saying the words while the therapist points to the correct picture. In selecting the target sounds for the minimal pairs, the child can produce one of the sounds chosen but the other is not in the child's inventory. If the target sound is stimulable, the child is probably able to contrast the minimal pair. If the target sound is not stimulable, which is typically the case, the child says one word in the pair incorrectly. For example, in the previous example, [f] and [p] were selected. The child could produce [p] but not [f]. If the child says [pɪn] for *pin* and [pɪn] for *fin*, the therapist points to *pin* both times; that is, the therapist points to a word not intended by the child. This communicative breakdown is hopefully an "aha" revelation for the child and is an important component of the training. If the child cannot articulate the sound correctly, a traditional motor approach could be implemented to achieve the sound at the *word level*. The word level is emphasized as the minimal unit. Immediate reinforcement should follow the correct sound production.

STEP 4: *Carryover training.* Once the target word can be articulated accurately, the following sequence is suggested:

Model	Example
"a" + word	a pig, a fig
"the" + word	the pig, the fig
"Touch the" + word	Touch the pig, Touch the fig
"Point to the" + word	Point to the pig, Point to the fig
longer expressions + word	That is a big pig, That is a big fig

Clinical Exercises You are setting up a program using minimal oppositions contrast therapy. Leo, age 4 years 0 months, has the following substitutions: t/s, d/z, w/l, w/ɹ, t/k, and d/g. Based on the outlined principles (and the child's age), which two phonemes would you target?

To consider: Leo is 4 years old. Although /s/ and /z/ are frequent sounds in General American English that would affect intelligibility, we might hesitate to begin s-therapy with a 4-year-old. If Leo is stimulable for /s/ or /z/, that would alter the picture. The same could be said for work on r-sounds, which are usually later sounds; however, again, if the r-sound is stimulable, it would be an excellent choice. Other earlier sounds to consider might be /k, g/.

Make a list of minimal pairs that you could use with this child.

Oppositions Approach

method, developed by Williams (1991, 2000a, 2000b), is an alternative to contrastive minimal pairs. The approach directly addresses the phonemes. For the child with extensive phoneme collapses, in which two or more words are pronounced alike but have This has a negative effect on intelligibility, and thus communications result. In the multiple oppositions approach, the child is presented simultaneously with several sounds that address that particular child's collapses contrasts. The supposition is that by treating more contrasts, several oppositions could be added to the child's system. This should result in length of treatment, improved intelligibility, and more efficient

OVERVIEW OF THE MULTIPLE OPPOSITIONS APPROACH. This treatment method, which is a variation of minimal oppositions contrast therapy, uses larger treatment sets. Instead of two sounds being opposed in minimal pairs, the multiple oppositions approach selects two to four sounds to be used in minimal word pairs of the error sounds versus the substitutions. The selection of targets is based on the individual child's phoneme collapses and generated rule sets. A distance metric is applied (refer to the section titled "How to Select Target Sounds for the Multiple Oppositions Approach"), which yields groups of sounds that are maximally distinct from the error sound and from each other. Thus, singletons are paired with consonant clusters, if possible, to establish one set of these contrasts.

The first step in selecting a set of treatment targets is to examine the child's phonemic inventory to determine the collapse of phonemic contrasts. Since singletons as well as consonant clusters can be targeted, the clinician will need to have a list of consonant clusters and their productions for the specific child. A list that can be used is contained in Appendix 10.1. Next, the clinician tries to find sets of sounds that are maximally distinct from the error and from each other. Typically, production features are used—for example, pairing a voiced alveolar fricative with a voiceless velar stop. Refer to the section titled "How to Select Target Sounds for the Multiple Oppositions Approach."

WHICH CHILDREN MIGHT BENEFIT FROM THE MULTIPLE OPPOSITIONS APPROACH? According to Williams (2000a), the multiple oppositions approach is used to treat severe speech sound disorders in children. The children included in research exhibited primarily moderate to severe phonological impairments (Williams, 2000b, 2006; Williams & Kalbfleish, 2001). This was defined as the exclusion of at least six sounds across three manner categories. The children in these studies were typically between 3 and 6 years of age, and their hearing and intelligence were considered to be typical, as were the structure and function of the speech mechanism. Thus, according to Dodd's (2013) classification, the children with consistent phonological disorder would benefit the most from this type of approach. Because this treatment protocol is specifically designed to treat the collapse of multiple phonemic contrasts, the children should definitely demonstrate a collapse of phonemic contrasts that incorporates several sounds.

Children who were treated using this method all demonstrated documented improvement. Although children who had more severe disorders required a longer time to reach the generalization stage, system-wide changes were especially noted in the children with the most severe disorders.

HOW TO SELECT TARGET SOUNDS FOR THE MULTIPLE OPPOSITIONS APPROACH. Selection of two to four treatment targets is based on the collapse of phonemic contrasts. Both maximal distinctions and maximal classifications are used to guide target selection. Maximal distinctions are those that are maximally different from a child's error. Maximal classifications indicate those targets that differ maximally in respect to place, manner, and voicing. In addition, a child's unique organizational structure is considered. Sounds that have potential for the greatest impact on the child's phonological reorganization should be targeted.

Rule sets for the specific child's collapses are first established. For example, Dillon, age 6 years 7 months, demonstrated the following:

k, g, s, θ, ʃ, ʧ, kj, kl, kɹ, ʃɹ, θɹ, sk, st, tɹ, tw → t
z, ð, ʤ, dɹ, gɹ, dw, gl → d

Dillon also had other errors, but we will use these to exemplify the process. It appears that Dillon collapses many phonemes to /t/. Let's choose /t/ as one of our target sounds. Typically two to four other sounds are used as a contrast. We need sounds that are maximally different from the error /t/. One option would be /g/, which is a voiced velar stop, contrasted to /t/, which is a voiceless alveolar stop. A second choice could include a consonant cluster. The cluster /ʃɹ/ would be a good option, as it is very different from /t/ and contains a postalveolar fricative and a voiced palatal approximant. Other consonant clusters might be options, although consonant clusters with /t/ probably should be eliminated, since they are not maximally different from /t/. As a third choice, the affricate /ʧ/ might be a good option. Now we have an affricate contrasted to a stop. Other options are possible. Possibly /s/ would be a good target due to its impact on intelligibility and the abundance of consonant clusters with /s/. However, for this example, let's choose the following:

/t/ contrasted to /g/, /ʃɹ/, and /ʧ/

We would now try to find minimal pairs that incorporate these sounds in the initial position. One set would be *till, gill, shrill,* and *chill*. Another might be *teak, geek, shriek,* and *cheek*. Williams (2000a, 2010) suggests that each set contain five different word pair examples. So, our example could look like this:

/t/	/g/	/ʃɹ/	/tʃ/
till	gill	shrill	chill
teak	geek	shriek	cheek
Ted	Ged	shred	Ched
two	goo	shrew	chew
tug	gug	shrug	chug

As can be noted, nonsense (nonwords) were also used to establish this list.

SELECTION OF TREATMENT TARGETS: JONAH. The following is summarized from Jonah, Figure 7.3, pages 202–203, and Table 7.2, page 206.

SUMMARY OF PHONEMIC COLLAPSES

Phonemes	Collapses to:
k, g, s, z, ʃ, θ, ð*, tʃ, ʤ	t
g, z, ð*, ʤ	d
l*. ɹ	w
θ*	f
f*	p
v*	b
j*	d

*Stimulable phones or those that are produced correctly on occasion: [j, l, f, v, θ, ð].

Phones Jonah does not have in his inventory: [k, g, s, z, ʃ, θ, ð, ɹ, tʃ, ʤ]

Prevocalic consonant clusters: Initial: kw, gɹ, sl, sw, kɹ, tɹ, st → t; dɹ, gl → d; sp, pl, fɹ, pɹ → p; bɹ, bl → b

Intervocalic consonant clusters: ŋk, nt, ŋg → n; ns → nt; bɹ → b; ʤt → t; kj → ∅

Postvocalic consonant clusters: nt → n

Jonah appears to have several phonemic contrasts that evidence a collapse. The collapse of several phonemes to /t/ is the most obvious. In addition to the singletons listed, the following consonant clusters demonstrate a reduction to /t/:

kw, gɹ, sl, sw, kɹ, tɹ, st → t

Let's go through the target selection using the error phoneme /t/. Sounds would be selected based on Jonah's collapse to /t/. Therefore, only those sounds

Video Example 10.1
In this video, Dr. Lynn Williams describes how to assist a child when using a contrast approach, such as multiple oppositions. Note the strategies she uses as examples.

https://www.youtube.com/watch?v=YYSTGcttnso

listed to the left of /t/ (/k, g, s, z, ʃ, θ*, ð*, tʃ, ʤ/) in the previous table would be considered as choices. First, a voiced sound would be a maximum contrast. We have /g/, /ð/, and /ʤ/. All three voiced consonants would be possibilities. Jonah is stimulable for /ð/, which might be advantageous. For this example, /g/ and /ð/ will be chosen. We need to choose one consonant cluster: If we eliminate clusters with /t/ (not a maximal distinction), our choices would be /kw, gɹ, sl, sw, kɹ/. Since /g/ is selected as a singleton, /gɹ/, /kɹ/, and /kw/ could possibly be eliminated, although the last two clusters are with /k/. Good cluster choices would be /sl/ or /sw/. The /l/ is stimulable, which might prove helpful. Our end result would be contrasting a voiceless alveolar stop /t/ to a voiced velar stop /g/, a voiced interdental fricative /ð/, and a consonant cluster with a fricative and an approximant /sl/.

A word set such as *toe—go—slow—though* would be a possibility, as would *tot—got—slot—Thott* (a magical character's name).

OVERVIEW OF MULTIPLE OPPOSITIONS THERAPY. Williams (2000a, 2003, 2010) outlines a progression of therapy for multiple oppositions that includes several phases. The following is a summary of these stages and steps:

PHASE 1: *Familiarization and initial production of contrasts.*

STEP 1: *Introduction to the rule set.* The child is introduced to the rule set, which includes the target and contrastive differences. This step includes learning how each sound differs from the others. The /t/ could be characterized as a short front sound, whereas the /g/ is a short, loud back sound.

STEP 2: *Familiarization with the pictures and vocabulary.* The clinician needs to be sure that the child can identify the pictures and the vocabulary represented by each of the words.

STEP 3: *Initial production of contrasts.* Imitation is used, and maximal cueing should be provided so that the child is successful. At this point, the goal is not a perfect production but rather that the child starts to somehow productionally differentiate the minimal word pairs.

PHASE 2: *Production of contrasts and interactive play.*

STEP 1: *Imitation.* In this step, the child produces each word after the clinician's model. According to this treatment protocol, the child should produce the minimal pairs approximately 40 times (20 times for each pair). Treatment data should be gathered during every session. If 70% accuracy is achieved for any minimal pair (e.g., the child now achieves 70% on the word "Joe"), that word is moved to the next step or phase.

STEP 2: *Spontaneous production.* The focus now shifts to the child achieving the necessary phonemic contrasts spontaneously. Feedback provided by the clinician should be used to signal any miscommunications. For example, if the child should say "slow" and says "toe," the clinician would point to the wrong picture or object.

STEP 3: *Interactive play.* In this step, the child engages in play with the new contrasts, which allows the child to be exposed to a more naturalistic context. It is hoped that practice with hearing the correct contrasts and using them may generalize to other contexts.

PHASE 3: *Contrasts within communicative contexts.* In this phase, the child begins to produce the targets spontaneously in the context of structured interactive games. Generalization probes, sets of words that are not being used in therapy (refer to Appendix 10.2) should be administered every third session.

PHASE 4: *Conversational recasts.* A conversational recast strategy will be used if the child reaches 90% accuracy on a specific target but is not using the sound accurately in conversational speech (in at least half of the opportunities presented). A recast strategy involves the clinician repeating the child's utterance in a correct manner.

Target Selection for Minimal Pair Therapy: Maximal Oppositions and the Complexity Approach

Maximal Oppositions

Elbert and Gierut (1986) introduced the concept of maximal oppositions training in response to their continuum of productive phonological knowledge. A series of investigations (Dinnsen & Elbert, 1984; Elbert, Dinnsen, & Powell, 1984; Gierut, 1985) examined the relationship between "most" and "least" phonological knowledge and the amount of generalization that occurred in the phonological system of children. The findings of one of these studies indicated that children treated in the order of least to most phonological knowledge showed generalization across the overall sound system (Gierut, 1985). In other words, if treatment focused first on sounds that the child could not produce (consistent "error" productions) and only later targeted sounds that appeared in some contexts (inconsistent "error" productions), the most generalization occurred. On the other hand, if the order of treatment proceeded from sounds that the child might be able to produce accurately in some contexts to unknown sounds, generalization was very limited. These findings led to the development of the maximal oppositions approach.

OVERVIEW OF THE MAXIMAL OPPOSITIONS APPROACH. This approach is a target selection method and does not include a specific therapy protocol such as those noted with minimal oppositions contrast therapy or the multiple oppositions approach. However, a clinician could use any number of therapy structures once the targets are selected. For this example, the author has chosen to use the therapy that was outlined in the research articles. The maximal oppositions approach is also based on minimal word pairs. However, in direct contrast to minimal oppositions contrast therapy, in which target sounds that may be similar in production are selected, the maximal oppositions approach chooses sounds that are very different. Differences in production were originally defined according to the number of variations in place, manner, or voicing between the two sounds (Elbert & Gierut, 1986; Gierut, 1989). Since then, the conceptual framework for this therapy has changed somewhat. As this concept evolved, the term *maximal oppositions* referred to differences in distinctive features. These differences vary along two dimensions: (1) the nature of the features—that is, whether differences represent major class features—and (2) the number of unique features that differentiate between the two phonemes. The Chomsky and Halle (1968) system, which defines major class features as consonantal, sonorant, and approximant, is used. Recall that the term *vocalic* has been replaced by *approximant.*

WHICH CHILDREN MIGHT BENEFIT FROM THE MAXIMAL OPPOSITIONS APPROACH?   The children in maximal oppositions research were between the ages of 3 years 6 months and 5+ years of age. They all demonstrated at least six sounds that were excluded from their inventory. In addition, large "gaps" in their phonemic inventory were noted. Based on this information, it appears that this approach is valuable for even younger children with a moderate to severe phonological disorder. Based on Dodd's (2013) classification, the children with consistent phonological disorder would benefit the most from this type of approach.

The maximal oppositions technique has been described in a number of research investigations in which its efficacy has been verified. For example, Gierut (1989) reported that after 3 different word pairs using maximal oppositions had been presented, the child learned 16 word-initial consonants and restructured his phonological system. Other studies (Gierut, 1990, 1991, 1992; Gierut & Neumann, 1992) supported these findings. When minimal oppositions and maximal oppositions approaches were therapeutically contrasted, more generalization was noted using maximal contrasts (Gierut, 1990). Also, if both sounds used to establish word pairs were *not* in the child's inventory, this proved to be as effective as, or at times even more effective than, teaching one sound the child could produce (a known sound) versus the substituted sound (an unknown sound). In the last of the series of investigations, word pairs comparing two previously unknown phonemes that differed by maximal number and major class features were found to be the preferred way to change the phonological system of the child (Gierut, 1992). Research findings seem to support the efficacy of maximal oppositions therapy.

HOW TO SELECT TARGET SOUNDS FOR THE MAXIMAL OPPOSITIONS APPROACH.   Between the earlier and the later versions of maximal oppositions therapy, the procedure for target selection changed (Elbert & Gierut, 1986; Gierut, 1989, 1992). Only the later selection procedures are outlined here.

The therapist selects two sounds not in the child's inventory (i.e., two unknown sounds). In addition, these two sounds should be maximally different according to their distinctive features. Two parameters are used to determine the maximum distinctive feature differences:

1. The nature of the features—that is, whether a major feature difference differentiates the two sounds (major class features = maximum feature distinction). The major class features are sonorant, consonantal, and approximant.
2. The number of distinctive features that differentiate the two sounds (more distinctive feature differences = maximum feature distinction). (Refer to Chapter 4 for more information on distinctive features.)

Box 10.1 provides an overview of the major class features and the distinctive feature differences.

To select targets, find:

1. Sounds that are not in the child's inventory.
2. Sounds that demonstrate a major class feature difference. First, note the sounds that are along the vertical axis, /ɹ, l, w, j, h/, to see if any of them are

Box 10.1

Major Class Features and Distinctive Feature Differences

Major Class Features

Sonorants	Consonantals	Approximants
vowels +	stops +	vowels +
glides +	fricatives +	liquids +
nasals +	affricates +	stops −
liquids +	nasals +	fricatives −
[h] +	liquids +	affricates −
stops −	vowels −	nasals −
fricatives −	glides −	[h] −
affricates −	[h] −	

Distinctive Feature Differences of + and − Sonorants

	p	b	t	d	k	g	f	v	s	z	ʃ	ʒ	θ	ð	tʃ	ʤ
ɹ	4	3	3	2	5	4	4	3	3	2	3	2	2	1	5	4
l	4	3	3	2	7	6	4	3	3	2	5	4	2	1	7	6
w	6	5	7	6	3	2	6	5	7	6	5	4	6	5	7	6
j	4	3	5	4	3	2	4	3	5	4	3	2	4	3	5	4
h	3	4	4	5	4	5	3	4	4	5	4	5	3	4	6	7

In the bottom table, the consonants have been separated into those that demonstrate major class features. Thus, the approximants (liquids and glides) and /h/ on the vertical axis represent the (+) sonorant features, whereas the horizontal axis shows the (−) sonorant features. The nasals have not been included in this display due to their infrequent use as targets. The number in each cell represents the total number of distinctive feature differences. For example, /l/ and /p/ have four distinctive feature differences, whereas /w/ and /p/ have six. In this approach, we are looking for two phonemes that demonstrate maximal distinctive feature differences; thus, we are looking for a higher number in the respective cells. *Note*: The major class feature differences have not been added to the numbers in this lower table.

not in the child's inventory. Second, look at the sounds along the horizontal axis, /p, b, t, d, k, g/, etc., to see which ones are not in the child's inventory. Third, compare the number of distinctive feature differences, looking for the highest number.

By following this procedure, you would locate two unknown sounds (two sounds that the child cannot produce) that demonstrate a major class feature difference and have the most distinctive feature contrasts. These two would be your targets.

SELECTION OF TREATMENT TARGETS: JONAH.   The following was noted for Jonah:

Phones not in his inventory: [k, g, s, z, ʃ, ɹ, ʧ, ʤ]

The /θ, ð, and l/ have been eliminated, as Jonah can produce those phones on occasion.

Looking at the vertical axis in the bottom table in Box 10.1, we find that /ɹ/ demonstrates a major class feature difference when compared to /k, g, s, z, ʃ, ʧ, ʤ/. Now we examine the feature differences to determine which one has the highest number relative to /ɹ/. The following can be noted from the bottom table in Box 10.1: Distinctive feature differences of /ɹ/ and /k/ = 5, /ɹ/ and /g/ = 4, /ɹ/ and /s/ = 3, /ɹ/ and /z/ = 2, /ɹ/ and /ʧ/ = 5, /ɹ/ and /ʤ/ = 4. For Jonah, the phoneme /ɹ/ versus either /k/ or /ʧ/ would be good selections as targets. For intelligibility, the /k/ would be a higher priority than /ʧ/. Therefore, in this example, /ɹ/ and /k/ would be chosen as targets for Jonah. These would be put in minimal word pairs such as:

rod versus *cod*	*ran* versus *can*	*rat* versus *cat*	*right* versus *kite*

Clinical Application

The following example (Subject 11 from Gierut, 1992) is given to illustrate the selection process used in maximum feature distinctions:

Inventory	Sounds Not in Inventory	Major Class Difference
m, n, ŋ,		
w, j, h,	ɹ, l	
p, b, t, d,	k, g	Yes, between ɹ, l versus k, g
f, v, ʧ, ʤ	s, z, ʃ, ʒ, θ, ð	Yes, between ɹ, l versus s, z, ʃ, ʒ, θ, ð

Major class differences are evidenced between /ɹ/ and /l/ and several other phonemes. Because both /ɹ/ and /l/ are [+ voice], the voiceless consonants [– voice] demonstrate one more distinctive feature difference than the voiced consonants. When feature differences for the noted voiceless consonants and /ɹ/ and /l/ are counted, the following number of distinctive feature differences emerges:

[ɹ] and [k] = 5	[l] and [k] = 7
[ɹ] and [s] = 3	[l] and [s] = 3
[ɹ] and [ʃ] = 3	[l] and [ʃ] = 5
[ɹ] and [θ] = 2	[l] and [θ] = 2

Therefore, considering both major class distinctions and the number of differences in distinctive features, for maximal oppositions /l/ and /k/ would be good selections for targets. These phonemes are then used to form minimal pairs such as *lane-cane, leg-keg,* and *lamp-camp.*

OVERVIEW OF MAXIMAL OPPOSITIONS THERAPY.   According to the research model, treatment included two phases, *imitation* and *spontaneous production,* for each sound pair. However, it should be noted that this treatment protocol originated from a research project that compared different word pairs and their impact on changes in the phonological systems of children. For clinical purposes, practitioners may want to implement additional activities to serve the needs of individual clients.

1. *Imitation phase.* Minimal pair picture cards are presented to the client, who is asked to repeat the clinician's model of the pictures. Several activities can be used to maintain interest, such as matching or sorting pictures during imitative production, moving a car around one space on a track each time the word is imitated, playing various card games with the pictures, and so on. This phase of treatment continues until the child achieves 75% imitative accuracy in two sessions. The maximal number of sessions in this phase is seven. During the imitation phase, the clinician can use cueing or phonetic placement to achieve the sound within the context of minimal word pairs. These aids should be faded as soon as possible.

2. *Spontaneous production phase.* Word pairs are now produced by the client without the clinician's model. Again, various activities can be found to keep the child's interest. This phase continues until 90% accurate production without a model for at least 3, with a maximum of 12 sessions is achieved.

The Complexity Approach

The complexity approach emerged from a series of studies that examined which types of treatment targets for children with speech sound disorders could promote the most generalization within a child's phonological system (e.g., Elbert et al., 1984; Gierut, 1985; Williams, 1991). It was found that by using more complex linguistic input (sounds that the child was not stimulable for and incorporating consonant clusters), more change occurred in a child's phonological system. The complexity approach focuses on *what* is targeted in intervention as opposed to *how* it is implemented within a therapy procedure. Target selection becomes a very important consideration.

OVERVIEW OF THE COMPLEXITY APPROACH. This approach, similar to maximal oppositions, is a target selection process. Conventional approaches to phonological treatment often recommend that targets are based on stimulability—in other words, a target the child can produce with some degree of accuracy (Hodson & Edwards, 1997). In addition to stimulability, targets are selected according to a developmental sequence, from earlier to later. However, according to some research findings, these recommendations result in only limited generalization (Rvachew & Nowak, 2001). Complex input consists of targeting sounds that are *not* stimulable and later developing. When this occurs, improvement of both treated and untreated sounds occurs (Gierut, Morrisette, Hughes, & Rowland, 1996). Complexity can also refer to consonant clusters versus singletons. Based on the complexity concept, training consonant clusters can result in generalization to singletons (e.g., Gierut, 1999, 2001; Tyler & Figurski, 1994). A specific ranking can be established that will provide guidance in determining which consonant clusters would be the most conducive to promoting overall phonological change. Several studies have documented that the use of consonant clusters in treatment demonstrated more widespread change than when only singletons were targeted (e.g., Gierut, 1998; Powell & Elbert, 1984).

WHICH CHILDREN MIGHT BENEFIT FROM THE COMPLEXITY APPROACH? This approach was designed for children with moderate to severe phonological impairments. According to Dodd's (2013) classification, children identified as having a consistent phonological disorder would be good candidates for this target selection approach. Based on several research investigations (e.g, Gierut, 1999; Miccio & Ingrisano, 2000), children's ages ranged from 2 years 8 months to 7 years 11 months, with most being around 4 years of age. Typically between five and seven sounds were excluded from their inventories across three manner categories. These were children with limited phonemic inventories. However, children who had phonemic structure difficulties (problems with stress, sequencing of sounds, and/or producing multiple syllables) were not considered to be good candidates for the complexity approach. Therefore, the complexity approach may not be the best possibility for children with mild speech sound disorders or for those with phonemic structure difficulties.

HOW TO SELECT TARGET SOUNDS FOR THE COMPLEXITY APPROACH: SELECTING SINGLETON CONSONANTS. When going through the steps for the complexity approach with singletons, two sounds are targeted, which are then used in minimal pairs. The following four principles are used to select singleton targets:

1. *Error patterns.* A list should be made of those sounds that are not in the child's inventory. If a child produces a sound in some contexts but not in others, put that sound in the category of sounds the child can produce.
2. *Stimulability.* Sounds that are not stimulable have priority in the complexity approach. Based on the results of your standardized speech assessment, error sounds should be probed for stimulability. Sounds that are not stimulable are targeted. Ideally, non-stimulability represents 0% accuracy in production.
3. *Implicational universals.* These universals were introduced in Chapter 4 (pages 86–87). These implicational universals are summarized in Table 10.2. According to this principle, the sound pairs [s, θ], [z, ð], and [l, ɹ] have priority as targets (Gierut & Hulse, 2010). Implicational universals suggest that the presence of affricates predicts the presence of fricatives, fricatives predict the presence of stops, and liquids predict the presence of nasals.
4. *Developmental norms.* Later-developing sounds have priority over earlier-developing ones. Later-acquired sounds are [s, z, ʃ, ʒ, θ, ð, l, ɹ, tʃ, dʒ].

Let's demonstrate this process with Billy, age 4 years 5 months. Billy does not have the following sounds in his inventory: [v, z, θ, ð, ʃ], [ɹ], [tʃ, dʒ]. However,

Table 10.2 Implicational Universals

Predicting Property	Imply →	The Presence of:
Pairs /s, θ/, /z, ð/, or /l, ɹ/		All manner categories
Affricates /tʃ, dʒ/		Fricatives /f, v, s, z, θ, ð, ʃ, ʒ/
Fricatives /f, v, s, z, θ, ð, ʃ, ʒ/		Stops /p, b, t, d, k, g/
Liquids /l, ɹ/		Nasals /m, n, ŋ/
Voiced obstruents /b, d, g, v, z, ð, ʒ, dʒ/		Voiceless obstruents /p, t, k, f, s, θ, ʃ, tʃ/

Source: Based on Gierut & Hulse (2010).

the following sounds are stimulable: [v, z]. If we examine implicational universals, we find that one sound of each of the sound pairs [s, θ], [z, ð], [l, ɹ] is either in Billy's inventory or stimulable. For example, [s] and [l] are in his inventory, and [z] is stimulable. Using implicational universals, affricates might be a good choice for Billy. They would predict fricatives. Finally, looking at developmental norms, we find that the affricates are within the later-developing sounds. Targeting two fricatives [ʃ, θ], or [ð] would not be as effective. The presence of fricatives implies stops, but Billy's inventory includes the stop consonants, or they are stimulable. The [ɹ], although it is a later sound, is not a good choice due to implicational universals. The only sound class that liquids imply is nasals. Nasals are already present in Billy's inventory. Thus, for singletons, the affricates [tʃ, dʒ] would be selected as targets.

HOW TO SELECT TARGET SOUNDS FOR THE COMPLEXITY APPROACH: SELECTING A CONSONANT CLUSTER.   To choose a consonant cluster, you would need to determine (1) the clusters not in the child's inventory, (2) which cluster has the smallest sonority difference between the individual members of that cluster, (3) the individual consonants that are not in the child's inventory, (4) whether three-element clusters would be a possibility. Also noted are clusters that the child produced but that were possibly used as substitutions for other consonant clusters, such as [fw] (as a substitute for [fɹ], for example) or [θw] (as a substitute for [ʃɹ]). Unlike the target selection for singletons, only one consonant cluster is selected for treatment.

1. *The clusters not in the child's inventory.* Difficulties with specific consonant clusters should be noted from your standardized speech assessment and spontaneous speech sample. To supplement this, a list of initial consonant clusters is contained in Appendix 10.1. Probe words contained in this list could be used to determine a list of clusters not in the child's inventory. Research from the complexity approach has used only initial clusters. However, final clusters could also be a target if they seem to affect intelligibility. If the child demonstrates *no* clusters in his or her inventory, *select a consonant cluster as a target* for the complexity approach (Taps Richard, Barlow, & Combiths, 2017).

2. *The smallest sonority difference demonstrated between consonants within a cluster.* Sonority was discussed in Chapter 4 (pages 107–110). As a brief review, sonority refers to the relative loudness of a sound. In General American English, the most sonority is demonstrated by the vowel nucleus of the syllable, while most of the time the sonority falls toward the edges of the syllable. The individual sonority values for consonants are contained in Table 10.3.

   To calculate the sonority difference of the consonant cluster, subtract the sonority of the consonant with the largest value from the other consonant. For example, [fl] would be 5 (voiceless fricative) − 2 (approximant [l]) = 3, and [dɹ] would be 6 (voiced plosive) − 2 (approximant [ɹ]) = 4. If a child uses a substitution, such as [pw] for "pl," then these sonority values could also be calculated. For [pw], the sonority would be 7 for [p] (voiceless plosive) − 1 for [w] (approximant [w]) = 6. When selecting a consonant cluster for a target, priority is given to clusters that have the *least* sonority difference. These are considered to be marked and, therefore, more complex. If there is a choice between several clusters, always select a cluster that has the least sonority. A cluster that is less by 1 or 2 sonority point differences is a good choice. Refer to Table 10.4 for sonority differences between various initial consonant clusters.

Table 10.3 Sonority Values of Individual Sounds

Sound Class	Steriade (1990) Values
Vowels	0
Approximants [w, j]	1
Approximants [ɹ, l]	2
Nasals	3
Fricatives	
Voiced fricatives	4
Voiceless fricatives	5
Plosives	
Voiced plosives	6
Voiceless plosives	7

Table 10.4 Initial Consonant Clusters That Could Be Targets, Ranked from Least to Most Sonority

Desirable targets are more complex (have least sonority).

Consonant Cluster	Sonority Calculation	Sonority Difference	Word Examples
sm	5 − 3 = 2	2	small, smell, smart, smoke, smile
sn	5 − 3 = 2	2	snow, snack, snail, snake, snap
sl	5 − 2 = 3	3	slow, sleep, slap, sled, slide
fl	5 − 2 = 3	3	fly, flow, flat, flag, flap
fɹ	5 − 2 = 3	3	fry, free, fruit, frog, from
θɹ	5 − 2 = 3	3	throw, three, threw, thread, threat
ʃɹ	5 − 2 = 3	3	shred, shrink, shrimp, shrub, shrug
bl	6 − 2 = 4	4	blue, blow, black, block, blink
bɹ	6 − 2 = 4	4	brain, brake, brick, bright, broom
dɹ	6 − 2 = 4	4	dry, draw, drum, dream, drink
gl	6 − 2 = 4	4	glue, glow, glad, glove, glide
gɹ	6 − 2 = 4	4	grow, grey, green, grape, group
pl	7 − 2 = 5	5	play, plow, plum, plant, plane
pɹ	7 − 2 = 5	5	prune, print, proof, proud, prove
tɹ	7 − 2 = 5	5	true, train, trick, trail, trap
kl	7 − 2 = 5	5	clay, clue, clap, clean, clock
kɹ	7 − 2 = 5	5	crow, cry, crab, crumb, crawl
dw	6 − 1 = 5	5	dwell, dwarf, dwelling
tw	7 − 1 = 6	6	twig, tweet, twin, twelve, twice
kw	7 − 1 = 6	6	quack, quick, quit, queen, quite

As noted in Chapter 4, there are clusters ([sp], [st], and [sk]) that do not follow the sonority sequencing principle. As such, they are not treated like true clusters and are labeled adjunct clusters. As adjunct clusters, they are considered to be unmarked—thus, easier for the child. These clusters are not targeted for treatment. Also, the clusters with [j] ([pj, kj, fj, bj, and mj]) are not considered treatment targets. However, if your child does produce one of these clusters, the sonority difference should be noted and used as a reference for the selection process.

The clusters [sm], [sn], and [sl], although being more marked clusters (less sonority difference), are also frequently not used as targets. If these clusters are produced in a similar way as the other s-clusters, they are excluded from target possibilities. For example, if they all show a reduction to one element, such as [m], [n], and [l], this would eliminate them from being a target. Or, if they all show reduction to [t], for example, they would not be considered good targets. As a general statement, the author would suggest that these clusters are not targeted or targeted only as an exception.

3. *The individual consonants that are not in the child's inventory.* Select one cluster as a target in which at least one but preferably two consonants are not present in the inventory and possibly not stimulable.

4. *Consider three-element clusters.* Three-element clusters consist of [skw], [spɹ], [stɹ], [skɹ], and [spl]. Using a three-element cluster in treatment was more effective if the child produced the second and third member of the cluster accurately but not the initial [s] (Morrisette, Farris, & Gierut, 2006). Therefore, for [spl], the child should be able to produce [p] and [l]; however, [s] as a singleton should not be a part of the child's inventory. At least *one* of the three-element cluster sounds should be in the child's inventory; ideally, the second and third sound of the three-element cluster should be in the inventory or stimulable (Gierut & Champion, 2001).

Let's use a clinical example with Cliff, age 5 years 9 months.

Cliff has the following sounds in his inventory: [p, b, t, d, m, n, ŋ, w, j, h, ʃ]. He does not have the following sounds in his inventory: [k, g, f, v, s, z, θ, ð, ɹ, l, tʃ, ʤ].
Initial probes indicate that Cliff has 0% accuracy and is not stimulable for: [g, f, v, s, z, θ, ð, ɹ, l].

Cliff's cluster inventory includes [tw, dw, pw, bw]. All other consonant clusters are reduced to one consonant. The sonority differences are as follows: [tw], [pw] $7 - 1 = 6$; [bw], [dw] $6 - 1 = 5$. Therefore, one should try to target a consonant cluster with a sonority difference of 4 or 3. If we look at Table 10.4, we find that there are several options for Cliff. If we choose clusters in which both elements are not stimulable and unknown, the following are possibilities we could use to continue the selection process: [gɹ, gl, θɹ, fɹ, sl].

The s-clusters, [sn], [sm], and [sl], are usually not good targets, and in this case, they also are not good targets. If a child uses a similar pattern across all s-clusters (which Cliff does, as he reduces them to one singleton consonant), then they are not acceptable targets. If we look at the consonant clusters with a sonority difference of 3 or 4, and also consider nonstimulability, we find that the following clusters could be potential targets: sonority difference of 4, [gɹ, gl]; sonority difference of 3, [fɹ, fl, θɹ]. Consonant clusters with a sonority difference of 3 would have priority. If /f, θ, ɹ, and l/ are all not stimulable, [fl] might be a good choice, as this cluster is fairly frequent and might lend itself fairly easily to production possibilities.

To use three-element clusters, the child should be able to produce the second and/or third element of the cluster. Cliff can do this with all of the three-element clusters: [skw, spr, str, skr, spl]. If we narrow this down to three-element clusters in which *both* the second and third element are stimulable, which is the ideal target possibility, we arrive at [skw].

To summarize for Cliff we find that we have several target options. If two-element clusters are selected then [fɹ, fl] and [θɹ] would be potential targets. For three-element clusters, [skw] is a good choice.

SELECTION OF TREATMENT TARGETS: JONAH.   Phones not in Jonah's inventory and those that are not stimulable include [k, g, s, z, ʃ, ɹ, tʃ, ʤ]. Jonah demonstrates no initial consonant clusters in his standardized assessment, nor in his spontaneous speech sample. According to the parameters outlined in this complexity approach, a consonant cluster would be targeted. However, to exemplify the process, let's go through the target selection for two singleton consonants.

> **Selecting singleton consonants.**   Based on Jonah's inventory and stimulability, Table 10.2 can be used to analyze implicational universals. The pairs /s, θ/, /z, ð/, or /l, ɹ/ can be eliminated, as Jonah is stimulable for one of each pair. The affricates /tʃ, ʤ/ are later sounds and would be good target possibilities. Affricates imply fricatives and therefore acquisition of affricates should create expansion of Jonah's fricative system.

> **Selecting a consonant cluster.**   If we choose a two-element cluster in which both elements are not in Jonah's inventory and are not stimulable, the following clusters are possibilities: /kɹ, gɹ, ʃɹ/. If we want the cluster with the least sonority difference, then /ʃɹ/, with a sonority difference of 3, would be our choice. Are there any three-element clusters that might be possible targets? Jonah does not have /s/ in his inventory. The best situation would be for him to have the other two members of the cluster in his inventory. The three-element cluster /spl/ is an ideal target, as Jonah has both /p/ and /l/ in his inventory but not /s/.

OVERVIEW OF COMPLEXITY THERAPY.   The complexity approach is a target selection procedure. It is not a specific treatment option such as multiple oppositions, for example. However, research on the complexity approach has systematically outlined the therapy process (e.g., Gierut, 1992, 2001). Nonwords were used in all studies. Nonwords (nonsense words) have been effective in the treatment of phonological disorders (Gierut, Morrisette, & Ziemer, 2010). For example, Gierut and colleagues (2010) found that nonwords, as opposed to real words, induced greater, more rapid generalization in the phonological system as a function of treatment. In addition, children exposed to nonwords sustained levels of performance even after treatment was discontinued. Nonwords also provide a means of controlling several factors in specific contexts and across children (Gierut, 1999).

For singletons, 8 word pairs—thus, 16 individual items—with the sound in the initial position were used as stimuli. The stimuli used a variety of vowels and some actually had two syllables. The only other consonants used in the nonwords were [m, n, b, d].

Based on the selection of one consonant cluster for treatment, 15 nonwords were established. The nonwords contained a variety of vowels and were otherwise structured as outlined in the previous paragraph: One- and two-syllable nonwords were used, and consonants within the word were limited to [m, n, b, d].

The first phase of treatment, *imitation*, was based on the clinician providing a model. During this phase, the clinician uses whatever feedback is necessary to achieve the sound. For example, sound placement, cueing, or successive approximations could be used. This phase continues until 75% accuracy is reached over at least two sessions. As many as seven sessions can be spent on this imitation phase. It is important to note that therapy within these research projects was individual therapy for 60 minutes each session. The concept of seven sessions could be adjusted accordingly.

Activities during this phase could consist of storytelling (the nonsense words could be the characters or some of the actions), sorting, matching, worksheets with the characters, and so forth.

The second phase, *spontaneous production*, was conducted until an accuracy level of 90% over 3 sessions, or maximally 12 sessions (i.e., 12 hours), was realized.

The concept of the complexity approach is to create a circumstance whereby change in the phonological system begins to occur. To that end, probes should be used at periodic time intervals. **Probe words** are not being targeted in therapy but contain the sound or sounds you are trying to achieve as well as other sounds that were not found in the child's inventory. At regular intervals, the child is asked to repeat the probes, and the sound in question is judged as being correct or incorrect. The same words are given to the child each time, so that a percentage correct can be calculated. A list of probe words is contained in Appendix 10.2. The words all have one syllable with either a Consonant-Vowel or a Consonant-Vowel-Consonant structure, which can be used to monitor generalization.

Minimal oppositions contrast therapy, multiple oppositions, maximal oppositions, and the complexity approach are all based on minimal pairs. Table 10.5 provides a summary of these four treatment methods.

Table 10.5 Comparisons of Minimal Pair Therapy Methods

	Minimal Oppositions	Multiple Oppositions	Maximal Oppositions	Complexity Approach
Age range	2 years 1 month to 10 years 5 months Children were usually between 4 and 5 years old.	Typically, children were between 3 and 6 years old.	2 years 8 months to 7 years 11 months Most children were around 4 years old.	2 years 8 months to 7 years 11 months Most children were around 4 years old.
Severity of disorder	Research supports the most efficacy if the child is in the mild to moderate range of phonological disorders.	Moderate to severe phonological disorders. Six sounds were in error across three manner categories.	Moderate to severe phonological disorders. At least six sounds were missing from the phonemic inventory.	Moderate to severe phonological disorders. At least six sounds were excluded across three manner categories.
Targets phonetically similar sounds	Yes Phonological processes are used to determine the word pair. Selection process is based on frequency of occurrence, effect on intelligibility, and age of child.	No Maximal distinctions (those maximally different from the child's error) and maximal classifications (those maximally different in respect to phonetic production characteristics) are used to guide target selection.	No Targets should be maximally different based on the presence of major class features and the total number of feature differences.	No Targets should be as complex as possible based on not being in the child's inventory, lack of stimulability, later-developing sounds, and, in the case of consonant clusters, smaller sonority differences.

(Continued)

Table 10.5 Comparisons of Minimal Pair Therapy Methods *(Continued)*

	Minimal Oppositions	Multiple Oppositions	Maximal Oppositions	Complexity Approach
Targets based on	A sound the child can make versus one that is a substitution.	Collapse of phonemic contrasts (i.e., one sound is used as a substitution for several different sounds). Up to four sounds that also differ in respect to singletons versus consonant clusters can be selected.	Sounds that demonstrate major class distinctions and as many distinctive feature differences as possible.	Lack of stimulability, implicational universals, and marked, later-developing consonants. Consonant clusters are also based on smaller sonority differences (indicating more complexity) between the elements of the cluster. Nonwords are used.
Necessary stimulability of sound	Yes Stimulable sounds have priority as targets.	This is not a deciding variable. The collapse of phonemic contrasts relative to the sound system has high priority.	No Nonstimulable sounds are preferred targets.	No Nonstimulable sounds are preferred targets.

Cycles Phonological Remediation Approach

This approach was developed by Hodson and Paden (1983, 1991). It is a phonological approach to the remediation of unintelligible speech in children. Cycles are time periods during which all selected patterns are treated in a sequence. A clinician begins with primary patterns and, if still necessary, moves to secondary and advanced target patterns. It appears that by using cycles training as treatment, unintelligible children can make progress in a relatively short time (Tyler et al., 1987).

OVERVIEW OF THE CYCLES PHONOLOGICAL REMEDIATION APPROACH. This approach is distinctive for several reasons. First, each cycle has no predetermined level of mastery for phonemes or phoneme patterns. Therefore, clients are not required to reach 75% or 90% accuracy on any phoneme or pattern realization to move to the next cycle. The targeted patterns in the cycle are used to stimulate the *emergence* of a specific sound or pattern, not the *mastery* of it. The premise for this procedure is based on the known observation that phonological acquisition is gradual. The cycles approach is an attempt to approximate closely the way phonological development normally occurs as a gradual process. Second, several phonemes or patterns are targeted within one cycle. Although some of the patterns from Cycle 1 might be "recycled" in the next phase, new patterns are also introduced. Third, this approach targets very specific clients: It is explicitly designed for highly unintelligible children. The goal of cycles training is to increase intelligibility in a relatively short time. A byproduct is the acquisition of certain phonemes and patterns.

WHICH CHILDREN MIGHT BENEFIT FROM THE CYCLES PHONOLOGICAL REMEDIATION APPROACH? This therapy targets highly unintelligible children: "This approach was *not* designed for children with mild speech disorders" (Hodson, 1989, p. 331). Although *highly unintelligible* is not explicitly defined, these children seem to be in the severe to profound range on the *Hodson Assessment of*

Phonological Processes–Revised (Hodson, 2004). Utterances of children in the profound category were characterized by extensive omissions, some phoneme substitutions, and a very restricted repertoire of consonants. Utterances of children in the severe category had fewer omissions but more substitutions, and consonant classes were limited (Hodson & Paden, 1991). Within the case studies and the research, the ages of the children varied from 2 years 9 months to 7 years. Cycles phonological remediation training can be used with very young children.

Is cycles training a viable therapy? According to the authors, it was developed, tested, and refined at experimental clinics in which this approach was used with more than 200 clients (Hodson & Paden, 1991). Hodson (1992) states that "most clients have been dismissed from our clinic as essentially intelligible in less than 1 year" (p. 252). Numerous case studies have been published using the cycles approach (e.g., Gordon-Brannan, Hodson, & Wynne, 1992; Hodson, 2007). This seems to indicate that the cycles approach is an effective treatment method.

HOW TO SELECT TARGETS FOR THE CYCLES PHONOLOGICAL REMEDIATION APPROACH. Targets are selected based on the presence and frequency of specific phonological processes. According to the protocol from the cycles approach, a phonological process should be present at least 40% of the time (the exceptions are glides and nasals, which should show a deficiency level of at least 60%).

The cycles approach orders treatment targets in a systematic way as those you begin with (labeled primary), then secondary target patterns, and finally, for older children, advanced target patterns. The clinician determines which of the primary target patterns the child does not use (i.e., which meet the percentage of phonological process criteria for inclusion) and puts that pattern into the first cycle. The cycles approach does not target patterns that the child is already producing, even if they are inconsistent. Also, if we find that the child is not stimulable for a specific pattern, we will come back to that pattern at a later cycle. Unacceptable targets include /ŋ/, /θ/, /ð/, the syllabic /l/, and weak syllable deletion.

The following are potential *primary target patterns* for Cycle 1 training.

1. *Syllableness.* This refers to two- and three-syllable, equal-stress word combinations such as *cowboy* or *cowboy hat*. The target here is the correct *number* of vowels or diphthongs in the word, not correct production of the consonants. For example, if the child says [ɑʊ.ɔɪ. æ] for "cowboy hat," the child does have syllableness.

2. *Singleton consonants.* The target pattern here relates to the word structure, such as CV, VC, CVC, and VCV. Again, it is not the correctness of the word production but whether the child does produce CVC structures, for example. This would also be a primary target if the child does not produce CV structures with the phonemes /m, n, p, b, t, d, w/. Postvocalic singletons are targeted if the child does not produce VC structures with /p, t/ and/or /k, m, n/. If the child uses only CV or VCV structures, a CVC syllable shape is an important Cycle 1 consideration.

3. *Posterior/anterior contrasts.* Trying to establish velar sounds, /k, g, h/, is a very common goal for children with unintelligible speech. When velars are deficient, they are typically targeted in Cycle 1. It appears that word-final position is easier than word-initial position with /k/ (Hodson & Paden, 1991). Avoid using the substitution, typically [t], in your word choices at first, and

Video Example 10.2
In this video, Dr. Barbara Hodson discusses evaluating and enhancing children's phonological skills. What are the advantages of the cycles phonological remediation program that she talks about?

https://www.youtube.com/watch?v=OjsM4GY_7QA

do not have two [k] sounds in one word. Therefore, "take" or "talk" would not be good initial words, nor would "cake" and "cook." Another possibility is to target /h/ for a back contrast. The goal is to establish a posterior-anterior contrast; targets will depend on the production possibilities of the child in question.

4. *Stridency deletion and /s/ clusters.* The reduction of consonant clusters in general and specifically of s-clusters is very prevalent in children with unintelligible speech. For the child who uses a [t] for [s] substitution, Hodson and Paden (1991) found that the /st/ cluster is very effective—more effective than just /s/. Words such as "stop" or "stay" are possibilities. For children who have alveolars but not velars, it would make sense to target /sp/, /sm/, or /sn/ but not /sk/. However, for the child who has velars but not alveolars, /sk/ might be a good starting point. Some children might find it easier to target /ts/ in the word-final position. A probe would be warranted to see if this is the case with your child.

5. *Liquids.* Many clinicians wait to target /ɹ/, the thought being that this is a later-developing sound. Hodson and Paden (1991) have a different view on targeting /ɹ/. They point out that /ɹ/ seems to be emerging in normally developing 2- or 3-year-old children—not mastered, but rather emerging (refer to Robb & Bleile, 1994). It is easier to elicit an approximation of /ɹ/ in 3- and 4-year-olds than to attempt this later with children who are 6 or 7 years old. The goal here is not a perfect production of liquids but an attempt to suppress the gliding process (/ɹ → w/). The first step might be to try to eliminate the lip rounding that is present on /w/. Although the resulting sound might not be a perfect /ɹ/, this would be a good first goal. In addition, the authors of the cycles approach break the words apart—for example, "red" becomes [ɝ] pause [ɛd]. If /l/ is not immediately stimulable, home practice with tongue clicking is recommended. Vowels that seem to be good with /l/ include /ɑ/ or /ʌ/. The rounded vowels /u/ and /o/ are to be avoided, as they possibly trigger /w/, with its characteristic lip rounding.

The following are potential secondary target patterns:

1. Palatals: glide /j/, sibilants /ʃ, ʒ, tʃ, dʒ/, vocalic /ɝ, ɚ/, word-medial /ɹ/. Singleton stridents, /f/, /s/ if not present
2. Word-medial and word-final /s/ + stop (e.g., rooster, mask)
3. Consonant clusters with sonorants: glide clusters /kw, kj/ and other liquid clusters /tɹ, sl/, for example
4. Voicing contrasts (prevocalic only)
5. Other consonant clusters, such as /skw/ or /stɹ/
6. Residual context-related processes (Hodson, 2011)

SELECTION OF TREATMENT TARGETS: JONAH. Jonah's inventory is contained in Chapter 7 (pages 202–203), and his errors according to phonological processes are on pages 215–216. Let's go through each of the primary target patterns for Jonah.

Syllableness: Jonah has syllableness consistently with two-syllable words (brother [bʌ.tə]) and inconsistently with three-syllable words (vegetable [bɛ.tə.po]). Therefore, syllableness is not a problem for Jonah.

Clinical Application

The following results are from Kathie, age 5 years 10 months, based on the *Hodson Assessment of Phonological Patterns* (HAPP-3) (Hodson, 2004). Kathie was considered unintelligible to most listeners.

Phonological Process	Percentage	Notes
Word/Syllable Structures (Omissions)		
Syllables	6	There was only one occurrence. She uses two- and three-syllable words (the vowels are present).
Consonant sequences/clusters	92	There was a high percentage of consonant cluster reduction.
Consonant singletons		
Prevocalic singletons	0	Substitutions but not omissions.
Intervocalic singletons	0	Substitutions but not omissions.
Postvocalic singletons	14	There were substitutions, not omissions.
Class Deficiencies		
Sonorants		
Liquids	94	No correct [ɹ] sounds, no [l] sounds.
Nasals	0	
Glides	0	
Obstruents		
Stridents	98	She produced one correct [f], but no [s] singletons or clusters.
Velars (e.g., fronting)	91	No correct [g] or [k] productions.
Anterior nonstridents (e.g., backing)	0	

Kathie has syllableness, and she does have singleton consonants and several CVC structures. Based on these percentages and looking at primary targets, it would appear that the following are needed: (1) posterior-anterior contrasts (either word-initial or word-final /k/ or word-initial /g/), (2) stridency deletion and s-clusters (stimulability would be probed for initial and/or final s-clusters), and (3) liquids (both /l/ and /ɹ/).

Singleton consonants: Jonah has many CVC structures with various consonants. Singleton consonants are not a problem for Jonah.

Posterior-anterior contrasts: Jonah does not produce /k/ or /g/ in any contexts. He does appear to have /h/. This would be a target area for Jonah.

Stridency deletion and s-clusters: Jonah does not produce /s/ or /z/. All consonant clusters with /s/ are reduced to a one-consonant sound—for example, /sp/ → /p/.

Liquids: Jonah can produce the liquid /l/, although /ɹ/ is not in his inventory. The liquid /ɹ/ should be a primary target for the first cycle.

To summarize, Jonah's first cycle would consist of (1) posterior-anterior contrasts, (2) stridency and s-clusters, and (3) liquid /ɹ/.

OVERVIEW OF CYCLES PHONOLOGICAL REMEDIATION THERAPY

Establishing a Cycle. Based on the frequency of occurrence of phonological processes, typically several patterns are targeted. Each pattern usually has several phoneme possibilities. For example, anterior-posterior contrasts include /k/ and /g/ or possibly /h/. Each phoneme in a pattern should be targeted for *60 minutes per cycle.* If therapy is 30 minutes per session twice a week, the first phoneme would be targeted for 1 week of therapy. After completion of the first phoneme, a second one is initiated for the next 60 minutes. Each phoneme is targeted for 1 hour; each pattern is targeted for 2 to 6 hours. For example, if our pattern is anterior-posterior contrasts, then, depending on the stimulability of the client, we might start with word-final /k/. That is done for 60 minutes. Then we could possibly move to word-initial /g/ for 60 minutes. We would want to evaluate at that point and see whether we would move on to a new pattern, such as liquids, or stay with anterior-posterior contrasts for additional time. All remaining phonemes are presented consecutively for 60 minutes each. If the goal is a specific phonological pattern rather than an individual phoneme, at least two exemplars of the pattern should be presented in two consecutive 60-minute time intervals before moving to the next phoneme or pattern. For example, if the pattern targeted is CVC structures, two different CVC word types should be used: CVCs with final voiced stops versus CVCs with final nasals. Only one phonological pattern or phoneme should be targeted during any *one* session. In Cycle 1, all patterns determined from the assessment should be presented consecutively. Typically, this cycle has between three and six different patterns or phonemes.

Preparing Word Cards for Therapy. Words are used as the minimal unit of production practice, so word cards that picture each of the chosen phonemes or patterns are developed. Chosen words should be monosyllabic and incorporate facilitative phonetic environments. For example, words with sounds produced at the same place of articulation as the substitute sound should be avoided. Thus, *cat, can, kite,* and *goat* should not be used if the child has a t/k substitution (Hodson, 1989). Object and action words are preferred. Obviously, the words should also be appropriate for the child's vocabulary level. Stimulability probes are used to determine the specific child's appropriate word cards. The child should be able to produce the words with near 100% accuracy. Therefore, the selection process is an important one. Approximately 10 words are selected for the initial 60 minutes of therapy.

Structuring the Remediation Session. Each therapy session should follow these steps:

1. *Review.* The child reviews the preceding session's word cards.

2. *Auditory bombardment.* Amplified auditory stimulation is provided for 1 to 2 minutes while approximately 20 words are provided that contain the target pattern for this session.

3. *Target word cards.* The child draws, colors, or pastes pictures of three to five target words on large index cards while repeating the words modeled by the clinician.

4. *Production practice through experiential play.* During experiential play (e.g., fishing, bowling), the clinician and the child take turns naming the pictures. The clinician provides models and/or tactile cues (such as touching the child's upper lip to indicate an alveolar sound or the child's throat to indicate a velar production), so that the child achieves 100% success on the target patterns. (This is why it is essential that target words are carefully selected.) The clinician also provides opportunities to engage in conversation to determine whether the pattern is beginning to emerge spontaneously.

5. *Stimulability probes.* The clinician assesses the child's stimulability for the next session's potential targets. For example, if /s/ clusters are prospects for the next session, the child is asked to model several words that contain different /s/ clusters. The most stimulable /s/ cluster is then targeted for the next session.

6. *Auditory bombardment.* Step 2 is repeated.

7. *Home program.* The parent or school aide participates in a home program that is 2 minutes per day. This program consists of reading the week's listening list (Step 2) and having the child name picture cards of the production practice words.

Inconsistent Speech Disorder and the Core Vocabulary Approach

This approach was originally developed as a response to a child who did not seem to improve with phonological contrast strategies that were successful in improving other children's speech (Dodd & Iacano, 1989). It was observed that this child had inconsistent productions of the same exact words; thus, many words demonstrated random changes from production to production. Because this child was not making progress in therapy, it was hypothesized that he might require a different approach. The child needed to produce the same word in the same way each time it was said. This child received 2 months of weekly intervention targeting consistent (although not necessarily completely accurate) production of highly functional words. After this time, consistency and accuracy increased (e.g., Crosbie, Holm, & Dodd, 2005).

OVERVIEW OF THE CORE VOCABULARY APPROACH. The core vocabulary approach is for children with an inconsistent speech disorder. According to the Dodd (2013) classification system (refer to Chapter 7, pages 216–218), children in this subgroup of speech sound disorders had the most severe speech problems. Also, these children demonstrated the highest percentage of additional involvement, including difficulties with receptive and expressive language, vocabulary, and phonological awareness.

Inconsistency is characterized by the unpredictable use of a large number of different phones with multiple error types (Dodd, Holm, Crosbie, & McIntosh, 2010). Children with an inconsistent speech disorder may produce the same word differently each time they say it. For example, one child in the Dodd and colleagues (2010) study produced "parrot" in the following ways: [kætoʊə], [kɑdɔwə], and [koʊtuə] (McIntosh & Dodd, 2008). When this occurs on a high percentage of words, it is labeled an inconsistent speech disorder.

To diagnose an inconsistent speech disorder, the child is asked to name 25 one-, two-, and three-syllable words on three separate trials within one session. (The core vocabulary authors use the Word Inconsistency Assessment in the *Diagnostic Evaluation of Articulation and Phonology* [DEAP; Dodd, Hua, Crosbie, Holm, & Ozanne, 2006]). If the child demonstrates 40% or more variability (10 or more of the 25 words), the child is diagnosed with an inconsistent speech disorder.

It is notable that there are certain similarities between children with an inconsistent speech disorder and those with childhood apraxia of speech (Dodd et al., 2010). For example, both groups demonstrate an increase in errors with increased length of utterance. However, the inappropriate oral movements during speech (such as groping and silent posturing) that affect prosody, rate, and fluency are not present in the child with an inconsistent speech disorder. In addition, although those with childhood apraxia of speech show more difficulty with imitation, the child with an inconsistent speech disorder is better with imitation than in spontaneous productions. However, it is important to rule out oral-motor difficulties before diagnosing a child with inconsistent speech disorder. There are several screeners available (refer to Chapter 11) that could be used for this purpose.

WHICH CHILDREN MIGHT BENEFIT FROM THE CORE VOCABULARY APPROACH? The core vocabulary intervention model for children with inconsistent speech disorders seems to be supported by research (e.g., Broomfield & Dodd, 2010; McIntosh & Dodd, 2008). It presents an option that can be used for a relatively short time until stabilization of the word forms occurs. After that, other methods can be used to decrease the noted error patterns. Also, this approach can be used for a rather wide age range of children. Children in the research studies have varied in age from 3 to 11 years old. However, Broomfield and Dodd (2010) note that children who made the most progress with core vocabulary were around 3 years old. Dodd and colleagues (2010) state that the core vocabulary approach could be used for any age child who is diagnosed with an inconsistent speech disorder. When therapy occurred two times per week, stabilization of word forms occurred in approximately 8 weeks (e.g., Crosbie et al.., 2005).

HOW TO SELECT TARGETS FOR THE CORE VOCABULARY APPROACH. The core vocabulary approach is a unique therapy method. It is unique in that its primary goal is to stabilize productions; decreasing the error patterns is a secondary feature and not the main goal. In addition, it is unique in that it is custom designed for the individual child. Thus, based on the child's immediate needs and environment, a vocabulary that will increase the child's functionality is selected.

The child, parents and caregivers, and the child's teacher generate a list of 50 to 70 functionally relevant words. Relevance is the key issue, not the phonemes the words contain. These words should be important and meaningful to the child. Therefore, if possible, the child should be actively involved in selecting this word list. These lists will vary from child to child but should contain items that are useful in the child's environment on a daily basis. For example, the words can include names (family members, other important people, pets), places (school, pool, grandma's house), functional words (please, thank you, good, sorry), and favorite things (football, ice cream, biking). It appears that lexical consistency generalizes after approximately 50 words, so this should be the minimal target word list.

SELECTION OF TREATMENT TARGETS: LORENZO. Jonah does not fit as a case study for the core vocabulary approach, since his productions are not inconsistent. For this case study, Lorenzo will be used.

Lorenzo, age 4 years 1 month, was referred to the speech-language specialist due to his lack of intelligibility. Although his rate of speech was a little slow, he did not show evidence of any oral-motor difficulties when given a screening test for oral-motor skills. After giving him a standardized speech assessment and listening to his conversational speech, which centered around his summer activities, the clinician noted variable productions of /s/, /z/, /f/, /v/, /l/, /k/, /g/, /ʃ/, /tʃ/, /dʒ/, /θ/, /ð/, and /ɹ/. He scored below the 1st percentile on the *Goldman-Fristoe Test of Articulation* (Goldman & Fristoe, 2015), and overall intelligibility was rated as poor. Errors seemed to increase with two- or more-syllable words. Lorenzo was given a consistency probe and demonstrated inconsistent productions on 18 of 25 words (72%). Due to this high percentage, he was classified as having an inconsistent speech disorder. Examples of his variable productions include "kangaroo" [tænhu], [tɑnu], [nəwu]; "thumb" [tʌm], [bʌm], [tɑ]; and "balloon" [bun], [wun], [ədun]. He helped formulate the word list by pointing to items, holding up his toys, and enlisting the aid of his parents to figure out the words he wanted. Lorenzo's preschool teacher also helped by noting specific items that he routinely asked for or were needed to help him function better with the other children. The core vocabulary items selected for Lorenzo are listed in Table 10.6.

OVERVIEW OF CORE VOCABULARY THERAPY. Once you have selected the core vocabulary words, you and the child's family and teacher will need to find pictures of these words. The word is written underneath the picture. Holm, Crosbie, and Dodd (2005) suggest using some type of storage bag or box, in which the picture

---

Table 10.6 Core Vocabulary Items for Lorenzo, Age 4 Years 1 Month

Vader (dog's name)	hungry	pajamas
Louis (brother's name)	chocolate	phone
Sid (best friend's name)	strawberry	dinosaur
Nancy (sister's name)	potty	go
swimming	give	house
banana	baseball	more
cereal	bat	car
ice cream	nose	color
please	mouth	crayons
thank you	hand	pencil
help	upstairs	water
shoes	candy	jacket
school	truck	bye-bye
cookie	ouch	pizza
that	game	burger
camping	play	french fries
bike	open	bathtub
outside	more	comb
juice	glass	brush
milk	bowl	teeth
park	want	football
thirsty	toast	beach
bed	sandwich	eat
apple		

cards are stored and can be picked out for the individual therapy sessions. The number of words practiced in a session can vary, but no more than 10 words is suggested (Holm et al., 2005).

Dodd and colleagues (2010) recommend that core vocabulary intervention occur two times a week in 30-minute individual sessions. There should be home practice between sessions. The total time for intervention is usually 6 to 8 weeks. During the first session of the week, the child's best production of a subset of core vocabulary words should be established. This is done by randomly choosing words (e.g., 10 cards) from the larger set of core vocabulary word cards.

To teach "best" production, first, pictures and the written representation are used for all targets. Second, it must be emphasized to the child that the primary goal is that she or he will produce the word in the same way each time. It does not need to be an error-free production, but it must be the same production. Third, production is drilled sound-by-sound as the child breaks the word into syllables and then reassembles them. Fourth, after reassembly, the word is practiced five times before moving on to the next target word. This method is hypothesized to teach phonological assembly, which is problematic for these children. If necessary, a number of production cues could be used, including an auditory model for immediate and delayed imitation, visual-phonetic cues, verbal-phonetic cues, manual tactile feedback, prosodic cueing, successive approximation or shaping, orthographic cues, metaphor use, the use of metaphonological information about the specific sound class or sound, and phonological awareness instruction (Holm, Crosbie, & Dodd, 2013).

The first session of each week focuses on the best production of approximately 10 words. The second session of the week focuses on massed practice. During this time, the clinician can still use various cueing techniques, but imitation should be kept to a minimum. Children with inconsistent speech disorders are better at imitating than at spontaneous productions. The child needs to learn to plan the sequence of phonological units in the word, not just imitate them. Dodd and colleagues (2010) state that the amount of practice during fun activities or games should be high; the child should attempt between 150 and 170 responses in 30 minutes. During the end of the second session, the 10 practice words are tested for consistency across three repetitions. Any words that are consistent (not necessarily accurate) are removed from the list. At the end of each week, any inconsistent words are retained for further therapy.

Between sessions, the parents and caregivers, family members, and teachers are involved in daily practice. These helpers should focus on the consistency of the child's productions. It must be emphasized to all individuals working with the child that the goal of intervention is that the child says the word in exactly the same way each time she or he attempts to say it. At this point, it is not necessarily a production without errors; it is a production without variability.

A generalization probe is used every 2 weeks to monitor consistency. This probe should be a 10-item list of words that are not being used in treatment. Once the untreated words become consistent, Dodd and colleagues (2010) recommend using the Inconsistency Subtest of DEAP (Dodd et al., 2006) or a similar measure to reconfirm consistency. If generalization has occurred (less than 40% variation in production), core vocabulary therapy as an intervention method can be terminated. At this point, it is reported that children's speech becomes more consistent *and* more accurate, and that their speech is now characterized by developmental, and not atypical, error patterns (Holm et al., 2005).

The Metaphon Approach

Metaphon therapy originated in the 1980s as a result of dissatisfaction with minimal pair management strategies for children with phonological disorders. In the experience of its developers, Janet Howell and Elizabeth Dean, the use of minimal pair contrasts was often not causing the necessary changes in children's phonological systems. This led to them questioning the metaphonological skills of these children. In other words, what do children with phonological disorders know about sounds?

OVERVIEW OF THE METAPHON APPROACH.   Similar to cycles training, metaphon therapy has evolved out of clinical experience and incorporates different approaches that are merged into two therapy phases. However, the framework established to guide therapy is obviously different from that proposed by other treatment protocols. Metaphon therapy is based on metalinguistic awareness. **Metalinguistic awareness** is the ability to think about and reflect on the nature of language and the way it functions. Specifically, metaphon therapy is structured to develop children's metaphonological skills. **Metaphonology** is defined as the ability to pay attention to and reflect on the phonological structure of language (Howell & Dean, 1991, 1994).

Is there evidence that supports the notion that children with phonological disorders have problems with metaphonological skills? Using different metaphonological tasks, several investigations have demonstrated that children with phonological disorders generally do not perform as well as normally developing children of a similar age (e.g., Bird & Bishop, 1992; Gillon, 2018; Hesketh, Dima, & Nelson, 2007; Magnusson, 1991).

Metaphon therapy also assumes that children with phonological disorders fail to realize the communicative significance of the phonological rule system. Their difficulties do not pertain to producing speech sounds in a normal manner but to their failure to acquire the rules of the phonological system. Howell and Dean (1991, 1994) postulate that the best way to help these children change their rule systems is to provide them with information that will encourage them to make their own changes and thus affect their speech output. The phases of metaphon therapy are constructed in an attempt to provide this knowledge.

WHICH CHILDREN MIGHT BENEFIT FROM THE METAPHON APPROACH?   Howell and Dean (1991, 1994) target preschool children because it is at this age that metaphonological knowledge is developing. In the existing case studies cited by Howell and Dean (1994), several common features can be noted: Most of the children presented had very restricted phonetic inventories; all of the children had unusual or idiosyncratic processes, such as initial consonant deletion; and all of the children had a wide variety of phonological processes operating in their speech. These results might indicate that metaphon therapy would be a good match for preschool children who have moderate to severe phonological disorders and who have at least two or three processes that predominate their speech patterns.

Does metaphon therapy work? Both the first and the second editions of Howell and Dean's book (1991, 1994) provide the results of an efficacy study that evaluated several aspects of metaphon therapy. Originally, 13 children participated in the study; in the second edition, the number of subjects increased to 50. Preliminary results indicate that metaphon therapy does indeed work. First, they indicate a reduction in the use of specific phonological processes pre- and post-treatment.

Second, changes in the phonological system were accelerated beyond the expected level according to chronological development. Because the children in this study were not divided into treatment versus no-treatment groups, two different measures of language were used to verify whether treatment, not development, was actually responsible for the changes. Pre- and post-treatment scores for phonological processes were compared to those obtained from a second nontreated language area that was measured by the British Picture Vocabulary Scale (Dunn, Dunn, & Styles, 2009). Although significant differences could be verified with pre- and post-treatment phonological process scores, the scores from the British Picture Vocabulary Scale remained the same, verifying that treatment, not development, had caused the noted changes. Third, some subjects demonstrated a reduction in the targeted phonological processes, but for others the change generalized, causing a reduction in processes that were unrelated to those specifically targeted in treatment. Based on these results, metaphon therapy appears to be a viable therapeutic option.

HOW TO SELECT TARGETS FOR THE METAPHON APPROACH.   Howell and Dean (1991, 1994) use the *Metaphon Resource Pack* (Dean, Howell, Hill, & Waters, 1990) as the basis for their assessment procedure. Seventy words (44 monosyllabic and 26 multisyllabic) are elicited, and 13 different phonological processes are identified.

Howell and Dean (1991, 1994) provide the following general considerations that influence the choice among the processes to be treated:

1. Those selected should not be the same as the ones seen in normally developing children of the same age.
2. Inconsistent use of a simplifying process, which might be evidence of spontaneous development in the child's phonological system, should be given priority in the selection process.
3. The effect the phonological process has on the intelligibility of the child is important. Processes that cause an increased loss of intelligibility, such as stopping of fricatives or atypical processes, should be given priority.
4. The sounds available to the child, both spontaneously and on an imitative basis, play a role in the selection process; sounds that are not in the inventory but can be imitated are usually given priority.

An example is a child, Vivian, age 3 years 4 months, who demonstrates the following processes with an occurrence of more than 50%:

Velar fronting	Word-initial and word-final positions
Stopping of fricatives	All positions
Stopping of affricates	All positions
Initial consonant deletion	Limited to fricatives
Initial consonant cluster reduction/deletion	All contexts
Phonetic inventory	[m, n, ŋ]
	[p, b, t, d, k, g]
	[w, j]
	[l]

Based on the child's age, the velar fronting, stopping of fricatives, and initial fricative deletion were all potential target processes. Consonant cluster reduction could be seen as a consequence of the child's lack of fricatives and of the limited phonetic inventory. Velar fronting was chosen as the first target because the child showed evidence of suppression of this process in some contexts. Initial fricative deletion was selected as the second target because the introduction of fricatives might generalize, eliminating the stopping of fricatives as well.

SELECTION OF TREATMENT TARGETS: JONAH.   Jonah is age 7 years 4 months, so way beyond the preschool age suggested for metaphon therapy. However, as an example, we will go through the phonological processes he demonstrated and the target selection for him.

A phonological process analysis form is filled out for Jonah on pages 215-216. He demonstrates a high number of instances of cluster reduction (almost all clusters are reduced to one element), stopping (of almost all fricatives), and fronting (of primarily /k/ and /g/). There is a limited number of occurrences of final consonant deletion (a total of seven). Applying the criteria, we find the following:

1. *Select processes that are not the same as the ones seen in normally developing children of the same age:* For Jonah, this would apply to all of the previously mentioned processes.
2. *Inconsistent use of a simplifying process has priority:* Jonah does produce /f/ and /v/ accurately on some occasions. These are the only fricatives in which stopping is not evidenced.
3. *The effect the phonological process has on the intelligibility of the child is important:* Stopping and consonant cluster reduction definitely affect intelligibility. Fronting is limited to velar fronting of /k/ and /g/.
4. *The sounds available to the child, both spontaneously and on an imitative basis, have priority:* Jonah can produce /f/ and /v/ correctly on occasion. He is also stimulable for /θ/ and /ð/.

Based on this information, consonant cluster reduction was selected as the first target area. This has a large impact on Jonah's intelligibility. We could possibly start with /f/ clusters (/fl/ might be a possibility, as Jonah can produce /l/) and then target word-final clusters, as Jonah has several sounds that could potentially be put into word-final clusters: -nt, -nd, -mp, -pt. There is one word-medial cluster that Jonah did produce correctly: [nf] in "french fries"; one could attempt /nf/ across syllable boundaries in words such as "info" or "bonfire." Stopping of /θ/ and /ð/ was selected as the second target. Although this will not have a large impact on intelligibility, Jonah is stimulable for both sounds.

OVERVIEW OF METAPHON THERAPY.   This therapy has two phases. Phase 1 is designed to develop an awareness of the properties of sounds. This is accomplished in a motivating setting where success is facilitated. Phase 1 is the most important phase because it forms the basis for the application to more realistic communicative settings emphasized in Phase 2.

Phase 1 Therapy: Developing Phonological Awareness.   The primary aim of Phase 1 is to capture the child's interest in sounds and the entire sound system. Although this is a natural activity of normally developing preschoolers, Howell and Dean (1991, 1994) believe that such awareness has not been possible for a child with a phonological disorder. The child and the clinician explore the properties of sounds together, how sounds differ from each other (i.e., place, manner, and voicing distinctions), and the importance of realizing these distinctions.

Phase 1 therapy is divided into four levels: concept level, sound level, phoneme level, and word level. Although the emphasis is somewhat different depending on whether the target selection is a substitution or a syllable structure process, every client moves through each of the levels with each process. Throughout Phase 1, the child remains a listener only.

Therapy for Substitution Processes

1. *Concept level.* During the discussion and exploration of sounds with a child, it is essential that there be a shared understanding of the vocabulary and concepts used. At the concept level, the child and the clinician play games that involve this vocabulary when talking about different classes of sounds. At this level, individual speech sounds are not contrasted; rather, some of their characteristics—such as long versus short, front versus back, and noisy versus whisper—are considered. The child plays games such as matching long and short socks, ribbons, or strings; putting bricks at the front or back of the house; and growling noisily and in a whisper. These activities are used to identify the respective characteristics as preparation for later place-manner-voicing comparisons of actual speech sounds. At this level, 100% success should be achieved. Therapy at this level may be brief, depending on the child's success.

2. *Sound level.* In this level, the previous achievements are transferred to the description of sounds in general. Games might involve musical instruments, noisemaking rattles, shakers, and vocalizations made by the therapist and child, such as lions "roaring" (supporting the "noisy" concept), people "singing" (supporting the "noisy," voicing concept), and girls "whispering" (supporting the "whisper," voiceless concept). The aim is to show that all sounds can be classified according to the dimensions specified in the concept level—that is, long–short, front–back, and noisy–whisper.

3. *Phoneme level.* After having achieved success at the first two levels, the child is now ready to move on to activities involving speech sounds. The child and clinician take turns producing a range of sounds that vary along the three dimensions previously indicated. Individual sounds are not yet the focus; rather, all sounds from one class are contrasted with sounds from another (e.g., different stops are contrasted with various fricatives). The respective speech sounds may be produced spontaneously or in response to a visual referent (a card with a mnemonic of the property in question). At this level, speech sound activities can also be paired with those introduced at the concept level—for example, first the matching of long and short strings and then the identification of long and short sounds.

4. *Word level.* After the phoneme level, minimal pairs of words containing the targeted contrast are introduced. A child is asked to make a judgment about whether the sound is, for example, long or short, front or back, or noisy or whispered. Although the child is only a listener at this level, some discussion about the sound properties is included. For example, a noisy (voiced) sound is identified, and then knowledge of other "noisy" sounds is questioned. Later, other minimal pairs can be introduced. In addition, visual referents used in

previous levels can be placed on the back of the card to provide additional feedback about the target item.

Therapy for Syllable Structure Processes

1. *Concept level.* For syllable structure processes, such as initial or final consonant deletion, other concepts are introduced, such as "beginning" and "end." These concepts could be exemplified by the engine at the beginning of a train and the caboose at the end or by the nose of the alligator at the beginning and its tail at the end. If cluster simplification is the target, suitable contrasts could consist of the concepts of one horse in front of the wagon, two engines pulling the train, or three dogs pulling the sled.

2. *Syllable level/word level.* At this level, syllables representing the targeted contrast are used. For initial consonant deletion, for example, V and CV structures with nonsense syllables could be introduced with the analogy of a train with no engine versus one with an engine. Because therapy may not be motivating if the clinician stays with nonsense syllables, some words might be selected as well.

Phase 2 Therapy: Developing Phonological and Communicative Awareness. The link between Phases 1 and 2 is established by incorporating Phase 1 activities into Phase 2. Phonological awareness needs to be well developed before Phase 2 can be successful. Both Phase 1 and Phase 2 activities are essential for the *core activity*.

The core activity is structured so that the clinician and the child take turns in producing minimal pair words. If the child says the word pictured on the card accurately, the clinician provides positive feedback and this feedback is expanded into a relevant discussion. For example: "Right, that was a noisy sound. I bet you know lots of other noisy sounds." If, however, the child produces one of the minimal pair words incorrectly, intending the other word, the clinician picks the word that was said, not the intended one. This might stimulate the child to produce a spontaneous repair. The clinician never comments directly on the child's inappropriate production of a particular word but draws the child's attention to the salient features of the contrast: "That was a noisy sound. Should it have been a whisper sound?" Phase 1 activities can be used before or after the core activity.

There are no instructions regarding a child who repeatedly does not produce the sound or sound pattern in question correctly. The assumption is that the child goes back to Phase 1 activities. Therefore, for children who are not stimulable for a particular sound and remain unstimulable throughout Phase 1, Phase 2 could prove to be frustrating. In a later portion of the text, Howell and Dean suggest that based on the child's increased metalinguistic awareness, a discussion of the reasons for the loss of contrast should be explored. "Referring to sounds in a way which allows children to discuss them allows specific exploration of the reasons why a child has failed to convey meaning" (Howell & Dean, 1994, p. 110).

The last activities move the minimal word pairs into sentences, such as "Put the picture of the pea/key in the box" and "Draw a picture of the pea/key on the board." Situations that facilitate communication and promote repairing communicative breakdowns are important variables. It is stressed that a supportive environment is an essential ingredient of this therapy.

Speech Sound Disorders with Concurrent Language Problems: The Treatment of Morphosyntax, Vocabulary, and the Child with Emerging Phonology

Speech sound disorders often co-occur with language disorders. Based on a variety of studies, the estimated co-occurrence rate was 35% to 60% (e.g., Botting & Conti-Ramsden, 2004; Shriberg, 2004). Thus, many children seen clinically for a speech sound disorder also demonstrate other language problems.

To address this co-occurrence of language and speech sound disorders, several approaches have attempted to link speech sound intervention to other language components. For example, Hoffman and Norris (2010) have supported a whole language approach in which phonological development is targeted at the same time as development of discourse structure, semantic, morphosyntactic, and letter-sound knowledge. In addition, the morphosyntax intervention approach (Haskill, Tyler, & Tolbert, 2001; Tyler & Haskill, 2011) focuses on structures that interface with phonology and are significant for language development. This approach targets as many as four grammatical morphemes in a cycle for approximately a week. This cycle can be repeated or alternated with direct speech intervention every other cycle. Singleton or final consonant clusters can be targeted in past tense (row<u>ed</u>, wal<u>ked</u>), third-person singular (he go<u>es</u>, she dri<u>nks</u>), or in a copula sentence (He <u>is</u> away, He <u>is</u> <u>m</u>ad). Specific studies have suggested that participants made significant gains in speech and morphosyntax (Tyler, Lewis, Haskill, & Tolbert, 2002, 2003). Although more research is needed on the interaction of phonology with other language areas, it is currently safe to say that (1) many children with phonemic-based disorders also demonstrate language difficulties, and (2) intervention needs to target both phonology and any additional deficient language areas. To achieve this, a specified amount of time could be allotted to each deficient area: phonology, morphosyntax, semantics, or pragmatics. Of course, it would be more time efficient if some language therapy goals could be unified. The following section, "Connecting Phonology to Morphosyntax: Morphosyntax Intervention," offers some suggestions on how specific phonological remediation goals could be combined with noted morphosyntactic problems.

Connecting Phonology to Morphosyntax: Morphosyntax Intervention

Various morphological problems in children with specific language impairment (SLI) have been observed (e.g., Bishop, 1994; Eyer & Leonard, 1994; Leonard, 1994; Leonard, McGregor, & Allen, 1992; Oetting & Horohov, 1997; Oetting & Rice, 1993; Rice & Oetting, 1993; Rice, Wexler, & Cleave, 1995). Based on the findings of several of these investigations, Leonard and colleagues (1992) summarized the grammatical morphemes that were used less frequently by children with SLI: Among others, these grammatical morphemes include plurals, regular and irregular past tense, possessives, third-person singular, and copula/auxiliary sentence forms.

Based on production difficulties, it becomes clear that children with speech sound disorders might have problems actually producing some of these grammatical morphemes. Plurality, past tense *-ed*, possessive, and third-person singular, for example, very often result in word-final consonant clusters. If a child deletes final consonants or reduces consonant clusters, the grammatical function of these morphemes will be lost. Even for a child who is displaying primarily substitution processes, these morphemes might not be realized accurately. To preserve morphemic contrasts, attention must be given to final consonants and consonant clusters when working with a child with a speech sound disorder and language difficulties.

Length and complexity of the utterance also need to be considered because syntactical complexity affects productional accuracy. The more complex the syntax is, the more likely a child is to demonstrate a breakdown in articulatory accuracy. Although one therapeutic goal could be to increase the length and complexity of a child's utterances, this should always be evaluated with respect to the interaction between production accuracy and syntactic complexity.

REMEDIATION SUGGESTIONS

1. If a therapy goal is the elimination of final consonant deletion, words that incorporate specific grammatical morphemes in contrasting word pairs could be targeted. The use of such pairs depends on the sounds in the client's inventory and the targeted sounds but could include, whenever possible, aspects of morphology, especially grammatical morphemes. The following are given as examples of words and phrases that incorporate grammatical morphemes that end in CVC structures:

Grammatical Morpheme	Examples
Plurality	toe-toes, key-keys, shoe-shoes
Possessive	Joe-Joe's, Ray-Ray's
Regular past tense	row-rowed, lay-laid, show-showed
Third-person singular	I go-he goes, I do—he does

2. If a therapy goal pertains to reducing consonant cluster reduction or deletion, contrastive word pairs such as the following incorporate grammatical morphemes in a word-final VCC structure:

Grammatical Morpheme	Examples
Plurality	boat-boats, cup-cups, wheel-wheels
Possessive	cat-cat's, Dad-Dad's, dog-dog's
Regular past tense	walk-walked, kiss-kissed
Third-person singular	I walk-he walks, I sip-he sips
Irregular past tense	drink-drank, hold-held

3. In sentences, minimal pair words could be used systematically to represent other grammatical morphemes:

Grammatical Morpheme	Examples
Copula	She is sad *versus* She is mad He is tall *versus* He is small
Auxiliary	He is shopping *versus* He is hopping She is kissing *versus* She is hissing

4. Subject and object pronouns could also be used in sentences:

	Examples
Subject pronouns	She is here *versus* He is here She opened the door *versus* Lee opened the door She has the tea *versus* He has the key He helped the man *versus* We helped the man
Object pronouns	Give it to Jim *versus* Give it to him The tea belongs to her *versus* The key belongs to him

Connecting Phonology to Semantics: Vocabulary Intervention

Most research on the semantic limitations of children with language impairments has focused on their use of nouns (Leonard, 1988; Rice, 1991). These studies have found that children with language impairment are slow in using their first words and that subsequent vocabulary development occurs at a slower rate than in normally developing children. Other literature has examined the use of verbs in children with language impairment (Conti-Ramsden & Jones, 1997; King & Fletcher, 1993; Paul, 1993; Rice, 1994; Rice & Bode, 1993; Rice et al., 1995; Watkins, Rice, & Moltz, 1993). These studies suggest that verbs and verb-related grammatical properties can be a particular problem for children with language impairments.

Clinical Exercises Lizbeth, age 4 years 0 months, has a /t/ for /k/ substitution. She is also delayed in language and has difficulty with subject-object pronouns. Can you suggest five sentences in which you could target /k/ versus /t/ and work on subject pronouns (he, she, it) and object pronouns (him, her)?

Marcus, age 5 years 11 months, is working on [s] and [z]. He also deletes the "s" ending of third-person singular forms (He walks, She thinks). Create eight sentences, four that work with [z] in word-final position as a singleton (e.g., "He goes") and four that are in word-final position as clusters with [s] or [z], that address third-person singular forms (e.g., "She hops").

REMEDIATION SUGGESTIONS

1. Although minimal pair words typically incorporate nouns ("things" are easier to picture), various verbs could also be targeted. These could be selected in accordance with the child's targeted sound or process. Some examples follow:

Velar fronting	[t/k] substitution
taught-caught, knot-knock, bait-bake	
Stopping of fricatives	[t/s]
tell-sell, tip-sip, talk-sock	

Final consonant deletion	CVC structures with final C
pay-paid, say-sail, show-shown	
Initial consonant deletion	CVC structures with initial C
eat-beat, aid-made, earn-burn	

2. When targeted sounds emerge in the child's speech, expand vocabulary with new words containing the target. Children appear to learn more new words easier and quicker when the words begin with consonants that the children have used previously in other words. Therefore, if a targeted sound is emerging in the child's speech, the clinician could try to use new practice words that also expand the child's vocabulary.

The Child with an Emerging Phonological System: Expanding the System and Vocabulary

As previously noted, the term *emerging phonological system* refers to a time period when sounds are beginning to be used to form conventional words—in other words, the emergence of expressive language. At approximately age 2, normally developing toddlers begin to combine single words into two-word utterances. However, this communicative development seems to lag behind in some 2-year-olds. Children whose comprehension abilities are considered normal but who fail to achieve a 50-word vocabulary and 2-word combinations by age 2 are referred to as "late talkers," toddlers with "slow expressive language development or delay" (Paul & Jennings, 1992; Reed, 2018; Rescorla & Schwartz, 1990), or children with "specific expressive language impairment" (Rescorla & Ratner, 1996). It has been estimated that approximately 10% to 15% of the total 2-year-old population meet these criteria (Rescorla, 1989). Half of them seem to outgrow this delay; the other half continues to demonstrate language problems at age 3 and beyond.

To evaluate a child's emerging phonological system, an independent analysis was suggested in Chapter 6. Such an analysis examines the child's productions of individual sounds; however, the sound productions are not compared to the adult model. At this point in the child's development, it is far more important to note the actual usage of specific sounds in words. To this end, two types of data need to be collected: (1) the inventory of speech sounds, and (2) the syllable shapes used.

General remediation strategies for children with slow emerging language development include developing expressive language skills—specifically, expanding the number of vocabulary items, the consonant inventory, and syllable shapes—and, finally, the use of two-word utterances (Paul, Norbury, & Gosse, 2018). At this stage of a child's development, therapy must represent a unified package. Therapy to promote phonological skills must be combined with increasing the child's lexicon. The use of specific syllable shapes is also a consideration when selecting which words to target. Remediation for the child with an emerging language system must account for the interdependencies that exist among all language areas.

The following suggestions provide some points to consider when choosing the first words for children with small expressive vocabularies. The *consonant inventory* and the *syllable shapes* the child uses are especially important variables in this selection process.

COMBINING PHONOLOGY WITH DEVELOPING A LEXICON

1. First, children's consonant inventories need to be considered. Early vocabularies are influenced by their phonological composition. Words that are easier for children to produce are more likely to be included in their early vocabularies. In addition, children appear to learn more easily and quickly new words that begin with consonants that they have used previously in other words. Therefore, new words that contain sounds already in a child's inventory should be targeted.

   An example: The child's inventory contains the following sounds:

   [m, n]
   [p, b, t, d]
   [h, j]

   Depending on the child's present lexicon, the following might be good word choices:

   me, no-no
   puppy, baby, bye-bye, teddy, toe
   happy, yay

2. The child's present use of syllable shapes needs to be considered. Early syllable shapes include V, CV, CVCV, and CVC. The therapist selects words with syllable shapes the child already uses, possibly including other early syllable shapes. In doing so, it should be kept in mind that the therapy goal is to *expand* the child's use of syllable shapes; therefore, early syllable shapes not in the child's repertoire should also be stimulated.

   An example: If the child primarily realizes V, CV, and CVCV syllable shapes:

   mama might be easier than *mom*
   papa might be easier than *dad*
   puppy or *doggie* might be easier than *dog*
   kittie might be easier than *cat*
   baby might be easier than *doll*

3. When expanding a child's consonant inventory, the normal developmental sequence should be the guiding principle. Children with slow emerging language seem to acquire consonants in the same order as normally developing children but at a slower rate (Paul & Jennings, 1992). Therefore, early sounds that are not yet in the child's inventory should be targeted. For the child with only a few expressive words, Paul and colleagues (2018) suggest introducing the sound by first using a babbling game activity rather than by putting it directly into words. The clinician begins by imitating the child's vocalizations. Once a reciprocal babbling exchange is established, the clinician introduces the new consonant into the babbling activity. The goal of this activity is not to get the child to produce that particular sound but to increase the consonant inventory. Therefore, any new consonant, even if it is not the one modeled by the clinician, should be rewarded.

4. New words should be similar to those used first by normally developing children. These include, for example, names of important people in the child's environment; names for objects the child directly acts on; labels for objects that move and change; and labels for actions, games, and routines in which the child is an active participant (Berko Gleason & Bernstein Ratner, 2017; Owens, 2016).

5. After having evaluated the child's inventory and use of syllable structures, words from a wide variety of grammatical classes should be selected. Although nouns dominate young children's early speech, children's vocabularies include words from a variety of grammatical classes from the beginning (Berko Gleason & Bernstein Ratner, 2017). Therefore, not only nouns should be targeted but also words that can be used to talk about the *relations* between objects. These relational words express more communicative functions and can be readily combined with other words into two-word utterances.

At this stage in the child's development, articulation patterns very seldom mirror adult pronunciation. However, the therapy focus for these children is on expanding the use of consonants, syllable shapes, and words, not on norm production. Therefore, any word approximations produced by the child should be rewarded, not corrected. For example, if the word is *down* and the child says [da] or [ta], the clinician should reward this word approximation. Even if the child produces the final [n] in another word, that does not mean the child can produce [n] under different coarticulatory conditions in a new word. The goal during this phase of therapy is to stimulate word production, not articulatory "correctness."

> **Clinical Exercises** Melody, age 2 years 2 months, is just beginning to say her first words. She says [mɑmi], [dæ.i] for "daddy," [ta] for "cat," [mi], [nono], [beɪbi], [dɑ] for "there," and [up] for "oops."
>
> Can you make a list of additional words that you might target using these sounds?
>
> Which sound(s) might you target for stimulation?

Treatment of Multiple Vowel Errors

An abundance of information about children's difficulties with consonant articulation and their remediation is available. In contrast, vowel problems have not received the same degree of attention. This generally has been justified by the fact that vowels are mastered at an early age in the child's development. Therefore, children with speech sound disorders probably show few vowel errors. However, this assumption stands in contrast to the documented vowel errors in many case studies and in the literature (e.g., Ball & Gibbon, 2002; Clark & Goldstein, 1996; Pollock & Keiser, 1990; Renfrew, 1966; Reynolds, 1990; Stoel-Gammon & Herrington, 1990).

Although vowels are normally among the earliest sounds acquired, it appears that some children with speech sound disorders demonstrate difficulties with regular vowel realizations. Using the Pollock and Keiser (1990) data as an estimate for the frequency of occurrence, 1 of their 15 children with phonemic-based problems (6.7%) had distinct difficulties with vowel productions. This child's speech showed that approximately half of the vowels were in error. Vowel difficulties could well belong to the clinical profile of some children with speech sound disorders.

A review of several studies containing vowel data from children with speech sound disorders seems to indicate that two patterns emerge (Stoel-Gammon &

Herrington, 1990). First, some children have extremely limited vowel inventories. These children's vowel productions seem to resemble those of the babbling period, with lax, non-high vowels predominating. A second group demonstrates relatively large vowel inventories but a high incidence of vowel errors—that is, a large number of vowel substitutions. The sequence of vowel acquisition in this group of children appeared to be similar to the one for younger, normally developing children. In both groups of children with vowel problems, the vowels represented by the corners of the vowel quadrilateral were mastered earlier.

How disordered should a vowel system be to warrant therapy? Three types of diagnostic information for vowel analysis are suggested: (1) the vowel inventory, (2) the accuracy of production, and (3) error patterns. Examination of the vowel inventory can determine whether the child has a limited or near-normal inventory. Data on the accuracy of vowel production are important when assessing children with a fairly complete vowel inventory but a high proportion of vowel substitutions. The third type of diagnostic information, error patterns, is especially valuable when planning therapy. Figure 10.1 is a matrix that can be used to record the child's vowel inventory. Accurate and irregular vowel realizations can be recorded directly on the matrix. This provides the inventory and the number of occurrences of accurate productions. Error patterns can also be identified by comparing the substitutions to the norm productions.

The Child with a Very Limited Vowel Inventory: Therapeutic Suggestions

According to the limited data available, it appears that the vowel system of these children is characterized by only two or three vowels. These vowels are lax and non-high vowels such as [ɑ], [ɛ], [æ], or [ʌ]. Such lax, non-high vowels are typical

---

Figure 10.1 Matrix for Recording Vowels

Put a + below the vowel sound if present and accurate in the inventory. Write in the error production if a substitution is noted.

Front Vowels					Back Vowels			
i	ɪ	eɪ	ɛ	æ	u	ʊ	oʊ	ɑ/ɔ/a

Central Vowels		Phonemic Diphthongs		
ʌ/ə	ɝ/ɚ	aɪ	aʊ	ɔɪ

in the babbling period. Stoel-Gammon and Herrington (1990) group vowel acquisition into three categories:

Group 1	
Vowels that are mastered relatively early	i, ɑ, u, o, ʌ
Group 2	
Vowels acquired somewhere between early and late (some investigations reported early acquisition, others later acquisition)	æ, ʊ, ɔ, ə
Group 3	
Vowels that are mastered relatively late	e, ɛ, ɪ, ɝ, ɚ

> **Clinical Exercises** Refer back to Melody (page 383). Based on her limited vocabulary, what is her vowel inventory?
>
> Are there "early" vowels that she does not have in her inventory? Can you identify four words that you could use in therapy to stimulate these vowels? Make sure that you also consider her consonant inventory.

USING ONE KNOWN AND ONE UNKNOWN VOWEL IN MINIMAL PAIRS

1. *The child's vowel inventory needs to be compared to those vowels that are mastered relatively early.* A vowel from Group 1 that is very different from one of the child's vowels is selected. For example, if the child has [ɑ], a lax, low-back vowel, a good candidate would be [i], the tense high-front vowel.

2. *The two vowels should be contrasted in minimal pairs.* Whenever possible, consonants from the child's inventory should be used. Examples follow:

Not in Inventory	In Inventory
me	ma
beet	bought
team	Tom
hee	haw

3. *Other early vowels in minimal contrasts with the original vowel are introduced.* Using the example with [ɑ], another distinct vowel is [u]. Examples follow:

Not in Inventory	In Inventory
moo	me, ma
boo	bee
moon	mean
new	knee

USING TWO UNKNOWN VOWELS IN MINIMAL PAIRS

1. *This variation uses two unknown vowels in minimal pairs.* Two vowels that are not in the child's inventory should be chosen from Group 3, if possible. The vowels should again be as different as possible. If the child's inventory includes [ɑ] and [ʌ], [ɪ] and [ɝ] might be selected. These sounds are placed in minimal pairs. Examples follow:

   bit-Burt
   bid-bird
   ill-Earl
   gill-girl

2. *Two different unknown vowels are then targeted.* The selection process should consider the complexity of the vowel and its lack of stimulability.

The Child with a High Proportion of Vowel Substitutions: Therapeutic Suggestions

Children with a high proportion of vowel substitutions usually show a relatively intact vowel inventory. An error pattern analysis can be helpful in selecting the target vowels.

This analysis procedure contrasts the target vowel to the substituted vowel. A list of all vowel substitutions with their relative percentage of occurrence is generated. One possible target could be inconsistent vowel substitutions (i.e., those vowels that are sometimes produced correctly but also have different substitutions). For example, the following are noted for /æ/:

   ɛ/æ, frequency of occurrence = 30%
   ɪ/æ, frequency of occurrence = 35%
   correct production of [æ], frequency of occurrence = 35%

One of the substitutions for [æ] would be selected as the second vowel. In addition, the substitution chosen should be as different as possible from the target. These two vowels would then be used as the vowel nuclei of minimally paired words. Using these criteria, [æ] and [ɪ] would be good choices. These two vowels are then placed in minimal word pairs. Examples follow:

   mat-mitt
   bag-big
   pan-pin
   ham-him

A second possibility is to target a vowel that is used as a substitution for several vowels. The following exemplifies this scenario:

Target Vowel	Substitution
i	ɪ
eɪ	ɑ
ɛ	ɑ
æ	ɑ
ʊ	u

In this case, [ɑ] is used as a substitution for [eɪ], [ɛ], and [æ]. Therefore, [ɑ] would be contrasted with either [eɪ], [ɛ], or [æ]. Clear production differences should be given priority when selecting the targeted vowel. Contrasting [ɑ], a low-back vowel, to [eɪ], a diphthong with a mid-high onglide, would provide such distinct differences. These two vowels would then be placed in minimal pairs. Examples follow:

tall-tail
cop-cape
top-tape

Therapy proceeds from vowels with dissimilar to more similar production features. In this example, [ɑ] and [ɛ] would be the next vowels targeted as the nuclei for minimal pairs.

Using a multiple oppositions approach, several different minimal pairs could be contrasted using the three substitutions of [eɪ], [ɛ], and [æ]. The following words would then be targeted simultaneously: bought – bait – bet – bat.

Summary

This chapter described several intervention approaches for the treatment of children with phonological disorders. Some of these remediation programs use minimal pair contrasts as the beginning unit of remediation—for example, minimal opposition contrasts, multiple oppositions, maximum oppositions, and the complexity approaches. Other remediation techniques are unique, such as cycles training, core vocabulary, and metaphon therapy. These last three therapy protocols, which have been developed and refined through actual clinical experience, together forge a combination of methods that can be effectively used to treat speech sound disorders in children.

Discussion of the treatment approaches has been structured according to specific parameters: (1) an overview of the treatment method, followed by (2) which children might benefit from this approach, (3) how to select targets for this approach, (4) selecting treatment targets for the case study, Jonah, and (5) an overview of the therapy protocol. Selecting targets and intervention methods were outlined in some detail to illustrate the use of each approach in a therapy setting.

The final part of this chapter explored and suggested some special applications of phonological therapy. Phonological remediation principles with children who display concurrent language difficulties and those with emerging phonological systems were discussed. The merging of phonological intervention strategies with other language areas such as morphology and semantics was attempted. Finally, treatment principles for children with disordered vowel systems were presented to demonstrate how minimal pair contrasts can be structured in a remediation program.

This chapter emphasized assessment results and their connection to therapy goals. Whenever possible, the assessment results outlined in Chapter 7 and the therapy procedures in this chapter were directly linked. Several clinical applications were provided to demonstrate the connection between assessment and treatment, which is essential for professional speech-language services.

Case Study

The following results are from *Hodson Assessment of Phonological Patterns* (HAPP-3) (Hodson, 2004) for Andrew, age 5 years 6 months.

1. basket	[bæ.tə]		26. shoe	[du]
2. boats	[boʊ]		27. slide	[jaɪd]
3. candle	[tæn.ə]		28. smoke	[boʊt]
4. chair	[teə]		29. snake	[deɪt]
5. clouds	[jaʊd]		30. soap	[doʊp]
6. cowboy hat	[taʊ.bo.æt]		31. spoon	[pun]
7. feather	[pɛ.də]		32. square	[twɛə]
8. fish	[pɪd]		33. star	[tɑə]
9. flower	[taʊ.ə]		34. string	[twɪŋ]
10. fork	[pot]		35. swimming	[twɪm.ɪn]
11. glasses	[jæ.tət]		36. television	[tɛ.də.bɪ.dən]
12. glove	[dʌb]		37. toothbrush	[tu.bət]
13. gum	[dʌm]		38. truck	[twʌt]
14. hanger	[hæn.də]		39. vase	[beɪd]
15. horse	[hoət]		40. watch	[wɑt]
16. ice cubes	[aɪt.jub]		41. yoyo	[jʌ.joʊ]
17. jumping	[dʌmp]		42. zip	[jɪp]
18. leaf	[jif]		43. crayons	[tweɪ.ən]
19. mask	[mæt]		44. black	[bæt]
20. music box	[mu.ɪt.bɑt]		45. green	[dwin]
21. page	[peɪd]		46. yellow	[jɛ.joʊ]
22. plane	[peɪn]		47. three	[twi]
23. queen	[twin]		48. thumb	[tʌm]
24. rock	[wɑt]		49. nose	[noʊd]
25. screwdriver	[dwu.dwaɪ.və]		50. mouth	[maʊf]

We have decided to use the cycles approach. The following process is used to determine which patterns to target. According to the protocol from the cycles approach, the selected phonological processes were present at least 40% of the time (the exceptions are glides and nasals, which should show a deficiency level of at least 60%).

1. *Early developing phonological patterns:*

   Syllableness. Andrew seems to demonstrate evidence of this in words such as *cowboy hat* and *ice cubes.*

   Word-initial singleton consonants. Andrew produces appropriate word-initial singleton consonants.

Word-final singleton consonants. Andrew uses appropriate consonants in the word-final position.

Other word structures. Andrew can produce CVC structures (e.g., *mouth*), CVCV structures (e.g., *yoyo*, *feather*), and CCVC structures ([dwin] for *green*).

2. *Posterior/anterior contrasts.* Velar sounds /k/ and /g/ are absent in Andrew's speech.
3. *Stridency and s-clusters.* Andrew does not seem to be able to produce /s/ as a singleton nor in clusters.
4. *Liquids.* Andrew does not demonstrate that he can produce the liquids /l/ and /ɹ/.

Patterns targeted: Based on stimulability, the following patterns could be targeted:

1. *Anterior-posterior contrasts.* The velar /k/ or /g/ would be targets for the first cycle.
2. *Stridency and s-clusters.* Hodson and Paden (1991) recommend that word-final s-clusters be targeted. The clinician should determine which one(s) might be stimulable.
3. *Liquids.* Andrew does not produce any liquids. Stimulability should be probed on both /l/ and /ɹ/. One or both of these could be used in the first cycle.

Think Critically

1. Based on the earlier case study featuring Andrew, age 5 years 6 months, we note that the following consonants are not in his inventory: /k, g, s, z, ʃ, θ, ð, ŋ, l, and ɹ/. If you were going to use maximal oppositions, which two sounds would you target? First, find the sounds that have major class feature differences. Second, find the two sounds that have the most distinctive feature differences.

2. Based on the earlier case study featuring Andrew, age 5 years 6 months, note the collapse of phonemic contrasts. For example, the consonants /k, s, f/ (one time in *flowers*), /ʃ, tʃ/, and /θ/ are all collapsed to /t/. What other neutralization of phonemic contrasts can be noted in Andrew's articulation test results? Use this information to establish treatment targets with the multiple oppositions approach.

 Chapter Quiz 10.1 Complete this quiz to check your understanding of chapter concepts.

Appendix 10.1 Probes for Initial Consonant Clusters That Could Be Targets

Consonant Clusters	Word Examples
sm	small, smell, smart, smoke, smile
sn	snow, snack, snail, snake, snap
sl	slow, sleep, slap, sled, slide
sp	spot, spin, spoon, speed, spade

st	stop, stick, stew, steam, stay
sk	ski, skip, skate, sky, scoop
sw	swat, swam, swim, sweet, swell
spɹ	spread, spring, sprain, spray, sprout
spl	splash, split, splint, splat, splurge
stɹ	string, strap, straw, straight, street, strike
skɹ	screw, screen, scratch, scrub, scrap
skw	square, squeak, squeeze, squash, squeal
fl	fly, flow, flat, flag, flap
fɹ	fry, free, fruit, frog, from
fj	few, fuel, furry, fume, fuming
θɹ	throw, three, threw, thread, threat
ʃɹ	shred, shrink, shrimp, shrub, shrug
bl	blue, blow, black, block, blink
bɹ	brain, brake, brick, bright, broom
bj	beauty
dɹ	dry, draw, drum, dream, drink
gl	glue, glow, glad, glove, glide
gɹ	grow, grey, green, grape, group
pl	play, plow, plum, plant, plane
pɹ	prune, print, proof, proud, prove
pj	puke, pure
mj	music, muse
tɹ	true, train, trick, trail, trap
kl	clay, clue, clap, clean, clock
kɹ	crow, cry, crab, crumb, crawl
dw	dwell, dwarf, dwelling
tw	twig, tweet, twin, twelve, twice
kw	quack, quick, quit, queen, quite
kj	cute, cupid, cutie
vj	view, viewer

Due to their infrequency of occurrence in words, the clusters [mj, pj, bj, kj, vj, and fj] are typically not selected for targets.

Appendix 10.2 Probes for Monitoring Generalization or Therapy Progress

[p]	[b]	[t]	[d]	[k]	[g]
paw	big	toe	do	key	go

pig	bite	two	day	comb	game
pea	bean	tan	deep	cow	get
pen	ball	tail	dime	cup	good
poke	boat	ten	down	can	gate
up	tub	bat	bad	back	bag
lip	cab	boot	bed	book	hog
top	knob	hot	hide	duck	dog
tape	mob	out	wood	look	dig
mop	web	nut	need	pack	leg

[m]	[n]	[ŋ]
mad	no	
man	now	
map	night	
me	knot	
mean	need	
came	pin	wing
dime	bone	long
name	down	hang
time	one	king
gum	pain	bang

[f]	[v]	[s]	[z]	[ʃ]	[ʒ]
fall	van	sew	zoom	shake	Jacques
fan	vote	sing	zoo	shoe	
fed	volt	sock	zip	show	
fig	vault	soup	zap	shut	
fight	veil	some	zing	ship	
beef	cave	bus	bees	cash	beige
cough	dive	face	boys	leash	rouge
half	five	gas	does	brush	
leaf	give	mess	is	wash	
tough	have	yes	noise	wish	

[θ]	[ð]	[tʃ]	[dʒ]
thank	that	chain	gym
think	the	cheap	jack
thick	they	chop	jam

thin	then	chin	jeep
thing	them	chick	jet
bath	smooth	beach	age
math	bathe	catch	cage
moth	breathe	peach	edge
tooth	clothe	match	huge
teeth	loathe	witch	fudge

[l]	[ɹ]	[j]	[w]	[h]
low	row	you	we	high
lamb	rain	yell	wet	have
like	road	yolk	week	hill
late	ring	young	wall	him
lap	rock	your	wide	home
ball	bear			
bull	four			
pail	her			
will	more			
fall	deer			

Chapter 11
Speech Sound Disorders in Selected Populations

 Learning Objectives

When you have finished this chapter, you should be able to:

11.1 Understand the definitions, general features, speech sound characteristics, assessment, and treatment options for childhood apraxia of speech.

11.2 Define cerebral palsy as a motor-speech disorder; describe its accompanying difficulties in respiration, phonation, resonation, and articulation; and understand the diagnostic and therapeutic possibilities.

11.3 Classify cleft palate features as well as the subsequent speech sound characteristics, assessment, and treatment guidelines.

11.4 Describe general features and note specific speech sound disorders of children with intellectual disabilities, including Down syndrome, as well as diagnostic and therapy options.

11.5 Recognize the definition, characteristics, speech sound difficulties, and assessment and treatment options for children with a hearing loss.

11.6 Categorize motor-speech disorders in adults—apraxia of speech and dysarthria—according to their general features, speech sound characteristics, and diagnostic and therapeutic measures.

Chapter Application: Case Study

Trish had just received her externship placement. She was going to be at a major hospital in Portland where she would be learning from the three speech-language pathologists working there. She was very excited, although also apprehensive. She would eventually be helping with the diagnosis and treatment of children with cleft palates, childhood apraxia of speech, and hearing impairments and adults in acute care, such as those with aphasia and dysarthria. She had learned

(Continued)

about these disorders in her classes but was not sure about the specifics of diagnosis and treatment. There were a lot of different disorders she needed to review and be prepared to evaluate and treat. How could she do that in a time-effective manner?

THIS CHAPTER provides an overview of the speech characteristics of selected populations in which speech sound problems are among the primary difficulties. Many comprehensive books have been written on each of these disorders. Therefore, the following synopses represent only selected aspects of the characteristics as well as diagnostic and treatment principles relative to the speech sound disorder. Each discussion is organized into four sections: (1) definition and general features, (2) speech sound characteristics, (3) clinical diagnostics, and (4) therapeutic implications. Many references are given throughout the chapter; these can be used to delve deeper into specifics for each of the disorders discussed.

This chapter does not reflect all the disorders that speech-language specialists assess and treat in clinical practice. It is also not within the scope of this book to examine all the techniques that are available when working with individuals who have these disorders. Instead, it provides an overview of the disorders, assessment possibilities, and treatment options directly related to the individual's speech sound difficulties.

Childhood Apraxia of Speech: A Disorder of Speech Motor Control

Definition and General Features

The term *developmental articulatory dyspraxia* was first used by Morley, Court, and Miller (1954) to describe a small subset of children with speech sound disorders that seemed to demonstrate different characteristics from those of other children with speech problems. Subsequently, over the years these children have been categorized as having developmental apraxia of speech, congenital articulatory apraxia, and developmental verbal apraxia, to mention a few labels. Currently, the preferred term is *childhood apraxia of speech (CAS)* (American Speech-Language-Hearing Association [ASHA], 2007a). The preferred use of *childhood apraxia of speech* distinguishes this disorder from being merely a "developmental" disorder that the child could outgrow under normal circumstances.

After surveying the literature, the Ad Hoc Committee on Childhood Apraxia of Speech (ASHA, 2007b) found that CAS occurs in children in three clinical contexts: known neurological etiologies (e.g., intrauterine stroke, infections, trauma), as a result of complex neurobehavioral disorders (e.g., genetic, metabolic), and as an idiopathic neurogenic disorder with no known neurological or complex behavioral disorders. To paraphrase the definition of the Ad Hoc Committee on Childhood Apraxia of Speech (ASHA, 2007b), it could be stated that CAS is a neurological childhood (pediatric) speech sound disorder in which the precision and consistency of movements underlying speech are impaired in the absence of neuromuscular deficits (e.g., abnormal reflexes, abnormal tone). The main difficulty appears to be in the planning and/or programming of spatiotemporal parameters of movement sequences, resulting in errors in speech sound production and prosody. The term *childhood apraxia of speech* implies shared core features (both speech and prosodic) regardless of the time of onset and whether it is congenital, acquired, or has a specific etiology. Definitions of CAS have universally described it as being based on a neurological deficit (as the ASHA [2007b] definition indicates); there is also agreement that whatever neuroanatomical sites or circuits are involved, they are clearly different from those underlying the dysarthrias.

An exact delineation of symptoms of childhood apraxia of speech is problematic. Early reports of symptoms were based on acquired apraxia of speech in adults. The specific articulatory problems noted in adults with acquired apraxia of speech and in children with so-called developmental apraxia of speech were compared. The most important similarity between these two groups of clients pertains to the lack of sequential volitional control of the oral mechanism. However, initial studies could never verify a neurological basis for comparable speech symptoms in children with apraxia of speech. Although verifiable neurological impairment can cause childhood apraxia of speech, by far most children who are diagnosed are in the group with no known neurological or behavioral disorders.

There remains a clinical necessity to delineate the speech characteristics of children with CAS from those evidenced by children with developmental speech sound disorders. Both groups of children have certain characteristics in common: The onset is early in the developmental period, and the course is long term, often extending into adulthood (Shriberg, Aram, & Kwiatkowski, 1997a). Review of the research literature indicates that, at present, there is no validated list of diagnostic features of CAS that differentiates this symptom complex from other types of childhood speech sound disorders, including those primarily caused by phonological delay or neuromuscular disorder (dysarthria) (ASHA, 2007b). Its estimated prevalence of occurrence is approximately 1 to 2 children per 1000, or 0.1% to 0.2% (Shriberg et al., 1997a). However, in a study by Delaney and Kent (2004), the prevalence noted for 12,000 to 15,000 children was much higher, or between 3.4% and 4.3%. Refer to Box 11.1 for additional information on the demographics of CAS.

Articulatory and Phonological Characteristics

Several studies have reported speech characteristics of children with suspected CAS. However, some of these reports refer to case studies describing only one or two children. Other investigations cannot be compared because uniform criteria

---

Box 11.1

Childhood Apraxia of Speech (CAS): Demographics

- More than 80% of children with CAS have at least one family member with reported speech and/or language disorders (Velleman, 2003).
- CAS demonstrates higher rates of family history than other speech sound disorders, which suggests a genetic basis in at least some cases (Lewis et al., 2004).
- Up to 3% to 4% of children with speech delay are given the diagnosis of CAS (Delaney & Kent, 2004).
- CAS symptoms are common among children with Down syndrome (Kumin & Adams, 2000).
- Approximately 60% of children with autism spectrum disorder have speech problems; about 13% report primarily symptoms of apraxia of speech (Marili, Andrianopoulos, Velleman, & Foreman, 2004).

were not used when selecting the subjects. Therefore, when interpreting the data of these reports, it should be remembered that methodological differences exist between the studies. With this in mind, the following speech characteristics are offered for children with CAS (ASHA, 2007a, 2007b; Hall, Jordan, & Robin, 1993).

According to ASHA's (2007a, 2007b) technical report and position statement, three segmental and suprasegmental features of apraxia of speech in children are consistent and have gained some consensus among investigators:

1. *Inconsistent errors on consonants and vowels in repeated productions of syllables or words.* If a child says a specific word or syllable in different contexts, variability of performance is noted. Although the child might say [fit] the first time, this could be [pit], [vit], or [fɪt] in a repeated performance.

2. *Lengthened and disrupted coarticulatory transitions between sounds and syllables.* The relatively smooth transitions between speech sounds that are noted in children with normally developing speech sound systems are problematic for children with CAS. These transitions could be slow, broken, or appear difficult to achieve.

3. *Inappropriate prosody, especially in the realization of lexical or phrasal stress.* Both word and sentence stress could be noticeably different. In a series of studies by Shriberg, Aram, and Kwiatkowski (1997a, 1997b, 1997c), inappropriate stress was found to be the only linguistic domain that differentiated children with CAS from those with delayed speech development.

The diagnostic challenge is to differentiate CAS from speech delay, a dysarthria, and a speech sound disorder that might be moderate to severe in nature. The following general behaviors have been studied: nonspeech motor, speech motor, prosody, speech perception, language difficulties, and metalinguistic/literacy variables.

Nonspeech Motor

1. *Impaired nonspeech oral volitional movements.* This behavior includes imitated or elicited postures and sequences, such as difficulties making the movements of "smile" versus "kiss" (e.g., Shriberg et al., 1997b).

2. *Groping behavior and silent posturing.* **Groping behavior** is an ongoing series of movements of the articulators in an attempt to find the desired articulatory position. **Silent posturing** refers to the positioning of the articulators for a specific articulation without sound production. Both groping behaviors and silent posturing have been noted in the speech of children with CAS (e.g., Davis, Jakielski, & Marquardt, 1998).

Speech Motor

3. *Difficulty sequencing speech sounds and syllables.* According to Hall and colleagues (1993), sequencing problems are central to this disorder. Difficulty with sequencing seems to increase as the complexity and/or length of the utterance increases (e.g., Davis et al., 1998). Also included in this category are poor performances on the maximum repetition of syllables and slow diadochokinetic rates (e.g., Nijland et al., 2002).

4. *More errors made in the sound classes involving more complex oral gestures.* Consonant clusters, fricatives, and affricates evidence a larger percentage of difficulty (e.g., Davis et al., 1998). These same sound classes are also troublesome for children with developmental phonological disorders.

5. *Unusual errors not typically found in children with speech sound disorders.* These include sound additions, prolongations of vowels and consonants, repetitions of sounds and syllables, and unusual substitutions, such as glottal plosives and bilabial fricatives (e.g., Lewis et al., 2004; McCabe, Rosenthal, & McLeod, 1998).

6. *A large percentage of omission errors.* Several investigators (e.g., Lewis et al., 2004) have found that sound and syllable omissions are the most frequent type of errors noted in children with CAS. This could be related to the complexity of the speech tasks. Polysyllabic words demonstrated more syllable omissions, whereas spontaneous speech included more sound omissions.

7. *Difficulty producing and maintaining appropriate voicing.* Children with CAS might voice unvoiced sounds and devoice voiced sounds (e.g., Lewis et al., 2004). These errors have also been verified by acoustic analyses (e.g., Nijland et al., 2002).

8. *Vowel and diphthong errors.* Several studies have identified these errors in children with CAS (e.g., Nijland et al., 2002). Pollock and Hall (1991) specifically describe the vowel errors of five school-age children with CAS. All of these children had difficulty with tense-lax vowel contrasts, and four of the five evidenced diphthong reduction.

Prosodic Characteristics

9. *Variable nasal resonance, pitch, loudness, and stress.* These characteristics have been reported in children with CAS. It appears that this group of children tends to use excessive equal stress (Shriberg et al., 1997a, 1997b, 1997c). Their inability to fully contrast stressed versus unstressed syllables gives the impression of inappropriate stress patterns.

10. *Prosodic impairment.* General and more specific difficulties with prosody have often been reported in the speech of children with CAS (e.g., Boutsen & Christman, 2002; Davis et al., 1998).

Speech Perception

11. *Difficulty in discriminating sound sequences in nonsense words.* This was noted by Bridgeman and Snowling (1988), as was poor discrimination of vowels (Maassen, Groenen, & Crul, 2003).

Language Difficulties

12. *Significant language delays.* These have been reported in children with CAS (e.g., Velleman & Strand, 1994). Lewis and colleagues (2004) reported that language impairments were more significant and persistent in these children. They found that gains in articulation did not eliminate the language deficits; both receptive and expressive language deficits were noted, as was a strong family history of language impairment in the families of children with CAS.

Metalinguistic/Literacy Characteristics

13. *Difficulty identifying rhymes and syllables.* Investigators (Marion, Sussman, & Marquardt, 1993; Marquardt, Sussman, Snow, & Jacks, 2002) have found that children with suspected CAS demonstrate problems with rhyming and syllabification. These disorders could be evidence of a more broad-based phonological or linguistic problem as opposed to motor-based difficulties alone (Velleman, 2003).

▶ Video Example 11.1

In this video, Jewel, age 4 years 9 months, has been diagnosed with childhood apraxia of speech. Note the difficulties she has with her speech. Review the video a second time, and based on her productions, try to guess the card she is looking at. How many were you able to get right?

https://www.youtube.com/watch?v=tYmm23EPXjU&list=PL122A3871DE5687FA

Although all of these error patterns have been reported in the speech of children with CAS, not all of them occur in all children. Inconsistency and variability of errors is probably the most frequent pattern that characterizes this disorder. Children with CAS are often highly unintelligible. Another common feature is the lack of progress these children make despite a considerable amount of therapy over a long period.

Clinical Implications: Diagnostics

Generally, a broad cluster of symptoms, including speech, nonspeech, and language deficits, is assumed to represent CAS. However, not all symptoms must be present, nor is there one characteristic or symptom that must be present. In addition, the typically reported symptoms are not exclusive to childhood apraxia of speech. Compounding the problem is the observation that children change over time. Therefore, assessment must be organized in a way that allows us to look at a wide range of symptoms.

In respect to assessing a child with CAS, the ASHA (2007b) technical report adopted the position that referrals to other professionals, including neurologists, occupational therapists, and physical therapists, are often appropriate for associated, nonspeech issues. It is the speech-language pathologist, however, who is responsible for making the primary diagnosis of CAS and for designing, implementing, and monitoring the appropriate individualized speech-language treatment program.

The following assessment procedures are recommended for the child who is suspected of demonstrating CAS:

- Hearing screening
- Language testing
- Thorough speech-motor assessment, including diadochokinetic rates
- Standardized speech assessment
- Language sample and language screening
- Tests to examine the sequencing of sounds and syllables as well as their consistency.

Hearing screening is a portion of every assessment; however, it should be verified that the child with suspected CAS does not have a hearing loss as the basis for the noted speech sound problems. Language testing is also an important dimension of the assessment process. Although some research studies have used the absence of receptive language problems as one criterion for inclusion in the group with suspected CAS, others report both expressive and receptive language difficulties co-occurring with CAS (e.g., Lewis et al., 2004). Formal and informal assessment of language should always be used to gain a more complete understanding of the language proficiency of children suspected of having this disorder.

A speech-motor assessment needs to include sequential volitional movements of the oral mechanism for both speech and nonspeech tasks. Oral diadochokinetic rates in nonspeech and speech activities should be evaluated as well (e.g., Love, 2000). Such information helps to document the structural and neuromuscular adequacy of the oral peripheral mechanism. Its functional adequacy for nonspeech and speech tasks should be described and compared. Refer to Chapter 6 for diadochokinetic rates (page 164) and Appendix 6.1 for specific structural and functional measures of the oral peripheral mechanism.

A standardized speech assessment and language sample can be used to appraise several speech parameters: types of errors, any unusual errors, voicing problems with consonants, vowel and diphthong errors, difficulties with nasality and nasal emission, and prosodic problems. Differences between productions of one-word responses and those requiring increased articulatory length or complexity need to be ascertained. Groping behavior and/or silent posturing are additional areas that require close observation.

Tests and protocols specifically designed to assess children with CAS are available. A study by McCauley and Strand (2008) reviewed several standardized tests of nonverbal oral and speech-motor performance in children according to very specific parameters. Tests published between 1990 and 2006 were selected; only 6 of the 22 tests reviewed met their parameters. These six tests are outlined in Table 11.1.

In addition, Gubiani, Pagliarin, and Keske-Soares (2015) investigated specific tools used to evaluate CAS. They analyzed 12 studies from 2003 to 2014 that examined the following assessment instruments: Verbal Motor Production Assessment for Children (VMPAC), Dynamic Evaluation of Motor Speech Skill (DEMSS), Orofacial

Table 11.1 Standardized Tests to Assess Nonverbal Oral and Speech-Motor Performance in Children

Test	Age Range	Oral Structure Assessed	Percentage of Nonverbal versus Speech Oral Motor Measures on Test	Provides Screening Measures	Used for a Complete Diagnosis	Aid in Treatment Planning	Assessment of Change over Time
The Apraxia Profile[1]	3 years 0 months to 13 years 11 months	No	Nonverbal, 10% Speech, 90%	No	Yes	Yes	No
Kaufman Speech Praxis Test for Children[2]	2 years 0 months to 6 years 0 months	No	Nonverbal, 10% Speech, 90%	No	Yes	Yes	No
Oral Speech Mechanism Screening Examination[3]	5 years 0 months to 7 years 8 months	Yes	Nonverbal, 40% Speech, 10% Oral structure, 50%	Yes	No	No	No
Screening Test for Developmental Apraxia of Speech[4]	4 years 0 months to 7 years 11 months	No	Nonverbal, 0% Speech, 100%	Yes	No	No	Yes
Verbal Dyspraxia Profile[5]	Not specified in manual but could be used for children and adults	No	Nonverbal, 75% Speech, 25%	No	Yes	Yes	No
Verbal Motor Production Assessment for Children[6]	3 years 0 months to 12 years 0 months	Yes	Nonverbal, <50% Speech, >50%	No	Yes	Yes	Yes

[1] Hickman, L. A. (1997).
[2] Kaufman, N. (1995).
[3] St. Louis, K. O., & Ruscello, D. (2000).
[4] Blakeley, R. W. (2001).
[5] Jelm, J. M. (2001).
[6] Hayden, D., & Square, P. (1999).

Praxis Test, Kaufman Speech Praxis Test for Children (KSPT), and Madison Speech Assessment Protocol (MSAP). Their conclusion was that the Dynamic Evaluation of Motor Speech Skills was the only tool with a study for validity and reliability. Two other assessment instruments, the Verbal Motor Production Assessment for Children and the Kaufman Speech Praxis Test for Children, had partial evidence of validity (content and criteria). Note that the Dynamic Evaluation of Motor Speech Skills has been recently (November, 2018) published by Brookes.

Clinical Implications: Therapeutics

An established set of therapeutic approaches for the treatment of CAS does not exist. This is not surprising when one considers the limited understanding of the cause, nature, and differential diagnostic markers for this disorder. Even after a careful diagnostic evaluation of the appraisal data, only *suspected* CAS can normally be assumed. Based on this assumption, many different remediation approaches have been suggested. The following is a synopsis of the treatment suggested by Hall and colleagues (1993) and the ASHA (2007b) technical report. It is based on the analysis of outcome measures from many different remediation programs as well as their clinical experience.

1. *Intensive services are needed.* Children with suspected CAS require an extraordinarily high amount of intensive therapy on an individual basis. This is also supported in a comprehensive review by Kaipa and Peterson (2016), who evaluated several studies of treatment intensity. A child, his or her caregivers, and the clinician must be dedicated to this concept. Hall and colleagues (1993) recommend a summer program in which the children are in residence for 6 weeks, receiving 4 hours of therapy per day, 5 days a week.

2. *Remediation should progress systematically through hierarchies of task difficulty.* Where to begin with remediation and how to progress depend on the assessment data from each child. Hall and colleagues (1993) evaluate the child's strengths and progress in very small, carefully manipulated steps. They analyze what the child can do successfully and proceed from there. Because of the variability of their developmental progress, therapy goals may need to be changed or modified (Bauman-Waengler & Garcia, 2011). Therefore, the consonant inventory, distribution, and syllable shapes provide important information when evaluating where to begin and how to continue with therapy. Speech sounds that can be articulated successfully are combined into syllable structures already present in the child's speech. These are then gradually expanded to include a few monosyllabic words of high utility and, possibly, carrier phrases.

3. *Remediation stresses sequences of movements.* Careful incremental increases in sequencing movements and the "memory" for such movements are important. Articulation "memory" should be based on internalized tactile-kinesthetic-proprioceptive information relating sounds that are heard to specific motor patterns.

4. *Many repetitions of speech movements are required in drill-oriented sessions.* Hall and colleagues (1993) use 3 to 10 repetitions of each stimulus. Stimuli range from CV utterances to multisyllabic words. Pausing is used between each set of repetitions so that the client can return to a neutral or resting position to reduce perseverative behavior.

5. *The clinician must determine the need for auditory discrimination tasks.* Not all children need enhancement of auditory discrimination skills. Based on assessment data, the clinician should determine whether an individual child needs work in this area.

6. *Remediation should emphasize self-monitoring.* Self-monitoring should be emphasized as early as possible within the remediation program. Some suggest that tactile and kinesthetic self-monitoring be trained (e.g., Square, Martin, & Bose, 2001).

7. *Input from multiple modalities is needed.* Multisensory input appears helpful to many children with suspected CAS. Various types of cueing have been introduced and can be used to meet the specific needs of these children. All of the cueing techniques represent visual and/or tactile cues used to help a child articulate certain sounds or sound sequences (refer to the "Clinical Application" below for sources).

8. *Remediation should include manipulation of prosodic features as an integral part of the total remedial program.* Whenever possible, rhythm, intonation, stress, and rate manipulation should be integrated into the therapy program from the beginning. The diagnostic data should reveal the areas that specifically need to be targeted. However, some children do not seem capable of manipulating articulatory and prosodic features simultaneously. In this case, an articulatory goal is established first and prosody is added later to articulation tasks that are relatively easy for the client.

9. *If necessary, the clinician should teach compensatory strategies.* Compensatory strategies include slowing the overall rate of speech, increasing the use of pauses between words and syllables, vowel prolongation, and the intrusion of a schwa vowel between consonants in a cluster. Hall and colleagues (1993) state that compensatory strategies could be a necessary part of therapeutic measures but generally should be seen as only a stage of remediation to facilitate a child's progress. When the compensatory strategies are no longer necessary, productions without them should become the goal.

10. *The clinician must provide successful experiences.* Treatment should begin at a level at which children can succeed. Therefore, it is important that the clinician understand a child's baseline level of articulatory functioning and the strengths that this individual demonstrates. Children with suspected CAS need success with speech goals to keep them motivated throughout the typically long and slow remediation process.

It is perhaps overwhelming for clinicians to read about all of the different therapy methods and to choose which might be best for a client who has been diagnosed with CAS. A valid concern relates to which of the many treatment protocols demonstrates verifiable efficacy. Murray, McCabe, and Ballard (2014) evaluated peer-reviewed published articles from 1970 to 2012 to identify treatment methods for CAS that were of good quality; defined the treatment procedures adequately; examined the treatment outcomes, especially maintenance and generalization of the behavior; and established a level of certainty for each treatment approach. Central to this review was treatment efficacy. Demonstration of efficacy extends beyond treatment effects but also requires assessing maintenance and generalization of the treatment effects and hopefully increased performance on untrained items that are somehow related to those trained items. Forty-two articles were reviewed and analyzed according to very specific parameters. Three approaches emerged as having sufficient evidence to be considered for interim clinical practice: (1) integral stimulation/dynamic temporal and tactile cueing, (2) rapid syllable transition treatment, and (3) integrated phonological awareness intervention. These three techniques are explained briefly in the "Clinical Application" below, and references are given. Keep in mind that this is based on a limited number of cases. However, it does point to the future need for maintenance and generalization measures to establish efficacy.

Clinical Application

Therapy Techniques That Demonstrated Treatment Efficacy (Murray, McCabe, & Ballard, 2014)

Integral Stimulation/Dynamic Temporal and Tactile Cueing

- **Brief Summary.** Integral stimulation involves repetition and imitation with visual and auditory models. Visual and tactile inputs, such as touches to the face or adjustments of the jaw and lip postures, are used at first. The therapist says the word or syllable with the child, and the child looks at the therapist as the word is pronounced while listening carefully. Dynamic temporal and tactile cueing is a variation of integral stimulation that was developed for children who cannot achieve a close approximation of consonants or vowels. The following stages are used: (1) imitation (to determine the severity of the disorder), (2) simultaneous production of lengthened vowels with a gradual reduction of lengthening to normal, (3) reduction of the therapist's vocal cueing to miming the sound, (4) the clinician's presentation of an auditory model that the child repeats, (5) a delayed response after presenting the model, and (6) spontaneous production. According to Murray and colleagues (2014), this approach works well with clients who have severe CAS.

- **Sample References.** Edeal & Gildersleeve-Neumann, 2011; Maas & Farinella, 2012; Strand & Debertine, 2000; Strand & Skinner, 1999.

Rapid Syllable Transition Treatment (ReST)

- **Brief Summary.** This method is based on principles of motor learning and attempts to address three core problem areas of childhood apraxia of speech (CAS): inconsistent sounds; transitions between sounds and syllables; and stressing difficulties, specifically lexical stress. The concept is that high-intensity, difficult targets with low-frequency knowledge should lead to long-term change in behavior. Items used are three-syllable nonwords, in which varying stress is placed on each of the syllables. An example would be the nonword "baguti" [bəguti]. Targets presented would be ['bɛguti] with stress on the first syllable; then [bə'guti], stress on the second syllable; and finally [bəgu'ti], stress on the third syllable. Consonants should be minimally stimulable, and targets are presented orthographically. The clinician begins by repeating the nonword, and the client attempts to say it until the word is recognized and produced correctly. There is immediate feedback on all trials. There are prepractice and practice phases. The prepractice phase uses 10 randomly selected treatment stimuli in a carrier phrase such as "He bought a ___." The practice phase consists of 10 to 12 treatment targets for a total of 100 to 120 trials. According to Murray and colleagues (2014), this approach seems to work better for children 7 to 10 years of age with mild to moderate CAS.

- **Sample References.** Ballard, Robin, McCabe, & McDonald, 2010; McCabe, Murray, Thomas, Bejjani, & Ballard, 2013.

Integrated Phonological Awareness Intervention

- **Brief Summary.** This approach targets three areas: speech production, phonological awareness, and printed-word decoding skills. Specifically targeted speech sound production practice, developing phonological awareness, and linking graphemes to phonemes are all parts of this approach and are trained in a block design. One speech error pattern was selected based on a phonological process analysis in which the children must demonstrate at least 40% usage of the pattern.

- *Speech Production.* A long "cycle" of intervention was used for each speech error pattern, consisting of 12 sessions over 6 weeks.

- *Phonological Awareness.* Different phoneme awareness tasks, such as phoneme segmentation or initial phoneme identification, were probed to determine whether the tasks were developmentally appropriate (refer to Chapter 5 for a developmental progression of these skills). The phoneme segmentation probe used 10 trained and 5 untrained words. As an example, for this task the child was required to segment the probe word into its components using colored blocks. All stimulus words for this task were taken from the child's target speech production task.

- *Linking Graphemes to Phonemes.* For the initial phoneme identification portion, the child was required to select one of three words with a target sound that corresponded to her or his target error pattern. This approach seems to work best with children 4 to 7 years of age.

- **Sample References.** Crosbie, Holm, & Dodd, 2005; McNeill, Gillon, & Dodd, 2009a, 2009b; Moriarty & Gillon, 2006.

Motor-Speech Disorders: Cerebral Palsy

Definition and General Features

Cerebral palsy (CP) is a nonprogressive disorder of motor control caused by damage to the developing brain during the prenatal, perinatal, or early postnatal period (Dillow, Dzienkowski, Smith, & Yucha, 1996; Hardy, 1994; Love, 2000). The condition results in a wide variety of motor disabilities, dysarthria among them. Approximately 400,000 children have cerebral palsy, making this disorder the most common developmental motor impairment (Best, Bigge, & Sirvis, 1994; Love, 2000), occurring in about 3 in 1000 births (Bigge, 1991). The lack of volitional speech-motor control is among its central clinical features. The cerebral palsy symptom complex, characterized by a host of neurological malfunctions, is far more than disordered articulation. In addition to general movement and coordination problems, primarily caused by spastic conditions of muscles and increased tendon reflexes, "these dysfunctions include disturbances in cognition, perception, sensation, language, hearing, emotional behavior, feeding, and seizure control" (Love, 2000, pp. 49–50).

The treatment of cerebral palsy requires a team approach to the problem, typically involving the cooperative effort of a physician specializing in such disorders, a physical and occupational therapist, a psychologist, a social worker, and a speech-language pathologist. Ferrari and Cioni (2005) provide guidelines for rehabilitation of children with cerebral palsy. They note the following based on experts' unanimous recommendations. Rehabilitation (1) may be affected by the child's communication disorder, (2) should be multidisciplinary and include speech-language pathologists, (3) should be individualized and target concrete realistic objectives, and (4) should include a functional assessment and prognosis.

Clinical management by the speech-language pathologist requires special considerations that differ considerably from those used in the treatment of other children with speech sound disorders. Clinical management can be effective only if the complexity of the disabling condition is understood. Among other important factors, this management involves being able to evaluate the intricate interrelationships between respiration, phonation, resonance, and articulation in individuals with cerebral palsy.

Articulatory and Phonological Characteristics

In addition to respiratory, phonatory, and articulatory problems, speech-related dysfunctions in cerebral palsy include prosodic abnormalities and velopharyngeal inadequacies (Bishop, Brown, & Robson, 1990; Dillow et al., 1996; Hardy, 1994; Love, 2000). Cerebral palsy encompasses many different types and degrees of speech-related problems. To facilitate an understanding of the various articulatory and phonatory characteristics, a distinction is usually made between three types of involvement commonly found in individuals with cerebral palsy: (1) spasticity, (2) dyskinesia, and (3) ataxia.

Among clients with cerebral palsy, spastic involvement is the most frequently found. Four major types of spastic involvement are recognized: (1) hemiplegia, (2) paraplegia, (3) diplegia, and (4) quadriplegia. With *spastic hemiplegia*, the arm and leg on one side of the body show signs of spastic paresis. *Spastic paraplegia*, which is relatively uncommon, is characterized by involvement of the legs only. *Spastic diplegia* affects all four limbs, but the lower limbs show more involvement than the upper ones. All four limbs are about equally involved in *spastic quadriplegia*. Individuals with spastic diplegia and quadriplegia are more likely to have speech disorders than are people who have hemiplegia or paraplegia. Respiratory, phonatory, resonatory, and articulatory symptoms of individuals with spasticity include the following:

Respiratory difficulties: Reduced vital capacity resulting in inadequate breath support for phonatory and articulatory purposes

Laryngeal dysfunction: Harsh voices and, when coupled with respiratory aberrations, short phrasing and prosodic disturbances

Velopharyngeal inadequacies: Hypernasality

Articulatory deficiencies: Difficulties with production of fricatives and affricates as well as an overall laborious, slow rate of speech; muscle weakness, articulatory instability, and inaccuracy in finding target articulation points are also noted (Love, 2000)

Dyskinesias in cerebral palsy are best exemplified by athetoid conditions marked by unilateral or bilateral disturbances of posture, tonus, and motion. They have been reported to be far less frequent than spastic involvement within this population, but their effects on speech performance are often severe. More often than not, the degree of limb dysfunction mirrors the impairments of the speech mechanism. Many clients with athetoid dysarthria show dysfunction of every physiological component contributing to speech:

Respiratory difficulties: Breathing might be rapid and irregular, showing a lack of thoracic respiratory movement or even "reverse breathing" in which the sternum is flattened instead of lifted during inspiration.

Laryngeal dysfunction: General hypertonicity, which can immobilize the phonatory process altogether, can be more pronounced than in spastic involvement. Voice is commonly marked by an especially strained quality, hard glottal onset, and reduced intensity and prosody realizations.

Velopharyngeal inadequacies: Slow velar activity often results in hypernasal effects.

Articulatory deficiencies: Distortions of consonants are possible, as are vowel productions. Positioning of the mandible during speech can somehow establish necessary differences in tongue height but not in anterior-posterior tongue movements for the production of front versus back vowels.

Ataxia is infrequent among clients with cerebral palsy. Its main symptom is lack of coordination of hypotonic muscle action. Based on clinical observation, the speech characteristics of individuals with ataxic cerebral palsy appear to be similar to those of adults with ataxic dysarthria but are more severe than in other children with dysarthria (Nordberg, Miniscalco, & Lohmander, 2014). The following characteristics are noted in children and adults with ataxia:

Respiratory difficulties: Shallow inspiration and lack of expiratory control.

Laryngeal dysfunction: Harsh voice productions, reduced range of prosodic feature realization.

Velopharyngeal inadequacies: Hypernasality is not typical.

Articulatory deficiencies: Imprecise consonants and vowel distortions, inconsistent sound substitutions and omissions, and a general dysrhythmia (Nordberg et al., 2014).

Refer to Table 11.2 for a summary of the three different types of cerebral palsy.

Table 11.2 Summary of Types of Cerebral Palsy

Type of Cerebral Palsy	Muscular Involvement	Speech Disorder
Spasticity		
1. Hemiplegia	Upper and lower limbs on one side demonstrate hypertonicity.	Speech is usually acceptable; a developmental delay is possible.
2. Paraplegia	Lower limbs and possibly torso musculature demonstrate hypertonicity.	Problems with respiration and breath control exist.
3. Diplegia	All four limbs are involved, although the lower limbs are more severely affected. Torso and neck muscles could also be involved.	Speech is variable depending on the extent of the neuromotor problem; prosodic and articulation difficulties could be present.
4. Quadriplegia	Spasticity in all four limbs occurs with equal degree.	Dysphonia and articulation difficulties depend on the severity of the disorder.
Athetosis	Impairment of voluntary movements results from extreme hypertonicity or extreme flaccidity; involuntary continuous muscle movements are present.	Speech difficulties can occur, although they vary in severity; speech is generally slow with poor articulation; and problems with phonation, stress, and rhythm are possible.
Ataxia	This is characterized by incoordination of movement with the inability to maintain posture and balance.	Speech problems are typically present; articulation and problems with rhythm are evident.

Milloy and Morgan-Barry (1990) describe the following phonological processes that relate to the speech errors of temporal and motor control:

Phonological Processes

Related to temporal coordination. Voicing difficulties, including devoicing initial consonants or voicing unvoiced sounds; variable realizations of voiced-voiceless cognates; prevocalic voicing; consonant cluster reductions; final consonant deletions; stopping of fricatives or frication of stops; and weak syllable deletions predominate.

Related to motor control, errors of phonetic placement. Fronting, backing, stopping, gliding, lateral realization of apical and coronal fricatives, vowelization of [l] and [ɹ], and nasalization have been noted.

Clinical Implications: Diagnostics

The primary communicative impairment of children with cerebral palsy is clearly motor-speech in nature. These children present a variety of clinical symptoms relating to both the type and the severity of involvement. However, all children with cerebral palsy share some common factors that directly relate to basic functions subserving speech—namely, problems with respiration, phonation, resonation, and articulation. It is important to assess the type and degree of interference that each of these systems could have on speech.

Problems with *respiration* could lead to difficulties in initiating vocalizations, difficulties in sustaining vocalizations, variations in loudness that could affect word and sentence stress, an inability to sustain vocalization for multisyllabic words or longer sentences, and a loss of expiratory support at the end of utterances.

Problems with *phonation* could result in interruptions in phonation, breathy voice, harsh voice, and pitch and intensity variations. There can also be problems coordinating voicing and articulation.

Problems with *resonation* could result in various degrees of hypernasality, variations in nasality within an utterance, and lack of intelligibility caused by nasality problems.

Problems with *articulation* could result in difficulties in achieving speech sound productions, sound distortions, and disorganized phonological systems, possibly leading to problems with language and learning to read.

When assessing children with cerebral palsy, it is essential to remember that the smooth integration of all systems subserving speech is a real problem. Therefore, the assessment and treatment of children with this disorder must account for far more than speech sound production difficulties.

The high diversity of possible involvements requires an encompassing evaluation. In addition to respiratory, phonatory, resonatory, and articulatory limitations and possibilities, data on the following areas should be obtained:

- Cognitive skills
- Sensory and perceptual abilities, beginning with an audiological evaluation
- Emotional behavior
- Feeding and eating characteristics
- Language competence.

Odding, Roebroeck, and Stam (2006) report that about 40% of the population with cerebral palsy shows some degree of cognitive impairment; the rest of these individuals demonstrate intelligence within normal limits. Impaired language development, learning difficulties, and academic problems often occur in these children (Rosenbaum et al., 2007).

Clinicians need to be very cautious when interpreting speech and language results obtained from children with cerebral palsy. In a review of research articles, O'Connor, Kerr, Shields, and Imms (2015) documented the assessment instruments for speech, language, and communication that were used with children with cerebral palsy in 14 studies from 2000 to 2015. Most of the assessment tools were age-standardized and norm-referenced; however, *none* demonstrated acceptable validity for use with children with cerebral palsy.

An audiological evaluation is necessary for children with cerebral palsy; those with athetosis, in particular, have higher auditory detection thresholds, poorer speech reception thresholds, and poorer speech discrimination than do children without cerebral palsy.

Often the speech-language pathologist becomes part of an early intervention team for infants who have been identified with cerebral palsy. As a member of this team, the speech-language pathologist could be asked to assess prespeech abilities as prerequisites for the development of articulation skills. These prerequisites include the following:

1. Head control with stability of the neck and shoulder girdle. Such stability provides later control and mobility of oral structures.
2. A coordinated pattern of respiration and phonation.
3. A variety of feeding experiences to enhance normal feeding patterns.
4. Babbling practice (Levin, 1999).

Clinical Implications: Therapeutics

As always, the selection of appropriate therapeutic measures to influence the communicative abilities of clients with cerebral palsy is a direct outgrowth of specific diagnostic results. Established methods for the treatment of various "types" of cerebral palsy only amount to guidelines for elementary orientation.

There are, nevertheless, general principles that apply to all remediation efforts with young clients who have cerebral palsy. First, some prespeech prerequisites must be met (the previously mentioned head control and the coordination of respiratory patterns with voice production, for example). The need for coordination between breathing and phonation for future articulation work is self-evident, but a certain degree of posture control is equally indispensable.

The next therapeutic phase with young children who have cerebral palsy pertains to communication and speech-language stimulation. In infants, this might start with vocal play and babbling practice. Chapter 6, pages 182–187, offers some considerations for speech therapy for children with emerging phonology.

For older children with cerebral palsy, a basic consideration is the facilitation of desired movements while inhibiting the abnormal reflex patterns. Before a speech-language clinician can address the coordination of respiration, phonation, resonation, and articulation, the child must be able to maintain some reflex-inhibiting postures that the physical therapist recommends. Because this is usually one of the primary goals of the early intervention team, the children should already have developed some skills in this area. If they can inhibit abnormal reflexes and realize certain movements required for speech, articulation training can be initiated.

Traditionally, therapy began by establishing temporal coordination and motor control of the speech musculature. The goals were to increase the speed, range, and accuracy of movement of the tongue, lips, and jaw (Gibbon & Wood, 2003). These goals were then integrated with the maintenance of body and head tonus as well as respiration, phonation, and resonation (Barlow & Farley, 1989). Selection of the target sound was guided by stimulability, consistency, visibility, and whether the sound developed early or late. Therefore, stimulable, visible sounds that in some contexts were produced accurately and were acquired early were normally given priority (Love, 2000).

However, some felt that groups of sounds, rather than a single sound, should be treated. Guidelines by Hardy (1994) and Crary (1993) include the following procedures:

1. *Consonants that are realized correctly in prevocalic positions but are misarticulated in postvocalic positions should be treated first.* Generally, postvocalic errors are more easily remedied if the child can produce the sound in a prevocalic position.

2. *Distortions should be treated before substitutions.* This includes distortions that fall short of the target because of motor involvement. Prognosis should be better if the child can produce the sound somewhat distorted rather than delete or use a substitute for the sound.

3. *Training articulatory omissions and substitutions that fall short of the target because of motor involvement should be delayed.* Compensatory articulatory efforts for sounds that are difficult to produce should be trained instead. Children usually have already developed some type of compensatory sound realization. The clinician's duty is to refine this production as much as possible. *A multiple auditory-visual stimulation approach should be used.* It is preferred over auditory stimulation alone.

4. *Voice–voiceless distinctions should be trained by slowing the speech process and then concentrating on the production of the sound's voicelessness.* This is important because these children have a tendency to substitute voiced for voiceless consonants.

5. *It is important to remember that some children with cerebral palsy cannot achieve "normal" articulation.* In these cases, *reasonable compensations* are the goal; they can be very efficient for communicative purposes.

Clinical Application

Augmentative and alternative communication (AAC) refers to an area of research as well as to a clinical and educational practice. AAC involves attempts to study and, when necessary, compensate for temporary or permanent impairments, activity limitations, and participation restrictions of individuals with severe disorders of speech-language production and/or comprehension, including spoken and written modes of communication. It is the position of the American Speech-Language-Hearing Association (ASHA) that communication is the essence of human life and that all people have the right to communicate to the fullest extent possible. No individuals should be denied this right, regardless of the type and/or severity of communication, linguistic, social, cognitive, motor, sensory, perceptual, and/or other disabilities they might present (ASHA, 2005).

Occasionally, the physical handicap in children with cerebral palsy is so severe that effective verbal communication cannot be achieved at all. If that is the case, *augmentative communication*—the use of other systems (gestural, boards with words or pictures, electronic devices) to promote meaningful communicative exchange—should be implemented. As an example, the following guidelines are offered from the New York State Department of Health (2006). They are based on information where a systematic review has not been done.

- When selecting a device, focus on the child's communication skills rather than on the child's skill in using the system.

- When selecting a communication system, consider the child's vision, hearing, and cognitive abilities; the intended audience; maintenance requirements; ease of use; modification flexibility; daily activities; motivation; and communication partners.

- Clinicians assessing communication for children between ages 6 months and 3 years with cerebral palsy should consider the child's use of gestures and other nonverbal communication attempts.

It should be noted that treatment efficacy is an issue for children with cerebral palsy. Pennington, Goldbart, and Marshall (2004) reviewed controlled studies that investigated the effectiveness of speech and language interventions in children with cerebral palsy. After reviewing 12 studies from 1996 to 2002, they stated, "It is not possible to conclude at the present time that speech and language therapy focusing on children with cerebral palsy or their communication partners is more effective than no intervention at all. However, no evidence has been found of any harmful effects of speech and language therapy for children with cerebral palsy and their families, and therapy has not been shown to be ineffective" (p. 12). On a more positive note, Novak and colleagues (2013) reviewed 166 studies, from the beginning of several databases until 2012. They grouped their findings into three categories: (1) Green—Findings were from strong, high-quality evidence, and the intervention was determined to be effective. Green interventions were classified as "do it." (2) Yellow—Findings were from moderate- to low-quality evidence requiring further research. Yellow interventions with moderate evidence were classified as "probably do it," but yellow interventions with low-quality evidence were classified as "probably do not do it." (3) Red—Findings were from little to no evidence, or the intervention was determined to be ineffective. Red interventions were classified as "do not do it." The following results emerged: Social stories and play therapy were classified as "probably do it" interventions for improved social skills (Yellow evidence). Oral motor treatment was classified as a "probably do not do it" intervention for communication and dysphagia (Yellow evidence). Dysphagia management (e.g., diet modification, positioning) and gastrostomy were classified as "probably do it" interventions (Yellow evidence).

Cleft Palate

Definition and General Features

Occurring in about 1 in 700 births (Grames, 2008), palatal and (upper) lip clefts are among the most frequent congenital anomalies (American Cleft Palate–Craniofacial Association and Cleft Palate Foundation, 1997). **Clefting** refers to a division of a continuous structure by a cleavage, a split prominently caused by a failure of the palate to fuse during fetal development (Shprintzen, 1995). Examples of clefting are cleft palate and cleft lip. Both the hard and soft palates and the lips form normally uninterrupted structures within their anatomical boundaries. If clefting occurs, a gap severs their unity, dividing the roof of the mouth (which also constitutes the floor of the nasal cavity) and/or the upper lip sagittally into separated left and right portions.

There are several etiologies that cause a failure of the regular median fusion of the embryo's oral-facial structures between the eighth and twelfth weeks of gestation. In addition, there is also the possibility of a rupture of already fused oral-facial elements (Kitamura, 1991). Contrary to common understanding, no single cause for clefting exists; "clefting is . . . a clinical outcome of many possible diseases" (Shprintzen, 1995, p. 5).

Although there are many classification systems, the recommendations made by the American Cleft Palate–Craniofacial Association have been adopted most frequently (Bzoch, 1997).

1. Clefts of the prepalate
   - *Cleft lip:* unilateral, bilateral, median, prolabium (central segment of upper lip), congenital scar
   - *Cleft of alveolar process:* unilateral, bilateral, median, submucous
   - *Cleft of prepalate:* any combination of types, prepalate protrusion, prepalate rotation, prepalate arrest (median cleft)
2. Clefts of the palate
   - *Clefts of soft palate:* extent, palatal shortness, submucous
   - *Clefts of hard palate:* extent, vomer attachment, submucous
3. Clefts of the prepalate and palate
4. Facial clefts other than of the prepalate and palate

Unilaterality or *bilaterality* of hard palate clefts refers to their presence on one or both sides of the hard palate; *median clefts* refers to their presence at the midline. These clefts are along a line where the lower edge of the nasal septum attaches to the palate. *Submucous clefts*, on the other hand, are characterized by an intact mucous membrane covering a cleft. This cleft could be separating muscular portions of the soft palate and/or a cleavage of the posterior bony portions of the hard palate. A V-shaped indentation in this area might be felt with the finger. Another sign of the probable existence of a submucous cleft is a divided uvula, a *bifid uvula*. Quite in contrast to unilateral and bilateral clefts, submucous clefts seldom cause feeding problems or abnormal speech.

Articulatory and Phonological Characteristics

Children with cleft palate may exhibit developmental and/or compensatory articulatory and phonological disorders (Bzoch, 1997; Pamplona, Ysunza, Gonzalez, Ramirez, & Patino, 2000; Whitehill, Francis, & Ching, 2003). Developmental speech-language delays are similar to those in children without cleft palates, but they occur more frequently in children with cleft palates (Schonweiler, Schonweiler, Schmelzeisen, & Ptok, 1995; Trost-Cardamone, 1990). Therefore, children with developmental delays are characterized by speech sound skills that resemble those of younger, normally developing children. Developmental delays cannot always be said to be completely independent of the underlying condition. Consonant cluster reductions, for example—a frequent occurrence in children with speech-language delays—can often be traced to placement or omission errors that are disorder specific in children with palatal clefts.

Compensatory errors pertain to specific errors in the placement of the articulators that could occur in patients who have inadequate closure of the velopharyngeal valve or a cleft or fistula in the hard palate (Witzel, 1995). They have also been described as "compensatory adjustments." These sound substitutions or distortions are produced more posteriorly and inferior in the vocal tract by posterior positioning of the tongue, associated true and false vocal fold adduction, or abnormal positioning of the arytenoid cartilage and epiglottis. Because of difficulties with velopharyngeal closure, these errors are thought to be a compensatory attempt to modify the airstream below the velopharyngeal valve. However, compensatory errors are not always a direct result of velopharyngeal incompetence. They could actually result from compensatory articulation caused by limited movements of the velopharyngeal valve during productions of specific sounds.

Although specific sound production difficulties have often been noted in the speech of children with cleft palate, these may not be entirely phonetic in nature. Children with cleft palate could also evidence difficulties with the organization of phonemes within their language system; that is, they might demonstrate phonological disorders (Broen & Moller, 1993; Chapman, 1993; Chapman & Hardin, 1992; Chapman, Hardin-Jones, & Halter, 2003). Early delays in phonological development include a high frequency of deletion of final consonants, syllable reduction, and backing. However, at the age of 4 to 5 years, these problems were less apparent.

Video Example 11.2
This video features a boy who has a repaired cleft palate but who still has severe articulation problems. Do you notice more substitutions or omissions in his speech? Listen to the word "truck." Does it seem plausible that he seems to correctly articulate the final [k]?
https://www.youtube.com/watch?v = -LR_YDBPW1Y

Clinical Implications: Diagnostic

Obviously, the initial diagnosis of clefting in a newborn—its nature, site, and extent—is a medical task. So is the beginning of its management, typically involving at least a pediatrician, an orthodontist, and an otolaryngologist. However, clefts are a matter of long-term care requiring a team of specialists for successful assessment and management. Speech-language pathologists are important members of this team. Their primary job is to assess the child's communicative status and development, a challenging task. Not only are all clefts different (including their various effects on verbal communication), but the personalities of the children and their caregivers vary regarding their ability to cope with the situation and its clinical consequences. However, the biggest diagnostic challenge might be the developmental aspects of the disorder—that is, the changing nature of the appraised findings. Today's status can differ from tomorrow's because of natural growth factors, necessary corrective measures of medical intervention, and compensatory prospects. Diagnostics involving children with clefts is a truly ongoing process.

The areas of diagnostic concern again underline the necessity of a team approach to the clinical management of children with cleft palate. For example, these children are all prone to intermittent middle ear infections and their concomitant conductive hearing loss. This means that an otolaryngologist and an audiologist must be involved to closely monitor the condition and hearing ability of all children with palatal clefts. The findings are important for the speech-language clinician because "evidence indicates that children with recurrent middle ear problems are slower to acquire speech production skills" (Broen & Moller, 1993, p. 230).

The central diagnostic issue pertaining to the phonatory, resonatory, and articulatory effects of velopharyngeal port incompetency (VPI) includes both structural abnormalities and neuromuscular inadequacies. Whereas structural abnormalities largely can be corrected by surgical and/or prosthetic measures, some functional deficits in respect to speech often remain, resulting in hypernasal resonance, nasal air emission, sound distortions, and sound substitutions. The latter two are characterized by *articulatory backing* in children with cleft palate. This is a compensatory measure to produce speech sounds more posteriorly in the oral cavity than is normally the case. Velopharyngeal incompetency impairs the intraoral pressure build-up necessary for the norm production of many speech sounds—primarily stops, fricatives, and affricates, the so-called pressure consonants. Nasals and semivowels such as [w] and [j] remain relatively intact.

One of the most striking features characterizing the speech of children with cleft palates with velopharyngeal incompetence is the substitution of glottal stops for stop-plosives. This compensatory articulatory behavior is triggered by the impossibility of accumulating the intraoral pressure required for the regular production of these so-called "pressure consonants." During this substitution, the standard positioning of the articulators is sometimes retained. For example, for [p], the lips are closed and suddenly opened simultaneously with the release of the glottal stop. This often results in an impression of a slightly distorted yet acceptable [p]-production.

In addition to the articulatory consequences of velopharyngeal incompetency, dental anomalies and problems with occlusion of the mandibular and maxillary arches often contribute to the aberrant articulation of children with cleft palate. These problems as well as their possible impact on specific consonant and vowel productions should be noted.

"The primary clinical task for the speech-language pathologist is to assess the child's phonological status and then infer the effects of structural deviations on the phonological behavior observed" (Trost-Cardamone & Bernthal, 1993, p. 317). This task differs considerably from child to child, primarily according to age, linguistic, and cognitive levels, but it always involves the following:

1. Speech sampling and analysis, including sound inventory and phonological pattern development
2. Stimulability probes
3. Intelligibility judgments
4. Oral-facial examination.

Each of these assessment areas has been discussed previously in some detail (refer to Chapters 6 and 7). The procedures do not differ significantly for children with cleft palate.

One important aspect of the diagnosis with these children is to find and distinguish between error patterns that are developmental in nature and those that, as a result of the cleft, have a structural or physiological basis. Some patterns are seen in children with cleft palate but are not typical for children with structurally and functionally intact oral and pharyngeal mechanisms. Trost-Cardamone and Bernthal (1993) provide the following list:

1. *Consonant distortions associated with nasal emissions.* Three error patterns are associated with nasal emission. It is important to distinguish between them because different interventions could be in order for each.

   - *Nasal emission caused by persistence of velopharyngeal inadequacy.* This is characterized by nasal emission during production of all pressure consonants and pervasive hypernasality accompanying production of vowels and the vocalic consonants [l], [ɹ], [j], and [w].

   - *Nasal emission caused by oronasal fistulae.* An oronasal fistula is an opening between the oral and nasal cavities. Although some fistulae can be eliminated surgically, others are too large for successful closure. There is a relationship between the location of the fistula and the consonants affected. Posteriorly located fistulae (near the juncture between the hard and soft palate) affect primarily [k] and [g] and have little influence on anteriorly produced consonants. When the fistula is anteriorly located, [t], [d], [s], [z], [p], and [b] are likely to be distorted.

- *Nasal emission that is speech sound specific.* This could occur in the absence of clefting or velopharyngeal impairment. It does not affect a class of sounds and is rarely associated with hypernasality. The nasal emission does not require surgical intervention; it is probably caused by faulty learning and can usually be treated with speech therapy if properly diagnosed (refer to pages 204–205).

2. *Vowel distortions secondary to hypernasality.* It is important for clinicians to differentiate between vowel distortions that could result from deviant articulatory placement and those that are deviations due to hypernasal resonance as the result of deficient velopharyngeal valving.

3. *Compensatory articulations.* There are several types of compensatory articulations. The clinician should differentiate between compensatory articulations that are used as substitutions and those that occur as coarticulations.

4. *Atypical backed articulation.* These articulations include back-velar substitutions for [l], [ɹ], and [n]. The posterior shifts could result from attempting to capture airflow or using the back of the tongue to help seal the velopharyngeal port. Such productions should be analyzed to determine whether they are part of a phonological pattern of backing or represent selective articulatory substitutions.

Clinical Application

Clinical Test Battery for Children with Cleft Palates

Bzoch (1997) recommends the following clinical test battery:

1. *Language testing.*
2. *Audiometric evaluation.*
3. *Nasal emission test.* A small mirrored surface or a headset listening device is sufficient to enhance the auditory and visual perceptions of nasal airflow. This test uses 10 two-syllable words, each containing two [p] or [b] sounds.
4. *Hypernasality test.* This measure uses 10 one-syllable words beginning with [b] and ending with [t]. The subject repeats each word twice. On the second repetition, the examiner pinches the nares closed. A perceptual judgment of hypernasality is indicated if words shift in quality between the first and second repetition.
5. *Hyponasality test.* This measure uses 10 one-syllable words beginning with [m] and ending with [t]. The subject repeats each word twice; on the second repetition, the examiner pinches the nares closed. On this test, there *should be a shift in quality* between the first and second repetition.
6. *Phonation test.* The subject prolongs [i], [ɑ], and [u] for 10 seconds. The examiner notes any aspirate or hoarse phonation. Also, failure of the client to sustain phonation for 10 seconds would indicate a habituated breathy voice. This can be confirmed by the conversational speech sample.
7. *Standardized speech assessment.* Special tests examining typical errors noted in the speech of children with cleft palate are available. These include, for example, the Iowa Pressure Test (Morris, Spriestersbach, & Darley, 1961),

(Continued)

the Bzoch Error Pattern Diagnostic Articulation Test (Bzoch, 1997), and the Great Ormond Street Speech Assessment (Sell, Harding, & Grunwell, 1994). However, older tests seem to not be used as frequently for assessing articulation. Most current standardized assessments are typically being used to examine errors in cleft palate speech (Mandulak, Baylis, & Thurmes, 2011).

8. *Screening nasometer test.* This test is used for children from 2 to 6 years of age. Procedures can be found in many sources. Two examples are found in Dalston (1997) and Dalston, Warren, and Dalston (1991).

Clinical Implications: Therapeutics

Many children with cleft palates undergo palate repair by the age of 18 months. They remain free of compensatory sound production errors such as glottal for oral stops and pharyngeal for oral fricatives. Other children require therapeutic intervention. Approximately 20% of children with repaired cleft palate will develop speech deficits that require additional intervention (Witt & D'Antonio, 1993).

To implement therapy with clients with cleft palates, four overall goals should be kept in mind:

1. Improve the placement of consonant productions by promoting a more forward place of articulation
2. Improve velopharyngeal valve function and decrease hypernasal resonance quality
3. Modify compensatory articulations
4. If developmental phonological errors exist, improve the child's phonological system (Van Demark & Hardin, 1990).

Improving the placement of consonant productions and modifying compensatory articulations are usually accomplished by direct work on the place of articulation—that is, through motor placement techniques. Glottal stops can easily be eliminated by using maneuvers such as gentle whispering, overaspiration, or the use of a sustained [h] that keeps the vocal folds apart (Golding-Kushner, 1995). Slight overaspiration by using a sustained [h] usually breaks the glottal pattern because it requires an open glottis. Voiceless oral stops are first introduced at the end of a prolonged [h]. In addition, the voiceless stop itself is overaspirated. If the word were *pie*, the production would sound similar to a prolonged [h] + [p] + *high*. Teaching voiceless homorganic oral fricatives before establishing oral stops is a good technique for breaking up compensatory coarticulations. Nasal occlusion and release help to eliminate nasal snorting and to establish stops and fricatives. By occluding the nares, clients quickly learn to direct the airstream orally.

Clinical Application

Case Study: JD

This case study is adapted from Albery and Russell (1990). JD was born with a cleft of the soft palate, which was repaired relatively late at age 2 years 6 months. In the United States, the trend for many years has been toward early closure of palatal clefts, typically between the ages of 6 and 18 months (Marsh & Lehman, 1988).

According to the authors, progression through the early speech stages with an open cleft had influenced JD's articulatory development. Therefore, his deviant and restricted inventory is not typical but does exemplify some of the compensatory articulation errors that can be noted in the speech of children with cleft palate.

JD's speech was highly unintelligible because the inventory restrictions resulted in the loss of numerous phonemic contrasts.

Phonetic Inventory

[m], [n], [w], [j], [h]		Articulated in a regular manner in the prevocalic, intervocalic, and, where applicable, postvocalic word positions.
[ʔp], [ʔb]		A glottal component accompanied the bilabial productions in the prevocalic word positions.
[p], [b], [t], [d], [k], [g], [f], [v], [ʃ], [ʒ], [θ], [ð], [tʃ], [dʒ]	[ʔ]	Stop-plosive productions (including [p] and [b] in intervocalic and postvocalic positions), most fricatives, and affricates were realized as glottal stops.
[s]	→ [ħ]	[s] was realized as a voiceless pharyngeal fricative [ħ] in all word positions.
[z]	→ [ʕ]	[z] was realized as a voiced pharyngeal fricative [ʕ] in all word positions.
[l]	→ [ĩ]	[l] was nasalized in the postvocalic word position.
[ɹ]	→ [w]	[ɹ] was realized as [w].

Sometimes, even after surgery, the velopharyngeal mechanism is only marginally adequate for articulatory function; hypernasality may persist to varying degrees. If further surgery and/or prosthodontic intervention is not indicated, improving velopharyngeal valve function and decreasing hypernasal resonance quality may then become a treatment goal. Several ways to improve velopharyngeal valve function have been suggested. The velum is massaged and electrically stimulated; various devices have been used to improve the effectiveness of these exercises (Starr, 1993). Behavioral approaches that provide feedback to clients are attempts to enhance their awareness and control of the velopharyngeal mechanism. Perceptual and acoustic feedback, visual feedback, and airflow and air pressure feedback have been offered with varying degrees of success (refer to Starr, 1993, for a review of these techniques). However, due to lack of clinical studies, outcome measures for these techniques remain unclear.

Decreasing hypernasal resonance could be another important therapy goal for these clients. Hypernasal resonance occurs in individuals with adequate and inadequate velopharyngeal competency. The following describes one such technique, increased mouth opening or orality (Boone, McFarlane, Von Berg, & Zraick, 2013). During sound articulation, varying degrees of velar activity occur. For example, stop-plosives require complete closure of the nasopharyngeal port for the necessary build-up of intraoral air pressure. Productions of [ɑ] or [w], on the other hand, do not demand the same degree of closure to prevent undue nasal resonance. Complete velopharyngeal closure is necessary only during the production of stops and sounds with little articulatory possibility for oral air escape, fricatives, and affricates, for example. With more "open" sounds, the same degree of closure is not required.

If open sounds require less velar activity to keep nasality effects from occurring, increasing the opening of the respective phoneme realizations should at least lessen, and possibly prevent, such consequences. Consider /i/ realizations as an example. They can be achieved in several ways without violating phonemic boundaries, specifically with a more or less restricted oral passageway. Under otherwise comparable conditions, more open oral productions put less demand on proper velar function than the more restricted oral ones and are therefore preferable for the purpose at hand. The task is to train the hypernasal child to systematically use the widest oral-articulatory posture for the sound in question. This posture should not interfere with the phoneme value the sound represents.

The following two protocols are examples of training for articulation errors. The first set of treatment options is offered by Mandulak and colleagues (2011).

1. Start therapy as soon as possible. The speech-language pathologist needs to establish at least some correct articulation placement very early on.
2. Start with the sounds that are causing the most negative impact on intelligibility or velopharyngeal closure due to compensatory errors.
3. Target sounds for which the child is stimulable. Keep developmental progression in mind, but don't be afraid to deviate from it.
4. Start with the sounds that are most visible (anterior sounds). Usually, it is easier to start with voiceless sounds before voiced ones (especially if glottal stops are present).
5. Use traditional articulation therapy. This is not phonological therapy or oral-motor therapy, but the focus is on phonetic-based approaches with perceptual training using auditory, tactile, visual cueing, and self-monitoring techniques. Also use motor learning principles (refer to Chapter 9).

Peterson-Falzone, Trost-Cardamone, Karnell, and Hardin-Jones (2017) offer the following treatment option:

1. Teach identity, location, and actions of oral structures, teeth, lips, and tongue. A picture, mirror, Mr. Potato, or Mighty-Mouth can be helpful.
2. Teach sounds and their corresponding structures; for example, [p]: lip sound, popping sound, poof sound; [t]: tongue sound or teeth sound; [s]: snake sound; [ʃ]: quiet or windy sound.
3. Get the target sounds into the inventory by using "easier" sounds to elicit new sounds (shaping). For example, shaping [w] or [m] to [p] or [b]; shaping [l] or [n] to [d], or [j] to [ʃ].
4. Provide auditory, visual, and tactile cues, and use nasal occlusion as needed.
5. Teach correct oral target versus error sound contrasts, emphasizing auditory discrimination and "old sound" versus "new sound." This includes establishing reliable self-monitoring.
6. Start by teaching most visible, anterior sounds such as [p, h, t], attempting voiceless sounds first.
7. Plug the nose to provide sensation of oral pressure.
8. Try [h] words with the target sound in the final position. If the target is [p], use "hoop" or "hop," for example, using overaspiration of air and whispering as needed.
9. Avoid words with nasal sounds or words that begin with vowels.

Intellectual Disability (Intellectual Developmental Disorder)

Definition and General Features

The various attempts to define intellectual disability reflect the different understandings of and attitudes toward the disorder at different times. At least 10 different "official" definitions of intellectual disability have existed since 1921. Changes to the American Psychiatric Association's *Diagnostic and Statistical Manual of Mental Disorders* (DSM) from the fourth edition (DSM-IV; American Psychiatric Association [APA], 2000) to the fifth edition (DSM-5; APA, 2013) include the use of the term *intellectual disability* (intellectual developmental disorder) to reflect the more common terminology that has been used for decades by professional and lay groups. The definition has stayed relatively the same from DSM-IV to DSM-5, noting that this mental disorder is characterized by significant limitations both in intellectual functioning and in adaptive behavior as expressed in conceptual, social, and practical adaptive skills.

In such a definition, three criteria stand out:

1. Limitations in adaptive skills
2. Subaverage intellectual functioning
3. Manifestation of a cognitive impairment before 18 years of age.

The term *adaptive skills* refers to functioning in three domains or areas of specified everyday living activities: the conceptual domain includes skills in language, reading, writing, math, reasoning, knowledge, and memory; the social domain refers to empathy, social judgment, interpersonal communication skills, the ability to make and retain friendships, and similar capacities; the practical domain relates to self-management in areas such as personal care, job responsibilities, money management, recreation, and organizing school and work tasks.

The individual must also show significant deficits in adaptive behavior relative to his or her own cultural group. This delineation is used to rule out linguistic and cultural differences that might limit the individual's functioning in a larger setting.

Subaverage intellectual functioning in this definition refers to approximately 2 standard deviations below the mean on suitable standardized intelligence quotient (IQ) tests, translating to an IQ score of about 70 or below. *Manifestation of a cognitive impairment before age 18* identifies such deficiencies as a developmental disorder beginning somewhere between the time of conception and official adulthood. This would eliminate individuals who in adulthood might show signs of dementia and demonstrate similar problems in adaptive behavior, for example.

Previously, the DSM-IV (APA, 2000) reported that 2% to 3% of individuals met the criteria for intellectual disability. This resulted from the diagnostic criterion that required an IQ score of approximately 70 or below. Statistically, 2 standard deviations below average (a score of 70) equal 2.5% of the population, thus the estimate of 2% to 3% of the population. However, DSM-5 (APA, 2013) has moved away from relying on specific IQ scores and estimates a prevalence rate of approximately 1%. The DSM-5 defines severity in terms of adaptive functioning, not IQ scores. The level of adaptive functioning determines the levels of support necessary. The DSM-5 further states that IQ scores are less valid in the lower end of the IQ range.

Specific associated problems could also affect the communicative behavior of this population. Both sensorineural and conductive hearing losses as well as abnormal middle ear function are prevalent in these individuals. Individuals with intellectual disability are at least 40 times more likely than the general population to have a hearing impairment (Carvill, 2001).

Articulatory and Phonological Characteristics: General Information

All subgroups of children with intellectual disabilities demonstrate a higher prevalence of speech problems. They tend to lack articulatory precision and appropriate pauses and phrasing. The phonological characteristics of this population can be summarized as follows (Kumin, 1998; Shriberg & Widder, 1990; Stoel-Gammon, 1998):

1. Speech sound errors are more common than in the normally developing population.
2. Deletion of consonants is the most frequent error.
3. Errors are typically inconsistent.
4. Patterns are similar to those of children who are not cognitively disabled but demonstrate a functional delay.

In general, individuals with cognitive impairments demonstrate the same phonological processes as normally developing children but with a higher frequency of occurrence. It has been hypothesized that individuals with intellectual disabilities might use these processes for other reasons than to simplify their speech. For example, Shriberg and Widder (1990) suggest that consonant deletions may reflect cognitive processing constraints in the motor assembly stage of speech production.

Down Syndrome: General Information

Down syndrome is a condition in which a person is born with an extra copy of chromosome 21. People with Down syndrome have physical problems as well as intellectual disabilities. It is important to remember that every person born with Down syndrome is different. People with Down syndrome may be born with heart disease, and they may have dementia, hearing problems, and/or problems with the intestines, eyes, thyroid, and skeleton (Bull & The Committee on Genetics, 2011). Even though people with Down syndrome may act and look similar, each person has different abilities. People with Down syndrome usually have a cognitive impairment in the mild to moderate range. Only rarely is Down syndrome associated with severe cognitive impairment. Common physical features of Down syndrome include the following:

- A flattened face, especially the bridge of the nose
- Almond-shaped eyes that slant upward
- A short neck
- Small ears
- A tongue that tends to stick out of the mouth
- Tiny white spots on the iris of the eye
- Small hands and feet
- A single line across the palm of the hand (palmar crease)
- Small pinky fingers that sometimes curve toward the thumb

- Poor muscle tone or loose joints
- Shorter height as children and adults.

Other common cognitive and behavioral problems include short attention span, poor judgment, impulsive behavior, slow learning, and delayed language and speech development.

Down Syndrome: Articulatory and Phonological Impairments

Children with Down syndrome show developmental patterns that are not just slower to emerge. In a review of articles from 1950 to 2012, Kent and Vorperian (2013) found that children with Down syndrome demonstrated both delayed and deviant phonological patterns.

In respect to babbling behavior, Kent and Vorperian (2013) concluded that (1) the age of onset of canonical babbling in infants with Down syndrome might be somewhat delayed, but this delay is much less than delays in gross motor skills such as crawling or walking; and (2) based on research findings, there may be a difference between the babbling behavior of children with Down syndrome and normally developing infants.

Vowel errors have been reported in children with Down syndrome (e.g., Bunton, Leddy, & Miller, 2007). Bunton and colleagues (2007) reported frequent errors with high versus low vowels and front versus back vowels. These errors may indicate anatomical factors and/or motor limitations.

Studies of both children and adults with Down syndrome point to a higher number of articulation errors in respect to consonants (e.g., Roberts et al., 2005). Both emergence and mastery of consonants seems to be an extended process with considerable variability between individuals. The emergence of phones does not seem to follow the order of typical "norms." Thus, the most frequently misarticulated sounds noted in older individuals with Down syndrome (15- to 22-year-old subjects) were /s, d, t, ɹ, z, l/, consonant clusters with /s/, and consonant clusters with /ɹ/, /n/, and /v/ (ranked from most to least frequent) (Sommers, Patterson, & Wildgen, 1988). Several of these errors, such as /d, t, n, v/, are not customarily noted in typically developing children. Although the most common phonological processes are reduction of consonant clusters and final consonant deletion, there is variable use of these processes in individuals with Down syndrome.

For more details, including a review of voice, fluency, prosody, and intelligibility in Down syndrome research, refer to Kent and Vorperian (2013).

Clinical Implications: Diagnostics

Individuals who have intellectual disabilities are a diverse group of people. Not only are individuals with cognitive disabilities quite different among themselves, but the boundaries between disabled and what is considered to be the norm are rather indistinct. That is not to say that individuals with intellectual disabilities are not different from individuals who are considered to be developing in a normal manner; they are. The cognitive development of children with intellectual disabilities is said to be generally similar to that of children without disabilities, only slower (Owens, 2009), and their cognitive skills have been proven to keep growing through adulthood. However, organizational and recall problems as well as difficulties in recognizing the significant features of a given situation distinguish children with intellectual disabilities from their normally developing peers.

With this group diversity in mind, assessment procedures largely depend on the age of the individual and the level of speech and language functioning. Some individuals with intellectual disabilities do not have speech at all, and alternative means of communication need to be explored. For the very young child who is beginning to develop first words, an independent analysis can examine the inventory of sounds being used. For older children and adults with more developed speech and language skills, the following assessment procedures could be used:

1. *Standardized speech assessment.* This determines the consonant and vowel inventory. Phonological patterns and the intelligibility of speech at the single-word level can also be analyzed.

2. *Spontaneous speech sample.* This determines the consonant and vowel inventory in conversational speech. Phonological patterns can be noted, as can the overall intelligibility in natural communicative situations. Differences in intelligibility between spontaneous speech and the standardized speech assessment should be evaluated.

3. *Motor-speech capabilities.* Oral structure and function should be assessed to determine the individual's motor capabilities.

4. *Hearing acuity and middle ear function.* Because of the large percentage of hearing losses and problems with middle ear function, having a complete understanding of the individual's current hearing realities is important.

5. *Language.* The client's language should be assessed to determine the level of linguistic functioning.

6. *Assessment of the environment.* The environment in which the individual lives and works will determine communicative needs. One of the major roles of a clinician is to assess the communicative environment in which the individual resides. This should provide information about the circumstances demanding communication of some type and the way in which the client is currently communicating to express needs, wants, and desires.

Although the diagnostic assessment of an individual with intellectual disabilities is conducted in a manner essentially similar to that used with normally developing clients, specific factors need to be kept in mind. Individual differences, such as age, level of cognitive functioning, level of speech and language functioning, and learning style, naturally alter the methods used.

Clinical Implications: Therapeutics

Each child with an intellectual disability presents a unique pattern of communicative abilities and difficulties that must be identified. Some guiding principles for clinicians can nevertheless be suggested within an intervention framework. The following principles have been suggested for the treatment of speech sound disorders in the population with intellectual disabilities (Owens, 2009; Swift & Rosin, 1990):

1. Use overlearning and repetition.
2. Train in the natural environment.
3. Begin as early as possible.
4. Follow developmental guidelines.
5. Concentrate more on overall intelligibility than on training individual sounds.
6. Enlist the help of the client's caregivers.

7. Direct all therapeutic activities to communication training serving the daily routine.

8. All intervention efforts should be commensurate with the client's ability to grasp and attend to the respective tasks. This typically translates to short, repetitive, reinforced activities that are meaningful to the situation and result in real, tangible consequences (Owens, 2009).

With very few exceptions, traditional motor approaches with these individuals have been of little value in the treatment of speech production problems. Therefore, a sound-by-sound approach using placement techniques is probably not a good choice. The cycles approach has been adapted for use with children with intellectual disabilities in classroom settings. In these cases, time allotments have been doubled for the children; thus, each phoneme or pattern is targeted for 2 hours rather than for 60 minutes (Hodson & Paden, 1991). A training period of 3 years or more might be required before substantial intelligibility gains are observed.

Many of the treatment programs for children and adults with intellectual disabilities target the increase of overall functional language skills. Although intelligibility often is a noted problem with these individuals, very little information on the treatment of the phonological systems is available. One possibility, developed by Swift and Rosin (1990), presents a remediation sequence for improving intelligibility of children with Down syndrome. Although this program was designed for a specific population of children, it could be adapted for other children with intellectual disabilities (in Swift and Rosin's study, the children were in the mild to moderate range of intellectual disability, with little evidence of hypotonicity).

Swift and Rosin (1990) offer the following summary: The early linguistic stage emphasizes single words and early two-word utterances. In structured sound play, the clinician selects objects and toys that should elicit intended sounds. For example, if bilabial sounds were targeted, *ball, baby, bye-bye*, and *moo* could be selected. Drill work is then used to increase the target behavior, attention, and syllable sequencing. In their program, they also use other techniques, such as melodic speech, visual cues, cued speech, auditory bombardment, and an auditory training unit. Overlearned phrases associated with frequently occurring situations (scripts) are trained as well. In addition, augmentative communication is recognized as a valid option within the oral language intervention program.

During the late linguistic stage, drill work and the learning of scripts continue. In addition, repair strategies that could aid overall speech intelligibility are taught. Repair strategies include a listener's request for clarification when a message is not understood, for example. Repair strategies from a speaker's point of view include repeating, rewording, and adapting the prosodic features (e.g., slowing the rate, adjusting phrasing, and using stress and inflection to enhance meaning). Throughout the program, communication should be as functional as possible.

In respect to augmentative communication, speech-language pathologists are often asked if implementation might delay or even arrest the development of oral communication skills in children with an intellectual disability. Millar, Light, and Schlosser (2006) reviewed 23 research studies from 1975 to 2003 in which the subjects (ages 2 to 60 years) were diagnosed with intellectual disabilities or autism. The AAC interventions involved instruction in manual signs or nonelectronic aided systems. None of the 27 cases demonstrated decreases in speech production as a result of AAC intervention; 11% showed no change, and the majority (89%) demonstrated gains in speech.

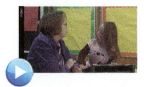

Video Tool Exercise 11.1

Articulation Therapy with Melinda

Complete the activity based on this video.

Clinical Application

Speech Goals and Activities for Facilitating the Development of Speech and Improving Intelligibility

Miller (1988) offered the following goals and suggestions. Although they were proposed for children with Down syndrome, they could be used with other children with intellectual disabilities who are in the *beginning stages* of speech and language development.

Speech Goals for the Child

1. *Increase the ability to respond to people and objects.* The more this skill can be promoted, the greater the opportunity for enhancing communication.
2. *Increase the frequency of vocal and verbal productions.* The more output, the more opportunity for modifying the quality of speech.
3. *Increase the production of sounds and the variety of sounds made.* This includes not only the actual production of speech sounds but also speaking rate, loudness, and intonation changes. These variables add to the child's intelligibility.
4. *Transition from babbling behavior to using words to represent objects and actions in the environment.* It appears that children who are intellectually disabled are trying to say words earlier than they are recognized by the caregivers in the children's environments. Their speech is often difficult to understand, and the words they use are simply labels and are not descriptive.

Clinical Exercises Pick one of the four speech goals for a child (from Miller [1988] in the Clinical Application above), and give three concrete examples noting how you could implement this in therapy.

You should treat in a natural environment (page 420)—that is, in situations the child encounters on a daily basis or using wants and needs that are part of the child's daily activities—and follow developmental guidelines. Lucas, age 5 years 6 months and who has an intellectual disability, has the following sounds: [p, b, t, d, w, h, and f]. According to developmental guidelines, which sounds would you target next?

List eight words that you could then target in a natural environment. What types of environments would you target?

SUGGESTIONS FOR CAREGIVERS

1. Identify situations and activities throughout the day in which a child is most vocal. List these over a week or two, noting the situation, the length of time the situation continues, and how many times it occurs during the day.
2. Document how much a child responds to people and things by looking, touching, or playing during a particular situation. Communication depends to a large degree on responsiveness.
3. Try to increase the time a child spends in these communication-enhancing situations (noted in speech goal 1 in the Clinical Application above).

4. Introduce a child to music at an early age. Children frequently respond enthusiastically to this stimulation. The type of music used depends on the child.

5. Speech activities should be a natural part of a child's day. Talk to the child about objects and activities during ordinary caregiving tasks. Introduce interactive games such as "pat-a-cake," "peek-a-boo," and "so big." These activities promote vocalizations and develop responsiveness to turn-taking and social interaction.

Based on a thorough assessment, the speech-language clinician can suggest sounds, sound patterns, and words that could be included in activities for a child's day. Suggestions offered in the section titled "The Child with an Emerging Phonological System: Expanding the System and Vocabulary" in Chapter 10 could also be incorporated here.

Hearing Impairment

Definition and General Features

Hearing loss (or **hearing impairment**) is a generic term for any diminished ability in normal sound reception. The different etiologies of hearing loss are only indirectly part of this definition. Commonly, hearing loss is described by type and degree of the particular auditory dysfunction (Northern & Downs, 2014). As far as the types of hearing impairments are concerned, conductive, sensorineural, and mixed dysfunctions are distinguished. The degree of hearing loss is categorized by reference to decibel (dB) levels, indicating the increase in intensity needed to make sound audible for the individual in question.

Conductive hearing loss refers to transmission problems affecting the travel of air-conducted sound waves from the external auditory canal to the inner ear. This affects the mechanical transfer of sound waves. A prominent medical condition that causes conductive hearing loss is otitis media. **Sensorineural hearing loss** occurs due to damage to the sensory end organ, the cochlear hair cells, or the auditory nerve. In these cases, air-conduction and bone-conduction thresholds are typically comparable. Mumps, among other medical conditions, can cause a sensorineural auditory dysfunction. If both a conductive and a sensorineural loss can be established, a *mixed hearing loss* exists.

The different degrees of hearing loss indicate the severity of the problem and are calculated according to the (approximate) threshold findings obtained. (*HL* stands for "hearing level.")

26 to 40 dB HL = mild hearing loss
41 to 55 dB HL = moderate hearing loss
56 to 70 dB HL = moderately severe hearing loss
71 to 95 dB HL = severe hearing loss
96+ dB HL = profound loss

Severity levels of hearing loss, which are determined by objective audiometric means, are not necessarily reliable indicators of speech-language function. Individuals deal differently with loss of hearing ability, especially within the context of communication. A 50 dB HL bilaterally in two children, for example, can have a notably different influence on their verbal communication. Such different effects of an objectively established hearing loss can become especially important when dealing with children in various phases of their speech-language development. Even relatively mild auditory dysfunctions with relatively minor communicative consequences for adult speakers and listeners can have lasting detrimental developmental effects in children. Nevertheless, the diminished ability to receive sound for comprehension is normally identified by the degree of hearing loss.

Articulatory and Phonological Characteristics

Speech production in an individual with hearing impairment is affected by the degree of hearing impairment and the frequencies involved. Generally, the greater the hearing loss, the more likely errors extend from consonant to vowel productions to errors in stress, pitch, and voicing (Hull, 2000). Children with bilateral hearing losses are usually described as having speech sound difficulties that are influenced by the amount and quality of acoustic information accessible through their hearing technology and by their listening experiences.

For children with mild to moderate degrees of hearing loss, speech is described as generally intelligible (Eisenberg, 2007). The most common errors involve the production of specific consonants, particularly affricates, fricatives, and consonant blends. In this group of children, consonant production is generally characterized by deletions and distortions. Vowel productions are generally accurate (Eisenberg, 2007; Elfenbein, Hardin-Jones, & Davis, 1994). Errors are typically described as resembling those of younger children.

In contrast, the speech of children with severe to profound hearing loss has been described as being less intelligible, particularly for those identified late or who receive hearing technology at a later age. These children have been described as having difficulties with respiration, phonation, speech rate, consonant production, vowels, suprasegmentals, coarticulatory movements, resonance, and voice quality (e.g., Culbertson, 2007; Ling, 2002). Speech sounds that are particularly difficult include affricates, fricatives, liquids, semivowels, plosives, and, in some cases, nasals (Abraham, 1989). Based on data obtained from 13 children with severe and profound hearing impairments, Abraham (1989) found that there was a marked difference in the accuracy of production word-initially versus word-finally. All sounds demonstrated a lower percentage of accuracy word-finally. Although the affricates were below 50% accuracy, consonants with even lower percentages of accuracy included [z] and [ð].

Children with hearing impairments have been found to use at least partially rule-governed phonological systems (e.g., Abraham, 1989; Buhler, DeThomasis, Chute, & DeCora, 2007). They use phonological processes similar to those of normally developing young children, although they use these processes more frequently. The overall intelligibility of speech is often reduced, particularly as linguistic complexity increases (Radziewicz & Antonellis, 1997). In a review of several investigations, Flipsen and Parker (2008) identified final consonant deletion, cluster reduction, devoicing of stops, stopping, fronting, liquid simplification, and gliding as the most common developmental processes of children with hearing losses. Among the idiosyncratic processes were initial consonant deletion, glottal stop substitutions, backing, vowel substitution, vowel neutralizations, and diphthong simplification. Final and initial consonant deletions were observed to be very frequent.

In children with cochlear implants, articulatory errors are generally described as being similar to those made by children with normal hearing at a younger age. Common phonological processes used by children with cochlear implants have been both developmental and idiosyncratic in nature. They include consonant cluster simplification, stopping, fronting, diphthong simplification, gliding, unstressed syllable deletion, initial consonant deletion, glottal replacement, vowel errors, and assimilation processes (e.g., Buhler et al., 2007; Eriks-Brophy, Gibson, & Tucker, 2013; Flipsen & Parker, 2008).

Clinical Implications: Diagnostics

In addition to audiometric results, the speech-language diagnostician assessing the impact of a client's impaired hearing on the speech sound status needs a host of appraisal data before any diagnostic conclusion can be reached. These include cause, age of onset, and identification of the impairment; its etiology and type; ages at which the hearing loss was identified and a hearing device was implemented; and length of previous intervention efforts. Speech intelligibility measures as well as results of formal and informal testing for language skills should also be included in the assessment data. Finally, the client's and caregivers' attitudes toward the disorder and the need for intervention give indications about the degree of motivation and possibly the impact of therapy.

Phonetic and phonological assessments must be completed for a child with a hearing impairment. Dunn and Newton (1994) outlined the following assessment procedures:

1. *Speech-motor assessment.* This is used to rule out any gross neurological or anatomical limitations that might interfere with speech sound production.
2. *Syllable imitation.* This tests the coordination of the speech mechanism during nonmeaningful speech.
3. *Administration of the Phonetic Level Evaluation (PLE).* This instrument (Ling, 2002) evaluates suprasegmental and segmental skills by imitation of non-sense syllables. The test provides a systematic, comprehensive hierarchy for the assessment of syllables with varied phonetic contexts. However, the PLE has specific shortcomings (refer to Dunn & Newton, 1994, pp. 130–132) and should not be used as the only evaluative measure for a child with hearing impairment.
4. *Spontaneous speech sample.* Depending on the age and developmental level of a child, this could be either single words or continuous speech. Ideally, the speech sample should include both.
5. *Analysis of the segmental and suprasegmental characteristics of the spontaneous speech sample.* Segmental analysis should include those procedures outlined in Chapter 7 (i.e., consonant and vowel inventory and distribution, syllable shape, and phonological pattern analysis). Suprasegmental analysis determines whether the child uses rate, pauses, stress, and intonational patterns appropriately. This can be done informally, with the clinician marking appropriate and inappropriate patterns. Dunn and Newton (1994) suggest a more formal measure developed at the National Technical Institute for the Deaf (Subtelny, 1980). This procedure provides rating scales for a variety of suprasegmental characteristics.

Clinical Implications: Therapeutics

With clients who are hearing impaired, the speech-language clinician's remedial task is mainly directed toward improving the client's speech intelligibility. "The term **'speech intelligibility'** may be defined generically as that aspect of oral speech-language output that allows a listener to understand what a speaker is saying" (Carney, 1994, p. 109; emphasis added). Above all, such a task involves structured work on speech sound errors and the selection of a suitable phonetic treatment program. Both of these objectives depend on the following two prerequisites (Dunn & Newton, 1994):

1. The improvement of residual hearing by speech signal amplification or cochlear implant and the methodical habituation of its application
2. The maximal use of the level of residual hearing for speech perception through systematic articulatory training.

The first prerequisite presupposes that a client wears an individualized hearing aid at all times and possibly uses auditory trainers during clinical sessions. For a child with a cochlear implant, this means implementing the device and providing training in an intervention program as soon as possible. A primary responsibility of the speech-language clinician called on to improve a client's intelligibility level is therefore to ensure constant proper amplification, not just amplification during therapy, and to facilitate the client's adjustment to the new hearing situation.

The maximal use of the client's residual hearing poses another challenge. Children with hearing impairments miss important information for the recognition of speech signals, which is the main reason for their lack of intelligibility. Essentially, these children produce what they are able to hear and leave out what they are unable to receive. In directing their attention systematically to specific oral-facial movements that accompany normal suprasegmental and segmental production, their residual hearing can be used more effectively, which in turn can positively influence intelligibility. In connection with suitable amplification, these efforts should increase speech intelligibility, especially in respect to voice, suprasegmental realization, and vowel production—three especially conspicuous problem areas for children who have hearing impairments.

However, children with hearing impairments also need systematic training on the phonetic and phonological levels. Dunn and Newton (1994) suggest a program that simultaneously teaches phonetic and phonological skills. The training sequence is as follows:

1. *Establish a suprasegmental base.* This is initially achieved through coordination of pitch, duration, and intensity with babbling or vocal play. Once this suprasegmental base is established, it should carry over to the various other stages of treatment. Dunn and Newton (1994) state that, in this context, "clinicians' eagerness to work on consonants before a suprasegmental base is established may result in many of the disordered patterns characteristic of deaf speech" (p. 140).
2. *Teach the segmental speech sounds.* This begins with basic vowel patterns. The patterns are first generated within any context the child can accurately produce, preferably a CV or VC syllable structure. For example, Ling (2002) provides procedures and strategies for achieving a new sound with people who are hearing impaired.
3. *Generalize a stable production by using different phonetic contexts and new syllable types.* Once a production is stable in one basic context, new contexts can be selected. Productions move from various other syllable types to monosyllabic words and, finally, to two-syllable words. With one- and two-syllable words, a child is responsible only for accurate production of the target sound. For example, if the target sound is [b] and the selected word is *boat,* [bo] would be considered an accurate production. Two-syllable words first begin with those containing reduplicated syllables, such as *bye-bye* and *boo-boo.* In this phase, acceptable speech sound production is applied to meaningful words. In addition, prosodic variation is practiced with these words.

Another approach, auditory-verbal therapy, has been used for a longer time with individuals who are deaf or hard of hearing. It is a method of working with a child who is hearing impaired or deaf and that child's family to develop spoken communication as the child's primary method of communication, regardless of the child's level of hearing impairment. This type of therapy is normally delivered by someone who is both a qualified teacher of the deaf and a speech-language therapist or audiologist and who is certified as an auditory verbal therapist by the Alexander Graham Bell Academy for Listening and Spoken Language (Alexander Graham Bell Academy for Listening and Spoken Language, 2017). The primary goal is for children with hearing impairments to reach the same level of expressive and receptive language as similar children who have typical hearing (Eriks-Brophy, Gibson, & Tucker, 2013). There are two reviews of this therapy and its efficacy with children who are deaf or hearing impaired. Kaipa and Peterson (2016) examined 14 studies using auditory-verbal therapy with individuals who are hearing impaired or deaf. Their conclusions suggest that auditory-verbal therapy can help children older than 3 years of age with receptive and expressive language, recognition of words in the presence of background noise, and successful mainstreaming. However, they caution that the evidence is limited due to the lack of well-designed studies in many cases. Bowers (2016) examined the efficacy of auditory-verbal therapy with children who are deaf in articles from 2000 to 2016. Again, the lack of well-designed studies made definitive conclusions limited; however, based on an analysis of these studies, the author noted that it does seem possible that children receiving auditory-verbal therapy from a certified individual can make gains in receptive and expressive language similar to those of their peers with normal hearing. The following principles of auditory-verbal therapy are outlined by the Alexander Graham Bell Academy for Listening and Spoken Language (2017).

1. Promote early diagnosis of hearing loss in all children, followed by immediate audiologic management of hearing technology and auditory-verbal therapy.

2. Recommend immediate assessment and use of state-of-the-art hearing technology to obtain the maximum benefits of auditory stimulation.

3. Coach parents to help their child use hearing as the primary sensory modality in developing spoken language.

4. Guide parents as they become the primary facilitators of their child's listening and spoken language development through active participation in individualized auditory-verbal therapy.

5. Direct parents to create environments that support listening for acquiring speech throughout the child's daily activities.

6. Show parents how to help their child integrate listening and spoken language into all aspects of the child's life.

7. Guide parents on how to use natural developmental patterns of audition, speech, language, cognition, and communication.

8. Show parents how to assist their child with self-monitoring skills of spoken language by listening.

9. Ongoing formal and informal diagnostic assessments should be used to develop individualized treatment plans, monitor progress, and evaluate the effectiveness of the plans for the child and family.

10. Promote education opportunities to mainstream the child in a regular school with peers who have typical hearing and to continue to provide appropriate services.

Video Example 11.3

In this short video, Henry, who is deaf and has bilateral hearing aids, works with a therapist. Which one of the principles of auditory-verbal therapy is the clinician trying to achieve?

https://www.youtube.com/watch?v=0GhjsBsmxIc

Motor-Speech Disorders in Adults

Acquired Apraxia of Speech

DEFINITION AND GENERAL FEATURES. The general term *apraxia* refers to a disorder in the execution of purposeful movements; reflexive or automatic motor actions remain largely intact. For example, as soon as an otherwise reflexive action is intended—on request, for example, or by one's own volition—gross execution difficulties occur. *Acquired apraxia of speech*, therefore, is the impaired volitional production of articulation and prosody (Ballard, Granier, & Robin, 2000). The primary clinical characteristics considered necessary for the diagnosis of apraxia of speech are (1) a slow rate of speech resulting in lengthened sound segments, (2) speech sound errors such as sound distortions or distorted sound substitutions, (3) errors that are inconsistent in type and location, and (4) disturbed prosody (McNeil, Robin, & Schmidt, 2009). These articulatory and prosodic aberrations do not result from muscle weakness or slowness but from impairment of the central nervous system's programming of oral movements. Apraxia of speech represents an inability to program and sequence articulatory requirements for volitional speech. Thus, **apraxia of speech** is a disorder of expressive communication resulting from brain damage that affects the normal realization of speech sounds, sound sequences, and prosodic features representing speech. Auditory comprehension, in principle, remains intact (Ballard et al., 2000; Duffy, 2005a).

Apraxia of speech is linked to cortical and/or subcortical damage in the language-dominant hemisphere of the brain, but researchers are still uncertain about the specific brain regions involved (e.g., Ogar et al., 2006).

Apraxia of speech should be separated from the dysarthrias, another type of motor-speech disorder that affects verbal expression. The following guidelines are given to differentiate between the two (e.g., Shipley & McAfee, 1998):

Apraxia of Speech	Dysarthria
Absence of any muscular weakness, paralytic condition, or discoordination	Presence of muscular weakness; change in muscular tone secondary to neurological involvement
Speech process of articulation primarily affected	All processes for speech affected: respiration, phonation, resonation, and articulation
Speech errors based on disruption of the central nervous system's programming of oral movements	Speech errors based on disruption of the central and peripheral nervous systems' control of muscular movements
Inconsistent articulatory errors	Consistent, predictable articulatory errors

Apraxia of speech differs from the aphasias by the language involvement noted in the aphasias. Apraxia of speech should also be distinguished from **oral (nonverbal) apraxia**, which is a disturbance in planning and executing volitional *nonspeech* movements of oral structures—that is, those movements not representing speech production. For example, a client who is asked to lick her or his lips might blow instead. The same client may be perfectly able to drink some juice, swallow the sip, and lick a drop off her or his lips. On request, though, this person cannot perform the same motor action, and attempts probably result in a series of laborious, bizarre trials. As might be expected, clients with apraxia of speech often suffer from oral (nonverbal) apraxia as well.

ARTICULATORY AND PHONOLOGICAL CHARACTERISTICS. The following characteristics of apraxia of speech have been noted (e.g., Croot, 2002; Haley, Ohde, & Wertz, 2000; McNeil et al., 2009):

1. *Effortful, trial-and-error groping of articulatory movements and attempts at self-correction.* This could result in equalization of syllabic stress patterns, slow rate of speech, and other prosodic alterations.
2. *Prosodic disturbances.*
3. *Difficulty initiating utterances.*
4. *Articulatory inconsistency on repeated production of the same utterance.* However, islands of clear, well-articulated speech exist.
5. *Predominance of sound substitution errors.* Additions and prolongations also occur; distortions and omissions are less frequent.
6. *Possible occurrence of sound or syllable transpositions.*
7. *Occasional articulatory errors that are complications rather than simplifications.* A consonant cluster could be substituted for a single consonant.
8. *Errors typically related to one another phonetically.* Substitutions, for example, could be related in place or manner of articulation to the intended sound.
9. *More errors on consonants that require more precise articulatory adjustments.* Examples are fricatives and affricates.
10. *Increased number of errors and articulatory struggle as words increase in length.*
11. *Speech comprehension and word recognition abilities often far better than speech production abilities.*
12. *Clients' recognition of their errors.* This could cause numerous retrials or self-correction attempts.
13. *Under otherwise comparable conditions, more sound production errors in stressed than in unstressed syllables.*

Video Example 11.4
Play the first 3 minutes of this video of an adult demonstrating apraxia of speech as he attempts oral nonverbal movements. Note the activities he has difficulties with. Does imitation seem to help his movements? Notice the differences between "bite your lower lip" with imitation versus "click your tongue."
https://www.youtube.com/watch?v=OPjDo03rUd0&list=PLuSyG9vYFwW9Cu2s3t-dEZi-5hcz4_LA96

Clinical Application

Formal and Informal Tests for Apraxia of Speech in Adults

Quick Assessment for Apraxia of Speech	Tanner and Culbertson, 1999
The Apraxia Profile	Hickman, 1997
Assessment of Apraxia of Speech	Duffy, 2005a
Assessment of Non-Verbal Oral Apraxia	Duffy, 2005b
Test of Oral and Limb Apraxia	Helm-Estabrooks, 1996
Dworkin-Culatta Oral Mechanism Examination	Dworkin and Culatta, 1980
Apraxia Battery for Adults	Dabul, 2000

Some of these tests can be used to evaluate the presence of oral and limb apraxia as well as specific characteristics of apraxia of speech. Others give the clinician information about a client's abilities to sequence words of varying length and complexity.

CLINICAL IMPLICATIONS: DIAGNOSTICS.   A diagnosis of apraxia of speech may not have been made before a clinician sees the client. Therefore, the following areas should be included in a thorough evaluation of a client with suspected apraxia of speech (Pindzola, Plexico & Haynes, 2016):

1. Aphasia test
2. Intelligence, cognitive, and memory tests, as needed
3. Apraxia battery
4. Speech-motor mechanism examination
5. Standardized speech assessment
6. Spontaneous speech sample

For the purpose at hand, this diagnostic section concentrates on testing procedures that involve only aspects of articulation and phonology—that is, on items 3 through 6 above.

The speech-motor assessment examines the structure and function of the articulators. Although their function is often assessed with one of the apraxia batteries, the oral mechanism examination can also be used to determine the presence of oral (nonverbal) apraxia. If the structure is intact but commands eliciting nonverbal movements such as "pucker your lips" or "stick out your tongue" result in laborious, bizarre movements, oral apraxia could be suspected.

Both the standardized speech assessment and the spontaneous speech sample should answer the following questions:

- *Does the client have difficulty initiating utterances?* Does this difficulty have a pattern? For example, is it better with words or sentences? Does the content of the message play a role?

- *Are there any islands of well-articulated speech?* These are usually automatic-reactive responses such as the days of the week or "I can't say that"; however, are there others?

- *Which sound errors occur?* Evaluate the differences between one-word standardized speech assessment results and spontaneous speech. Also note errors that occur as the complexity of the word or utterance increases. Furthermore, register substitutions, additions, prolongations, transpositions, distortions, and omissions.

- *Do sound errors have a pattern?* Errors are typically related to the target sound. An analysis based on the articulatory features of place of articulation, manner of articulation, and voicing could demonstrate which patterns are occurring. Observations should include if the client has any difficulties with fricatives, affricates, and consonant clusters, all typical problems for the individual with apraxia of speech.

- *Which prosodic aberrations occur?* Stress realizations (stressed versus unstressed syllables), intonation, rate of speech, and pausing should be observed and analyzed.

CLINICAL IMPLICATIONS: THERAPEUTICS.   In apraxia of speech, the client's ability to program and sequence articulatory requirements for volitional speech is impaired. This impairment ranges from mild to severe; each client demonstrates a different clinical picture. Some could have difficulty only in sequencing certain multisyllabic words or with specific clusters; others could have extreme problems sequencing a simple CV word. Obviously, such varying degrees of impairment influence the selection of therapeutic measures. In addition, certain aspects of motor production affect the error patterns of speakers with apraxia (Duffy, 2013; Knock, Ballard, Robin, & Schmidt, 2000; Wambaugh, Martinez,

McNeil, & Rogers, 1999). The following general guidelines can be used when structuring therapy:

1. *Articulatory accuracy is better for meaningful than for nonmeaningful utterances.* Therefore, avoid nonsense syllables; all treatment stimuli should be meaningful.

2. *Errors increase as words increase in length.* Determine the level at which the client demonstrates accurate production most of the time, and then build on that level. For example, if the assessment reveals that the client can produce CV, CVC, and VC words fairly accurately, start with this level of functioning and slowly build to CVCV structures or "easier" two-syllable words.

3. *Errors increase as the distance between successive points of articulation increases.* Evaluate your word material. Organize it so that this factor is taken into consideration. If you are working on consonant clusters, [st] should be easier than [sk]. If you are structuring words, *toilet* should be easier than *shopping*.

4. *Errors increase on consonants that require more precise articulatory adjustments.* Fricatives, affricates, and consonant clusters are extremely difficult for some clients with apraxia of speech. Begin with other sound classes until more volitional control is achieved.

After an extensive review of the treatment literature on apraxia of speech (Wambaugh, Duffy, McNeil, Robin, & Rogers, 2006), the following main categories of treatment for apraxia of speech were noted: (1) articulatory kinematic, (2) rate and/or rhythm, (3) augmentative and alternative communication, and (4) intersystemic facilitation and reorganization. The following is a brief overview of the articulatory kinematic approach.

1. *Motoric practice.* Stimulation is provided by the clinician, and the client responds with verbal production. Most of these techniques relied on modeling and repetition to elicit productions. A variation was integral stimulation that involved instructing the client to "watch me, listen to me, and say it with me." Repeated practice with limited verbal feedback has been shown to result in improved articulation with persons with chronic apraxia of speech (Wambaugh, Nessler, Cameron, & Mauszycki, 2010).

2. *Use of articulatory placement cues.* This method is used to communicate specific information about sound production. Placement cues have been provided for sounds produced in error and have taken the form of drawings, videotaped models, verbal instructions, and visual modeling. These cues have been used in conjunction with phonetic placement and sound modification techniques.

3. *Use of Prompts for Restructuring Oral Muscular Phonetic Targets (PROMPT; Square, Martin, & Bose, 2001).* This technique provides direct instruction for speech production with a combination of auditory, visual, tactile, and kinesthetic cues that are actively involved in providing sensory input regarding the place of articulatory contact, extent of jaw opening, and presence and manner of articulation and/or coarticulation. The cues focus on classes of speech movements and can be applied to isolated sound production gradating to sentence level. This technique has also been used with childhood apraxia of speech, children with cerebral palsy, and adults with dysarthria. Because of the relative complexity of the cues provided in the application of PROMPT, therapist training appears to be necessary for correct application. A list of workshops and dates are posted on the PROMPT website.

In addition, McNeil and colleagues (2017), in their review of recent developments in treatment of apraxia of speech, note that there is a clear trend to incorporate principles of motor learning. Bislick, Weir, Spencer, Kendall, and Yorkston (2012) conducted a systematic review of five studies that used motor learning strategies. Their goal was to see whether principles of motor learning did in fact enhance the acquisition and generalization of speech skills. Only one investigation (with two participants) showed consistent results that supported the use of principles of motor learning in treatment of apraxia of speech. Bislick and colleagues (2012) concluded that further research is necessary before any conclusions can be made. Refer to Bislick and colleagues (2012) and Maas and colleagues (2008) for discussions of motor learning principles as they apply to the treatment of motor speech disorders.

There is also an increased use of instrumentation or computer-based technologies in treatment of apraxia of speech. Approximately one-third of recent investigations have used these technologies. They include (1) kinematic biofeedback (McNeil et al., 2010), (2) telerehabilitation (e.g., Lasker, Stierwalt, Spence, & Cavin-Root, 2010), (3) computerized therapy (e.g., Whiteside et al., 2012), and (4) transcranial direct current stimulation (Marangolo et al., 2011). However, these technologies have not been evaluated to determine their treatment efficacy.

Clinical Exercises For the adult with apraxia of speech, *errors increase as the distance between successive points of articulation increases* and *errors increase on consonants that require more precise articulatory adjustments.*

If you are working on consonant clusters, list five CC clusters that should be relatively easy for an adult with apraxia of speech and five CC clusters that would be relatively difficult.

The Dysarthrias

DEFINITION AND GENERAL FEATURES. The word "articulation" has its origin in the Greek root *arthr-*, referring to the jointed connection between the many different parts of the speaking process. *Dys-arthr-ia*, therefore, literally means "disordered articulation." To be sure, in this context, "articulation" is to be understood in the broadest possible sense—that is, as signifying all articulated movements that result in speech. The technical term *dysarthria*, on the other hand, denotes a rather explicit group of articulation disorders, namely, those caused by neurogenic abnormalities and more specifically by the impairment of a single portion or several portions of the central and/or peripheral nervous systems that control and coordinate speech. **Dysarthrias** are neuromuscular speech disorders.

Dysarthrias have many different causes. Accident-induced trauma, tumors, cerebrovascular accidents (strokes), congenital conditions, and infectious and degenerative neurogenetic diseases are prominent among them. Each of these events can bring about more or less pronounced paralytic conditions and coordination impairments of the voluntary musculature required for speech production. The result is dysarthrias.

ARTICULATORY AND PHONOLOGICAL CHARACTERISTICS. It is customary to classify the dysarthrias into five main types according to the locus of the damage and its neuropathic consequences:

1. Spastic
2. Ataxic

3. Hypokinetic
4. Hyperkinetic
5. Flaccid

In addition, any simultaneous occurrence of characteristics of several types is categorized as:

6. Mixed

Each main type has a cluster of speech-impairing phonetic and articulatory production features (Duffy, 2013). These are summarized in Table 11.3.

Table 11.3 Features of the Dysarthrias

Type	Features
Spastic Dysarthria	
(Resulting from upper motor neuron system disorders. Example: pseudobulbar palsy)	
Respiration	Low respiratory frequency with shallow inspiration and lack of expiratory control
Phonation	Strained, harsh, low-pitched voice; reduced pitch and loudness ranges
Resonation	Hypernasality; nasal air emission
Articulation	Slow, labored, imprecise phoneme realization, especially of consonants
Ataxic Dysarthria	
(Resulting from cerebellar lesions. Example: cerebellar ataxia)	
Respiration	Shallow inspiration and lack of expiratory control; rapid, irregular, forced breathing patterns
Phonation	Forced, hoarse-breathy, trembling voice; generally reduced (but sometimes excessive) use of pitch and loudness
Resonation	Normal
Articulation	Slow, imprecise phone realization, especially of consonants; sound prolongations; irregular pausing between words, syllables, and sounds
Hypokinetic Dysarthria	
(Resulting from disorders of the extrapyramidal system. Example: parkinsonism)	
Respiration	Frequent respirations with shallow inspiratory phases and lack of expiratory control
Phonation	Harsh, tremorous voice; reduced pitch and loudness levels
Resonation	Normal
Articulation	Fluctuating, imprecise articulation; articulatory bursts; low intelligibility
Hyperkinetic Dysarthria	
(Resulting from disorders of the extrapyramidal system. Examples: athetosis, chorea)	
Respiration	Frequent respirations with shallow inspirations and incomplete expirations; lack of respiratory control
Phonation	Strained, tremorous voice; uncontrolled but generally reduced ranges in the expressive use of pitch and loudness
Resonation	Alternating hypernasality
Articulation	Variable imprecision of sounds, especially consonant realization

(Continued)

Table 11.3 Features of the Dysarthrias *(Continued)*

Type	Features
Flaccid Dysarthria	
(Resulting from lower motor neuron system disorders. Example: bulbar palsy)	
Respiration	Shallow, audible inspirations; uneven, incomplete expirations; low respiratory frequency; low expiratory air pressure
Phonation	Breathy, hoarse voice lacking expressive pitch and loudness variation
Resonation	Marked hypernasality with nasal air emission
Articulation	Slow, imprecise phone realization, especially of consonants

Source: Data from Dworkin, J. P. (1991). *Motor speech disorders: A treatment guide.* St. Louis, MO: Mosby Year Book; and Duffy, J. R. (2013). *Motor speech disorders: Substrate, differential diagnosis, and management* (3rd ed.). St. Louis, MO: Elsevier Mosby.

Summaries such as the one presented in Table 11.3 are helpful, but any division of dysarthric characteristics into just five subtypes suggests more group uniformity than is actually the case. Although some within-group similarities can probably serve as general guidelines, several across-group features overlap considerably. Several of the deficiencies mentioned belong in some measure simply to the clinical picture of most dysarthrias, including the following:

Respiration. Irregular, generally shallow breathing patterns may suddenly be interrupted by some deep breaths, rapid inspiration, incomplete expiration phases, waste of expiratory air during speaking, and lack of respiratory support.

Phonation. Strained voice is characteristic, including deviations from suitable loudness levels (either too loud or too soft) and voice quality (either too harsh or too "breathy," aphonic).

Resonation. Hypernasality and nasal air emission are consequences of incomplete velopharyngeal closure, distorting all speech sounds with the exception of nasals.

Articulation. Labored, indistinct sound production, especially of consonants, resulting in distortions or substitutions. Consonant errors might affect whole sound classes; fricatives, for example, might be realized as homorganic stops. Also, second and third elements of consonant clusters might be deleted; rate of speech is usually slower than normal (bradylalia), but bursts of fast speech (tachylalia) might occur as well; qualitative distortions of vowels are also noticeable.

Prosody. Characteristics include a narrow range of intonational configurations ("monopitch") and often greatly reduced varieties of expressive loudness levels ("monoloudness"). This generally reduced range of prosodic elements is sometimes interrupted by exaggerated stress and intonation patterns (Dworkin, 1991; Patel, 2002).

The physiological basis for all of these characteristics is a striking imbalance in the constant and subtle changes between phases of (relative) muscular tension and relaxation leading to normal speech events. The delicate synergism between the interaction of individual muscles and whole muscle groups to produce speech is in all cases of dysarthria disturbed. A disproportionate influence of agonistic and antagonistic forces determines dysarthric speech motor activity, distorting its normally smooth flow into effortful, poorly controlled speech production.

Common characteristics such as these exist across and within the main groups of dysarthrias. However, individual clients medically diagnosed with a specific type of dysarthria often show significant deviations from the noted group features. These individual differences are especially important in the assessment and intervention process. The speech-language clinician always needs to find the specific deviations from norm that each individual client displays.

CLINICAL IMPLICATIONS: DIAGNOSTICS. Most clients with dysarthrias are referred to speech-language clinicians by physicians or medical institutions. As a rule, an official diagnosis has already been established, usually down to the subtype the client belongs to medically (e.g., spastic dysarthria). What, then, remains for speech-language pathologists to assess and evaluate? Actually, quite a lot.

Even in the appraisal section of the assessment process, speech-language clinicians need to go far beyond the initial (mainly medical) information available. As mentioned earlier, dysarthric subtype characteristics are somewhat vague and indeterminate and therefore constitute little more than a point of departure for any appropriate collection of clinical data. They are both helpful and insufficient for clinical purposes. They are helpful because they indicate what to suspect and what to look for. They are insufficient because individual cases more often than not show considerable deviations from average, book-based descriptions. That is why *all* dysarthric symptoms contributing to abnormal voice and speech production need to be appraised as precisely as possible.

One possible aid to precise appraisal is the use of instrumentation. There is certainly no scarcity of instruments available to objectify the data. The problem does not lie in a lack of suitable instrumentation but in its proper application to the task at hand. Many clinicians are not trained well enough in instrumentation to feel comfortable with its use, or they do not have easy access to instrumentation. Another reason for the rare use of instruments in a clinical setting is a time concern: Clinicians feel too pressed for time to engage in the use of instruments to make their appraisal data more objective and verifiable.

A second way to make the appraisal of clients with dysarthrias more comparable, reliable, and precise is the use of a suitable protocol. Such a protocol might look like the one in Appendix 11.1.

Clinical Application

Protocols for Appraising the Speech Characteristics of Clients with Dysarthria

Frenchay Dysarthria Assessment (FDA-2)	Enderby and Palmer, 2008
Dysarthria Examination Battery	Drummond, 1993
Intelligibility Testing in Dysarthria	Kent, Weismer, Kent, and Rosenbek, 1989
Quick Assessment for Dysarthria	Tanner and Culbertson, 1999
Assessments of Intelligibility of Dysarthric Speech	Yorkston and Beukelman, 1981
Robertson Dysarthria Profile	Robertson, 1982

Some of these assessment instruments give profiles for the various diagnostic categories, whereas others provide severity ratings.

After having identified the type and severity of the dysarthric disturbances within the main subsystems contributing to speech, speech-language clinicians are ready to interpret and evaluate them in their totality; that is, they could draw a composite picture of the problem at hand, or make a diagnosis, in the narrow sense of the term. Diagnoses lead directly into therapy planning and form the basis for the professional selection of appropriate intervention measures.

CLINICAL IMPLICATIONS: THERAPEUTICS. The speech-language clinician's main therapeutic goal is improvement of the client's intelligibility. Thus, therapy can be restorative and is aimed at improving or restoring impaired function. Restorative approaches focus on increasing speech intelligibility, improving prosody and naturalness, and increasing efficiency of speech production. Compensatory approaches focus on improving the ability to understand the speaker by increasing the speaker's use of specific communicative strategies, improving listeners' skills and capacity, and attempting to alter the communication environment so that the individual can function adequately. Because the established deficits are caused by central and/or peripheral nervous system damage, the use of compensatory measures is extremely important. The diagnostic results should provide the necessary information about the type and degree of shortcomings in the various subsystems constituting normal speech production (i.e., respiration, phonation, resonation, and articulation). This information becomes the basis for therapy planning.

Most therapy plans are based on the principle of treating disordered facets of the subsystems contributing to speech thoroughly and methodically (e.g., Dworkin, 1991; McHenry, 2003; Rosenbek & Jones, 2009; Yorkston, 1996). Because speech results from cumulative effects of secondary physiological functions, the primary functions of structures in which speech is rooted must be considered as well. Thus, speech breathing has to evolve out of systematically modified breathing patterns for vital silent breathing; articulatory functions out of natural conditions of lip, tongue, and jaw movements; and the voicing and unvoicing of sound segments and suitable intonation patterning out of previously normalized voice production. In this way, an elaborate system of suitable exercises is created and diligently practiced. If aspects of different subsystems need to be combined—as in the case of respiratory preconditions for specific voice effects such as changes in pitch, loudness, and quality—matters can quickly become complicated. Planning and tenacity as well as flexibility during the implementation of the program are prerequisites for the successful treatment of practically all clients with dysarthria. A general guideline for this task pertains to the observance of certain sequences. For example, postural adjustments precede every specific measure, and respiratory and resonatory dysfunctions must be addressed before phonatory, articulatory, and prosodic ones.

Rosenbek and Jones (2009) summarized the following general treatment goals:

1. *Help the person become a productive patient.* Clinician and client have agreed on the necessity and value of treatment, what is to be accomplished, and the treatment procedures.
2. *Modify abnormalities of posture, tone, and strength.*
3. *Modify respiration.*
4. *Modify phonation.*
5. *Modify resonation.*
6. *Modify articulation.*
7. *Modify prosody.*
8. *If indicated, provide alternative or augmentative modes of communication.*

Dworkin (1991) provides a procedure based on a specific order of speech subsystems. The first-order subsystems consist of resonation and respiration, the second order is phonation, and the third order consists of articulation and prosody. First-order subsystems are treated first, second-order subsystems are treated next, and third-order subsystems are last in the treatment sequence. Inhibition and facilitation techniques probably need to precede the specific subsystem treatments. Inhibition techniques are implemented for increased tone and any associated weakness and paresis, hyperactive reflexes, hyperkinesia, and hypersensitivity. On the other hand, facilitation techniques are introduced to improve functioning of any of the following abnormal features: decreased tone and associated weakness and paresis, hypoactive reflexes, and hyposensitivity.

Dworkin (1991) provided the following general treatment objectives:

1. Promote adequate orofacial postures.
2. Promote integration of orofacial reflexes.
3. Improve orofacial muscle tone and strength.
4. Improve range, speed, timing, and coordination of orofacial muscle activities.

These general goals must be based on a treatment hierarchy that includes first-, second-, and third-order subsystems. Detailed exercises for each of the subsystems are included in Dworkin (1991).

The following overview of treating speech production subsystems is provided by ASHA in their Practice Portal (ASHA, n.d.-a).

Subsystem: Respiration

1. Make postural adjustments before treatment begins to improve breath support for speech. If in a hospital setting, the client should sit as upright as possible. Do not try to conduct speech therapy with your client lying down.
2. Have the client inhale deeply before beginning a speech utterance (known as *preparatory inhalation*).
3. Use specified breath groups when speaking. For each breath, have the client produce only the number of syllables that can be articulated comfortably. If speaking from a written text, this could be designated by lines marking where to take a breath. (Make sure that these are natural pauses and not inappropriate ones.)
4. Use expiratory muscle strength to assist expiration.
5. Use inspiratory muscle strength to improve inspiration.
6. Use maximum vowel prolongation tasks to improve duration and loudness of speech.

Subsystem: Phonation

1. The Lee Silverman Voice Treatment (Ramig, Bonitati, Lemke, & Horii, 1994) has been used successfully in therapy (refer to also Palmer and Enderby [2007] for an efficacy review). This program is intensive and targets high phonatory effort to improve loudness and intelligibility.
2. The Pitch Limiting Voice Treatment (De Swart, Willemse, Maassen, & Horstink, 2003) is also a program used to increase vocal loudness without increasing pitch.
3. Use effortful techniques to assist the adduction of the vocal folds by having the client pull upward on the chair seat or squeeze the palms of the hands together.
4. Improve timing of phonation by focusing on the initiation of phonation at the beginning of expiration.

Subsystem: Articulation

1. Use phonetic placement techniques to assist the positioning of the mouth, tongue, lips, or jaw during speech.

2. Use overarticulation to emphasize phonetic placement and increase precision.

3. Use minimal pair contrasts to emphasize production differences that are necessary to differentiate one phoneme from another.

4. Use intelligibility drills in which the individual reads words, phrases, or sentences and attempts to repair content that is not understood by the listener according to specific parameters that appear to work for this client.

5. Use rate modification to facilitate articulatory precision. Strategies include pausing at natural linguistic boundaries (e.g., using printed script marked at natural pauses); using external pacing methods such as pacing boards, hand or finger tapping, and alphabet boards; using auditory feedback such as a metronome; using visual feedback with computerized voice programs; and using other techniques that reduce speech rate, such as increasing the loudness level, accentuating the pitch variation, and modifying phrasing or breath patterns.

Summary

Several communication disorders have articulatory and phonological deficits as one of their central characteristics. This chapter provided an overview of the most prominent among them. First discussed were the disorders that are characteristically noted in children: (1) childhood apraxia of speech, (2) cerebral palsy, (3) cleft palate, (4) cognitive impairment, and (5) hearing impairment. Acquired communication disorders with articulatory deficits that commonly occur in adults were then represented by (1) apraxia of speech and (2) the dysarthrias. Each of these disorders has been defined, and general characteristics have been listed. This outline served as a foundation for the subsequent discussion of specific articulatory

and phonological problems found in these populations. Assessment principles for the respective speech problems have been identified, followed by selected therapeutic measures for the treatment of individuals within these seven populations.

For each of the disorders discussed, an impressive list of specialized literature exists. References have been given throughout the chapter to guide interested students and practitioners to more in-depth information. Each disorder represents a complex entity, including many important variables and involving several groups of professionals. This chapter briefly summarized basic considerations of articulatory and phonological features and their clinical intervention.

Case Study

The following results are from the Hodson Assessment of Phonological Patterns (HAPP-3) (Hodson, 2004) for Dillon, age 7 years 6 months. Dillon has been diagnosed with childhood apraxia of speech.

1. basket	[bæ.ə]	4. chair	[teə]
2. boats	[boʊ]	5. clouds	[daʊ]
3. candle	[dæ.nə]	6. cowboy hat	[taʊ.bə.æt]

7. feather	[bɛ.də]	29. snake	[deɪt]
8. fish	[bɪt]	30. soap	[doʊp]
9. flower	[daʊ.ə]	31. spoon	[bun]
10. fork	[fot]	32. square	[dɛ.ə]
11. glasses	[dæ.ət]	33. star	[dɑə]
12. glove	[dʌb]	34. string	[twɪn]
13. gum	[dʌm]	35. swimming	[tɪ.mɪn]
14. hanger	[æn.ə]	36. television (TV)	[tɛ.bi]
15. horse	[oət]	37. toothbrush	[tu.bət]
16. ice cubes	[aɪ.tu]	38. truck	[tjʌk]
17. jumping	[dʌm]	39. vase	[beɪd]
18. leaf	[jit]	40. watch	[wɑt]
19. mask	[mæt]	41. yoyo	[joʊ.joʊ]
20. music box	[mu.ɪt.bɑ]	42. zip	[jɪp]
21. page	[beɪt]	43. crayons	[deɪ.ə]
22. plane	[beɪn]	44. black	[bæt]
23. queen	[din]	45. green	[din]
24. rock	[wɑ]	46. yellow	[jɛ.joʊ]
25. screwdriver	[du.daɪ.ə]	47. three	[ti]
26. shoe	[du]	48. thumb	[dʌm]
27. slide	[daɪt]	49. nose	[noʊd]
28. smoke	[moʊt]	50. mouth	[maʊf]

Although Dillon appears to have a fairly complete vowel inventory with the exception of central vowels with r-coloring, his consonant repertoire is extremely limited. There are no fricatives, affricates, or lateral or central approximants represented in this sample. At age 7 years 6 months, Dillon was considered highly unintelligible.

Think Critically

1. Refer to the case study of Dillon, age 7 years 6 months. Which consonants does he have in the prevocalic, intervocalic, and postvocalic positions? Given that most children demonstrate a much larger inventory of consonants in the prevocalic position, what comments could you make about Dillon's inventory?

2. Which syllable shapes are present in Dillon's speech sample? Do you see any evidence of CC structures?

3. Note the collapse of phonemic contrasts in Dillon's speech. Do you see any sound preferences?

Chapter Quiz 11.1 Complete this quiz to check your understanding of chapter concepts.

Appendix 11.1 Protocol for Assessing Respiration, Phonation, Resonation, and Articulation of Dysarthric Speech

1. Rate the degree of normal, near-normal, or abnormal behavior on a scale from 1 to 5 by marking the dotted line at the judged value.

	Normal		⟶		Abnormal
	1	2	3	4	5
Respiration					
Silent breathing					
Speech breathing					
Inspiration					
Expiration					
Breath support					
Shouting					
Shortness of breath					
Resonation					
Nasality					
Quality of prolonged vowels (check one)					
Constant ☐					
Intermittent ☐					
Phonation					
Voice					
Pitch					
Volume					
Lips					
Appearance in resting position					
Lip protrusion					
Movement during speaking					
Jaw					
Appearance in resting position					
Movement during speaking					
Tongue					
Appearance in resting position					
Protrusion					
Elevating tip of tongue					
Lowering tip of tongue					
Lateral movements					

During speaking

Strength

Articulation

Vowels

Quality

Duration

Consonants

Clusters

Prosody

Stress

Intonation

Tempo

Rhythm

----

2. Itemize the most salient characteristic in each of the categories with a rating of 3 or more.

3. Repeat the rating process at least one more time on a different day.

Glossary

acoustic phonetics   Study of the transmission properties of speech.

addental [s]   A frequent s-sound distortion marked by an articulatory variation in which the tongue approaches the upper incisors, causing the resulting s-sound to lose its regular stridency, giving a "dull" or "flat" sound impression.

adduct   Closing the vocal folds; moving the vocal folds toward the midline of the glottis.

advanced tongue position   Diacritic for vowels that indicates a tongue position that is too far forward for a normal production of the vowel in question.

affricate   Single, uniform speech sounds characterized by a slow release of a stopping phase into a homorganic (hom = same) friction element. Example: [tʃ].

allophones   Variations in phoneme realizations that do not change the meaning of a word when they are produced in various contexts.

alveolar pressure   The pressure within the lungs.

alveolar ridge   Prominent ridge-like structure formed by the alveolar process, which is a thickened portion of the maxilla (upper jaw) housing the teeth.

appraisal   Collection of data to be interpreted and evaluated in the diagnostic phase.

approximant   A manner of articulation in which the articulators come close to each other (they approximate each other), but the constriction is far less than for the fricatives. The opening is wider, and there is a much broader passage of air. Example: [w], [j].

apraxia of speech   Disorder of expressive communication as a result of brain damage affecting the normal realization of speech sounds, sound sequences, and prosodic features representing speech.

articulation   The totality motor movements involved in production of the actual sounds that comprise speech.

articulation disorder   A subcategory of a speech disorder, which is the atypical production of speech sounds characterized by substitutions, omissions, additions, or distortions that may interfere with intelligibility. Articulation-based disorders are phonetic in nature. *See:* phonological disorder.

articulators   Anatomical structures used to generate speech sounds.

articulatory phonetics   Production features of speech sounds, their categorization, and classification according to specific details of their production.

aspiration of plosives   The strong burst of breath that accompanies the release of the articulatory closure in plosives.

assessment   Clinical evaluation of a client's disorder.

assimilation   Adaptive articulatory change by which one speech sound becomes similar, sometimes identical, to a neighboring sound segment.

assimilatory process   Natural consequences of normal speech production by which one speech sound becomes similar, sometimes identical, to a neighboring sound. Also called harmony process. A process that occurs in the early development of children's speech.

auditory phonetics   Study of speech (sound) perception.

augmentative and alternative communication (AAC)   Means of compensation for temporary or permanent impairments, activity limitations, and participation restrictions of individuals with severe disorders of speech-language production and/or comprehension, including spoken and written modes of communication.

backing   A substitution in which the place of articulation is more posteriorly located than the intended sound.

bifid uvula   Uvula that is medially divided into two portions, a split uvula (uvula bifida).

bilabial fricative   The lips approximate one another so that a horizontally long but vertically narrow passageway is left between them for the voiceless or voiced breath stream to pass.

443

binary system   In this context a methodology using a plus (+) and minus (−) system to signal the presence (+) or absence (−) of certain features.

broad transcription   Based on the phoneme system of the particular language in which each symbol represents a phoneme.

canonical babbling   Term for the reduplicated and nonreduplicated babbling stages.

categorical perception   Ability of listeners to perceive speech sounds varied along a continuum according to the phonemic categories of their native language.

cavity features   Term used in distinctive features (Chomsky & Halle, 1968) to refer to the place of articulation for distinguishing between phonemes.

centering diphthong   A diphthong in which the offglide, or less prominent element, is the central vowel [ə] or [ɚ]. Examples: bar [bɑɚ] or wear [wɛɚ].

central auditory processing disorder   Deficits resulting in difficulties with information processing of auditory signals that are not related to impaired sensitivity of the auditory system.

cerebral palsy (CP)   Nonprogressive disorder of motor control caused by damage to the developing brain during pre-, peri-, or early postnatal periods.

changes in tongue placement for vowels   Diacritics used to denote nonstandard tongue placement (along vertical or horizontal dimensions) in vowel articulation.

checked syllable   *See:* closed syllable.

childhood apraxia of speech (CAS)   Neurological childhood (pediatric) speech sound disorder in which the precision and consistency of movements underlying speech are impaired in the absence of neuromuscular deficits (e.g., abnormal reflexes, abnormal tone). The main difficulty appears to be the planning and/or programming of spatiotemporal parameters of movement sequences that results in errors in speech sound production and prosody.

citing   Giving a single-word test response. Example: naming a picture.

clefting   Dividing a continuous structure by a cleavage or splitting prominently caused by a failure of the palate to fuse during fetal development.

closed syllable   Checked syllable. A syllable that has a coda. Example: *stop.*

coarticulation   Concept that the articulators are continually moving into position for other segments over a stretch of speech.

coda   All sound segments of a syllable following its peak.

code mixing   In this developmental process, speakers alternate between L1 and L2. This may occur within a phrase or between sentences.

code switching   Changing back and forth between varieties of dialects, in this case, specifically between African American Vernacular English and General American English; also referred to as *code mixing.*

coding   Translating stimuli from one form to another. Example: from auditory to written form or from written to auditory.

cognate   Similarity between two sounds; can refer to similar vowels, such as [i] and [ɪ] being i-type vowels, or consonants that differ only in voicing features, for example [p] and [b] are cognates.

communication   Sharing information between individuals; any act in which information is given to or received from another person concerning that person's needs, desires, perceptions, knowledge, or affective states.

communication disorder   Impairment in the ability to receive, send, process, and comprehend concepts including verbal, nonverbal, and graphic symbol systems.

comprehensive evaluation   Activities and tests that allow a more detailed and complete collection of data than screenings.

conductive hearing loss   Transmission problem affecting the travel of air-conducted sound waves from the external auditory canal to the inner ear.

consonant   Speech sound with a significant constriction in the vocal tract, mainly in the oral and pharyngeal cavities, foremost along the oral cavity's sagittal midline.

constraint   Any patterns noted that seem to limit or restrict the productional possibilities of our clients.

contact assimilation   Adaptive process modifying immediately adjacent sounds; also called *contiguous assimilation.*

contextual testing   The use of specific phonetic contexts to facilitate possibly correct speech sound production.

contiguous assimilation   *See:* contact assimilation.

contoid   Nonphonemic consonant-like sound production.

culture   Way of life developed by a group of individuals to meet psychosocial needs; consists of values, norms, beliefs, attitudes, behavioral styles, and traditions that can impact a dialect.

deep structure   *See:* underlying form.

dentalization   Nonstandard articulatory variation in the production of nondental consonants: use of the dental place of articulation for a nondental consonant. Example: [s̪] for [s].

derhotacization   Loss of r-coloring during the production of [ɹ] and rhotacized central vowels.

developmental apraxia of speech (DAS)   *See:* childhood apraxia of speech (CAS).

developmental verbal dyspraxia (DVD)   *See:* childhood apraxia of speech (CAS).

deviant speech sound development   Speech sound errors that are not typically observed in the development of most young children.

diacritics   Marks added to sound transcription symbols to give them a particular phonetic value.

diadochokinetic rates   Maximum repetitions of the syllables [pʌ], [tʌ], and [kʌ] alone and in various combinations.

diagnosis   Result of studying and interpreting of data collected during an appraisal.

dialect   Neutral label that refers to any variety of a language that is shared by a group of speakers.

diphthong   Vowel sound that demonstrates articulatory movement during its production resulting in a change in quality.

distinctive feature   Phonetic constituent that distinguishes between phonemes.

distribution of speech sounds   Where the norm and aberrant articulations occurred in a word; in this context pre-, inter- or postvocalic positions.

dorsum   Body of the tongue.

duration symbols   Diacritics that mark the length of speech sounds.

dysarthrias   Neuromuscular speech disorders.

emerging phonology   The time span during childhood in which conventional words begin to appear as a means of communication.

epenthesis   Syllable structure process marked by the insertion of a sound segment into a word, primarily (but not always) a schwa insertion between two consonants. Example: [pəliz] for *please*.

ethnic dialects   Language variations that are generally related to ethnic background.

ethnicity   Commonalities such as religion, nationality, and region that can affect a dialect.

extrinsic muscles of the larynx   Those having at least one attachment to structures outside the larynx; responsible for support and fixation of the larynx.

feature geometry   Group of nonlinear phonological theories that have adopted the tiered representation of features used in autosegmental phonology; an attempt to explain why some features are affected by assimilation processes (known as *spreading* or *linking* of features), whereas others are affected by neutralization or deletion processes (known as *delinking*).

first word   An entity of relatively stable phonetic form that is produced consistently by a child in a particular context and that is recognizably related to the adult-like word form of a particular language.

flap   Occurs when plosives are preceded and followed by vowels, as in *city* or *butter*, and is articulated with a single tap of the tongue tip against the alveolar ridge or possibly just with a movement of the tongue tip in the direction of the alveolar ridge.

Formal Standard English   Language type that applies primarily to written language (and based on it) and the most formal spoken language situations; exemplified in guides of usage or grammar texts.

fricative   Consonant characterized by an audible friction noise established by forcing expiratory air through a constricted passage in the oral cavity.

fundamental frequency   The average number of glottal openings per second.

generative phonology   The application of principles of generative (or transformational) grammar to phonology.

glide   Manner of articulation; a shift in movement of the articulators from a narrower to a wider consonantal constriction. Examples: [w] and [j].

glossing   Repeating with normal pronunciation what a client has just said for easier identification later.

glottal stop   Produced when a closed glottis (i.e., the space between the vocal folds) is suddenly released after a buildup of subglottal air pressure.

groping behavior   Ongoing series of movements of the articulators in an attempt to find the desired articulatory position.

harmony process   *See:* assimilation process.

hearing impairment Impaired auditory sensitivity; individuals are typically classified as hard of hearing or deaf.

hearing loss Generic term for any diminished ability in normal sound reception.

hearing screening Used to identify children who may require a more comprehensive hearing assessment and/or medical management.

implicational universals Describe sound properties in which one property is, according to theoretical constructs, predictive of another. In this case, the presence of certain sound classes is predictive of another sound class.

inconsistent phonological disorder The phonological systems of these children demonstrate variability of production on the same item.

inconsistent speech disorder *See:* inconsistent phonological disorder.

independent analysis Assessment that considers only the client's productions without comparing them to the adult norm model.

individual sound approach Traditional or motor method referring to the treatment of individual speech sounds in sequence. *See:* motor approach.

Informal Standard English Based on the assessment by members of the American English-speaking community as they judge the "standardness" of other speakers; relative to a continuum between formal English and vernacular English.

intelligibility Individual's ability to be understood determined by a listener based on how much of an utterance can be recognized.

interference Impact of an individual's first language (L1) on English (L2); L2 error results from the direct influence of L1.

intrinsic muscles of the larynx Those having both attachments within the larynx.

inventory of speech sounds List of speech sounds that the client can articulate within normal limits.

item learning Acquisition of word forms as unanalyzed units and as productional wholes.

jargon Stage characterized by strings of babbled utterances that are modulated primarily by intonation, rhythm, and pausing.

labialization Consonant productions that normally occur without lip rounding are produced with lip rounding. Example: [s^{w}up] for [sup].

language Complex and dynamic system of conventional symbols used in various modes for thought and communication.

language disorder Impaired comprehension and/or use of spoken, written, and/or other symbol systems.

lateralization Any consonant production, other than [l], in which the air is released laterally.

limitation A concept in natural phonology which occurs when differences between a child's and an adult's systems become *limited* to only specific sounds, sound classes, or sound sequences.

limited English proficient Terminology for any individual between the ages of 3 and 21 who is enrolled or preparing to enroll in an elementary or secondary school, who was not born in the United States, or whose native language is a language other than English. Individuals who are Native Americans or Alaska Natives and come from an environment where a language other than English has had a significant impact on the individuals are also included in this definition. The difficulties in speaking, writing, or understanding the English language compromise the individual's ability to successfully achieve in classrooms, where the language of instruction is English, or to participate fully in society (PL107-110, The No Child Left Behind Act of 2001).

linear phonologies Phoneme theories characterized by an assumption that all meaning-distinguishing sound segments are serially arranged.

liquid Group term for the consonant categories laterals [l] and rhotics [ɹ].

lowered tongue position Diacritic used to mark a tongue position for a specific vowel that is too low.

major class features Term used in distinctive features (Chomsky & Halle, 1968) to characterize and distinguish among three sound production possibilities that result in different basic sound classes: consonantal, approximant, and sonorant.

manner of articulation Type of constriction or narrowing that occurs between the articulators for the realization of a particular consonant.

manner of articulation features Term used in distinctive features (Chomsky & Halle, 1968) regarding the way the articulators act jointly to produce sound classes, signaling differences between stops and fricatives, for example.

markedness (of phonemes) Sound that is relatively difficult to produce and less frequent in languages.

metalinguistic awareness   The ability to think about and reflect on the nature of language and how it functions.

metaphonology   Conscious awareness of the sounds in a particular language. The ability to pay attention to and reflect on the phonological structure of language.

metaphon therapy   Treatment approach marked by the systematic training of phonological awareness, especially the awareness of sound properties.

metathesis   Transposition of sounds in an utterance.

minimal opposition contrast therapy   Treatment that uses pairs of words that differ by one phoneme only.

minimal pair   Set of words that differ in only one phoneme value among their sound constituents. Example: *book* versus *cook*.

monophthong   Vowel that remains qualitatively the same throughout its entire production; a pure vowel.

morpheme   Smallest meaningful unit of a language. Examples: "hits" consists of two morphemes, "hit" and "s".

morphology   Study of the structure of words, analyzes how words can be divided into units labelled as morphemes.

morphophonemic function   Role of phonemes to signal grammatical units. For example, /s/ is a phoneme of the English language as demonstrable by the minimal pair *sick* versus *thick*. However, /s/ also signals plurality, *book* versus *books*, a morphological function.

morphophonology   Study of the different allomorphs of the morpheme and the rules governing their use.

motor approach   Procedure that treats individual sounds based on the placement of the articulators for normal speech sound production. *See:* individual sound approach.

multiple-sound approach   Therapy technique in which several error sounds are simultaneously treated.

narrow transcription   Recording of sound units with as much production detail as possible; encompasses the use of both the broad classification system noted in the International Phonetic Alphabet and extra symbols that can give a particular phonetic value.

nasal   Manner of articulation in which consonants are produced with the velum lowered so that the expiratory air can pass freely through the nasal cavity. Example: [m].

nasal cavities   Nose area, consists of two narrow chambers that begin at the soft palate and end at the exterior portion of the nostrils.

nasality symbols   Diacritics to mark the passing/nonpassing of expiratory air through the nasal cavity. Only nonnasal sounds can be nasalized, only nasals denasalized.

nasal "s"   Irregular s-productions marked by nasal airflow due to incomplete nasal-pharyngeal closure.

naturalness (of phonemes)   Designates (1) the relative simplicity of a sound production and (2) the sound's high frequency of occurrence in languages.

natural phonology   Theory that incorporates features of naturalness and was specifically designed to explain the development of a child's phonological system.

near-minimal pairs   Sets of two words that differ by more than one phoneme; the vowel preceding or following the target sound remains constant in both words.

nonaspiration of plosives   Plosives that are normally aspirated are produced without aspiration.

noncontiguous assimilation   *See:* remote assimilation.

nonlabialization   Consonants that are normally articulated with lip rounding are produced without lip rounding.

nonlinear phonologies   Group of theories that regards phoneme segments being governed by more complex linguistic dimensions.

nonphonemic diphthong   Vowel that can be realized in its onset only without a change in word meaning. Example: [heɪ] or [he] for *hay*.

non-reduplicated babbling   Stage of prelinguistic development that demonstrates variation of both consonants and vowels from syllable to syllable.

obstruents   Consonants characterized by a complete or narrow constriction between the articulators hindering the expiratory airstream; includes the stop-plosives, the fricatives, and the affricates.

offglide   End portion of a diphthong. Example: [ɪ] in [eɪ].

one-tap trill   *See:* flap.

onglide   Beginning portion of a diphthong. Example: [e] in [eɪ].

onset All sound segments of a syllable prior to its peak.

open syllable A syllable that does not contain a coda. Example: *do. See* unchecked syllable.

optimality theory Constraint-based approach, which is one nonlinear (multilinear) theory of phonology.

oral cavity Mouth area, extends from the lips to the soft palate.

oral muscle pattern disorder Excessive anterior tongue movement during swallowing and a more anterior tongue position during rest.

oral (nonverbal) apraxia Disturbance of the planning and execution of volitional *nonspeech* movements of oral structures.

ordering A concept of natural phonology that occurs when substitutions that appeared unordered and random become more organized.

palatal fricative Fricative produced with a palatal place of constriction of the articulators.

partial assimilation Adaptive influence of one sound segment on another, which results in a higher degree of similarity between the respective sound segments.

peak Most prominent, acoustically intense part of a syllable; usually a vowel.

perceptual constancy Ability to identify the same sound across different speakers, pitches, and other changing environmental conditions.

perceptual saliency Refers to the conspicuousness, or noticeability, of the error sound to listeners.

persistent speech disorder Errors that persist past the typical age of acquisition (9 years old).

pharyngeal cavity A muscular and membranous tubelike structure, extends from the epiglottis to the soft palate.

phone Physical sound realities; they are end products of articulatory motor processes. *See:* speech sound.

phoneme Smallest linguistic unit that is able, when combined with other such units, to establish word meanings between words.

phonemic awareness An understanding that words are composed of individual sounds.

phonemic-based disorder Impaired comprehension and/or use of the sound system of a language and the rules that govern the sound combinations.

phonemic diphthong Meaning would change in a particular word if only the vowel onglide was produced. Example: [mas] versus [maʊs].

phonemic error Replacement of one General American English phoneme with another.

phonemic inventory Repertoire of phonemes used contrastively by an individual.

phonemic transcription Transcription based on the phoneme system of the particular language; each symbol represents a phoneme. *See:* broad transcription.

phonetically consistent form *See:* proto-word.

phonetic context Segmental, suprasegmental, and phonotactic environment in which a given speech sound occurs.

phonetic inventory Repertoire of speech sounds for a particular client, including all the characteristic production features the client uses.

phonetic motor approach Therapy method that treats each error sound individually, one after the other; also referred to as *traditional-motor approaches*.

phonetic placement method Procedure in which a clinician instructs a client how to position the articulators to produce a norm production.

phonetic problem Any misarticulation based on phonetic production difficulties.

phonetic representation In generative phonology the surface level form or representation.

phonetics Study of speech emphasizing the description and classification of speech sounds according to their production, transmission, and perceptual features.

phonetic transcription *See:* narrow transcription.

phonetic variability Instability of pronunciations of a child's first 50 words.

phonetic variation Actual realization of a phoneme; also called *allophonic variation*.

phonological awareness The individual's awareness of the sound structure or phonological structure of a spoken word in contrast to written words.

phonological development Acquisition of speech sound form and function in a language system.

phonological disability Indicates a serious difficulty that impacts the child's or person's functioning in society.

phonological disorder   Impaired comprehension and/or use of the sound system of a language and the rules that govern the sound combinations.

phonological idiom   Accurate sound productions that are later replaced by inaccurate ones; also called *regression.*

phonological impairment   Typically used synonymously with phonological disorder.

phonological memory   The coding of phonological information in working memory.

phonological process   "Mental operation that applies in speech to substitute for a class of sounds or sound sequences presenting a common difficulty to the speech capacity of the individual" (Stampe, 1979, p. 1). They are innate and universal; therefore, all children are born with the capacity to use the same system of processes.

phonological processing   Refers to the use of sounds in one's language in processing written and oral language. Phonological processing requires working and long-term memory.

phonological representation   In generative phonology the underlying form or deep structure of the representation.

phonological rules   Notations used to demonstrate the relationship between the underlying (phonological) and the surface (phonetic) forms; in generative phonological analysis, formalized statements about the patterns of sound substitutions and deletions.

phonology   Study of the sound system of a language; examines the sound units of that particular language, how these units are arranged, and their systematic organization and rule system.

phonotactic constraints   Any patterns that are noted which seem to limit or restrict the productional possibilities of our clients.

phonotactics   Study of the allowed combinations of phonemes in a particular language.

place of articulation   Where the constriction or narrowing occurs for the various consonant productions.

pleural linkage   The mechanism by which the two pleurae, one covering the outer surface of the lungs and one covering the inner surface of the thorax and the top portion of the diaphragm, are linked together to support the movements of the rib cage which are transmitted to the lungs so that lungs can increase and decrease volume.

plosive   Manner of articulation resulting from a complete occlusion at some point in the vocal tract; the sudden release phase of a stop.

pragmatics   Study of language used to communicate in various social situational contexts, including, among other things, the reasons for talking, conversational skills, and the flexibility to modify speech for different listeners and social situations.

prelinguistic behavior   Vocalizations prior to the first actual words.

primary functions   Life-supporting roles of particular anatomical structures; in this case, the speech mechanism.

primary stress   The order of prominence of syllables in a word is actualized by differences in loudness, pitch, and duration, the loudness differences being the most striking of the three. The loudest syllable of a word.

primary target patterns   In the cycles approach, treatment targets that are assessed at the beginning of therapy to see which ones you would start with.

probe words   Words not being targeted in therapy but contain the sound or sounds you are trying to achieve as well as other sounds that were not found in the child's inventory.

progressive assimilation   The articulatory influence of a preceding sound on a following sound segment; also called *perseverative assimilation.*

prosodic features   Characteristics of large linguistic units, elements that occur across segments, influencing what an individual says.

prosody   Variations in stress (loudness), pitch (intonation), and duration (rate) that occur across segments.

proto-word   Vocalization used consistently by a child in particular contexts but without a recognizable adult model. Also called *vocables, phonetically consistent forms,* and *quasi-words.*

quasi-word   *See:* proto-word.

race   Biological label defined in terms of observable physical features (such as skin color, hair type and color, head shape and size) and biological characteristics (such as genetic composition).

raised tongue position   Tongue position for the production of the vowel in question that is too high.

reduplicated babbling   Prelinguistic stage marked by similar strings of consonant–vowel productions.

regional dialects   Forms of a language corresponding to various geographical locations.

regression *See:* phonological idiom.

regressive assimilation Adaptation of a sound's phonetic production characteristics under the influence of a following consonant. Example: [ɪʃi] for *is she;* also called *anticipatory assimilation.*

remote assimilation Adaptive process modifying a speech sound separated by at least one other segment; also called *noncontiguous assimilation.*

resonance The selective reinforcement and absorption of sound energy at specific frequencies.

retracted tongue position Diacritic for vowels indicating a tongue position that is too far back for a normal production of the vowel in question.

rhotic Relating to the manner of articulation characterized by r-coloring.

rhotic diphthong Vowel in which the offglide is the central vowel with r-coloring [ɚ]. *See also:* centering diphthong.

rhythm How stressed and unstressed syllables are distributed over time.

rime Linguistic term for the nucleus (vowel) and the coda (the arrest) of a syllable.

rising diphthong During production of these vowels, portions of the tongue move from a lower onglide to a higher offglide position; thus, relative to the palate, the tongue moves in a rising motion.

rounding of vowels Lip rounding of vowels which characteristically do not show lip rounding.

sagittal midline The median plane of the vocal tract that divides the vocal tract into right and left halves.

screening Activity or test that identifies individuals for further evaluation.

secondary functions Anatomical physiological tasks, including articulation of speech sounds, that occur in addition to the life-supporting ones.

secondary stress The order of prominence is actualized by differences in loudness, pitch, and duration, the loudness differences being the most striking of the three; the second loudest syllable in a word.

segmental Referring to the discrete, sequentially arranged speech segments of vowels and consonants.

semantics Study of linguistic meaning that includes the meaning of words, phrases, and sentences.

semivowels Sonorants, especially the glides among them, as productionally characterized by an articulatory movement from a sagitally more constricted to a sagitally more open oral cavity.

sensorineural hearing loss Hearing loss that occurs as a consequence of damage to the sensory end organ, the cochlear hair cells, or the auditory nerve.

sibilant Fricative sound characterized by a higher amplitude and pitch due to the presence of high-frequency components. Examples: [s], [z], [ʃ], and [ʒ].

silent period Time frame that might occur when English language learners are very quiet, speaking very little as they focus on understanding the new language.

silent posturing Positioning of the articulators for a specific articulation without sound production.

social dialects Particular forms of a language that are generally related to socioeconomic status.

sonorant Group of vowels and specific consonants that demonstrate increased sonority or more relative loudness in relationship to other sounds with the same length, stress, and pitch.

sonorant consonants Classes of speech sounds, including the nasals, glides, and liquids produced with a relatively open expiratory passageway.

sonority Sound's loudness relative to that of other sounds with the same length, stress, and pitch.

sonority value difference A calculation based on subtracting the sonority rank of each of the individual consonants of a cluster from one another. Used in the complexity approach for target selection.

sound modification method Therapy technique based on deriving the target sound from a phonetically similar sound that a client can accurately produce.

source features Term used in distinctive features (Chomsky & Halle, 1968) to refer to subglottal air pressure, voicing, and stridency.

speech Communication or expression of thoughts in spoken words; that is, in oral, verbal communication.

speech disability Would indicate a serious speech sound difficulty that impacts the child's or person's functioning in society.

speech disorder Oral, verbal communication that is so deviant from the norm that it is noticeable or interferes with communication.

speech impairment   Typically used synonymously with speech disorder.

speech intelligibility   "That aspect of oral speech language output that allows a listener to understand what a speaker is saying" (Carney, 1994, p. 109).

speech mechanism   The structures that are involved in producing speech.

speech sound delay   A category that is typically used in young children to denote a mismatch between the child's speech sound acquisition and what is considered to be a norm reference.

speech sound development   The gradual articulatory mastery of speech sound forms in a given language.

speech sound disorder   Difficulties making certain sounds that continue past a certain age. ASHA (n.d.-b) states that a speech sound disorder can impact the form of speech sounds (customarily referred to as articulation disorders) and/or the function of speech sounds (phonemes) within a language system (traditionally referred to as phonological disorders).

speech sounds   Real physical sound entities used in speech; end products of articulatory motor processes.

stimulability testing   Examining a client's ability to produce a misarticulated sound in an appropriate manner when "stimulated" by a clinician to do so.

stop   Manner of articulation resulting from a complete occlusion at some point in the vocal tract based on the action of the articulators; closure preceding the buildup of expiratory airstream pressure.

stress markers   Diacritics that indicate different levels of syllable prominence in an utterance.

strident [s]   Irregular s-production named after the auditory impression it creates; that is, a shrill, irritating, often whistle-like sound component.

subglottal air pressure   The pressure below the vocal folds.

substitution process   Describes those sound changes in which one sound or sound class is replaced by another.

suppression   Reduction of the use of one or more phonological processes as children move from the innate speech patterns to the adult norm production.

suprasegmental   Relating to intonation, stress, juncture, tempo, and rhythm as speech characteristics "added to" speech sound components.

surface-level representation   In generative grammar the actual end products of production.

syllabic   Relating to a consonant that functions as a syllable nucleus.

syllabification   Unit of spoken language that is a division of a (spoken or written) word.

syllable arresting sounds   *See:* coda.

syllable boundaries   Indicating the division between spoken syllables. Using diacritics this is marked as a period between the syllables.

syllable nucleus   "Core" of a unit of spoken language carrying its highest intensity and prosodic features, typically a vowel.

syllable releasing sounds   *See:* onset.

syllable shape   Structure of the units of spoken language within a word.

syllable structure process   Sound changes that affect the structure of a unit of spoken language.

syntax   Study of organizational rules denoting word, phrase, and clause order; sentence organization and the relationship between words, word classes, and other sentence elements.

system learning   Knowledge of phonemic principles that apply to a specific phonological system.

tap   *See:* flap.

tiers   Separable and independent levels that represent a sequence of gestures or a unified set of acoustic features.

timbre   The tonal quality that differentiates two sounds of the same pitch, loudness, and duration.

tone-unit   An organizational part imposed on prosodic data.

tongue thrust   Excessive anterior tongue movement during swallowing and a more anterior tongue position during rest.

tongue thrust swallow   Excessive anterior tongue movement during swallowing and a more anterior tongue position during rest. *See:* tongue thrust.

total assimilation   Influence of a sound segment on another by which all the phonetic properties of the influenced sound are changed, the changed segment and the source of the influence become identical.

traditional motor approaches   *See:* phonetic approaches.

transfer   Incorporation of language features into a nonnative language based on the occurrence of similar features in a native language.

trill   Sound produced by the vibratory action of the tongue tip against the alveolar ridge.

unchecked syllable   *See:* open syllable.

underlying form   Purely theoretical concept that is thought to represent a mental reality behind the way people use language.

unmarked   More natural phonemes that are found more frequently in languages around the world.

unreleased plosives   When the articulatory closure is maintained and not—as usual—released.

unrounding of vowels   Unrounding of vowels typically produced with lip rounding.

unstressed syllable deletion   A syllable structure process marked by the elimination of the unstressed syllable of a multisyllable word; also called *weak syllable deletion.*

uvular plosive   A plosive produced with the articulators coming together at the level of the uvula (further back than for [k] and [g]).

variegated babbling   *See:* nonreduplicated babbling.

velar fricative   The tongue is raised toward the velum similar to [k] and [g] but there is a narrow opening, not a complete closure.

velarization   A more posterior tongue placement (in the direction of the velum) for palatal sounds.

velopharyngeal mechanism   Consists of the structures and muscles of the velum (soft palate) and those of the pharyngeal walls.

velopharyngeal port   The passage that connects the oropharynx and the nasopharynx.

vernacular dialects   Varieties of spoken General American English that are considered outside the continuum of Informal Standard English.

vocable   *See:* proto-word.

vocal tract   Consists of all speech-related systems above the vocal folds.

vocoid   Nonphonemic vowel-like sound production.

voice symbols   Diacritics that mark the voicing of an unvoiced or the unvoicing of a voiced consonant.

vowel   Speech sound formed without significant constriction of the oral and pharyngeal cavities, especially along the sagittal midline of the oral cavity; normally it is the syllable nucleus.

References

Aase, D., Hovre, C., Krause, K., Schelfhout, S., Smith, J., & Carpenter, L. J. (2000). *Contextual Test of Articulation.* Eau Claire, WI: Thinking Publications.

Abercrombie, D. (1967). *Elements of general phonetics.* Chicago, IL: Aldine.

Abraham, S. (1989). Using a phonological framework to describe speech errors of orally trained, hearing-impaired school-agers. *Journal of Speech and Hearing Disorders, 54*, 600–609.

Abrams, D. A., Chen, T., Odriozola, P., Cheng, K. M., Baker, A. E., Padmanabhan, A., . . . Menon, V. (2016). Neural circuits underlying mother's voice perception predict social communication abilities in children. *Proceedings of the National Academy of Science, 113*, 6295–6300.

Albery, E., & Russell, J. (1990). Cleft palate and orofacial abnormalities. In P. Grunwell (Ed.), *Developmental speech disorders* (pp. 63–82). New York, NY: Churchill Livingstone.

Alexander Graham Bell Academy for Listening and Spoken Language. (2017). *The AG Bell Academy for Listening and Spoken Language certification handbook.* Washington, DC: Author.

Altaha, F. (1995). Pronunciation errors made by Saudi University students learning English: Analysis and remedy. *I.T. L. Review of Applied Linguistics,* 109–123.

American Cleft Palate–Craniofacial Association and Cleft Palate Foundation. (1997). *About cleft lip and cleft palate.* Chapel Hill, NC: Author.

American Psychiatric Association. (2000). *Diagnostic and statistical manual of mental disorders* (4th ed.). Arlington, VA: American Psychiatric Publishing.

American Psychiatric Association. (2013). *Diagnostic and statistical manual of mental disorders* (5th ed.). Arlington, VA: American Psychiatric Publishing.

American Speech-Language-Hearing Association. (n.d.-a). *Dysarthria in adults* (Practice Portal). Retrieved 7/6/2018 from https://www.asha.org/PRPSpecificTopic.aspx?folderid = 85899 43481&section = Overview

American Speech-Language-Hearing Association. (n.d.-b). *Speech sound disorders: Articulation and phonology* (Practice Portal). Retrieved from http://www.asha.org/Practice-Portal/Clinical-Topics/Articulation-and-Phonology

American Speech-Language-Hearing Association. (1989). Report of the ad hoc committee on labial-lingual posturing function. *ASHA, 31*, 92–94.

American Speech-Language-Hearing Association. (1991). The role of the speech-language pathologist in management of oral myofunctional disorders. *ASHA, 33*-(Suppl. 5), 7.

American Speech-Language-Hearing Association. (1993). *Definitions of communication disorders and variations* [Relevant Paper]. Retrieved from http://www.asha.org/policy

American Speech-Language-Hearing Association. (2003). *American English dialects* [Technical Report]. Retrieved from http://www.asha.org/policy

American Speech-Language-Hearing Association. (2004). *Preferred practice patterns for the profession of speech-language pathology.* Retrieved from https://www.asha.org/policy/PP2004-00191/#sec1.3.15

American Speech-Language-Hearing Association. (2005). *Roles and responsibilities of speech-language pathologists with respect to augmentative and alternative communication* [Position Statement]. Retrieved from http://www.asha.org/policy

American Speech-Language-Hearing Association. (2006). *Preferred practice patterns for the profession of audiology* [Preferred practice patterns]. Retrieved from http://www.asha.org/policy

American Speech-Language-Hearing Association. (2007a). *Scope of practice in speech-language pathology* [Scope of Practice]. Retrieved from http://www.asha.org/policy

American Speech-Language-Hearing Association. (2007b). *Childhood apraxia of speech* [Position Statement]. Retrieved from http://www.asha.org/policy

American Speech-Language-Hearing Association. (2008). *Communication facts: Incidence and prevalence of communication disorders and hearing loss in children-2008 edition.* http://www.asha.org/research/reports/children.htm

American Speech-Language-Hearing Association. (2013). Report Ad Hoc Committee on the Feasibility of the Standards of the Clinical Doctorate in Speech-Language Pathology. Retrieved from http://www.asha.org

American Speech-Language-Hearing Association. (2014). *Speech sound disorders: Articulation and phonological processes.* Retrieved from http://www.asha.org/public/speech/disorders/speechsounddisorders.htm

American Speech-Language-Hearing Association. (2017). *Issues in ethics: Cultural and linguistic competence.* Retrieved from http://www.asha.org/Practice/ethics/Cultural-and-Linguistic-Competence

American Speech-Language-Hearing Association Ad Hoc Committee on Service Delivery in the Schools. (1993). Definitions of communication disorders and variations. *ASHA, 35*(Suppl. 10), 40–41.

American Speech-Language Hearing Association Committee on Language. (1983). Definition of language. *ASHA, 25*, 44.

Andrews, N., & Fey, M. E. (1986). Analysis of the speech of phonologically impaired children in two sampling conditions. *Language, Speech, and Hearing Services in Schools, 17*, 187–198.

Anthony, J. L., Lonigan, C. J., Burgess, S. R., Driscoll Bacon, K., Phillips, B. M., & Cantor, B. G. (2003). Structure of preschool phonological sensitivity: Overlapping sensitivity to rhyme, words, syllables, and phonemes. *Journal of Experimental Child Psychology, 82*, 65–92.

Archangeli, D. (1988). Aspects of under-specification theory. *Phonology, 5*, 183–207.

Archangeli, D., & Langendoen, D. (1997). *Optimality theory: An overview.* Oxford, UK: Blackwell.

Archangeli, D., & Pulleyblank, D. (1994). *Grounded phonology*. Cambridge, MA: MIT Press.

Arciuli, J., & Ballard, K. J. (2017). Still not adult-like: Lexical stress contrastivity in word productions of eight- to eleven-year-olds. *Journal of Child Language, 44*, 1274–1288.

Arlt, P. B., & Goodban, M. T. (1976). A comparative study of articulatory acquisition as based on a study of 240 normals, aged three to six. *Language, Speech, and Hearing Services in Schools, 7*, 173–180.

Aslin, R. N. (2014). Infant learning: Historical, conceptual, and methodological challenges. *Infancy, 19*, 2–27.

Augustyn, M., & Zuckerman, B. (2007). From mother's mouth to infant's brain. *Archives of Disease in Childhood, Fetal, and Neonatal Education, 92*, F82.

Ayyad, H., & Bernhardt, B. M. H. (2007). *Phonological patterns in the speech of an Arabic-speaking Kuwaiti child with hearing impairment compared with a bilingual Arabic-English 2-year-old*. Paper presented at the Child Phonology Conference, Seattle, WA.

Baker, E. (2006). Management of speech impairment in children: The journey so far and the road ahead. *Advances in Speech-Language Pathology, 8*, 156–163.

Baker, E. (2010). Minimal pair intervention. In A. L. Williams, S. McLeod, & R. J. McCauley (Eds.), *Interventions for speech sound disorders in children* (pp. 41–72). Baltimore, MD: Brookes.

Baker, E. (2013). Polysyllable Preschool Test (POP). Sydney, Australia: Author.

Baker, E. (2016). *Children's independent and relational phonological analysis (CHIRPA): General American English*. Sydney, Australia: Author.

Ball, M. J. (2002). Clinical phonology of vowel disorders. In M. J. Ball & F. E. Gibbon (Eds.), *Vowel disorders* (pp. 187–216). Boston, MA: Butterworth-Heinemann.

Ball, M. J. (2016). *Principles of clinical phonology: Theoretical approaches*. New York, NY: Routledge.

Ball, M. J., & Gibbon, F. E. (2002). *Vowel disorders*. Boston, MA: Butterworth-Heinemann.

Ball, M. J., & Rahilly, J. (1999). *Phonetics: The science of speech*. London, UK: Arnold.

Ballard, K. J., Djaja, D., Arciuli, J., James, D. G., & van Doorn, J. (2012). Developmental trajectory for production of prosody: Lexical stress contrastivity in children ages 3 to 7 years and in adults. *Journal of Speech, Language, and Hearing Research, 55*, 1822–1835.

Ballard, K., Granier, J., & Robin, D. (2000). Understanding the nature of apraxia of speech: Theory, analysis, and treatment. *Aphasiology, 14*, 969–995.

Ballard, K. J., Robin, D. A., McCabe, P., & McDonald, J. (2010). A treatment for dysprosody in childhood apraxia of speech. *Journal of Speech, Language, and Hearing Research, 53*, 1227–1245.

Bankson, N. W. (1990) *Bankson Language Screening Test* (2nd ed.). Austin, TX: PRO-ED.

Bankson, N. W., & Bernthal, J. E. (1990). *Bankson-Bernthal test of phonology*. Chicago, IL: Riverside Press.

Barlow, J. A. (2001). Case study: Optimality theory and the assessment and treatment of phonological disorders. *Language, Speech, and Hearing Services in Schools, 32*, 242–256.

Barlow, J. A., & Gierut, J. A. (2002). Minimal pair approaches to phonological remediation. *Seminars in Speech and Language, 23*, 57–67.

Barlow, J., Taps Richard, J., & Storkel, H. (2010). *Phonological assessment and treatment target selection*. Seminar presented at the national convention of the American Speech-Language-Hearing Association, San Diego, CA.

Barlow, S., & Farley, G. (1989). Neurophysiology of speech. In D. P. Kuehn, M. L. Lemme, & J. M. Baumgartner (Eds.), *Neural bases of speech, hearing, and language* (pp. 146–200). Boston, MA: Little, Brown.

Baudouin de Courtenay, J. (1895). *Versuch einer Theorie phonetischer Alternationen: Ein Capitel aus der Psychophonetik*. Translation in E. Stankiewicz (Ed.), *Selected writings of Baudouin de Courtenay*. Bloomington: Indiana University Press.

Bauman, J. A., & Waengler, H.-H. (1977). Measurements of sound durations in the speech of apraxic adults. *Hamburger Phonetische Beiträge* (Monograph No. 23). Hamburg, Germany: H. Buske Verlag.

Bauman-Waengler, J. A. (1991). Phonological processes in three groups of preschool children: A longitudinal study. *Proceedings from the XII International Congress of Phonetic Sciences, Aix-en-Provence, 3*, 354–357.

Bauman-Waengler, J. A. (1993a). *Dialect versus disorder: Articulation errors in African American preschool children*. Presentation at the state convention of the Pennsylvania Speech-Language-Hearing Association, Harrisburg, PA.

Bauman-Waengler, J. A. (1993b). *Language testing of African American children: Assessing assessment instruments*. Seminar presented at the state convention of the Pennsylvania Speech-Language-Hearing Association, Harrisburg, PA.

Bauman-Waengler, J. A. (1994). *Phonetic phonological features in the speech of African American preschoolers*. Paper presented at the national convention of the American Speech-Language-Hearing Association, New Orleans, LA.

Bauman-Waengler, J. A. (1995). *Articulatory differences between two groups of African American preschoolers*. Paper presented at the national convention of the Canadian Association of Speech-Language Pathologists and Audiologists, Ottawa, Canada.

Bauman-Waengler, J. A. (1996). *Problems in assessing African American children with phonological disorders*. Seminar presented at the national convention of the Black American Speech Language-Hearing Association, Milwaukee, WI.

Bauman-Waengler, J. A. (2009). *Introduction to phonetics and phonology: From concepts to transcription*. Boston, MA: Pearson.

Bauman-Waengler, J. A., & Garcia, D. (2011). Case 10: Matthew: The changing picture of childhood apraxia of speech—from initial symptoms to diagnostic and therapeutic modifications. In S. S. Chabon & E. R. Cohn (Eds.), *The communication disorders casebook: Learning by example* (pp. 71–81). Boston, MA: Pearson.

Bauman-Waengler, J. A., & Garcia, D. (2020). *Phonological treatment of speech sound disorders in children: A practical guide*. San Diego, CA: Plural.

Bauman-Waengler, J. A., & Waengler, H.-H. (1988). *Phonological process analysis in three groups of preschool children*. Paper presented at the national convention of the American Speech-Language-Hearing Association, Boston, MA.

Bauman-Waengler, J. A., & Waengler, H.-H. (1990). *Individual variation in phonologically disordered preschoolers: A longitudinal study*. Paper presented at the national convention of the American Speech-Language-Hearing Association, Seattle, WA.

Berko Gleason, J., & Bernstein Ratner, N. (Eds.). (2017). *The development of language* (9th ed.). Boston, MA: Pearson.

Bernhardt, B. (1992). Developmental implications of nonlinear phonological theory. *Clinical Linguistics and Phonetics, 6,* 259–281.

Bernhardt, B. M. H., Bacsfalvi, P., Gick, B., Radanov, B., & Williams, R (2005). Exploring the use of electropalatography and untrasound in speech habilitation. *Journal of Speech-Language Pathology and Audiology, 29,* 160–182.

Bernhardt, B. M., Bopp, K. D., Daudlin, B. B., Edwards, S. M., & Wastie, S. E. (2010). Nonlinear phonological intervention, In A. L. Williams, S. McLeod, & R. J. McCauley (Eds.), *Interventions for speech sound disorders in children* (pp. 315–332). Baltimore, MA: Paul H. Brookes.

Bernhardt, B. M. H., Brooke, M., & Major, E. (2003). *Acquisition of structure versus features in nonlinear phonological intervention.* Poster presented at the Child Phonology Conference, University of British Columbia, Vancouver, Canada.

Bernhardt, B., & Holdgrafer, G. (2001). Beyond the basics I: The need for strategic sampling for in-depth phonological analysis. *Language, Speech, and Hearing Services in Schools, 32,* 18–27.

Bernhardt, B., & Stemberger, J. P. (1998). *Handbook of phonological development from the perspective of constraint-based nonlinear phonology.* San Diego, CA: Academic Press.

Bernhardt, B., & Stoel-Gammon, C. (1994). Nonlinear phonology: Introduction and clinical application: Tutorial. *Journal of Speech and Hearing Research, 37,* 123–143.

Bernthal, J. E., Bankson, N. W., & Flipsen, P., Jr. (2017). *Articulation and phonological disorders* (8th ed.). Boston, MA: Allyn & Bacon.

Best, C., & McRoberts, G. (2003). Infant perception of non-native consonant contrasts that adults assimilate in different ways. *Language and Speech, 3,* 183–216.

Best, C., McRoberts, G., & Goodell, E. (2001). Discrimination of non-native consonant contrasts varying in perceptual assimilation to the listener's native phonological system. *Journal of the Acoustic Society of America, 109,* 775–794.

Best, S., Bigge, J., & Sirvis, B. (1994). Physical and health impairments. In N. Haring, L. McCormick, & T. Haring (Eds.), *Exceptional children and youth: An introduction to special education* (pp. 300–341). New York, NY: Merrill.

Bigge, J., (1991). *Teaching individuals with physical and multiple disabilities.* New York, NY: Merrill.

Bird, J., & Bishop, D. V. (1992). Perception and awareness of phonemes in phonologically impaired children. *European Journal of Disorders of Communication, 27,* 289–311.

Bird, J., Bishop, D. V., & Freeman, N. H. (1995). Phonological awareness and literacy development in children with expressive phonological impairments. *Journal of Speech and Hearing Research, 38,* 446–462.

Bishop, D. (1994). Grammatical errors in specific language impairment: Competence or performance limitations. *Applied Psycholinguistics, 15,* 507–550.

Bishop, D., & Adams, C. (1990). A prospective study of the relationship between specific language impairment, phonological disorders, and reading retardation. *Journal of Child Psychology and Psychiatry, 31,* 1027–1050.

Bishop, D., Brown, B., & Robson, J. (1990). The relationship between phoneme discrimination, speech production, and language comprehension in cerebral-palsied individuals. *Journal of Speech and Hearing Research, 33,* 210–219.

Bishop, D., & Robson, J. (1989). Unimpaired short-term memory and rhyme judgment in congenitally speechless individuals: Implications for the notion of "articulatory coding." *Quarterly Journal of Experimental Psychology, 41A,* 123–140.

Bislick, L. P., Weir, P. C., Spencer, K., Kendall, D., & Yorkston, K. M. (2012). Do principles of motor learning enhance retention and transfer of speech skills? A systematic review. *Aphasiology, 26,* 709–728.

Blache, P. (2000). Constraints, linguistic theories, and natural language processing. In D. N. Christodoulakis (Ed.), *Natural Language Processing — NLP 2000. NLP 2000. Lecture Notes in Computer Science, 1835.* Berlin, Heidelberg, Germany: Springer.

Blache, S. (1978). *The acquisition of distinctive features.* Baltimore, MD: University Park Press.

Blache, S. (1989). A distinctive feature approach. In N. Creaghead, P. Newman, & W. Secord (Eds.), *Assessment and remediation of articulatory and phonological disorders* (2nd ed., pp. 361–382). New York, NY: Macmillan.

Blachman, B. A. (2000). Phonological awareness. In M. L. Kamil, P. B. Mosenthal, P. D. Pearson, & R. Barr (Eds.), *Handbook of reading research* (pp. 483–502). Mahwah, NJ: Erlbaum.

Blakeley, R. W. (2001). *Screening test for developmental apraxia of speech* (2nd ed.). Austin, TX: Pro-Ed.

Bleile, K. M. (1996). *Articulation and phonological disorders: A book of exercises* (2nd ed.). San Diego, CA: Singular.

Bleile, K. M. (2002). Evaluating articulation and phonological disorders when the clock is running. *American Journal of Speech-Language Pathology, 11,* 243–249.

Blockcolsky, V., Frazer, J., & Frazer, D. (1987). *40,000 selected words.* Tucson, AZ: Communication Skill Builders.

Bloom, L. (1973). *One word at a time: The use of single word utterances before syntax.* The Hague: Mouton.

Bogliotti, C. (2003). *Relation between categorical perception of speech and reading acquisition.* Proceedings of the 15th International Congress of Phonetic Sciences, Barcelona, Spain.

Boone, D. R., & McFarlane, S. C., Von Berg, S. L., & Zraick, R. I. (2013). *The voice and voice therapy.* Boston, MA: Allyn & Bacon.

Booth, T., & Ainscow, M. (2002). *Index for Inclusion.* Bristol, UK: Centre for Studies on Inclusive Education.

Botting, N., & Conti-Ramsden, G. (2004). Characteristics of children with specific language impairment. In L. Verhoeven & H. van Balkom (Eds.), *Classification of developmental language disorders: Theoretical issues and clinical implications* (pp. 23–38). London, UK: Lawrence Erlbaum.

Boutsen, F., & Christman, S. (2002). Prosody in apraxia of speech. *Seminars in Speech and Language, 23,* 245–255.

Bowen, C. (2009). *Children's speech sound disorders.* Chichester, UK: Wiley-Blackwell.

Bowen, C. (2011). Table 3: Elimination of Phonological Processes. Retrieved from http://www.speech-language-therapy.com/ on 9/10/2018.

Bowers, L. M. (2016). Auditory-verbal therapy as an intervention approach for children who are deaf: A review of the evidence. *EBP Briefs, 11*, 1–8.

Bowers, L., & Huisingh, R. (2018). *LAT-NU Linguisystems Articulation Test – Normative Update.* Austin, TX: Linguisystems – PRO-ED.

Boysson-Bardies, B., de (2001). *How language comes to children: From birth to two years* (M. DeBevoise, Trans.). Cambridge, MA: NET Press.

Boysson-Bardies, B., de, & Vihman, M. (1991). Adaptation to language. *Language, 67*, 297–339.

Bradley, L., & Bryant, P. (1983). Categorizing sounds and learning to read: A causal connection. *Nature, 301*, 419–421.

Brady, N., Marquis, J., Fleming, K., & McLean, L. (2004). Prelinguistic predictors of language growth in children with developmental disabilities. *Journal of Speech, Language, and Hearing Research, 47*, 663–677.

Bridgeman, E., & Snowling, M. (1988). The perception of phoneme sequence: A comparison of dyspraxic and normal children. *British Journal of Disorders of Communication, 23*, 245–252.

Broen, P. A., & Moller, K. T. (1993). Early phonological development and the child with cleft palate. In K. T. Moller & C. D. Starr (Eds.), *Cleft palate: Interdisciplinary issues and treatment* (pp. 219–249). Austin, TX: PRO-ED.

Broomfield, J., & Dodd, B. (2004). The nature of referred subtypes of primary speech disability. *Child Language Teaching and Therapy, 20*, 135–151.

Broomfield, J., & Dodd, B. (2010). Epidemiology of speech disorders. In B. Dodd (Ed.), *Differential diagnosis and treatment of children with speech sound disorders* (2nd ed.) West Sussex, UK: Whurr.

Browman, C., & Goldstein, L. (1992). Articulatory phonology: An overview. *Phonetica, 49*, 155–180.

Browman, C., & Goldstein, L. (1995). Dynamics and articulatory phonology. In R. Port & T. van Gelder (Eds.), *Mind as motion: Exploration in the dynamics of cognition* (pp. 175–193). Cambridge, MA: MIT Press.

Brown, R. (1973). *A first language: The early stages.* Cambridge, MA: Harvard University Press.

Brutten, G. J., & Dunham, S. L. (1989). The communication attitude test: A normative study of grade school children. *Journal of Fluency Disorders, 14*, 371–377.

Buckingham, H. W., & Christman, S. S. (2006). Phonological impairments: Sublexical. In K. Brown (Ed.), *Encyclopedia of language and linguistics* (2nd ed., pp. 509–518). Oxford, UK: Elsevier.

Buckingham, H. W., & Christman, S. S. (2008). Disorders of phonetics and phonology. In B. Stemmer & H. A. Whitaker (Eds.), *Handbook of neuroscience of language* (Chapter 12, pp. 127–136). London, UK: Elsevier.

Buhler, H., DeThomasis, B., Chute, P., & DeCora, A. (2007). An analysis of phonological process use in young children with cochlear implants. *The Volta Review, 107*, 55–74.

Bull, M. J., & the Committee on Genetics. (2011). Health supervision for children with Down syndrome. *Pediatrics, 128*, 393–406.

Bunton, K., Leddy, M., & Miller, J. (2007). Phonetic intelligibility testing in adults with Down syndrome. *Down Syndrome Research & Practice: The Journal of the Sarah Duffen Centre/University of Portsmouth, 12*, 230–239.

Butcher, A. (1990). The uses and abuses of phonological assessment. *Child Language Teaching and Therapy, 6*, 262–276.

Bybee, J. (2001). *Phonology and language use.* Cambridge, UK: Cambridge University Press.

Bzoch, K. (1997). Clinical assessment, evaluation, and management of 11 categorical aspects of cleft palate speech disorders. In K. R. Bzoch (Ed.), *Communication disorders related to cleft lip and palate* (4th ed., pp. 261–311). Austin, TX: PRO-ED.

Camp, B., Burgess, D., Morgan, L., & Zerbe, G. (1987). A longitudinal study of infant vocalizations in the first year. *Journal of Pediatric Psychology, 12*, 321–331.

Carney, A. E. (1994). Understanding speech intelligibility in the hearing impaired. In K. G. Butler (Ed.), *Hearing impairment and language disorders* (pp. 109–121). Gaithersburg, MD: Aspen.

Carrow-Woolfolk, E. (2017). *Comprehensive Assessment of Spoken Language,* 2nd ed. (CASL-2). Torrance, CA: Western Psychological Corporation.

Carterette, E., & Jones, M. (1974). *Informal speech: Alphabetic and phonemic texts with statistical analyses and tables.* Berkeley, CA: University of California Press.

Caruso, A. J., & Strand, E. A. (1999). Motor speech disorders in children: Definitions, backgrounds, and a theoretical framework. In A. J. Caruso & E. A. Strand (Eds.), *Clinical management of motor speech disorders in children* (pp. 1–27). New York, NY: Thieme.

Carver, C. M. (1987). Dialects. In S. Flexner & L. C. Hauck (Eds.), *The Random House dictionary of the English language* (2nd ed.) (pp. xxv–xxvi). New York, NY: Random House.

Carvill, S. (2001). Sensory impairment, intellectual disability, and psychiatry. *Journal of Intellectual Disability Research, 45*, 467–483.

Catts, H. (1993). The relationship between speech-language impairments and reading disabilities. *Journal of Speech and Hearing Research, 36*, 948–958.

Catts, H., Fey, M., & Zhang, X. (2001). Estimating the risk of future reading difficulties in kindergarten children: A research-based model and its clinical implementation. *Language, Speech, and Hearing Services in Schools, 32*, 38–50.

Catts, H., & Kamhi, A. (1999). Causes of reading disabilities. In H. Catts & A. Kamhi (Eds.), *Language and reading disabilities* (pp. 95–127). Boston, MA: Allyn & Bacon.

Chan, A., & Lee, D. (2000). English and Cantonese phonology in contrast: Explaining Cantonese ESL learners' English pronunciation problems. *Language, Culture, and Curriculum, 13*, 67–85.

Chapman, K. L. (1993). Phonological processes in children with cleft palate. *Cleft Palate-Craniofacial Journal, 30*, 64–71.

Chapman, K. L., & Hardin, M. A. (1992). Phonetic and phonologic skills of two-year-olds with cleft palate. *Cleft Palate-Craniofacial Journal, 29*, 435–443.

Chapman, K. L., Hardin-Jones, M., & Halter, K. (2003). The relationship between early speech and later speech and language performance for children with cleft lip and palate. *Clinical Linguistics & Phonetics, 17*, 173–197.

Chen, H. P., & Irwin, O. C. (1946). Infant speech: Vowel and consonant types. *Journal of Speech Disorders, 11*, 27–29.

Cheng, L. L. (1994). Asian/Pacific students and the learning of English. In J. Bernthal & N. Bankson (Eds.), *Child phonology: Characteristics, assessment, and intervention with special populations* (pp. 255–274). New York, NY: Thieme.

Chomsky, N., & Halle, M. (1968). *The sound pattern of English.* New York, NY: Harper & Row.

Christensen, M., & Hanson, M. (1981). An investigation of the efficacy of oral myofunctional therapy as a precursor to articulation therapy for pre-first-grade children. *Journal of Speech and Hearing Disorders, 46,* 160–165.

Christian, D., Wolfram, W., & Nube, N. (1988). *Variation and change in geographically isolated communities: Appalachian English and Ozark English.* Tuscaloosa: University of Alabama Press.

Clark, M. C., & Goldstein, B. (1996). *Analysis of vowel error patterns in children with phonological disorders.* Paper presented at the annual convention of the American Speech-Language Hearing Association, Seattle, WA.

Cohen, L., & Cashon, C. (2003). Infant perception and cognition. In R. Lerner, M. Easterbooks, & J. Mistry (Eds.), *Comprehensive handbook of psychology. Volume 6: Developmental psychology* (pp. 65–90), Hoboken, NJ: John Wiley and Sons.

Compton, A. J. (1976). Generative studies of children's phonological disorders: Clinical ramifications. In D. Morehead & A. Morehead (Eds.), *Normal and deficient child language* (pp. 61–96). Baltimore, MD: University Park Press.

Connolly, J. H. (1986). Intelligibility: A linguistic view. *British Journal of Disorders of Communication, 21,* 371–376.

Conti-Ramsden, G., & Jones, M. (1997). Verb use in specific language impairment. *Journal of Speech and Hearing Research, 40,* 1298–1313.

Coplan, J., & Gleason, J. R. (1988). Unclear speech: Recognition and significance of unintelligible speech in preschool children. *Pediatrics, 82,* 447–452.

Cornwall, A. (1992). The relationship of phonological awareness, rapid naming, and verbal memory to severe reading and spelling disability. *Journal of Learning Disabilities, 25,* 532–538.

Crary, M. A. (1983). Phonological process analysis from spontaneous speech: The influence of sample size. *Journal of Communication Disorders, 16,* 133–141.

Crary, M. A. (1993). *Developmental motor speech disorders.* San Diego, CA: Singular.

Croot, K. (2002). Diagnosis of AOS: Definition and criteria. *Seminar in Speech and Language, 23,* 267–280.

Crosbie, S., Holm, A., & Dodd, B. (2005). Intervention for children with severe speech disorder: A comparison of two approaches. *International Journal of Language and Communication Disorders, 40,* 467–491.

Cruttenden, A. (1985). Intonation comprehension in 10-year-olds. *Journal of Child Language, 12,* 643–661.

Crystal D. (1982). *Profiling linguistic disability.* Cambridge, UK : Cambridge University Press.

Crystal, D. (1986). Prosodic development. In P. Fletcher & M. Garman (Eds.), *Language acquisition* (2nd ed., pp. 174–197). Cambridge, UK: Cambridge University Press.

Crystal, D. (2010). *The Cambridge encyclopedia of language* (3rd ed.). Cambridge, UK: Cambridge University Press.

Culatta, R., Page, J. L., & Wilson, L. (1987). *Speech rates of normally communicative children.* Paper presented at the annual convention of the American Speech-Language-Hearing Association, New Orleans, LA.

Culbertson, D. (2007). Language and speech of the deaf and hard of hearing. In R. Schow & M. Nerbonne (Eds.), *Introduction to audiologic rehabilitation* (5th ed., pp. 197–244). Boston, MA: Allyn and Bacon.

Cummings, A. E. (2009). *Brain and behavior in children with phonological delays: Phonological, lexical, and sensory system interaction.* Unpublished doctoral dissertation, University of California, San Diego.

Dabul, B. (2000). *Apraxia battery for adults* (2nd ed.). Tigard, OR: C. C. Publications.

Dalston, R. (1997). The use of nasometry in the assessment and remediation of velopharyngeal inadequacy. In K. R. Bzoch (Ed.), *Communication disorders related to cleft lip and palate* (4th ed., pp. 331–346). Austin, TX: PRO-ED.

Dalston, R., Warren, D., & Dalston, E. (1991). Use of nasometry as a diagnostic tool for identifying patients with velopharyngeal impairment. *Cleft Palate-Craniofacial Journal, 28,* 184–189.

Darley, F. (1991). A philosophy of appraisal and diagnosis. In F. Darley & D. C. Spriestersbach (Eds.), *Diagnostic methods in speech pathology* (2nd ed., pp. 1–23). New York, NY: Harper & Row.

Davis, B. L., Jacks, A., & Marquardt, T. P. (2005). *Vowel patterns in developmental apraxia of speech: Three longitudinal case studies, 19,* 249–274.

Davis, B. L., Jakielski, K., & Marquardt, T. (1998). Developmental apraxia of speech: Determiners of differential diagnosis. *Clinical Linguistics and Phonetics, 12,* 25–45.

Davis, B. L., & MacNeilage, P. F. (1990). Acquisition of correct vowel production: A quantitative case study. *Journal of Speech and Hearing Research, 33,* 16–27.

Dean, E., Howell, J., Hill, A., & Waters, D. (1990). *Metaphon resource pack.* Windsor, UK: NFER Nelson.

Delaney, A., & Kent, R. (2004). *Developmental profiles of children diagnosed with apraxia of speech.* Paper presented at the annual meeting of the American Speech-Language-Hearing Association, Philadelphia, PA.

Denes, P. B., & Pinson, E. N. (1973). *The speech chain.* Garden City, NY: Anchor Press.

De Swart, B. J., Willemse, S. C., Maassen, B. A. M., & Horstink, M. W. I. M. (2003). Improvement of voicing in patients with Parkinson's disease by speech therapy. *Neurology, 60,* 498–500.

Dewey, G. (1923). *Relative frequency of English speech sounds.* Cambridge, MA: Harvard University Press.

Dillow, K. A., Dzienkowski, R. C., Smith, K. K., & Yucha, C. B. (1996). Cerebral palsy: A comprehensive review. *The Nurse Practitioner, 21,* 45–61.

Dinnsen, D. A. (1997). Nonsegmental phonologies. In M. J. Ball & R. D. Kent (Eds.), *The new phonologies* (pp. 77–125). San Diego, CA: Singular.

Dinnsen, D. A., & Elbert, M. (1984). On the relationship between phonology and learning. In M. Elbert, D. Dinnsen, & G. Weismer (Eds.), *Phonological theory and the misarticulating child, ASHA Monograph, 22* (pp. 59–68). Rockville, MD: ASHA.

Dinnsen, D. A., & O'Connor, K. M. (2001). Typological predictions in developmental phonology. *Journal of Child Language, 28,* 597–618.

Dodd, B. (1995). *Differential diagnosis and treatment of children with speech disorder.* London, UK: Whurr.

Dodd, B. (2005). *Differential diagnosis and treatment of children with speech disorder* (2nd ed.). London, UK: Whurr.

Dodd, B. (2011). Differentiating speech delay from disorder. Does it matter? *Topics in Language Disorders, 31,* 96–111.

Dodd, B. (2013). *Differential diagnosis and treatment of children with speech disorder* (2nd ed. ebook). London, UK: Whurr.

Dodd, B., Crosbie, S., McIntosh, B., Teitzel, T., & Ozanne, A. (2003). *Pre-Reading Inventory of Phonological Awareness (PIPA)*. San Antonio, TX: Harcourt Assessment.

Dodd, B., Gillon, G., Oerlemans, R., Russell, T., Syrmis, M., & Wilson, H. (1995). Phonological disorder and the acquisition of literacy. In B. Dodd (Ed.), *Differential diagnosis and treatment of children with speech disorder* (pp. 125–146). London, UK: Whurr.

Dodd, B., Holm, A., Crosbie, S., & McCormack, P. (2013). Differential diagnosis of phonological disorders. In B. Dodd (Ed.), *Differential diagnosis and treatment of children with speech disorder* (2nd ed. ebook, pp. 44–70). Hoboken, NJ: John Wiley & Sons.

Dodd, B., Holm, A., Crosbie, S., & McIntosh, B. (2010). Core vocabulary intervention. In A. L. Williams, S. McLeod, & R. J. McCauley (Eds.), *Interventions for speech sound disorders* (pp. 117–136). Baltimore, MD: Paul H. Brookes.

Dodd, B., Hua, Z., Crosbie, S., Holm, A., & Ozanne, A. (2006). *Diagnostic Evaluation of Articulation and Phonology (DEAP)*. San Antonio, TX: Psych Corp of Harcourt Assessment.

Dodd, B., & Iacano, T. (1989). Phonological disorders in children: Changes in phonological process use during treatment. *British Journal of Disorders of Communication, 24,* 333–351.

Donegan, P. J., & Stampe, D. (1979). The study of natural phonology. In D. A. Dinnsen (Ed.), *Current approaches to phonological theory* (pp. 126–173). Bloomington: Indiana University Press.

Dore, J. (1975). Holophrases, speech acts and language universals. *Journal of Child Language, 3,* 22–39.

Dore, J., Franklin, M. B., Miller, R. T., & Ramer, A. L. (1976). Transitional phenomena in early language acquisition. *Journal of Child Language, 3,* 13–29.

Drummond, S. S. (1993). *Dysarthria examination battery.* Austin, TX: PRO-ED.

Duffy, J. R. (2005a). Assessment of apraxia of speech. *Neuromotor exam form.* Rochester, MN: Mayo Clinic.

Duffy, J. R. (2005b). Assessment of non-verbal oral apraxia. *Neuromotor exam form.* Rochester, MN: Mayo Clinic.

Duffy, J. R. (2013). *Motor speech disorders: Substrate, differential diagnosis, and management* (3rd ed.). St Louis, MO: Elsevier Mosby.

Duncan, L., & Johnston, R. (1999). How does phonological awareness relate to nonword reading amongst poor readers? *Reading and Writing: An Interdisciplinary Journal, 11,* 405–439.

Dunn, C., & Newton, L. (1994). A comprehensive model for speech development in hearing-impaired children. In K. G. Butler (Ed.), *Hearing impairment and language disorders* (pp. 122–143). *Topics in language disorders series.* Gaithersburg, MD: Aspen.

Dunn, L. M., Dunn, D. M., & Styles, B. (2009). *British picture vocabulary scales.* London, UK: GL Assessment.

Dworkin, J. P. (1991). *Motor speech disorders: A treatment guide.* St. Louis, MO: Mosby Year Book.

Dworkin, J. P., & Culatta, R. A. (1980). *Dworkin-Culatta oral mechanism examination.* Nicholasville, KY: Edgewood Press.

Dyson, A. T., & Amayreh, M. M. (2007). Chapter 34: Jordanian Arabic speech acquisition. In S. McLeod (Ed.), *The international guide to speech acquisition* (pp. 472–482). Clifton Park, NY: Thomson Delmar Learning.

Edeal, D. M., & Gildersleeve-Neumann, C. E. (2011). The importance of production frequency in therapy for childhood apraxia of speech. *American Journal of Speech-Language Pathology, 20,* 95–110.

Edwards, H. T. (2003). *Applied phonetics: The sounds of American English* (3rd ed.). San Diego, CA: Singular.

Edwards, J., Beckman, M. E., & Munson, B. (2004). The interaction between vocabulary size and phonotactic probability effects on children's production accuracy and fluency in nonword repetition. *Journal of Speech, Language, and Hearing Research, 47,* 421–436.

Edwards, M. L. (1992). Clinical forum: Phonological assessment and treatment. In support of phonological processes. *Language, Speech, and Hearing Services in Schools, 23,* 233–240.

Ehren, T. (2010). *What /R/ you doing? Correcting /R/.* Paper presented at the American Speech Language Hearing Association Convention, Philadelphia, PA.

Eisenberg, L. (2007). Current state of knowledge: Speech recognition and production in children with hearing impairment. *Ear and Hearing, 28,* 766–772.

Eisenberg, S. L., & Hitchcock, E. R. (2010). Using standardized tests to inventory consonant and vowel production: A comparison of 11 tests of articulation and phonology. *Language, Speech, and Hearing Services in Schools, 41,* 488–503.

Elbers, L. (1982). Operating principles in repetitive babbling: A cognitive approach. *Cognition, 12,* 45–63.

Elbert, M. (1992). Clinical forum: Phonological assessment and treatment. Consideration of error types: A response to Fey. *Language, Speech, and Hearing Services in Schools, 23,* 241–246.

Elbert, M., Dinnsen, D., & Powell, T. (1984). On the prediction of phonologic generalization learning patterns. *Journal of Speech and Hearing Disorders, 49,* 309–317.

Elbert, M., & Gierut, J. (1986). *Handbook of clinical phonology: Approaches to assessment and treatment.* San Diego, CA: College-Hill Press.

Elfenbein, J., Hardin-Jones, M., & Davis, J. (1994). Oral communication skills of children who are hard of hearing. *Journal of Speech and Hearing Research, 37,* 216–226.

Elliott, L. L. (1979). Performance of children aged 9–17 years on a test of speech intelligibility in noise using sentence material with controlled word predictability. *Journal of the Acoustical Society of America, 66,* 651–653.

Elliott, L. L., Connors, S., Kille, E., Levin, S., Ball, K., & Katz, D. (1979). Children's understanding of monosyllabic nouns in quiet and in noise. *Journal of the Acoustical Society of America, 66,* 12–21.

Enderby, P., & Palmer, R. (2008). *Frenchay Dysarthria Assessment (FDA-2)–2nd edition.* Austin, TX: PRO-ED.

Eriks-Brophy, A. (2004). Outcomes of auditory-verbal therapy: A review of the evidence and a call for action. *Volta Review, 104,* 21–35.

Eriks-Brophy, A., Gibson, S., & Tucker, S.-K. (2013). Articulatory error patterns and phonological process use of preschool children with and without hearing loss. *The Volta Review, 113,* 87–126.

Eyer, J., & Leonard, L. (1994). Learning past tense morphology with specific language impairment: A case study.

Child Language Teaching and Therapy, *10,* 127–138.

Faircloth, S. R., & Faircloth, M. A. (1973). *Phonetic science: A program of instruction.* Englewood Cliffs, NJ: Prentice-Hall.

Fasold, R., & Wolfram, W. (1975). Some linguistic features of Negro dialect. In P. Stoller (Ed.), *Black American English* (pp. 49–87). New York, NY: Deli.

Fasolo, M., Majorano, M., & D'Odorico, L. (2008). Babbling and first words in children with slow expressive development. *Clinical Linguistics and Phonetics, 22,* 83–94.

Ferguson, C. A. (1976). Learning to pronounce: The earliest stages of phonological development in the child. In F. D. Minifie & L. L. Floyd (Eds.), *Communicative and cognitive abilities: Early behavioral assessment* (pp. 273–297). Baltimore, MD: University Park Press.

Ferguson, C. A., & Farwell, C. (1975). Words and sounds in early language acquisition: English initial consonants in the first fifty words. *Language, 51,* 419–439.

Ferguson, C. A., & Garnica, O. (1975). Theories of phonological development. In E. Lenneberg & E. Lenneberg (Eds.), *Foundation of language development* (Vol. 1, pp. 153–180). New York, NY: Academic Press.

Fernald, A., & Mazzie, C. (1991). Prosody and focus in speech to infants and adults. *Developmental Psychology, 27,* 209–221.

Ferrari, A., Cioni, G. (2005). Guidelines for Rehabilitation of Children with Cerebral Palsy. *Europa Medicophysica, 41,* 243–260.

Fey, M. E. (1992). Clinical forum: Phonological assessment and treatment. Articulation and phonology: Inextricable constructs in speech pathology. *Language, Speech, and Hearing Services in Schools, 23,* 225–232. (Reprinted from *Human Communication Canada, 1985, 9,* 7–16.)

Firth, J. R. (1948). Sounds and prosodies. *Transactions of the Philological Society.* Oxford, UK: Blackwell.

Fletcher, S. G. (1972). Time-by-count measurement of diadochokinetic syllable rate. *Journal of Speech and Hearing Research, 15,* 763–770.

Fletcher, S. G. (1978). *Time-by-count measurement of diadochokinetic syllable rate.* Austin, TX: PRO-ED.

Fletcher, S. G. (1992). *Articulation. A physiological approach.* San Diego, CA: Singular.

Fletcher, S. G., Casteel, R., & Bradley, D. (1961). Tongue-thrust swallow, speech articulation, and age. *Journal of Speech and Hearing Disorders, 26,* 201–208.

Flipsen, P., Jr. (2010). *Measuring intelligibility in children: Why and how.* Poster presented at the national convention of the American Speech-Language-Hearing Association, San Diego, CA.

Flipsen, P., Jr., & Parker, R. G. (2008). Phonological patterns in the speech of children with cochlear implants. *Journal of Communication Disorders, 41,* 337–357.

Fluharty, N. B. (2000) *Fluharty Preschool Speech and Language Screening* (2nd ed.). Austin, TX: Linguisystems – PRO-ED.

Fox, A. V., Howard, D., & Dodd, B. (2002). Risk factors for speech disorders in children. *International Journal of Language and Communication Disorders, 37,* 117–131.

Foy, J., & Mann, V. (2012). Speech production deficits in early readers: Predictors of risk. *Reading and Writing, 25,* 799–830.

French, A. (1989). The systematic acquisition of word forms by a child during the first-fifty-word stage. *Journal of Child Language, 16,* 69–90.

Froeschels, E. (1931). *Lehrbuch der Sprachheilkunde* (3rd ed.). Leipzig, Vienna: Deuticke.

Froeschels, E. (1937). Über das Wesen der multiplen Interdentalität. *Acta Oto-laryngologica, 25,* 341.

Frost, J., Madsbjerg, S., Niedersøe, J., Olofsson, A., & Sørensen, P. M. (2005). Semantic and phonological skills in predicting reading development: From 3–16 years of age. *Dyslexia, 11,* 79–92.

Fudala, J. B., & Stegall, S. (2017). *Arizona articulation proficiency scale* (4th ed.). Torrance, CA: Western Psychological Services.

Garn-Nunn, P., & Lynn, J. (2004). *Calvert's descriptive phonetics* (3rd ed.). New York, NY: Thieme.

Geambaşu, A., Scheel, M., & Levelt, C. C. L. (2016). Cross-linguistic patterns in infant babbling. In J. Scott & D. Waughtal (Eds.). *Proceedings of the 40th Annual Boston University Conference on Language Development,* (pp. 151–168). Somerville, MA: Cascadilla Press.

Gibbon, F. (2002). Personal correspondence.

Gibbon, F., & Wood, S. (2003). Using electropalatography (EPG) to diagnose and treat articulation disorders associated with mild cerebral palsy: A case study. *Clinical Linguistics and Phonetics, 17,* 365–374.

Gierut, J. (1985). *On the relationship between phonological knowledge and generalization learning in misarticulating children.* Bloomington: Indiana University Linguistics Club.

Gierut, J. (1989). Maximal opposition approach to phonological treatment. *Journal of Speech and Hearing Disorders, 54,* 9–19.

Gierut, J. (1990). Differential learning of phonological oppositions. *Journal of Speech and Hearing Research, 33,* 540–549.

Gierut, J. (1991). Homonymy in phonological change. *Clinical Linguistics and Phonetics, 5,* 119–137.

Gierut, J. (1992). The conditions and course of clinically induced phonological change. *Journal of Speech and Hearing Research, 35,* 1049–1063.

Gierut, J. (1998). Treatment efficacy: Functional phonological disorders in children. *Journal of Speech, Language, and Hearing Research, 41,* S85–S100.

Gierut, J. (1999). Syllable onsets: Clusters and adjuncts in acquisition. *Journal of Speech, Language, and Hearing Research, 42,* 708–726.

Gierut, J. A. (2001). Complexity in phonological treatment: Clinical factors. *Language, Speech and Hearing Services in Schools, 32,* 229–241.

Gierut, J. A. (2007). Phonological complexity and language learnability. *American Journal of Speech-Language Pathology, 16,* 6–17.

Gierut, J., & Champion, A. H. (2001). Syllable onsets II: Three-element clusters in phonological treatment. *Journal of Speech, Language and Hearing Research, 44,* 886–904.

Gierut, J., & Hulse, L. E. (2010). Evidence-based practice: A matrix for predicting phonological generalization. *Clinical Linguistics and Phonetics, 24,* 323–334.

Gierut, J. A., & Morrisette, M. L. (2005). The clinical significance of optimality theory for phonological disorders. *Topics in Language Disorders, 25,* 266–280.

Gierut, J., Morrisette, M. L., Hughes, M. T., & Rowland, S. (1996). Phonological treatment efficacy and developmental norms. *Language, Speech, and Hearing Services in Schools, 27*, 215–230.

Gierut, J., Morrisette, M. L., & Ziemer, S. M. (2010). Nonwords and generalization in children with phonological disorders, *American Journal of Speech-Language Pathology, 19*, 167–177.

Gierut, J., & Neumann, H. (1992). Teaching and learning /θ/: A nonconfound. *Clinical Linguistics and Phonetics, 6*, 191–200.

Gillon, G. (2000). The efficacy of phonological awareness intervention for children with spoken language impairment. *Language, Speech, and Hearing Services in Schools, 31*, 126–141.

Gillon, G. (2002). Follow-up study investigating benefits of phonological awareness intervention for children with spoken language impairment. *International Journal of Language and Communication Disorders, 37*, 381–400.

Gillon, G. (2018). *Phonological awareness: From research to practice* (2nd ed.). New York, NY: Guilford.

Golding-Kushner, K. J. (1995). Treatment of articulation and resonance disorders associated with cleft palate and VPI. In R. J. Shprintzen & J. Bardach (Eds.), *Cleft palate speech management. A multidisciplinary approach* (pp. 327–351). St. Louis, MO: Mosby Year Book.

Goldman, R., & Fristoe, M. (2015). *Goldman-Fristoe test of articulation* (3rd ed.). Boston, MA: Pearson.

Goldstein, B. A. (2007). Chapter 33: Spanish-influenced English speech acquisition. In S. McLeod (Ed.), *The international guide to speech acquisition* (pp. 277–287). Clifton Park, NY: Thomson Delmar Learning.

Golinkoff, R. M., Can, D. D., Soderstrom, M., & Hirsh-Pasek, K. (2015). (Baby) Talk to me: The social context of infant-directed speech and its effects on early language acquisition. *Current Directions in Psychological Science, 24*, 339–344.

González, G. (1988). Chicano English. In D. Bixler-Marquez & J. Ornstein-Galicia (Eds.), *Chicano speech in the bilingual classroom. Series VI, Vol. 6* (pp. 71–89). New York, NY: Lang.

Gordon-Brannan, M., & Hodson, B. W. (2000). Intelligibility/severity measurements of prekindergarten children's speech. *American Journal of Speech-Language Pathology, 9*, 141–150.

Gordon-Brannan, M., Hodson, B. W., & Wynne, M. K. (1992). Remediating unintelligible utterances of a child with a mild hearing loss. *American Journal of Speech-Language Pathology, 1*, 28–38.

Goswami, U., & Bryant, P. (2016). *Phonological skills and learning to read.* Psychology Press Classic Editions. New York, NY: Routledge.

Gozzard, H., Baker, E., & McCabe, P. (2006). Children's productions of polysyllables. *Acquiring Knowledge in Speech, Language and Hearing, 8*, 113–116.

Grames, L. M. (2008). Advancing into the 21st century: Care for individuals with cleft palate or craniofacial differences. *The ASHA Leader.* Retrieved from http://www.asha.org/Publications/leader/2008/f080506a/#1

Grunwell, P. (1987). *Clinical phonology* (2nd ed.). Baltimore, MD: Williams & Wilkins.

Grunwell, P. (1997). Developmental phonological disability: Order in disorder. In B. W. Hodson & M. L. Edwards (Eds.), *Perspectives in Applied Phonology* (pp. 61–104). New York, NY: Aspen.

Gubiani, M. B., Pagliarin, K. C., & Keske-Soares, M. (2015). Revisões Sistemáticas Instrumentos para avaliação de apraxia de fala infantile (Tools for the assessment of childhood apraxia of speech). *CoDAS, 27*, 610–615.

Günther, T., & Hautvast, S. (2010). Addition of contingency management to increase home practice in young children with a speech sound disorder. *International Journal of Language and Communication Disorders, 45*, 345–353.

Gutzmann, A. (1895). *Die Gesundheitspflege der Sprache.* Breslau: F. Hirt.

Ha, S., Johnson, C. J., & Kuehn, D.P. (2009). Characteristics of Korean phonology: Review, tutorial, and case studies of Korean children speaking English. *Journal of Communication Disorders, 42*, 163–179.

Haelsig, P. C., & Madison, C. L. (1986). A study of phonological processes exhibited by 3-, 4-, and 5-year-old children. *Language, Speech, and Hearing Services in Schools, 17*, 107–114.

Hageman, C. (2018). Motor learning guided therapy. In K. Bleile, *The late eight* (3rd ed., pp. 107–128). San Diego, CA: Plural.

Haley, K., Ohde, R., & Wertz, R. (2000). Precision of fricative production in aphasia and apraxia of speech: A perceptual and acoustic study. *Aphasiology, 14*, 619–634.

Hall, P. K., Jordan, L. S., & Robin, D. A. (1993). *Developmental apraxia of speech: Theory and clinical practice.* Austin, TX: PRO-ED.

Halliday, M. A. (1975). *Learning how to mean: Explorations in the development of language.* New York, NY: Elsevier.

Halliday, M. A. K., & Matthiessen, C. M. I. (2004). *An introduction to functional grammar* (3rd ed.). London, UK: Routledge.

Hanson, M. L. (1988). Orofacial myofunctional therapy: Guidelines for assessment and treatment. *International Journal of Orofacial Myology, 14*, 27–32.

Hanson, M. L., & Barrett, R. H. (1988). *Fundamentals of orofacial myology.* Springfield, IL: Charles C. Thomas.

Hardy, J. C. (1994). Cerebral palsy. In W. A. Secord, G. H. Shames, & E. Wiig (Eds.), *Human communication disorders: An introduction* (4th ed., pp. 562–604). New York, NY: Merrill.

Harlor, A. D., Jr., & Bower, C. (2009). Hearing assessment in infants and children: Recommendations beyond neonatal screening. *Pediatrics, 124*, 1252–1263.

Harrison, P. L., Kaufman, A. S., Kaufman, N. L., Bruininks, R. H., Rynders, J., Ilmer, S., . . . Cicchetti, D. V. (1990). AGS Early Screening Profiles. *Journal of Psychoeducational Assessment, 13*, 101–104.

Haskill, A. M., Tyler, A. A., & Tolbert, L. C. (2001). *Months of morphemes: A theme-based cycles approach.* Eau Claire, WI: Thinking Publications.

Haspelmath, M., & Sims, A. D. (2010). *Understanding morphology.* London, UK: Hodder.

Hayden, D., & Square, P. (1999). *Verbal Motor Production Assessment for Children.* San Antonio, TX: The Psychological Corporation.

Health Insurance Portability and Accountability Act of 1996, Pub. L. No. 104-191. "Recommendations With Respect to Privacy of Certain Health Information," [CFR164.514(b)(2)].

Hecht, S., Burgess, S., Torgesen, J., Wagner, R., & Rashotte, C. (2000). Explaining social class differences in growth of reading skills from beginning kindergarten through fourth-grade: The role of phonological awareness, rate of access, and print knowledge. *Journal of Reading and Writing, 12,* 99–128.

Heffner, R.-M. S. (1975). *General phonetics.* Madison, WI: University of Wisconsin Press.

Heilmann, J. J., Nockerts, A., & Miller, J. F. (2010). Language sampling: Does the length of the transcript matter? *Language, Speech, and Hearing Services in Schools, 41,* 393–404.

Helm-Estabrooks, N. (1996). *Test of oral and limb apraxia (TOLA).* Chicago, IL: Applied Symbols.

Hesketh, A. (2010). Metaphonological intervention: Phonological awareness therapy. In A. L. Williams, S. McLeod, & R. J. McCauley (Eds.), *Interventions for speech sound disorders in children* (pp. 247–274). Baltimore, MD: Paul H. Brookes.

Hesketh, A., Dima, E., & Nelson, V. (2007). Teaching phoneme awareness to pre-literate children with speech disorder: A randomized controlled trial. *International Journal of Language and Communication Disorders, 42,* 251–271.

Hewlett, N., Gibbon, F., & Cohen-McKenzie, W. (1998). When is a velar an alveolar? *International Journal of Language and Communication Disorders, 33,* 162–176.

Hickman, L. A., (1997). *The apraxia profile.* San Antonio, TX: Psychological Corporation.

Hidalgo, M. (1987). On the question of "standard" versus "dialect": Implications for teaching Hispanic college students. *Hispanic Journal of Behavioral Sciences, 9,* 375–395.

Hilton, L. (1984). Treatment of deviant phonological systems: Tongue thrust. In W. Perkins (Ed.), *Phonological-articulatory disorders* (pp. 47–54). New York, NY: Thieme-Stratton.

Himmelmann, N. P. (2000). Tagalog. In G. Booij, C. Lehmann, J. Mugdan, & S. Skopeteas (Eds.), *Morphology: An international handbook on inflection and word formation* (pp. 1473–1490). Berlin, Germany: de Gruyter.

Hislop, A., Wigglesworth, J., & Desai, R. (1986). Alveolar development in the human fetus and infant. *Early Human Development, 13,* 1–11.

Hodson, B. W. (1989). Phonological remediation: A cycles approach. In N. A. Creaghead, P. W. Newman, & W. A. Secord (Eds.), *Assessment and remediation of articulatory and phonological disorders* (2nd ed., pp. 323–333). New York, NY: Macmillan.

Hodson, B. W. (1992). Clinical forum: Phonological assessment and treatment, applied phonology: Constructs, contributions, and issues. *Language, Speech, and Hearing Services in Schools, 23,* 247–253.

Hodson, B. W. (1994). Helping individuals become intelligible, literate, and articulate: The role of phonology. *Topics in Language Disorders, 14*(2), 1–16.

Hodson, B. W. (2004). *Hodson assessment of phonological patterns (HAPP-3).* Greenville, SC: Super Duper.

Hodson, B. W. (2007). Identifying phonological patterns and projecting remediation cycles: Expediting intelligibility gains of a 7-year-old Australian child. *Advances in Speech-Language Pathology, 8,* 257–264.

Hodson, B. W. (2011). Enhancing phonological patterns of young children with highly unintelligible speech: *The ASHA Leader, 16,* 16–19.

Hodson, B. W., & Edwards, M. L. (1997). *Perspectives in applied phonology.* Gathersburg, MD: Aspen.

Hodson, B. W., & Paden, E. P. (1981). Phonological processes which characterize unintelligible and intelligible speech in early childhood. *Journal of Speech and Hearing Disorders, 46,* 369–373.

Hodson, B. W., & Paden, E. P. (1983). *Targeting intelligible speech: A phonological approach to remediation.* San Diego, CA: College-Hill Press.

Hodson, B. W., & Paden, E. P. (1991). *Targeting intelligible speech: A phonological approach to remediation* (2nd ed.). San Diego, CA: College-Hill Press.

Hodson, B. W., Scherz, J. A., & Strattman, K. H. (2002). Evaluating communicative abilities of a highly unintelligible preschooler. *American Journal of Speech-Language Pathology, 11,* 236–242.

Hoffman, P. R., & Norris, J. A. (2010). Dynamic systems and whole language intervention. In A. L. Williams, S. McLeod, & R. J. McCauley (Eds.), *Interventions for speech sound disorders in children.* Baltimore, MD: Paul Brookes.

Holm, A., Crosbie, S., & Dodd, B. (2005). Treating inconsistent speech disorders. In B. Dodd (Ed.), *Differential diagnosis and treatment of children with speech disorder* (2nd ed., pp. 182–201). London, UK: Whurr.

Holm, A., Crosbie, S., & Dodd, B. (2013). Treating inconsistent speech disorders. In B. Dodd (Ed.), *Differential diagnosis and treatment of children with speech disorder* (3rd ed., pp. 182–201). Hoboken, NJ: John Wiley and Sons.

Holmgren, K., Lindblom, B., Aurelius, G., Jalling, B., & Zetterstrom, R. (1986). On the phonetics of infant vocalization. In B. Lindblom & R. Zetterstrom (Eds.), *Precursors of early speech* (pp. 51–63). New York, NY: Stockton Press.

Houston, D. M., & Jusczyk, P. W. (2000). The role of talker-specific information in word segmentation by infants. *Journal of Experimental Psychology, 26,* 1570–1582.

Howell, J., & Dean, E. (1991). *Treating phonological disorders in children: Metaphon-theory to practice.* San Diego, CA: Singular.

Howell, J., & Dean, E. (1994). *Treating phonological disorders in children: Metaphon-theory to practice* (2nd ed.). London, UK: Whurr.

Hsu, H. C., & Fogel, A. (2001). Infant vocal development in a dynamic mother–infant communication system. *Infancy, 2,* 87–109. Retrieved from http://www.nccp.org/publications/pub_948.html

Hull, R. (2000). *Aural rehabilitation: Serving children and adults* (4th ed.). Clifton Park, NY: Thomson-Delmar.

Hurford, D., Darrow, L., Edwards, T., Howerton, C., Mote, C., Schauf, J., et al. (1993). An examination of phonemic processing abilities in children during their first-grade year. *Journal of Learning Disabilities, 26,* 167–177.

Huthaily, K. (2003). *Contrastive phonological analysis of Arabic and English.* Unpublished master's thesis, University of Montana.

Hwa-Froelich, D. A. (2007) Chapter 55: Vietnamese speech acquisition. In S. McLeod (Ed.), *The international guide to speech acquisition* (pp. 580–591). Clifton Park, NY: Thomson Delmar Learning.

Iglesias, A., & Anderson, N. (1995). Dialectal variations. In J. E. Bernthal & N. W. Bankson (Eds.), *Articulation and phonological disorders* (3rd ed., pp. 147–161). Boston, MA: Allyn & Bacon.

Ingram, D. (1974). Phonological rules in young children. *Journal of Child Language, 1,* 49–64.

Ingram, D. (1976). *Phonological disability in children.* New York, NY: Elsevier.

Ingram, D. (1989a). *First language acquisition: Method, description, and explanation.* Cambridge, UK: Cambridge University Press.

Ingram, D. (1989b). *Phonological disability in children: Studies in disorders of communication* (2nd ed.). London, UK: Cole & Whurr.

Ingram, D. (2002). The measurement of whole-word productions. *Journal of Child Language, 29,* 713–733.

Ingram, D. (2008). Chapter 38 Cross-linguistic phonological acquisition. In: M. J. Ball, M. R. Perkins, & N. Müller (Eds.), *The Handbook of Clinical Linguistics* (pp. 626-640). Malden, MA: Blackwell.

Ingram, D. (2010) The holophrastic stage. In P. C. Hogan (Ed.), *The Cambridge Encyclopedia of the Language Sciences* (pp. 364–366). Cambridge, UK: Cambridge University Press.

Ingram, D., Christensen, L., Veach, S., & Webster, B. (1980). The acquisition of word-initial fricatives and affricates in English by children between 2 and 6 years. In G. H. Yeni-Komshian, J. F. Kavanagh, & C. A. Ferguson (Eds.), *Child phonology: Vol. I. Production* (pp. 169–192). New York, NY: Academic Press.

Ingram, D., & Ingram, K. (2001). A whole-word approach to phonological analysis and intervention. *Language, Speech, and Hearing Services in Schools, 32,* 271–283.

International Phonetic Association: International Phonetic Alphabet Chart. (2015). Retrieved from http://www.langsci.ucl.ac.uk/ipa/ipachart.html

Irwin, O. C. (1945). Reliability of infant speech sound data. *Journal of Speech Disorders, 10,* 227–235.

Irwin, O. C. (1946). Infant speech: Equations for consonant-vowel ratios. *Journal of Speech Disorders, 11,* 177–180.

Irwin, O. C. (1947a). Infant speech: Consonant sounds according to place of articulation. *Journal of Speech and Hearing Disorders, 12,* 397–401.

Irwin, O. C. (1947b). Infant speech: Consonant sounds according to manner of articulation. *Journal of Speech and Hearing Disorders, 12,* 402–404.

Irwin, O. C. (1948). Infant speech: Development of vowel sounds. *Journal of Speech and Hearing Disorders, 13,* 31–34.

Irwin, O. C. (1951). Infant speech: Consonantal position. *Journal of Speech and Hearing Disorders, 16,* 159–161.

Irwin, O. C., & Chen, H. P. (1946). Infant speech: Vowel and consonant frequency. *Journal of Speech and Hearing Disorders, 11,* 123–125.

Irwin, J. V., & Wong, S. P. (Eds.). (1983). *Phonological development in children 18 to 72 months.* Carbondale: Southern Illinois University Press.

Jakobson, R. (1949). On the identification of phonemic entities. *Travaux du Cercle Linguistique de Prague, 5,* 205–213.

Jakobson, R. (1962). Zur Struktur des Phonems (pp. 280–310). *Selected Writings I. Vol. 1, Phonological studies.* The Hague: Mouton.

Jakobson, R. (1968). *Child language, aphasia and phonological universals.* The Hague: Mouton. (Original work published 1941)

Jakobson, R., Fant, G., & Halle, M. (1952). *Preliminaries to speech analysis: The distinctive features and their correlates.* Cambridge, MA: MIT Press.

Jakobson, R., & Halle, M. (1956). *Fundamentals of language.* The Hague: Mouton.

James, D. G. H. (2001). An item analysis of Australian English words for an articulation and phonological test for children aged 2 to 7 years. *Clinical Linguistics and Phonetics, 15,* 457–485.

James, D. G. H. (2006). *Hippopotamus is so hard to say: Children's acquisition of polysyllabic words.* Unpublished PhD thesis, University of Sydney, Australia. Retrieved from http://ses.library.usyd.edu.au/handle/2123/1638

James, D. G. H. (2009). The relationship between the underlying representation and surface form of long words. In C. Bowen (Ed.), *Children's speech sound disorders* (pp. 329–334). Oxford, UK: Wiley-Blackwell.

James, D. G. H., van Doorn J., & McLeod, S. (2008). The contribution of polysyllabic words in clinical decision making about children's speech. *Clinical Linguistics and Phonetics, 22,* 345–353.

James, D. G. H., van Doorn, J., & McLeod, S., & Esterman, A. (2008). Patterns of consonant deletion in typically developing children aged 3 to 7 years. *International Journal of Speech-Language Pathology, 10,* 179–192.

Jelm, J. M. (2001). *Verbal Dyspraxia Profile.* DeKalb, IL: Janelle.

Johnson, W., & Reimers, P. (2010). *Patterns in child phonology.* Edinburgh, UK: Edinburgh University Press.

Jones, D. (1938). Concrete and abstract sounds. *Proceedings of the 3rd International Congress of Phonetic Sciences.* Ghent, Belgium.

Jones, D. (1950). *The phoneme: Its nature and use.* Cambridge, UK: Heffer.

Jusczyk, P., & Luce, P. (2002). Speech perception and spoken word recognition: Past and present. *Ear and Hearing, 23,* 2–40.

Justice, L. M., & Redle, E. E. (2014). *Communication sciences and disorders: A clinical evidence-based approach* (3rd ed.). Boston, MA: Pearson.

Kaipa, R., & Peterson, A. M. (2016). A systematic review of treatment intensity in speech disorders. *International Journal of Speech-Language Pathology, 18,* 507–520.

Kamhi, A. G. (1992). Clinical forum: Phonological assessment and treatment. The need for a broad-based model of phonological disorders. *Language, Speech, and Hearing Services in Schools, 23,* 261–268.

Kamhi, A. G., Minor, J. S., & Mauer, D. (1990). Content analysis and intratest performance profiles on the Columbia and the TONI. *Journal of Speech and Hearing Research, 33,* 375–379.

Kantner, C., & West, R. (1960). *Phonetics* (Rev. ed.). New York, NY: Harper & Brothers.

Kaufman, N. (1995). *Kaufman speech praxis test for children.* Detroit, MI: Wayne State University Press.

Keating, D., Turrell, G., & Ozanne, A. (2001). Childhood speech disorders: Reported prevalence, comordity, and socioeconomic profile. *Journal of Pediatric and Child Health, 37,* 149–171.

Kehoe, M. M. (2001). Prosodic patterns in children's multisyllabic word productions. *Language, Speech, and Hearing Services in Schools, 32,* 284–294.

Kenney, M. K., Barac-Cikoja, D., Finnegan, K., Jeffries, N., & Ludlow, C. L. (2006). Speech perception and short-term memory deficits in persistent developmental speech disorder. *Brain and Language, 96,* 178–190.

Kent, R. D. (1997). *The speech sciences.* San Diego, CA: Singular.

Kent, R. D., & Bauer, H. R. (1985). Vocalizations of one-year-olds. *Journal of Child Language, 13,* 491–526.

Kent, R. D., Kent, J. F., & Rosenbeck, J. C. (1987). Maximum performance tests of speech production. *Journal of Speech and Hearing Disorders, 52,* 367–387.

Kent, R. D., Miolo, G., & Bloedel, S. (1994). The intelligibility of children's speech: A review of evaluation procedures. *American Journal of Speech-Language Pathology, 3*(2), 81–95.

Kent, R. D., & Vorperian, H. K. (2013). Speech impairments in Down Syndrome: A review. *Journal of Speech, Language, Hearing Research, 56,* 178–210.

Kent, R. D., Weismer, G., Kent, J. F., & Rosenbek, J. C. (1989). Toward phonetic intelligibility testing in dysarthria. *Journal of Speech and Hearing Disorders, 54,* 482–499.

Kercher, M. B., & Bauman-Waengler, J. (1992). *Performances of Black English speaking children on standardized language tests.* Presentation at the national convention of the American Speech-Language-Hearing Association, San Antonio, TX.

Khan, L. M. (2002). The sixth view: Assessing preschoolers' articulation and phonology from the trenches. *American Journal of Speech-Language Pathology, 11,* 250–254.

Khan, L. M., & Lewis, N. P. (2015). *Khan-Lewis Phonological Analysis* (3rd ed.). Boston, MA: NCS Pearson.

Kharma, N., & Hajjaj, A. (1989). *Errors in English among Arabic speakers: Analysis and remedy.* London, UK: Longman International Education.

Kim, M., & Pae, S. (2007). Korean speech acquisition. In S. McLeod (Ed.), *The international guide to speech acquisition* (pp. 472–482). Clifton Park, NY: Thomson Delmar Learning.

King, G., & Fletcher, P. (1993). Grammatical problems in school-age children with specific language impairment. *Clinical Linguistics and Phonetics, 7,* 339–352.

Kiparsky, P. (1982). From cyclic phonology to lexical phonology. In H. van der Hulst & H. Smith (Eds.), *The structure of phonological representations* (Vol. II, pp. 131–176). Dordrecht, the Netherlands: Foris.

Kiparsky, P., & Menn, L. (1977). On the acquisition of phonology. In J. Macnamara (Ed.), *Language learning and thought* (pp. 47–78). New York, NY: Academic Press.

Kirk, C. (2008). Substitution errors in the production of word-initial and word-final consonant clusters. *Journal of Speech, Language and Hearing Research, 51,* 35–48.

Kisilevsky, B. S., Hains, S. M. J., Jacquet, A.-Y., Grannier-Deferre, C., & Lecanuet, J. P. (2004). Maturation of fetal responses to music. *Developmental Science, 7,* 550–559.

Kitamura, H. (1991). Evidence for cleft palate as a postfusion phenomenon. *Cleft Palate Journal, 28,* 195–211.

Klein, E. S. (1996). *Clinical phonology: Assessment and treatment of articulation disorders in children and adults.* San Diego, CA: Singular.

Klein, H. B., Lederer, S. H., & Cortese, E. E. (1991). Children's knowledge of auditory/articulatory correspondences: Phonologic and metaphonologic. *Journal of Speech and Hearing Research, 34,* 559–564.

Klieve, S. A. (1998). *Perception of prosody assessment* (Unpublished master's thesis). University of Melbourne, Australia.

Knock, T., Ballard, K., Robin, D., & Schmidt, R. (2000). Influence or order of stimulus presentation on speech motor learning: A principled approach to treatment for apraxia of speech, *Aphasiology, 14,* 653–668.

Krueger, B. I., & Storkel, H. L. (2017). The effect of speech sound disorders on the developing language system: Implications for treatment and future directions in research. In M. G. Gaskell & J. Mirkovic (Eds.), *Current issues in the psychology of language: Speech perception and spoken word recognition.* United Kingdom: Psychology Press.

Kuhl, P., Conboy, B., Padden, D., Nelson, T., & Pruitt, J. (2005). Early speech perception and later language development: Implications for the "critical period." *Language Learning and Development, 1,* 237–264.

Kuhl, P., Stevens, E., Hayashi, A., Deguchi, T., Kiritani, S., & Iverson, P. (2006). Infants show a facilitation effect for native language phonetic perception between 6 and 12 months. *Developmental Science, 9,* F13–F21.

Kumin, L. (1998). Speech and language skills in children with Down syndrome, *Mental Retardation and Developmental Disabilities Research Reviews, 2,* 109–115.

Kumin, L., & Adams, J. (2000). Developmental apraxia of speech and intelligibility in children with Down syndrome. *Down Syndrome Quarterly, 5,* 1–6.

Kussmaul, A. (1885). Die Störungen der Sprache. In H. V. Ziemsson (Ed.), *Handbuch der Speciellen Pathologie und Therapie: Volume 12* (pp. 1–299). Leipzig, Germany: F. C. W. Vogel.

Labov, W. (1991). The three dialects of English. In P. Eckert (Ed.), *New ways of analyzing sound change* (pp. 1–44). New York, NY: Academic Press.

Labov, W. (1994). *Principles of linguistic change. Volume 1: Internal factors.* Oxford, UK: Blackwell.

Labov, W. (1996). *The phonological atlas of North America.* Philadelphia, PA: Linguistics Laboratory of the University of Pennsylvania.

Labov, W., Ash, S., & Boberg, C. (2005). *Atlas of North American English.* Berlin, Germany: Mouton de Gruyter.

Labov, W., Yaeger, M., & Steiner, R. (1972). *A quantitative study of sound change in progress.* Philadelphia, PA: U.S. Regional Survey.

Ladefoged, P., & Johnson, K. (2014). *A course in phonetics* (7th ed.). Boston, MA: Cengage Learning.

Ladefoged, P., & Maddieson, I. (1996). *The sounds of the world's languages.* Oxford, UK: Blackwell.

Lagerberg, T. B., Åsberg, J., Hartelius, L., & Persson, C. (2014). Assessment of intelligibility using children's spontaneous speech: Methodological aspects. *International Journal of Language and Communication Disorders, 49,* 228–239.

Larrivee, L., & Catts, H. (1999). Early reading achievement in children with expressive phonological disorders. *American Journal of Speech-Language Pathology, 8,* 137–148.

Lasker, J. P., Stierwalt, J. A. G., Spence, M., & Cavin-Root, C. (2010). Using webcam interactive technology to implement treatment for severe apraxia: A case example. *Journal of Medical Speech-Language Pathology, 18,* 71–76.

Leafstedt, J., Richards, C., & Gerber, M. (2004). Effectiveness of explicit phonological-awareness instruction for at-risk English learners. *Learning Disabilities Research and Practice, 19,* 252–261.

Lee, H. B. (1999). Korean. In *Handbook of the International Phonetic Association* (pp. 120–122). Cambridge, UK: Cambridge University Press.

Lee, L., Koenigsknecht, R., & Mulhern, S. (1975). *Interactive language development teaching*. Evanston, IL: Northwestern University Press.

Lehiste, I. (1970). *Suprasegmentals*. Cambridge, MA: Massachusetts Institute of Technology.

Leitao, S., Hogben, J., & Fletcher, J. (1997). Phonological processing skills in speech and language impaired children. *European Journal of Disorders of Communication, 32*, 73–93.

Leonard, L. (1988). Lexical development and processing in specific language impairment. In R. Schiefelbusch & L. Lloyd (Eds.), *Language perspectives: Acquisition, retardation, and intervention* (2nd ed., pp. 69–87). Austin, TX: PRO-ED.

Leonard, L. (1994). Some problems facing accounts of morphological deficits in children with specific language impairments. In R. Watkins & M. Rice (Eds.), *Specific language impairments in children* (pp. 91–106). Baltimore, MD: Brookes.

Leonard, L., & McGregor, K. (1991). Unusual phonological patterns and their underlying representations: A case study. *Journal of Child Language, 18*, 261–271.

Leonard, L., McGregor, K., & Allen, G. (1992). Grammatical morphology and speech perception in children with specific language impairment. *Journal of Speech and Hearing Research, 35*, 1076–1085.

Leonard, L., Newhoff, M., & Mesalam, L. (1980). Individual differences in early child phonology. *Applied Psycholinguistics, 1*, 7–30.

Leopold, W. F. (1947). *Speech development of a bilingual child: A linguist's record*. Evanston, IL: Northwestern University Press.

Lepschy, G. C. (1970). *A survey of structural linguistics*. London, UK: Faber and Faber.

Levin, K. (1999). Babbling in infants with cerebral palsy. *Clinical Linguistics and Phonetics, 13*, 249–267.

Lewis, B., Freebairn, L., Hansen, A., Taylor, H., Iyengar, S., & Shriberg, L. (2004). Family pedigrees of children with suspected childhood apraxia of speech. *Journal of Communication Disorders, 37*, 157–175.

Lewis, B., Freebairn, L., & Taylor, H. (2000). Correlates of spelling abilities in children with early speech sound disorders. *Reading and Writing: An Interdisciplinary Journal, 15*, 389–407.

Li, C., & Thompson, S. (1987). Chinese. In B. Comrie (Ed.), *The world's major languages* (pp. 811–833). New York, NY: Oxford University Press.

Liberman, I. Y., & Shankweiler, D. (1985). Phonology and the problems of learning to read and write. *Topical Issues: Remedial and Special Education, 6*, 8–17.

Ling, D. (2002). *Speech and the hearing-impaired child: Theory and practice* (2nd ed.). Washington, DC: Alexander Graham Bell Association for the Deaf.

Lippke, B., Dickey, J., Selmar, J., & Soder, A. L. (1997). *PAT-3: Photo articulation test* (3rd ed.). Austin, TX: PRO-ED.

Lipsitt, L. (1966). Learning processes of human newborns. *Merrill-Palmer Quarterly, 12*, 45–71.

Lipski, J. (2000). The linguistic situation of Central Americans. In S. McKay & S. Wong (Eds.), *New immigrants in the United States* (pp. 189–215). Cambridge, UK: Cambridge University Press.

Lisman, A. L., & Sadagopan, N. (2013). Focus of attention and speech motor performance. *Journal of Communication Disorders, 46*, 281–293.

Local, J. (1983). How many vowels in a vowel? *Journal of Child Language, 10*, 449–453.

Locke, J. L. (1980a). The inference of speech perception in the phonologically disordered child. Part I: A rationale, some criteria, the conventional tests. *Journal of Speech and Hearing Disorders, 45*, 431–434.

Locke, J. L. (1980b). The inference of speech perception in the phonologically disordered child. Part II: Some clinically novel procedures, their use, some findings. *Journal of Speech and Hearing Disorders, 45*, 435–468.

Locke, J. L. (1983). *Phonological acquisition and change*. Orlando, FL: Academic Press.

Locke, J. L. (1990). Structure and stimulation in the ontogeny of spoken language. *Developmental Psychobiology, 23*, 621–643.

Lof, G. L. (2002). Two comments on this assessment series. *American Journal of Speech-Language Pathology, 11*, 255–256.

Lonigan, C., Burgess, S., & Anthony, J. (2000). Development of emergent literacy and early reading skills in preschool children: Evidence from a latent-variable longitudinal study. *Developmental Psychology, 36*, 596–613.

Lonigan, C., Burgess, S., Anthony, J., & Barker, T. (1998). Development of phonological sensitivity in 2- to 5-year-old children. *Journal of Educational Psychology, 90*, 294–311.

Lonigan, C. J., Wagner, R. K., Torgesen, J. K., & Rashotte, C. A. (2002). *Preschool Comprehensive Test of Phonological and Print Processing*. Tallahassee, FL: Author.

Love, R. J. (2000). *Childhood motor speech disability* (2nd ed.). Boston, MA: Allyn & Bacon.

Lowe, R. J. (1986). *Assessment link between phonology and articulation: ALPHA*. Moline, IL: LinguiSystems.

Lowe, R. J. (1994). *Phonology: Assessment and intervention applications in speech pathology*. Baltimore, MD: Williams & Wilkins.

Lowe, R. J. (1996). *Assessment link between phonology and articulation: ALPHA* (Rev. ed.). Mifflinville, PA: Speech and Language Resources.

Lowe, R. J., Knutson, P., & Monson, M. (1985). Incidence of fronting in preschool children. *Language, Speech, and Hearing Services in Schools, 16*, 119–123.

Lund, N. J., & Duchan, J. F. (1993). *Assessing children's language in naturalistic contexts* (3rd ed.). Englewood Cliffs, NJ: Prentice-Hall.

Lyytinen, H., Ahonen, T., Eklund, K., Guttorm, T., Laakso, M., Leinonen, S., et al. (2001). Developmental pathways of children with and without familial risk for dyslexia during the first years of life. *Developmental Neuropsychology, 20*, 535–554.

Maas, E., Butalla, C. E., & Farinella, K. A. (2012). Feedback frequency in treatment for childhood apraxia of speech. *American Journal of Speech-Language Pathology, 21*, 239–257.

Maas, E., & Farinella, K. A. (2012). Random versus blocked practice in treatment for childhood apraxia of speech. *Journal of Speech, Language, and Hearing Research, 55*, 561–578.

Maas, E., Robin, D. A., Hula, S. N. A., Freedman, S. E., Wulf, G., Ballard, K. J., & Schmidt, R. A. (2008). Principles of motor learning in treatment of motor speech disorders. *American Journal of Speech-Language Pathology, 17*, 277–298.

Maassen, B., Groenen, P., & Crul, T. (2003). Auditory and phonetic perception of vowels in children with apraxic speech disorders. *Clinical Linguistics and Phonetics, 17*, 447–467.

Maclean, M., Bryant, P., & Bradley, L. (1987). Rhymes, nursery rhymes and reading in early childhood. *Merrill-Palmer Quarterly, 33*, 255–282.

Maddieson, I. (1984). *Patterns of sounds.* Cambridge, UK: Cambridge University Press. (Paperback reprint 2009)

Magnusson, E. (1991). Metalinguistic awareness in phonologically disordered children. In M. Yavas (Ed.), *Phonological disorders in children: Theory, research and practice* (pp. 87–120). London, UK: Routledge.

Malabonga, V., & Marinova-Todd, S. (2007). Chapter 38: Filipino speech acquisition. In S. McLeod (Ed.), *The international guide to speech acquisition* (pp. 340–350). Clifton Park, NY: Thomson Delmar Learning.

Mampe, B., Friederici, A. D., Christophe, A., & Wermke, K. (2009). Newborns' cry melody is shaped by their native language, *Current Biology, 19*, 1994–1997.

Mandulak, K., Baylis, A., & Thurmes, A. (2011). *Cleft palate and velopharyngeal dysfunction: Evaluation, treatment, and problem-solving.* American Speech-Language-Hearing Association National Convention, San Diego, CA.

Marangolo, P., Marinelli, C. V., Bonifazia, S., Fiori, V., Ceravoloa, M. G., Provinciali, L., & Tomaiuolod, F. (2011). Electrical stimulation over the left inferior frontal gyrus (IFG) determines long-term effects in the recovery of speech apraxia in three chronic aphasics. *Behavioural Brain Research, 225*, 498–504.

Marcos, H. (2001). Introduction: Early pragmatic development. *First Language, 21*, 209–218.

Mareschal, D., & French, R. (2000). Mechanisms of categorization in infants. *Infancy, 1*, 59–76.

Marili, J., Andrianopoulos, K., Velleman, M., & Foreman, C. (2004). *Incidence of motor speech impairment in autism and Asperger's disorders.* Paper presented at the annual convention of the American Speech-Language-Hearing Association, Philadelphia, PA.

Marion, M. J., Sussman, H. M., & Marquardt, T. P. (1993). The perception and production of rhyme in normal and developmentally apraxic children. *Journal of Communication Disorders, 26*, 129–160.

Marquardt, T. P., Sussman, H. M., Snow, T., & Jacks, A. (2002). The integrity of the syllable in developmental apraxia of speech. *Journal of Communication Disorders, 35*, 31–49.

Marsh, J. L., & Lehman, J. A. (1988). *Cleft care in 1986: An ACPA survey* [abstract]. American Cleft Palate–Craniofacial Annual Meeting, Williamsburg, VA.

Martin, J. (2017). *How to calculate speech intelligibility.* Retrieved from http://jacimartin.weebly.com/uploads/2/8/7/2/28728745/jminstructions.pdf on 5/16/2018

Martinet, A. (1960). *Elements de linguistique général I.* [Elements of general linguistics I]. Paris, France: Armand Colin.

Masso, S., McLeod, S., Baker, E., & McCormack, J. (2016). Polysyllable productions in preschool children with speech sound disorders: Error categories and the framework of polysyllable maturity. *International Journal of Speech-Language Pathology, 18*(3), 272–287.

Masterson, J., Bernhardt, B., & Hofheinz, M. (2005). A comparison of single words and conversational speech in phonological evaluation. *American Journal of Speech-Language Pathology, 14*, 229–241.

Matisoff, J. (1991). Sino-Tibetan linguistics: Present state and future prospects. *Annual Review of Anthropology, 20*, 469–504.

Maye, J., & Weiss, D. (2003). Statistical cues facilitate infants' discrimination of difficult phonetic contrasts. In B. Beachley, A. Brown, & F. Conlin (Eds.), *Proceedings of the 27th Boston University Conference on Language Development* (pp. 508–518). Somerville, MA: Cascadilla Press.

Maye, J., Werker, J., & Gerken, L. (2002). Infant sensitivity to distributional information can affect phonetic discrimination. *Cognition, 82*, B101–B111.

McCabe, P., Rosenthal, J. B., & McLeod, S. (1998). Features of developmental dyspraxia in the general speech impaired population? *Clinical Linguistics and Phonetics, 12*, 105–126.

McCabe, T., Murray, E., Thomas, D., Bejjani, L., & Ballard, K. (2013). *A new evidence-based treatment for childhood apraxia of speech: ReST.* Paper presented at the national convention of the American Speech-Language-Hearing Association, Tampa, FL.

McCarthy, J. (1988). Feature geometry and dependency: A review. *Phonetics, 43*, 84108.

McCarthy, J. J., & Prince, A. S. (1995). Faithfulness and reduplicative identity. In *Papers in optimality theory: University of Massachusetts occasional papers in linguistics 18* (pp. 249–384). Amherst, MA: Graduate Linguistics Student Association.

McCauley, R. J., & Strand, E. A. (2008). A review of standardized tests of nonverbal oral and speech motor performance in children. *American Journal of Speech-Language Pathology, 17*, 81–91.

McCune, L., & Vihman, M. M. (2001). Early phonetic and lexical development: A productivity approach. *Journal of Speech, Language, and Hearing Research, 44*, 670–684.

McCurdy, S. (2010). *Hmong learners' deletion and replacement of syllable-final consonants in English.* Unpublished master's thesis, Hamline University, St. Paul, Minnesota.

McDonald, E. T. (1964). *A deep test of articulation—Picture form.* Pittsburgh, PA: Stanwix.

McGee, C. (2006). *Phonological awareness skills of children with autism spectrum disorder.* Unpublished master's thesis, University of British Columbia, Vancouver, British Columbia, Canada.

McHenry, M. (2003). The effect of pacing strategies on the variability of speech movement sequences in dysarthria. *Journal of Speech, Language, and Hearing Research, 46*, 702–710.

McIntosh, B., & Dodd, B. (2008). Evaluation of core vocabulary intervention for treatment of inconsistent phonological disorder: Three treatment case studies. *Child Language and Teaching Therapy, 25*, 9–30.

McLeod, S. (2004). Speech pathologists' application of the ICF to children with speech impairment. *International Journal of Speech-Language Pathology, 6*, 75–81.

McLeod, S., & Arciuli, J. (2009). School-aged children's production of /s/ and /r/ consonant clusters. *Folia Phoniatrica et Logopaedica, 61*, 336–241.

McLeod, S., & Baker, E. (2017). *Children's speech: An evidence-based approach to assessment and intervention.* Boston, MA: Pearson.

McLeod, S., Crowe, K., Masso, S., Baker, E., McCormack, J., Wren, X., . . . Howland, C. (2017). Profile of Australian preschool children with speech sound disorders at risk for literacy difficulties. *Australian Journal of Learning Difficulties, 6*, 1–19.

McLeod, S., van Doorn, J., & Reed, V. (2001). Consonant cluster development in two-year-olds: General trends and individual difference. *Journal of Speech, Language, and Hearing Research, 44,* 1144–1171.

McNeil, M. R., Ballard, K. J., Duffy, J. R., Wambaugh, J. U., van Lieshout, P., Maassen, B., & Terband, H. (2017). Apraxia of speech theory, assessment, differential diagnosis, and treatment: Past, present, and future. In P. van Liesout, B. Maassen, & H. Terband (Eds.), *Speech motor control in normal and disordered speech: Future developments in theory and methodology,* (pp. 195–221). Rockville, MD: American Speech-Language-Hearing Association.

McNeil, M. R., Fossett, T. R., Katz, W. F., Garst, D., Carter, G., Szuminsky, N., & Doyle, P. J. (2010). Effects of on-line kinematic feedback treatment for apraxia of speech. *Brain and Language, 103,* 223–225.

McNeil, M. R., Katz, W. F., Fossett, T, R. D., Garst, D. M., Szuminsky, N. J., Carter, G., & Lim, K. Y. (2010). Effects of online augmented kinematic and perceptual feedback on treatment of speech movements in apraxia of speech. *Folia Phoniatrica et Logopedica, 62,* 127–133.

McNeil, M. R., Robin, D. A., & Schmidt, R. A. (2009). Apraxia of speech: Definition, differentiation, and treatment. In M. R. McNeil (Ed.), *Clinical management of sensorimotor speech disorders* (2nd ed., pp. 249–268). New York, NY: Thieme.

McNeill, B. C., Gillon, G. T., & Dodd, B. (2009a). Effectiveness of an integrated phonological awareness approach for children with childhood apraxia of speech (CAS). *Child Language Teaching and Therapy, 25,* 341–366.

McNeill, B. C., Gillon, G. T., & Dodd, B. (2009b). A longitudinal case study of the effects of an integrated phonological awareness program for identical twin boys with childhood apraxia of speech (CAS). *International Journal of Speech-Language Pathology, 11,* 482–495.

McReynolds, L. V., Engmann, D., & Dimmitt, K. (1974). Markedness theory and articulation errors. *Journal of Speech and Hearing Disorders, 39,* 93–103.

McReynolds, L. V., & Engmann, D. (1975). *Distinctive features analysis of misarticulations.* Baltimore, MD: University Park Press.

Mealings K. T., Cox, F., & Demuth, K. (2013). Acoustic investigations into the delayed acquisition of the syllabic *-es* plural in 2-year-olds' speech. *Journal of Speech Language and Hearing Research, 56,* 1260–1271.

Mealings K. T., Demuth, K. (2014). Cluster reduction and compensatory lengthening in the acquisition of possessives. *Journal of Child Language, 41.* 690–714.

Melby-Lervåg, M., Lyster, S. A.-H., & Hulme, C. (2012). Phonological skills and their role in learning to read: A meta-analytic review. *Psychological Bulletin, 138,* 322–352.

Menn, L. (1971). Phonotactic rules in beginning speech. *Lingua, 26,* 225–251.

Menn, L. (1976). *Pattern, control and contrast in beginning speech: A case study in the development of word form and word function.* Unpublished doctoral dissertation, University of Illinois, Urbana–Champaign.

Menn, L. (1978). *Pattern, control and contrast in beginning speech: A case study in the development of word form and word function.* Bloomington: Indiana University Linguistics Club.

Menn, L., & Velleman, S. (2010). *Framework for decision making in clinical phonology.* Paper presented at the American Speech-Language-Hearing Association, Philadelphia, PA.

Menyuk, P. (1980). The role of context in misarticulations. In G. Yeni-Komshian, J. Kavanagh, & C. Ferguson (Eds.), *Child phonology: Vol. 1. Production* (pp. 211–226). New York, NY: Academic Press.

Miccio, A. W. (2002). Clinical problem solving: Assessment of phonological disorders. *American Journal of Speech-Language Pathology, 11,* 221–229.

Miccio, A. W., & Elbert, M. (1996). Enhancing stimulability: A treatment program. *Journal of Communication Disorders, 29,* 335–351.

Miccio, A. W., Elbert, M., & Forrest, K. (1999). The relationship between stimulability and phonological acquisition in children with normally developing and disordered phonologies. *American Journal of Speech-Language Pathology, 8,* 347–363.

Miccio, A. W., & Ingrisano, D. R. (2000). The acquisition of fricatives and affricates: Evidence from a disordered phonological system. *American Journal of Speech-Language Pathology, 9,* 214–229.

Migration Policy Institute. (2016). State immigration data profiles. Migration Policy Institute tabulations of the U.S. Bureau of the Census' American Community Survey (ACS) and Decennial Census. Washington, D.C. Retrieved from https://www.migrationpolicy.org/data/state-profiles/state/demographics/US on 5/26/2018

Millar, D. C., Light, J. C., & Schlosser, R. W. (2006). The impact of augmentative and alternative communication intervention on the speech production of individuals with developmental disabilities: A research review. *Journal of Speech, Language, and Hearing Research, 49,* 248–264.

Miller, J. F. (1988). Facilitating speech and language. In C. Tingey (Ed.), *Down syndrome. A resource book* (pp. 119–133). Boston, MA: College-Hill Press.

Milloy, N., & Morgan-Barry, R. (1990). Developmental neurological disorders. In P. Grunwell (Ed.), *Developmental speech disorders* (pp. 109–132). New York, NY: Churchill Livingstone.

Mines, M., Hanson, B., & Shoup, J. (1978). Frequency of occurrence of phonemes in conversational English language and speech. *Language and Speech, 21,* 221–241.

Mitchell, P. R., & Kent, R. (1990). Phonetic variation in multisyllable babbling. *Journal of Child Language, 17,* 247–265.

Moran, M. (1993). Final consonant deletion in African American children speaking Black English: A closer look. *Language, Speech, and Hearing Services in the Schools, 24,* 161–166.

Moriarty, B., & Gillon, G. (2006). Phonological awareness intervention for children with childhood apraxia of speech. *International Journal of Language & Communication Disorders, 41,* 713–734.

Morley, M. E., Court, D., & Miller, H. (1954). Delayed speech and developmental aphasia. *British Medical Journal, 2,* 463–467.

Morris, H. L., Spriestersbach, D. C., & Darley, F. L. (1961). An articulation test for assessing competency of velopharyngeal closure. *Journal of Speech and Hearing Research, 4,* 48–55.

Morris, S. R. (2010). Clinical application of the mean babbling level and syllable structure level. *Language, Speech, and Hearing Services in Schools, 41,* 223–230.

Morrisette, M. L., Farris, A. W., & Gierut, J. A. (2006). Applications of learnability theory to clinical phonology. *International Journal of Speech-Language Pathology, 8,* 207–219.

Morrison, J., & Shriberg, L. (1992). Articulation testing versus conversational speech sampling. *Journal of Speech and Hearing Research, 35,* 259–273.

Mortensen, D. (2004). *Preliminaries to Mong Leng (Hmong Njua) phonology.* Retrieved from http://ist-socrates. berkeley.edu/~dmort/mong_leng_phonology.pdf

Mortimer, J. (2007). *Effects of speech perception, vocabulary, and articulation skills in morphology and syntax in children with speech sound disorders.* Unpublished doctoral dissertation, McGill University, Montreal, Canada.

Mosher, J. (1929). *The production of correct speech sounds.* Boston, MA: Expression.

Moskowitz, A. (1971). *Acquisition of phonology.* Unpublished doctoral dissertation, University of California, Berkeley.

Müller, N., Ball, M. J., & Rutter, B. (2006). A profiling approach to intelligibility problems. *Advances in Speech-Language Pathology, 8,* 176–189.

Munson, B., Edwards, J., & Beckman, M. (2005a). Phonological knowledge in typical and atypical speech-sound development. *Topics in Language Disorders. Clinical Perspectives on Speech Sound Disorders, 25,* 190–206.

Munson, B., Edwards, J., & Beckman, M. E. (2005b). Relationship of nonword repetition accuracy and other measures of linguistic development in children with phonological disorders. *Journal of Speech, Language and Hearing Research, 47,* 61–78.

Murray, E., McCabe, P., & Ballard, K. J. (2014). A systematic review of treatment outcomes for children with childhood apraxia of speech. *American Journal of Speech-Language Pathology, 13,* 1–19.

Mysak, E. D. (1959). A servomodel for speech therapy. *Journal of Speech and Hearing Disorders, 24,* 144–149.

Nakazima, S. A. (1962). A comparative study of the speech developments of Japanese and American English in childhood (1): A comparison of the developments of voices at the prelinguistic period. *Studia Phonologica, 2,* 27–46.

Nathani, S., Ertmer, D., & Stark, R. (2006). Assessing vocal development in infants and toddlers. *Clinical Linguistics and Phonetics, 20,* 351–369.

National Center for Children in Poverty: Brief on English language proficiency, family economic security, and child development. (2010). *Mailman School of Public Health.* New York, NY: Columbia University.

National Joint Committee for the Communication Needs of Persons with Severe Disabilities. (2010). *Communication services for individuals with severe disabilities: FAQs and discussion.* American Speech-Language-Hearing Association, Philadelphia, PA.

Neilson, R. (2003). *Sutherland Phonological Awareness Test-Revised.* NSW, Australia: Author.

Nelson, K. (1973). Structure and strategy in learning to talk. *Monographs of the Society of Research in Child Development, 38*(149). Chicago, IL: University of Chicago Press.

Nemoy, E. M. (1954). *Speech correction through story telling units.* Magnolia, MA: Expression.

Nemoy, E. M., & Davis, S. (1937). *The correction of defective consonant sounds.* Boston, MA: Expression.

Newborg, J. (2005). *Battelle Developmental Inventory Screening Test* (2nd ed.), Itasca, IL: Riverside.

Newman, D. (2002). The phonetic status of Arabic within the world's languages: The uniqueness of the lughat al-daad. *Antwerp Papers in Linguistics, 100,* 65–75.

New York State Department of Health. (2006). *Clinical practice guideline: Report of the recommendations. Motor disorders, assessment and intervention for young children (age 0-3 years)* (Publication No. 4962). Albany, NY: Author.

Nijland, L., Maassen, B., van der Meulen, S., Gabreëls, F., Kraaimaat, F. W., & Schreuder, R. (2002). Coarticulation patterns in children with developmental apraxia of speech. *Clinical Linguistics and Phonetics, 16,* 461–483.

Nordberg, A., Miniscalco, C., & Lohmander, A. (2014) Consonant production and overall speech characteristics in school-aged children with cerebral palsy and speech impairment. *International Journal of Language & Communication Disorders, 16,* 386–395.

Northern, J. L., & Downs, M. P. (2014). *Hearing in children* (6th ed.). San Diego, CA: Plural.

Novak, I., McIntyre, S., Morgan, C., Campbell, L., Dark, L., Morton, N., . . . Goldsmith, S. (2013). A systematic review of interventions for children with cerebral palsy: State of the Evidence. *Developmental Medicine & Child Neurology, 55,* 885–910.

O'Connor, B., Kerr, C., Shields, N., & Imms, C. (2015) A systematic review of evidence-based assessment practices by allied health practitioners for children with cerebral palsy. *Developmental Medicine and Neurology, 58,* 332–347.

Odding, E., Roebroeck, M. E., & Stam, H. J. (2006). The epidemiology of cerebral palsy: Incidence, impairments and risk factors. *Disability and Rehabilitation, 28,* 183–191.

Oetting, J., & Horohov, J. (1997). Past tense marking by children with and without specific language impairment. *Journal of Speech and Hearing Research, 40,* 62–74.

Oetting, J., & Rice, M. (1993). Plural acquisition in children with specific language impairment. *Journal of Speech and Hearing Research, 36,* 1236–1248.

Ogar, J., Willock, S., Baldo, J., Wilkins, D., Ludy, C., & Dronkers, N. (2006). Clinical and anatomical correlates of apraxia of speech. *Brain and Language, 97,* 343–350.

O'Grady, W. D., & Archibald, J. (2012). *Contemporary linguistic analysis: An introduction* (7th ed.). Toronto, Canada: Pearson Longman.

Oller, D. K. (1980). The emergence of the sounds of speech in infancy. In G. Yeni-Komshian, J. Kavanagh, & C. A. Ferguson (Eds.), *Child phonology: Vol. I. Production* (pp. 93–112). New York, NY: Academic Press.

Oller, D., Eilers, R., Neal, A., & Schwartz, G. (1999). Precursors to speech in infancy: The prediction of speech and language disorders. *Journal of Communication Disorders, 32,* 223–245.

Olmsted, D. (1971). *Out of the mouth of babes: Earliest stages in language learning.* The Hague: Mouton.

Osberger, M. J., Robbins, A. M., Todd, S. L., & Riley, A. I. (1994). Speech intelligibility of children with cochlear implants. *The Volta Review, 96,* 169–180.

Otheguy, R., Garcia, O., & Roca, A. (2000). Speaking in Cuban: The language of Cuban Americans. In S. McKay & S. Wong (Eds.), *New immigrants in the United States* (pp. 165–188). Cambridge, UK: Cambridge University Press.

Owens, R. E. (2009). Mental retardation/mental disability. In D. K. Bernstein & E. Tiegerman-Farber (Eds.), *Language and communication disorders in children* (6th ed., pp. 246–313). Boston, MA: Allyn & Bacon: Pearson.

Owens, R. E. (2016). *Language development: An introduction* (9th ed.). Boston, MA: Allyn & Bacon.

Ozanne, A. (2013). Childhood apraxia of speech. In B. Dodd (Ed.), *Differential diagnosis and treatment of children with speech disorder* (2nd ed. ebook, pp. 71–82). Hoboken, NJ: John Wiley & Sons.

Paavola, L., Kunnari, S., & Moilanen, I. (2005). Maternal responsiveness and infant intentional communication: Implications for the early communicative and linguistic development. *Child: Care, Health and Development, 31,* 727–735.

Palmer, R., & Enderby, P. (2007). Methods of speech therapy treatment for stable dysarthria: A review. *Advances in Speech Language Pathology, 9,* 140–153.

Pamplona, M., Ysunza, A., Gonzalez, M., Ramirez, E., & Patino, C. (2000). Linguistic development in cleft palate patients with and without compensatory articulation disorder. *International Journal of Pediatric Otorhinolaryngology, 54,* 81–91.

Panagos, J., & Prelock, P. (1982). Phonological constraints on the sentence production of language disordered children. *Journal of Speech and Hearing Research, 25,* 171–177.

Parker, F., & Riley, K. (2010). *Linguistics for non-linguists: Primer with exercises* (5th ed.). Boston, MA: Allyn & Bacon.

Patel, R. (2002). Prosodic control in severe dysarthria. *Journal of Speech, Language, and Hearing Research, 45,* 858–870.

Patel, R., & Brayton, J. T. (2009). Identifying prosodic contrasts in utterances produced by 4-, 7-, and 11-year-old children. *Journal of Speech, Language, and Hearing Research, 52,* 790-801.

Paul, R. (1993). Patterns of development in late talkers: Preschool years. *Journal of Childhood Communication Disorders, 15,* 7–14.

Paul, R., & Jennings, P. (1992). Phonological behavior in toddlers with slow expressive language development. *Journal of Speech and Hearing Research, 35,* 99–107.

Paul, R., Norbury, C., & Gosse, C. (2018). *Language disorders from infancy through adolescence: Assessment and intervention* (5th ed.). St. Louis, MO: Mosby Year Book.

Peña-Brooks, A., & Hegde, M. N. (2000). *Assessment and treatment of articulation and phonological disorders in children.* Austin, TX: PRO-ED.

Pence Turnbull, K. L., & Justice, L. M. (2017). *Language development from theory to practice* (3rd ed.). Upper Saddle River, NJ: Pearson Education.

Pennington, L., Goldbart, J., & Marshall, J. (2004). Speech and language therapy to improve the communication skills of children with cerebral palsy, *Cochrane Database of Systematic Reviews, 3,* CD003466.

Peppé S, & McCann J. (2003). Assessing intonation and prosody in children with atypical language development: The PEPS-C test and the revised version. *Clinical Linguistics and Phonetics,* 345–354.

Perez, E. (1994). Phonological differences among speakers of Spanish-influenced English. In J. Bernthal & N. Bankson (Eds.), *Child phonology: Characteristics, assessment, and intervention with special populations* (pp. 245–254). New York, NY: Thieme.

Peterson-Falzone, S. J., Trost-Cardamone, J. E., Karnell, M. P., & Hardin-Jones, M. (2017). *The clinician's guide to treating cleft palate speech* (2nd ed.). St. Louis, MO: Elsevier.

Pharr, A., Ratner, N., & Rescorla, L. (2000). Syllable structure development of toddlers with expressive specific language impairment. *Applied Psycholinguistics, 21,* 429–449.

Pike, K. L. (1943). *Phonetics.* Ann Arbor: University of Michigan Press.

Pindzola, R. H., Plexico, L. W., & Haynes, W. O. (2016). *Diagnosis and evaluation in speech pathology* (9th ed.). Boston, MA: Pearson.

Polka, L., Colantonio, C., &, Sundara, M. (2001). A cross-language comparison of /d/-/th/ perception: Evidence for a new developmental pattern. *Journal of the Acoustic Society of American, 109,* 2190–2201.

Pollock, K. E. (2013). Identification of vowel errors: Methodological issues and preliminary data from the Memphis vowel project. In M. J. Ball & F. E. Gibbon (Eds.), *Vowel disorders* (pp. 83–113). Boston, MA: Butterworth-Heinemann.

Pollock, K. E., & Berni, M. C. (2001). Transcription of vowels. *Topics in Language Disorders, 21,* 22–40.

Pollock, K. E., & Berni, M. C. (2003). Incidence of non-rhotic vowel errors in children: Data from the Memphis Vowel Project. *Clinical Linguistics and Phonetics, 17,* 393–401.

Pollock, K., & Hall, P. K. (1991). An analysis of the vowel misarticulations of five children with developmental apraxia of speech. *Clinical Linguistics and Phonetics, 5,* 207–224.

Pollock, K., & Keiser, N. (1990). An examination of vowel errors in phonologically disordered children. *Clinical Linguistics and Phonetics, 4,* 161–178.

Poole, I. (1934). Genetic development of articulation of consonant sounds in speech. *Elementary English Review, 11,* 159–161.

Powell, T. W., & Elbert, M. (1984). Generalization following the remediation of early- and later-developing consonants clusters. *Journal of Speech and Hearing Disorders, 49,* 211–218.

Powell, T. W., Elbert, M., & Dinnsen, D. A. (1991). Stimulability as a factor in the phonologic generalization of misarticulating preschool children. *Journal of Speech and Hearing Research, 34,* 1318–1328.

Power, T. (2003). Practice for Arabic language backgrounds. Retrieved from http://www.btinternet.com/-ted.power/11arabic.html

Prather, E. M., Hedrick, D., & Kern, C. (1975). Articulation development in children aged two to four years. *Journal of Speech and Hearing Disorders, 40,* 179–191.

Preisser, D. A., Hodson, B. W., & Paden, E. P. (1988). Developmental phonology: 18–29 months. *Journal of Speech and Hearing Disorders, 53,* 125–130.

Preston, J. L., Hull, M., & Edwards, M. L. (2013). Preschool speech error patterns predict articulation and phonological awareness outcomes in children with histories of speech-sound disorders. *American Journal of Speech-Language Pathology, 22,* 173–184.

Preston, J. L., McCabe, P., Rivera-Campos, A., Whittle, J. L., Landry, E., & Maas, E. (2014). Ultrasound visual feedback treatment and practice variability for residual speech sound errors. *Journal of Speech, Language, and Hearing Research, 57,* 2102–2115.

Prince, A. S., & Smolensky, P. (1993). Optimality theory: Constraint interaction in generative grammar. *RUCCs Technical Report #2.* New Brunswick, NJ: Rutgers University Center for Cognitive Science.

Privacy Policy (2003) Health Insurance Reform: Security Standards; 45 [CFR Parts 160, 162, and 164]. Retrieved from https://www.hhs.gov/sites/default/files/ocr/privacy/hipaa/administrative/securityrule/securityrulepdf.pdf?language=es

Pulleyblank, D. (1986). Underspecification and low vowel harmony in Okpe2. *Studies in African Linguistics, 17,* 119–153.

Radziewicz, C., & Antonellis, S. (1997). Considerations and implications for habilitation of hearing impaired children. In D. K. Bernstein & E. Tiegerman (Eds.), *Language and communication disorders in children* (4th ed., pp. 574–603). Boston, MA: Allyn & Bacon.

Ramig, L. O., Bonitati, C., Lemke, J., & Horii, Y. (1994). Voice treatment for patients with Parkinson disease: Development of an approach and preliminary efficacy data. *Journal of Medical Speech-Language Pathology, 2,* 191–209.

Ramsdell, H. L., Oller, D. K., Buder, E. H., Ethington, C. A., & Chorna, L. (2012). Identification of prelinguistic phonological categories. *Journal of Speech, Language, Hearing Research, 55,* 1626–1639.

Ratliff, M. (1992). *Meaningful tone: A study of tonal morphology in compounds, form classes, and expressive phrases in White Hmong* (Monograph No. 27, Southeast Asia). De Kalb: Northern Illinois University Center for Southeast Asian Studies.

Reed, V. (2018). *Introduction to children with language disorders* (5th ed.). Boston, MA: Pearson.

Renfrew, C. (1966). Persistence of the open syllable in defective articulation. *Journal of Speech and Hearing Disorders, 31,* 370–373.

Rescorla, L. (1989). The Language Development Survey: A screening tool for delayed language in toddlers. *Journal of Speech and Hearing Disorders, 54,* 587–599.

Rescorla, L., Mirak, J., & Singh, L. (2000). Vocabulary growth in late talkers: Lexical development from 2;0 to 3;0. *Journal of Child Language, 27,* 293–311.

Rescorla, L., & Schwartz, E. (1990). Outcome of toddlers with expressive language delay. *Applied Psycholinguistics, 11,* 393–407.

Reynolds, J. (1990). Abnormal vowel patterns in phonologically disordered children: Some data and a hypothesis. *British Journal of Disorders of Communication, 25,* 115–148.

Reynolds, J. (2013). Recurring patterns and idiosyncratic systems in some English children with vowel disorders. In M. J. Ball & F. E. Gibbon (Eds.), *Handbook of vowels and vowel disorders* (pp. 229–259). East Sussex, UK: Psychological Press.

Rice, M. (1991). Children with specific language impairment: Towards a model of teachability. In N. Krasnegor (Ed.), *Biological and behavioral determinants of language development* (pp. 447–480). Hillsdale, NJ: Lawrence Erlbaum.

Rice, M. (1994). Grammatical categories of children with specific language impairments. In R. Watkins & M. Rice (Eds.), *Specific language impairment in children* (pp. 69–90). Baltimore, MD: Brookes.

Rice, M., & Bode, J. (1993). Gaps in the verb lexicons of children with specific language impairment. *First Language, 13,* 113–131.

Rice, M., Wexler, K., & Cleave, P. (1995). Specific language impairment as a period of extended optional infinitive. *Journal of Speech and Hearing Research, 38,* 850–863.

Richardson, U., Leppaenen, P., Leiwo, M., & Lyytinen, H. (2003). Speech perception of infants with high familial risk for dyslexia differ at the age of 6 months. *Developmental Neuropsychology, 23,* 385–397.

Rivera-Gaxiola, M., Silva-Pereyra, J., & Kuhl, P. K. (2005). Brain potentials to native and non-native speech contrasts in 7- and 11-month-old American infants. *Developmental Science, 8,* 162–172.

Robb, M. P., & Bleile, K. M. (1994). Consonant inventories of young children from 8 to 25 months. *Clinical Linguistics & Phonetics, 8,* 295–320.

Robbins, J., & Klee, T. (1987). Clinical assessment of oropharyngeal motor development in young children. *Journal of Speech and Hearing Disorders, 52,* 271–277.

Roberts, A. (1965). *A statistical linguistic analysis of American English.* The Hague: Mouton.

Roberts, J. E., Burchinal, M., & Footo, M. (1990). Phonological process decline from 2½ to 8 years. *Journal of Communication Disorders, 23,* 205–217.

Roberts, J., Long, S. H., Malkin, C., Barnes, E., Skinner, M., Hennon, E. A., & Anderson, K. (2005). A comparison of phonological skills of boys with fragile X syndrome and Down syndrome. *Journal of Speech, Language, and Hearing Research, 48,* 980–995.

Roberts, S., Fyfield, R., Baibazarova, E., van Goozen, S., Culling, J. F., & Hay, D. F. (2013). Parental speech at 6 months predicts joint attention at 12 months. *Infancy, S1,* E1–E5.

Roberts, T. (2005). Articulation accuracy and vocabulary size contributions to phonemic awareness and word reading in English language learners. *Journal of Educational Psychology, 97,* 601–616.

Robertson, C., & Salter, W. (2007). *The Phonological Awareness Test -2 (PAT-2).* East Moline, IL: Linguisystems, ProEd.

Robertson, S. J. (1982). *Robertson dysarthria profile.* San Antonio, TX: Communication Skill Builders.

Roca, I. (1994). *Generative phonology.* London, UK: Routledge.

Rose, Y., & MacWhinney, B. (2014). The PhonBank Project: Data and software assisted methods for the study of phonology and phonological development. In J. Durand, U. Gut, & G. Kristoffersen (Eds.), *The Oxford handbook of corpus phonology* (pp. 308-401). Oxford, UK: Oxford University Press.

Roseberry-McKibbon, C. (2007). *Language disorders in children: A multicultural and case perspective.* Boston, MA: Pearson Education.

Roseberry-McKibbon, C., & Brice, A. (2010). *Acquiring English as a second language: What's "normal," and what's not.* American Speech-Language Hearing Association. Retrieved from http://www.asha.org/public/speech/-development/easl.htm

Rosenbaum, P., Paneth, N., Leviton, A., Goldstein, M., Bax, M., & Jacobsson, B. (2007). A report: The definition and classification of cerebral palsy. *Developmental Medicine & Child Neurology, 109,* 8–14.

Rosenbek, J. C., & Jones, H. N. (2009). Principles of treatment for sensorimotor speech disorders. In M. R. McNeil (Ed.), *Clinical management of sensorimotor speech disorders* (2nd ed., pp. 269–288). New York, NY: Thieme.

Rosner, J. (1971). The Auditory Analysis Test: An initial report. *Journal of Learning Disabilities, 4,* 384–392.

Rothgaenger, H. (2003). Analysis of the sounds of the child in the first year of age and a comparison to the language. *Early Human Development, 75,* 55–69.

Ruhlen, M. (1976). *Guide to the languages of the world.* San Diego, CA: Los Amigos Research Associates.

Ruscello, D. M. (2008). *Treating articulation and phonological disorders in children.* St Louis, MO; Elsevier.

Rvachew, S., & Nowak, M. (2001). The effect of target-selection strategy on phonological learning. *Journal of Speech, Language, and Hearing Research, 44,* 610–623.

Rvachew, S., Rafaat, S., & Martin, M. (1999). Stimulability, speech perception skills, and the treatment of phonological disorders. *American Journal of Speech-Language Pathology, 8,* 33–43.

Saben, C., & Costello-Ingham, J. (1991). The effects of minimal pairs treatment on the speech-sound production of two children with phonologic disorders. *Journal of Speech and Hearing Research, 34,* 1023–1040.

Sagey, E. (1986). *The representation of features and relations in non-linear phonology.* Unpublished doctoral dissertation, MIT, Cambridge, MA.

Salmoni, A. W., Schmidt, R. A., & Walter, C. B. (1984). Knowledge of results and motor learning: A review and critical appraisal. *Psychological Bulletin, 95,* 322–386.

Sander, E. K. (1972). When are speech sounds learned? *Journal of Speech and Hearing Disorders, 37,* 55–63.

Sapir, E. (1921). *Language: An introduction to the study of speech.* New York, NY: Harcourt, Brace and World.

Sapir, E. (1925). Sound patterns in language. *Language, 1,* 37–51.

Saussure, F., de. (1959). *A course in general linguistics* (J. Cantineau, Trans.). London, UK: Owen. (Original work published 1916)

Schmauch, V., Panagos, J., & Klich, R. (1978). Syntax influences the accuracy of consonant production in language-disordered children. *Journal of Communication Disorders, 11,* 315–323.

Schmidt, R. A., & Lee, T. D. (2005). *Motor control and learning: A behavioral emphasis* (4th ed.). Champaign, IL: Human Kinetics.

Schneider, W., Roth, E. & Ennemoser, M. (2000). Training phonological skills and letter knowledge in children at-risk for dyslexia: A comparison of three kindergarten intervention programs. *Journal of Educational Psychology, 92,* 284–295.

Schonweiler, R., Schonweiler, B., Schmelzeisen, R., & Ptok, M. (1995). The language and speech skills in 417 children with cleft formations. *Fortschritte in der Kieferorthopädie, 56,* 1–6.

Schwartz, R. (1992). Nonlinear phonology as a framework for phonological acquisition. In R. Chapman (Ed.), *Processes in language acquisition and disorders* (pp. 108–124). St. Louis, MO: Mosby Year Book.

Scripture, E. W. (1902). *Elements of experimental phonetics.* New York, NY: Charles Scribner's Sons.

Scripture, M., & Jackson, E. (1919). *A manual of exercises for the correction of speech disorders.* Philadelphia, PA: Davis.

Secord, W. (1981a). *C-PAC: Clinical probes of articulation consistency.* Sedona, AZ: Red Rock Education.

Secord, W. (1981b). *Eliciting sounds: Techniques for clinicians.* San Antonio, TX: Psychological Corporation.

Secord, W. (1989). The traditional approach to treatment. In N. A. Creaghead, P. W. Newman, & W. A. Secord (Eds.), *Assessment and remediation of articulatory and phonological disorders* (2nd ed., pp. 129–158). New York, NY: Macmillan.

Secord, W. A., & Donohue, J. S. (2002). *Clinical Assessment of Articulation and Phonology.* Greenville, SC: Super Duper Publications.

Secord, W. A., & Shine, R. E. (2003). *S-CAT: Secord Contextual Articulation Test.* Greenville, SC: Super Duper Publications.

Selby, J. C., Robb, M. P., & Gilbert, H. R. (2000). Normal vowel articulations between 15 and 36 months of age, *Clinical Linguistics & Phonetics, 14,* 255–265.

Sell, D., Harding, A., & Grunwell, P. (1994). A screening assessment of cleft palate speech (Great Ormond Street Speech Assessment). *European Journal of Disordered Communication, 29,* 1–15.

Semel, E., Wiig, E. H., & Secord, W. A. (2004). *Clinical evaluation of language fundamentals, (4th ed.).— Screening test (CELF-4 screening test).* Toronto, Canada: The Psychological Corporation/A Harcourt Assessment Company.

Seymour, H., Green, L., & Hundley, R. (1991). *Phonological patterns in the conversational speech of African American children.* Paper presented at the national convention of the American Speech-Language-Hearing Association, Atlanta, GA.

Seymour, H., & Miller-Jones, D. (1981). Language and cognitive assessment of Black children. *Speech Language: Advances in Basic Research and Practice, 6,* 203–255.

Shibamoto, J., & Olmsted, D. (1978). Lexical and syllabic patterns in phonological acquisition. *Journal of Child Language, 5,* 417–456.

Shipley, K. G., & McAfee, J. G. (1998). *Assessment in speech-language pathology: A resource manual* (2nd ed.). San Diego, CA: Singular Thomson Learning.

Shprintzen, R. J. (1995). *Cleft palate speech management. A multidisciplinary approach.* St. Louis, MO: Mosby Year Book.

Shriberg, L. D. (1980). Developmental phonological disorders. In T. J. Hixon, L. D. Shriberg, & J. S. Saxman (Eds.), *Introduction to communication disorders* (pp. 262–309). Englewood Cliffs, NJ: Prentice-Hall.

Shriberg, L. D. (1991). Directions for research in developmental phonological disorders. In J. F. Miller (Ed.), *Research on child language disorders: A decade of progress* (pp. 267–276). Austin, TX: PRO-ED.

Shriberg, L. D. (1993). Four new speech and prosody-voice measures for genetics research and other studies in developmental phonological disorders. *Journal of Speech and Hearing Research, 36,* 105–140.

Shriberg, L. D. (2004). *Diagnostic classification of five subtypes of childhood speech sound disorders (SSD) of currently unknown origin.* Paper presented at the International Association of Logopedics and Phoniatrics, Brisbane, Queensland, Australia.

Shriberg, L. D. (2010). Childhood speech sound disorders: From postbehaviourism to the postgenomic era. In R. Paul & P. Flipsen Jr. (Eds.), *Speech sound disorders in children: In honour of Lawrence D. Shriberg* (pp. 1–33). San Diego, CA: Plural.

Shriberg, L. D., Aram, D. M., & Kwiatkowski, J. (1997a). Developmental apraxia of speech: I. Descriptive and theoretical perspectives. *Journal of Speech, Language, and Hearing Research, 40,* 273–285.

Shriberg, L. D., Aram, D. M., & Kwiatkowski, J. (1997b). Developmental apraxia of speech: II. Toward a diagnostic marker. *Journal of Speech, Language, and Hearing Research, 40*, 286–312.

Shriberg, L. D., Aram, D. M., & Kwiatkowski, J. (1997c). Developmental apraxia of speech: III. A subtype marked by inappropriate stress. *Journal of Speech, Language, and Hearing Research, 40*, 313–337.

Shriberg, L. D., Austin, D., Lewis, B., McSweeny, J. L., & Wilson, D. L. (1997). The percentage of consonants correct (PCC) metric: Extensions and reliability data. *Journal of Speech, Language, and Hearing Research, 40*, 708–722.

Shriberg, L. D., Fourakis, M., Hall, S. D., Karlsson, H. B., Lohmeier, H. I., McSweeny, J. L., . . . Wilson, D. (2010). Extensions to the speech disorders classification system (SDCS). *Clinical Linguistics and Phonetics, 24*, 795–824.

Shriberg, L. D., Kent, R. D., McAllister, T., & Preston, J. L. (2019). *Clinical phonetics* (5th ed.). Boston, MA: Pearson.

Shriberg, L. D., & Kwiatkowski, J. (1982a). Phonological disorders II: A conceptual framework for management. *Journal of Speech and Hearing Disorders, 47*, 242–256.

Shriberg, L. D., & Kwiatkowski, J. (1982b). Phonological disorders III: A procedure for assessing severity of involvement. *Journal of Speech and Hearing Disorders, 47*, 256–270.

Shriberg, L. D., Kwiatkowski, J., & Rasmussen, C. (1990). *The prosody-voice screening profile.* Tucson, AZ: Communication Builders.

Shriberg, L. D., & Lof, G. L. (1991). Reliability studies in broad and narrow transcription. *Clinical Linguistics and Phonetics, 5*, 225–179.

Shriberg, L. D., Tomblin, J., & McSweeney, J. (1999). Prevalence of speech delay in 6-year-old children and comorbidity with language impairment. *Journal of Speech, Language, and Hearing Research, 42*, 1461–1481.

Shriberg, L. D., & Widder, C. J. (1990). Speech and prosody characteristics of adults with mental retardation. *Journal of Speech and Hearing Research, 33*, 627–653.

Simons, G. F., & Fennig, C. D. (Eds.). (2018). Ethnologue: Languages of the world, twenty-first edition. Dallas, TX: SIL International. Retrieved from http://www.ethnologue.com

Skahan, S. M., Watson, M., & Lof, G. L. (2007). Speech-language pathologists' assessment practices for children with suspected speech sound disorders: Results of a national survey. *American Journal of Speech-Language Pathology, 16*, 246–259.

Skelton, S. L. (2004). Concurrent task sequencing in single-phoneme phonologic treatment and generalization. *Journal of Communication Disorders, 37*, 131–155.

Sloat, C., Taylor, S., & Hoard, J. (1978). *Introduction to phonology.* Englewood Cliffs, NJ: Prentice-Hall.

Small, L. (2020). *Fundamentals of phonetics: A practical guide for students* (5th ed.). Boston, MA: Pearson.

Smit, A. (1986). Ages of speech sound acquisition: Comparisons and critiques of several normative studies. *Language, Speech, and Hearing Services in Schools, 17*, 175–186.

Smit, A. B. (1993a). Phonologic error distributions in the Iowa-Nebraska Articulation Norms Project: Word-initial consonant clusters. *Journal of Speech and Hearing Research, 36*, 931–947.

Smit, A. B. (1993b). Phonologic error distributions in the Iowa-Nebraska Articulation Norms Project: Consonant singletons. *Journal of Speech and Hearing Research, 36*, 533–547.

Smit, A. B., & Bernthal, J. E. (1983). Voicing contrasts and their phonological implications in the speech of articulation-disordered children. *Journal of Speech and Hearing Research, 26*, 486–500.

Smit, A. B., Hand, L., Freilinger, J., Bernthal, J., & Bird, A. (1990). The Iowa Articulation Norms Project and its Nebraska replication. *Journal of Speech and Hearing Disorders, 55*, 779–798.

Smith, B. L. (1979). A phonetic analysis of consonant devoicing in children's speech. *Journal of Child Language, 6*, 19–28.

Smith, B. L., Brown-Sweeney, S., & Stoel-Gammon, C. (1989). A quantitative analysis of reduplicated and variegated babbling. *First Language, 9*, 175–189.

Smith, N. V. (1973). *The acquisition of phonology: A case study.* Cambridge, UK: Cambridge University Press.

Snow, D. (1998a). Children's imitations of intonation contours: Are rising tones more difficult than falling tones? *Journal of Speech, Language and Hearing Research, 41*, 576–587.

Snow, D. (1998b). A prominence account of syllable reduction in early speech development: The child's prosodic phonology of tiger and giraffe. *Journal of Speech, Language, and Hearing Research, 41*, 1171–1184.

Snow, D. (2000). The emotional basis of linguistic and nonlinguistic intonation: Implications for hemispheric specialization. *Developmental Neuropsychology, 17*, 1–27.

Snow, D. (2017). Gesture and intonation are "sister systems" of infant communication: Evidence from regression patterns of language development. *Language Science, 59*, 180–191.

Snowling, M., Bishop, D., & Stothard, S. (2000). Is preschool language impairment a risk factor for dyslexia? *Journal of Child Psychology and Psychiatry, 41*, 587–600.

Snowling, M., Goulandris, N., & Stackhouse, J. (1994). Phonological constraints on learning to read: Evidence from single case studies of reading difficulty. In C. Hulme & M. Snowling (Eds.), *Reading development and dyslexia* (pp. 86–104). London, UK: Whurr.

Sommers, R. K., Patterson, J. P., & Wildgen, P. L. (1988). Phonology of Down syndrome speakers, ages 13-22. *Communication Disorders Quarterly, 12*, 65-91.

Song, J. Y., Demuth, K., & Morgan, J. (2010). Effects of the acoustic properties of infant-directed speech on infant word recognition. *Journal of the Acoustical Society of America, 128*, 389–400.

Square, P., Martin, N., & Bose, A. (2001). The nature and treatment of neuromotor speech disorders in aphasia. In R. Chapey (Ed.), *Language intervention strategies in aphasia and related neurogenic communication disorders* (pp. 847–884). Baltimore, MD: Lippincott, Williams, & Wilkins.

Stackhouse, J. (1982). An investigation of reading and spelling performance in speech disordered children. *British Journal of Disorders of Communication, 17*, 53–60.

Stackhouse, J. (1993). Phonological disorder and lexical development: Two case studies. *Child Language Teaching and Therapy, 9*, 230–241.

Stackhouse, J. (1997). Phonological awareness: Connecting speech and literacy problems. In B. W. Hodson & M. L. Edwards (Eds.), *Perspectives in applied phonology* (pp. 157–196). Gaithersburg, MD: Aspen.

Stampe, D. (1969). The acquisition of phonetic representation. *Proceedings of* the *Fifth Regional Meeting of the Chicago Linguistic Circle*, 443–454.

Stampe, D. (1972). On the natural history of diphthongs. *Chicago Linguistic Society* (8th Regional Meeting), 578–590.

Stampe, D. (1973). *A dissertation on natural phonology*. Unpublished doctoral dissertation, University of Chicago.

Stampe, D. (1979). *A dissertation on natural phonology*. New York, NY: Garland.

Stanovich, K. (2000). *Progress in understanding reading: Scientific foundations and new frontiers*. New York, NY: Guilford.

Stark, R. (1980). Stages of speech development in the first year of life. In G. Yeni-Komshian, J. Kavanagh, & C. A. Ferguson (Eds.), *Child phonology: Vol. I. Production* (pp. 73–92). New York, NY: Academic Press.

Stark, R. E. (1981). Infant vocalization: A comprehensive view. *Infant Mental Health Journal, 2*, 118-128.

Stark, R. (1986). Prespeech segmental feature development. In P. Fletcher & M. Garman (Eds.), *Language acquisition. Studies in first language development* (pp. 149–173). Cambridge, UK: Cambridge University Press.

Starr, C. D. (1993). Behavioral approaches to treating velopharyngeal closure and nasality. In K. T. Moller & C. D. Starr (Eds.), *Cleft palate: Interdisciplinary issues and treatment* (pp. 337–356). Austin, TX: PRO-ED.

Stathopoulos, E. T., & Sapienza, C. (1993). Respiratory and laryngeal measures of children during vocal intensity variation. *Journal of the Acoustical Society of America, 94*, 2531–2543.

Steriade, D. (1990). *Greek prosodies and the nature of syllabification*. Doctoral dissertation, Massachusetts Institute of Technology. New York, NY: Garland Press.

St. Louis, K. O., & Ruscello, D. M. (2000). *Oral speech mechanism screening examination (OSMSE)* (3rd ed.). Austin, TX: PRO-ED.

Stockman, I. (1996a). Phonological development and disorders in African American children. In A. Kamhi, K. Pollock, & J. Harris (Eds.), *Communication development and disorders in African American children: Research, assessment, and intervention* (pp. 117–154). Baltimore, MD: P. H. Brookes.

Stockman, I. (1996b). The promises and pitfalls of language sample analysis as an assessment tool for linguistic minority children. *Language, Speech, and Hearing Services in Schools, 27*, 355–366.

Stoel-Gammon, C. (1985). Phonetic inventories, 15–24 months: A longitudinal study. *Journal of Speech and Hearing Research, 28*, 505–512.

Stoel-Gammon, C. (1987a). Phonological skills of two-year-olds. *Language, Speech, and Hearing Services in Schools, 18*, 323–329.

Stoel-Gammon, C. (1987b). Language production scale. In L. Olswang, C. Stoel-Gammon, T. Coggins, & R. Carpenter (Eds.), *Assessing prelinguistic and early linguistic behaviors in developmentally young children* (pp. 120–150). Seattle: University of Washington Press.

Stoel-Gammon, C. (1998). Phonological development in Down syndrome. *Mental Retardation and Developmental Disabilities Research Reviews, 3*, 300–306.

Stoel-Gammon, C. (2011). Relationships between lexical and phonological development in young children. *Journal of Child Language, 38*, 1–34.

Stoel-Gammon, C., & Cooper, J. A. (1984). Patterns of early lexical and phonological development. *Journal of Child Language, 11*, 247–271.

Stoel-Gammon, C., & Dunn, C. (1985). *Normal and disordered phonology in children*. Baltimore, MD: University Park Press.

Stoel-Gammon, C., & Herrington, P. (1990). Vowel systems of normally developing and phonologically disordered children. *Clinical Linguistics and Phonetics, 4*, 145–160.

Stoel-Gammon, C., & Menn, L. (1997). Phonological development: Learning sounds and sound patterns. In J. Berko Gleason (Ed.), *The development of language* (4th ed., pp. 69–121). Boston, MA: Allyn & Bacon.

Stoel-Gammon, C., & Otomo, K. (1986). Babbling development of hearing-impaired and normally hearing subjects. *Journal of Speech and Hearing Disorders, 51*, 33–41.

Storkel, H., & Morrisette, M. L. (2002). The lexicon and phonology: Interactions in language acquisition. *Language, Speech, and Hearing Services in Schools, 33*, 24–37.

Strand, E. A., & Debertine, P. (2000). The efficacy of integral stimulation intervention with developmental apraxia of speech. *Journal of Medical Speech-Language Pathology, 8*, 295–300.

Strand, E. A., & Skinner, A. (1999). Treatment of developmental apraxia of speech: Integral stimulation methods. In A. J. Caruso & E. A. Strand (Eds.), *Clinical management of motor speech disorders in children* (pp. 109–148). New York, NY: Thieme.

Subtelny, J. D. (1980). *Speech assessment and speech improvement for the hearing impaired*. Washington, DC: Alexander Graham Bell Association for the Deaf.

Swift, E., & Rosin, P. (1990). A remediation sequence to improve speech intelligibility for students with Down syndrome. *Language, Speech, and Hearing Services in Schools, 21*, 140–146.

Swingley, D., & Aslin, R. N. (2000). Spoken word recognition and lexical representation in very young children. *Cognition, 76*, 147-166.

Tang, G., & Barlow, J. (2006). Characteristics of the sound system of monolingual Vietnamese-speaking children with phonological impairment. *Clinical Linguistics and Phonetics, 8*, 235–255.

Tanner, D., & Culbertson, W. (1999). *Caregiver-administered communication inventory*. Oceanside, CA: Academic Communication Associates.

Taps Richard, J., & Barlow, J. A. (2011). *Phonological assessment and treatment target selection*. Paper presented at the American Speech-Language-Hearing Association, San Diego, CA.

Taps Richard, J., Barlow, J. A., & Combiths, P. N. (2017). *Applying phonological complexity in the schools: Insights from 32 case studies*. Paper presented at the national convention of the American Speech-Language-Hearing Association, Los Angeles, CA.

Tattersall, P. J., & Dawson, J. I. (2016). *Structured Photographic Articulation Test–III* (3rd ed.). DeKalb, IL: Janelle Publications.

Templin, M. (1957). *Certain language skills in children: Their development and interrelationships* (Institute of Child Welfare, Monograph No. 26). Minneapolis: University of Minnesota Press.

Terrell, S., & Terrell, F. (1993). African American cultures. In D. Battle (Ed.), *Communication disorders in multicultural populations* (pp. 3–37). Boston, MA: Andover Medical.

Thal, D., Oroz, M., & McCaw, V. (1995). Phonological and lexical development in normal and late-talking toddlers. *Applied Psycholinguistics, 16,* 407–424.

Thelwall, R., & Akram Sa'Adeddin, M. (1999). Arabic. In International Phonetic Association, *Handbook of the International Phonetic Association* (pp. 51–54). Cambridge, UK: Cambridge University Press.

Thiessen, E. D. (2007). The effect of distributional information on children's use of phonemic contrasts. *Journal of Memory and Language, 56,* 16–34.

Thiessen, E. D., & Pavlik, P. I., (2016). Modeling the role of distributional information in children's use of phonemic contrasts. *Journal of Memory and Language, 88,* 117–132.

Thiessen, E. D., & Yee, M. N. (2010). Dogs, bogs, labs, and lads: What phonemic generalizations indicate about the nature of children's early word-form representations. *Child Development, 81,* 1287–1303.

Thurlbeck, W. (1982). Postnatal human lung growth, *Thorax, 37,* 465–571.

To, C. K. S., Cheung, P. S. P., & McLeod, S. (2013). A population study of children's acquisition of Hong Kong Cantonese consonants, vowels, and tones. *Journal of Speech, Language, and Hearing Research, 56,* 103–122.

Tomas, E., Demuth, K., Smith-Lock, K. M., & Petocz, P. (2015). Phonological and morphophonological effects on grammatical development in children with specific language impairment. *International Journal of Language and Communication Disorders, 50,* 516–528.

Toppelberg, C., Shapiro, M., & Theodore, M. (2000). Language disorders: A 10-year research update review. *Journal of the American Academy of Child and Adolescent Psychiatry, 39,* 143–152.

Torgesen, J. (2000). Individual differences in response to early interventions in reading: The lingering problem of treatment resisters. *Learning Disabilities Research and Practice, 15,* 55–64.

Torgesen, J. K., & Bryant, B. R. (2004). *Test of Phonological Awareness – Second Edition: PLUS (TOPA 2+).* Austin, TX: Pro-Ed.

Torgesen, J., Wagner, R., Rashotte, C., Burgess, S., & Hecht, S. (1997). Contributions of phonological awareness and rapid automatic naming ability to the growth of word-reading skills in second- to fifth-grade children. *Scientific Studies of Reading, 1,* 161–185.

Torgesen, J., Wagner, R., Simmons, K., & Laughon, P. (1990). Identifying

phonological coding problems in disabled readers: Naming counting, or span measures? *Learning Disability Quarterly, 13,* 236–243.

Trost-Cardamone, J. E. (1990). The development of speech: Assessing cleft palate misarticulations. In D. A. Kernahan & S. W. Rosenstein (Eds.), *Cleft lip and palate: A system of management* (pp. 227–235). Baltimore, MD: Williams & Wilkins.

Trost-Cardamone, J. E., & Bernthal, J. E. (1993). Articulation assessment procedures and treatment decisions. In K. T. Moller & C. D. Starr (Eds.), *Cleft palate. Interdisciplinary issues and treatment* (p. 307 ff.). Austin, TX: PRO-ED.

Trubetzkoy, N. S. (1931). Gedanken über Morphophonologie. *Travaux du Cercle Linguistique de Prague, 4,* 160 ff.

Trubetzkoy, N. S. (1969). *Grundzüge der Phonologie.* Prague, Czechoslovakia: TCLP, 4. (Original work published 1939)

Tsao, F.-M., Liu, H.-M., & Kuhl, P. (2004). Speech perception in infancy predicts language development in the 2nd year of life: A longitudinal study. *Child Development, 75,* 1067–1084.

Ttofari Eecen, K., Reilly, S., & Eadie, P. (2007, May). *Parent concern and parent report of speech sound development at 12 months of age.* Paper presented at the Speech Pathology Australia National Conference, Sydney, Australia.

Tyler, A. A., Edwards, M. L., & Saxman, J. H. (1987). Clinical application of two phonologically based treatment procedures. *Journal of Speech and Hearing Disorders, 52,* 393–409.

Tyler, A. A., & Figurski, G. R. (1994). Phonetic inventory changes after treating distinctions along an implicational hierarchy. *Clinical Linguistics & Phonetics, 8,* 91–107.

Tyler, A., & Haskill, A. M. (2011). Morphosyntax intervention. In A. L. Williams, S. McLeod, & R. J. McCauley (Eds.), *Interventions for speech sound disorders in children.* Baltimore: Paul H. Brookes.

Tyler, A., & Langsdale, T. (1996). Consonant–vowel interactions in early phonological development. *First Language, 16,* 159–191.

Tyler, A., Lewis, K. E., Haskill, A. M., & Tolbert, L. C. (2002). Efficacy and cross-domain effects of a morphosyntax and a phonology intervention. *Language,*

Speech, and Hearing Services in Schools, 33, 52–66.

Tyler, A., Lewis, K. E., Haskill, A. M., & Tolbert, L. C. (2003). Outcomes of different speech and language goal attack strategies. *Journal of Speech, Language, and Hearing Research, 46,* 1077–1095.

Tyler, A., & Tolbert, L. (2002). Speech-language assessment in the clinical setting. *American Journal of Speech-Language Pathology, 11,* 215–220.

Ukrainetz, T. (2015). *Phonemic awareness therapy.* Paper presented at the convention of California Speech-Language-Hearing Association, Long Beach, CA.

United States Census Bureau (2011). *American Community Survey.* Washington, DC: United States Department of Commerce. Retrieved from https://www.census.gov/programs-surveys/acs/guidance/comparing-acs-data/2011.html

United States Census Bureau. (2012). *Statistical Abstract of the United States: 2012* (131st ed.). Washington, DC: United States Department of Commerce. Retrieved from http://www.census.gov/compendia/statab

United States Census Bureau. (2016). *American Community Survey (ACS), Table B05006, Place of Birth for the Foreign-Born Population.* Washington, DC: United States Department of Commerce. Retrieved from https://factfinder.census.gov/faces/tableservices/jsf/pages/productview.xhtml?src=bkmk on 5/26/2018

United States Department of Commerce. (2017). *Yearbook of immigration statistics.* Springfield, VA: National Technical Information Service.

United States Department of Education, Office of English Language Acquisition, Language Enhancement, and Academic Achievement for Limited English Proficient Students. (June, 2013). *The biennial evaluation report to Congress on the implementation of the Title III State Formula Grant Program for school years 2008–2012.* Retrieved from https://www2.ed.gov/about/offices/list/oela/resources.html

Val Barros, A.-M. (2003). *Pronunciation difficulties in the consonant system experienced by Arabic speakers when learning English after the age of puberty.* Master's thesis, University of West Virginia, Wheeling.

Van Demark, D. R., & Hardin, M. A. (1990). Speech therapy for the child with cleft lip and palate. In J. Bardach & H. L. Morris (Eds.), *Multidisciplinary management of cleft lip and palate.* Philadelphia, PA: W. B. Saunders.

Van Keulen, J. E., Weddington, G. T., & DeBose, C. E. (1998). *Speech, language, learning, and the African American child.* Boston, MA: Allyn & Bacon.

Van Riper, C. (1939a). Ear training in the treatment of articulation disorders. *Journal of Speech Disorders, IV,* 141–142.

Van Riper, C. (1939b). *Speech correction: Principles and methods.* Englewood Cliffs, NJ: Prentice-Hall.

Van Riper, C. (1978). *Speech correction: Principles and methods* (6th ed.). Englewood Cliffs, NJ: Prentice-Hall.

Van Riper, C., & Emerick, L. (1984). *Speech correction: An introduction to speech pathology and audiology* (7th ed.). Englewood Cliffs, NJ: Prentice-Hall.

Van Riper, C., & Irwin, J. (1958). *Voice and articulation.* Englewood Cliffs, NJ: Prentice-Hall.

Velleman, S. (2003). *Childhood apraxia of speech: Resource guide.* Clifton Park, NY: Thomson Delmar Learning.

Velleman, S. (2016). *Speech sound disorders.* Philadelphia, PA: Wolters Kluwer.

Velleman, S., & Strand, K. (1994). Developmental verbal dyspraxia. In J. E. Bernthal & N. W. Bankson (Eds.), *Child phonology: Characteristics, assessment, and intervention with special populations* (pp. 110–139). New York, NY: Thieme Medical Publishers.

Velten, H. (1943). The growth of phonemic and lexical patterns in infant language. *Language, 19,* 281–292.

Vihman, M. M. (1992). Early syllables and the construction of phonology. In C. A. Ferguson, L. Menn, & C. Stoel-Gammon (Eds.), *Phonological development: Models, research, implications* (pp. 393–422). Timonium, MD: York Press.

Vihman, M. M. (2004). Early phonological development. In J. E. Bernthal & N. W. Bankson (Eds.), *Articulation and phonological disorders* (5th ed., pp. 63–112). Boston, MA: Allyn & Bacon.

Vihman, M. M., Ferguson, C. A., & Elbert, M. (1986). Phonological development from babbling to speech: Common tendencies and individual differences. *Applied Psycholinguistics, 7,* 3–40.

Vihman, M. M., & Greenlee, M. (1987). Individual differences in phonological development: Ages one through three years. *Journal of Speech and Hearing Research, 30,* 503–521.

Vihman, M. M., Macken, M. A., Miller, R., Simmons, H., & Miller, J. (1985). From babbling to speech: A reassessment of the continuity issue. *Language, 61,* 397–445.

Waengler, H.-H., & Bauman-Waengler, J. A. (1984). *Phonetische Logopädie, Lieferung 2: S-Lautbildungen und ihre Störungen.* Berlin, Germany: Marhold Verlag.

Waengler, H.-H., & Bauman-Waengler, J. A. (1989). *Phonological development of normal and speech/language disordered 4-year-olds.* Paper presented at the national convention of the American Speech-Language-Hearing Association, St. Louis, MO.

Wagner, R. K., Torgesen, J. K., & Rashotte, C. A. (1994). Development of reading-related phonological processing abilities: New evidence of bi-directional causality from a latent variable longitudinal study. *Developmental Psychology, 30,* 73–87.

Wagner, R. K., Torgesen, J. K., Rashotte, C. A., & Pearson, N. A. (2013). *Comprehensive Test of Phonological and Print processing (2nd ed.), (CTOPP-2).* Austin, TX: PRO-ED.

Walton, P. D., Walton, L. M., & Felton, K. (2001). Teaching rime analogy or letter recoding reading strategies to pre-readers: Effects on prereading skill and word reading. *Journal of Educational Psychology, 93,* 160–180.

Wambaugh, J. L., Duffy, J. R., McNeil, M. R., Robin, D. A., & Rogers, M. (2006). Treatment guidelines for acquired apraxia of speech: Treatment descriptions and recommendations. *Journal of Medical Speech-Language Pathology, 14,* 35–97.

Wambaugh, J., Martinez, A., McNeil, M., & Rogers, M. (1999). Sound production treatment for apraxia of speech: Overgeneralization and maintenance effects. *Aphasiology, 13,* 821–837.

Wambaugh, J. L., Nessler, C., Cameron, R., & Mauszycki, S. (2010). *Effects of repeated practice and practice plus pacing control on sound production accuracy in acquired apraxia of speech.* Presentation at the annual Clinical Aphasiology Conference, Isle of Palms, SC.

Ward, I. (1923). *Defects of speech.* New York, NY: E. P. Dutton.

Waring, R., & Knight, R. (2013). How should children with speech sound disorders be classified? A review and critical evaluation of current classification systems. *International Journal of Language and Communication Disorders, 48,* 25–40.

Washington, J. (1998). *African American English research: A review and future directions.* Retrieved from http://www.rcgd.isr.umich.edu/prba/perspectives/spring1998/jwashington.pdf

Washington, J. A., & Craig, H. K. (1994). Dialectal forms during discourse of poor, urban, African American preschoolers. *Journal of Speech and Hearing Research, 37,* 816–823.

Watkins, R., Rice, M., & Moltz, C. (1993). Verb use by language-impaired and normally developing children. *First Language, 13,* 133–143.

Watson, J. (2002). *The phonology and morphology of Arabic.* Oxford, UK: Oxford University Press.

Watson, M. M., & Scukanec, G. P. (1997). Profiling the phonological abilities of 2-year-olds: A longitudinal investigation. *Child Language Teaching and Therapy, 13,* 3–14.

Webb, J. C., & Duckett, B. (1990). *The RULES phonological evaluation.* Vero Beach, FL: The Speech Bin.

Webster, P. E., & Plante, A. S. (1992). Effects of phonological impairment on word, syllable, and phoneme segmentation and reading. *Language, Speech, and Hearing Services in Schools, 23,* 176–182.

Webster, P. E., Plante, A. S., & Couvillion, L. (1997). Phonologic impairment and prereading: Update on a longitudinal study. *Journal of Learning Disabilities, 30,* 365–375.

Webster, R., Majnemer, A., Platt, R., & Shevell, M. (2005). Motor function at school age in children with a preschool diagnosis of developmental language impairment. *Journal of Pediatrics, 146,* 80–85.

Weiner, F. (1979). *Phonological process analysis.* Baltimore, MD: University Park Press.

Weiner, F. (1981). Treatment of phonological disability using the method of meaningful minimal contrast: Two case studies. *Journal of Speech and Hearing Disorders, 46,* 97–103.

Weiner, F., & Bankson, N. (1978). Teaching features. *Language, Speech, and Hearing Services in Schools, 9,* 29–34.

Weinert, H. (1974). *Die Bekämpfung von Sprechfehlern*. Berlin, Germany: VEB Verlag Volk und Gesundheit.

Weismer, G. (1997). The role of stress in language processing and intervention. *Topics in language disorders, 17*, 41–52.

Wellman, B. L., Case, I. M., Mengert, I. G., & Bradbury, D. E. (1931). Speech sounds of young children. *University of Iowa Studies in Child Welfare, 5*. Iowa City: University of Iowa Press.

Wells, B., Peppé, S., & Goulandris, N. (2004). Intonation development from five to thirteen. *Journal of Child Language, 31*, 749–778.

Wells, B., Stackhouse, J., & Vance, M. (1996). A specific deficit in onset-rhyme assembly in a 9-year-old child with speech and literacy difficulties. In T. W. Powell (Ed.), *Pathologies of speech and language: Contributions of clinical phonetics and linguistics*. New Orleans, LA: International Clinical Phonetics and Linguistics Association.

Werker, J., & Fennell, C. (2004). Listening to sounds versus listening to words: Early steps in word learning. In D. Hall & S. Waxman (Eds.), *Weaving a lexicon* (pp. 79–110). Cambridge, MA: MIT Press.

Werker, J., & Tees, R. (2005). Speech perception as a window for understanding plasticity and commitment in language systems of the brain. *Developmental Psychobiology, 46*, 233–251.

Wesseling, R., & Reitsma, P. (2000). The transient role of explicit phonological recoding for reading acquisition. *Journal of Reading and Writing, 13*, 313–336.

West, R., & Ansberry, M. (1968). *The rehabilitation of speech* (4th ed.). New York, NY: Harper & Row.

West, R., Kennedy, L., & Carr, A. (1937). *The rehabilitation of speech*. New York, NY: Harpers.

Whitehill, T., Francis, A., & Ching, C. (2003). Perception of place of articulation by children with cleft palate and posterior placement. *Journal of Speech, Language, and Hearing Research, 46*, 451–461.

Whitehurst, G., Smith, M., Fischel, J., Arnold, D., & Lonigan, C. (1991). The continuity of babble and speech in children with specific expressive language delay. *Journal of Speech and Hearing Research, 34*, 1121–1129.

Whiteside, S. P., Inglis, A. L., Dyson, L., Roper, A., Harbottle, A., Ryder, J., . . . Varley, R. A. (2012). Error reduction therapy in reducing struggle and grope behaviours in apraxia of speech. *Neuropsychological Rehabilitation, 22*, 267–294.

Wiig, E. H., & Secord, W. A. (2011). *HearBuilder Phonological Awareness Test (H-PAT)*. Greenville, SC: SuperDuper Publications.

Wiig, E. H., Semel, E., & Secord, W. A. (2013). *Clinical Evaluation of Language Fundamentals* (5th ed.). Bloomington, MN: NCS Pearson.

Wilcox, K. A., Schooling, T. L., & Morris, S. R. (1991). *The preschool intelligibility measure (P-SIM)*. Paper presented at the annual convention of the American Speech-Language-Hearing Association, Atlanta, GA.

Williams, A. L. (1991). Generalization patterns associated with training least phonological knowledge. *Journal of Speech and Hearing Research, 34*, 722–733.

Williams, A. L. (2000a). Multiple oppositions: Theoretical foundations for an alternative contrastive intervention approach. *American Journal of Speech-Language Pathology, 9*, 282–288.

Williams, A. L. (2000b). Multiple oppositions: Case studies of variables in phonological intervention. *American Journal of Speech-Language Pathology, 9*, 289–299.

Williams, A. L. (2003). *Speech disorders resource guide for preschool children*. Clifton Park, NY: Thomson Delmar Learning.

Williams, A. L. (2006). A systematic perspective for assessment and intervention: A case study. *Advances in Speech-Language Pathology, 8*, 245–256.

Williams, A. L. (2010). Multiple oppositions intervention. In A. L. Williams, S. McLeod, & R. J. McCauley (Eds.), *Interventions for speech sound disorders in children*. Baltimore, MD: Brookes.

Williams, A. L. (2012). Intensity in phonological intervention: Is there a prescribed amount? *International Journal of Speech-Language Pathology, 14*, 456–461.

Williams, A. L., & Kalbfleish, J. (2001, August). *Phonological intervention using multiple oppositions*. Poster session presented at the 25th World Congress of the International Association of Logopedics and Phoniatrics, Montreal, Canada.

Winitz, H. (1969). *Articulation acquisition and behavior*. New York, NY: Appleton-Century-Crofts.

Winitz, H. (1975). *From syllable to conversation*. Baltimore, MD: University Park Press.

Winitz, H. (1984). Auditory considerations in articulation training. In H. Winitz (Ed.), *Treating articulation disorders: For clinicians by clinicians*. Baltimore, MD: University Park Press.

Winitz, H. (1989). Auditory considerations in treatment. In N. Creaghead, P. Newman, & W. Secord (Eds.), *Assessment and remediation of articulatory and phonological disorders* (2nd ed., pp. 243–264). New York, NY: Macmillan.

Winitz, H., & Irwin, O. C. (1958). Syllabic and phonetic structure of infants' early words. *Journal of Speech and Hearing Research, 1*, 250–256.

Wise, C. M. (1958). *Introduction to phonetics.* Englewood Cliffs, NJ: Prentice-Hall.

Witt, P. D., & D'Antonio, L. L. (1993). Velopharyngeal insufficiency and secondary palatal management. A new look at an old problem. *Clinics in Plastic Surgery, 20*, 707–721.

Witzel, M. A. (1995). Communicative impairment associated with clefting. In R. J. Schprintzen & J. Bardach (Eds.), *Cleft palate speech management: A multidisciplinary approach*. St. Louis, MO: Mosby.

Wolfram, W. (1989). Structural variability in phonological development: Final nasals in vernacular Black English. In R. Fasold & D. Schiffren (Eds.), *Current issues in linguistic theory: Language change and variation* (pp. 301–332). Amsterdam, the Netherlands: John Benjamin.

Wolfram, W. (1994). The phonology of a sociocultural variety: The case of African American Vernacular English. In J. Bernthal & N. Bankson (Eds.), *Child phonology: Characteristics, assessment, and intervention with special populations* (pp. 227–244). New York, NY: Thieme.

Wolfram, W., & Schilling-Estes, N. (2006). *American English: Dialects and variation* (2nd ed.). Malden, MA: Blackwell.

Wolk, L., & Meisler, A. (1998). Phonological assessment: A systematic comparison of conversation and picture naming. *Journal of Communication Disorders, 31*, 291–313.

World Health Organization. (2001). *ICF: International classification of functioning, disability and health*. Geneva, Switzerland: Author.

World Health Organization (WHO). (2014). *Health topics 2014*. Retrieved from http://www.who.int/topics/disabilities/en/

Wren, Y., Roulstone, S., & Miller, L. L. (2012). Distinguishing groups of children with persistent speech disorder: Findings from a prospective population study. *Logopedics, Phoniatrics and Vocology, 37, 1*, 1–10.

Yeni-Komshian, G., Flege, J., & Liu, S. (2000). Pronunciation proficiency in the first and second languages of Korean-English bilinguals. Bilingualism: Language. *Cognition, 3*, 131–150.

Yorkston, K. (1996). Treatment efficacy: Dysarthria. *Journal of Speech and Hearing Research, 39*, S42–S57.

Yorkston, K. M., & Beukelman, D. R. (1981). Communication efficiency of dysarthric speakers as measured by sentence intelligibility and speaking rate. *Journal of Speech and Hearing Disorders, 46*, 296–301.

Young, E. H., & Hawk, S. S. (1955). *Moto-kinesthetic speech training.* Palo Alto, CA: Stanford University Press.

Zeltner, T., Caduff, J., Gehr, P., Pfenninger, J., & Burri, P. (1987). The postnatal growth and development of the human lung I. *Morphometry Respiratory Physiology, 67*, 247–267.

Zemlin, W. R. (1998). *Speech and hearing science: Anatomy and physiology* (4th ed.). Englewood Cliffs, NJ: Prentice-Hall.

Zentella, A. C. (1997). *Growing up bilingual.* Malden, MA: Blackwell.

Zentella, A. (2000). Puerto Ricans in the United States: Confronting the linguistic repercussions of colonialism. In S. McKay & S. Wong (Eds.), *New immigrants in the United States* (pp. 137–164). Cambridge, UK: Cambridge University Press.

Zgonc, Y. (2000). *Sounds in action.* Peterborough, NH: Crystal Springs Books.

Zimmerman, I. L., Steiner, V. G., & Pond, R. E. (2011). *PLS-5: Preschool Language Scales* (5th ed.). Boston, MA: Pearson.

Index